LAVIN'S

Radiography for Veterinary Technicians

LAVIN'S

Radiography for Veterinary Technicians

Seventh Edition

Marg Brown, RVT, BEd Ad Ed

Formerly of Seneca College of Applied Arts and Technology King City, Ontario;
Formerly of Penn Foster College, Scranton, Pennsylvania;
Active Member:
Ontario Association of Veterinary Technicians
Association of Veterinary Technician Educators
National Association of Veterinary Technicians in America

Lois C. Brown, RTR (Can/USA), ACR, MSc, P.Phys

President
Xray Imaging Consultants Ltd.
Orangeville, Ontario, Canada

ELSEVIER

Elsevier
3251 Riverport Lane
St. Louis, Missouri 63043

LAVIN'S RADIOGRAPHY FOR VETERINARY TECHNICIANS, SEVENTH EDITION   ISBN: 978-0-323-76370-7
Copyright © 2022 by Elsevier, Inc. All rights reserved.

No part of this publication may be reproduced or transmitted in any form or by any means, electronic or mechanical, including photocopying, recording, or any information storage and retrieval system, without permission in writing from the publisher. Details on how to seek permission, further information about the Publisher's permissions policies and our arrangements with organizations such as the Copyright Clearance Center and the Copyright Licensing Agency, can be found at our website: www.elsevier.com/permissions.

This book and the individual contributions contained in it are protected under copyright by the Publisher (other than as may be noted herein).

Notice

Practitioners and researchers must always rely on their own experience and knowledge in evaluating and using any information, methods, compounds or experiments described herein. Because of rapid advances in the medical sciences, in particular, independent verification of diagnoses and drug dosages should be made. To the fullest extent of the law, no responsibility is assumed by Elsevier, authors, editors or contributors for any injury and/or damage to persons or property as a matter of products liability, negligence or otherwise, or from any use or operation of any methods, products, instructions, or ideas contained in the material herein.

Previous editions copyrighted 2018, 2014, 2007, 2003, 1999, and 1994.

Library of Congress Control Number: 2021939951

Director, Content Development: Laurie Gower
Senior Content Strategist: Brandi Graham
Content Strategist: Melissa Rawe
Content Development Specialist: Brooke Kannady
Publishing Services Manager: Deepthi Unni
Senior Project Manager: Manchu Mohan
Design Direction: Amy Buxton

Printed in India

Last digit is the print number: 9 8 7 6 5 4 3

Working together
to grow libraries in
developing countries

www.elsevier.com • www.bookaid.org

To my contributors and reviewers:
Susan McNeal, RVT, Ashley Jenner, RVT, BSc, VTS-DI,
Lorelei D'Avolio, LVT, VTS (Exotics), CVPM, Shana Lemmenes, CVT, VTS-EVN, and
Julia Bitan, RVT. Thank you for your expertise and dedication in making this a
valuable resource.
To all our students and the veterinary profession: may you never stop learning.
To Phil, Alina, Jacquie and Tylor: love always.
Marg Brown

To my contributors.
Darryl Bonder, DVM;
Stephanie Holowka, MRT(R), MRT, (MR) MRSO, (MRSC TM)
Bob Hylands, DVM;
Lori Ponte, Animal Health Partners, Toronto
Arvind Singh, HND Mech (UK) Raymax Medical Corporation;
This would be a very thin book without your expertise. Thank you for your prompt
and enthusiastic presentations.
Lois C. Brown

Contributors

Darryl Bonder, DVM, RSO
Nuclear Medicine, Ontario Equine Hospital
Mississauga, Ontario

Stephanie Holowka, MRT(R), MRT(MR), MRSO (MRSC™)
Lead Technologist, MEG and 3-Dimensional Imaging
Diagnostic Imaging
The Hospital for Sick Children
Toronto, Ontario

Robert F. Hylands, DVM
Westbridge Veterinary Hospital
Mississauga, Ontario

Susan MacNeal, RVT, CVDT, BSc
Coordinator, Veterinary Technician
Georgian College
Orillia, Ontario

Reviewers

Laura L. Black, LVT, BAAS
Associate Professor of Veterinary Technology
Veterinary Technology Distance Learning Program
San Juan College
Farmington, New Mexico

Lorelei D'Avolio, LVT, VTS (Exotics), CVPM
Practice Manager
The Center for Avian and Exotic Medicine
New York, New York

Lynda Forgie, RVT
Professor, Veterinary Technician
Georgian College
Orillia, Ontario

Jennifer V. Freese, DVM
Program Director
Veterinary Technology
University of Maine at Augusta
Bangor, Maine

Michelle E. Goodnight, DVM, MS, DACVECC
Instructor, Veterinary Technology
Gwinnett Technical College
Lawrenceville, Georgia

Susan Guttschow, DVM
Program Director/Instructor
Veterinary Science
Gateway Technical College
Elkhorn, Wisconsin

Amanda Hackerott, RVT
Program Director, Health Sciences
WSU Tech College of Applied Sciences and Technology
Wichita, Kansas

Ashley Jenner, BSc, RVT, VTS-DI
Diagnostic Imaging
Toronto Veterinary Emergency
Toronto, Ontario

Shana Lemmenes, CVT, VTS-EVN
Large Animal Technician
University of Minnesota
St. Paul, Minnesota

Shauna Lesick, RVT
RVT Instructor, Animal Studies
Northern Alberta Institute of Technology
Edmonton, Alberta

George W. McCommon, DVM
Chair/Professor
Veterinary Science and Public Health
Fort Valley State University
Fort Valley, Georgia

Sarah Meyer-Paterson, CVT, AAS
Program Director, Veterinary Technology
Pensacola State College
Pensacola, Florida

Gordon Smok, DVM, BA, AS
Program Chair Veterinary Technology
City College
Gainesville, Florida

We are excited to present the seventh edition of *Lavin's Radiography for Veterinary Technicians*. This text continues to focus on teaching the science of imaging used for veterinary medicine and veterinary technology education and referencing. The purpose of the book is to instill a working knowledge of radiologic science as it applies to producing a diagnostic quality image, to prepare radiography students in veterinary technology programs for the certification exam, to assist in the training of veterinary medicine students, and to provide a base from which practicing veterinary radiographers can make informed decisions about technical factors and diagnostic image quality in the workplace.

This text is divided into two major parts: the technical side of diagnostic imaging, and radiographic positioning and related anatomy. Part One puts theory into practice, and each of the chapters in Part Two have been expanded to include not only essential positioning information but also anatomic references to support the technician in understanding normal anatomic features so that accurate images for diagnosis are produced. This text is a mainstay for teaching radiographic anatomy and positioning of all common species.

Each chapter is unique, yet succinct, so that all important information is available and easy to understand without the need to reference other sources. This is a valuable reference for both technicians and veterinarians when they have finished their training. This seventh edition provides a thorough yet practical level of imaging and positioning coverage to equip individuals with the knowledge they need to produce high-quality images on the first attempt with a focus on radiation safety.

Photographs, radiographs, and a consistent style of color line drawings, along with tables and boxes, have been updated. Numerous images are scattered throughout the text, with many chapters ending in an image gallery for further observation. Application information and technician notes boxes continue to provide practical information to help prepare the veterinary technician for on-the-job challenges. Review questions are included in the textbook at the end of each chapter. Further review questions can be found in the accompanying Evolve website in the Student Resources. A comprehensive glossary in which key words and other terms are defined has been rewritten and is also now included in the text.

Features of Part One

The world of diagnostic imaging continues to evolve with better and clearer images in all aspects of the science. In this,

the seventh edition of the text, we have once again rewritten large sections and modified other parts of the chapters.

Information on film processing, both automatic and manual, has been included in this edition. There are still many facilities that use film/screen technology and for this reason, it is presented here.

The computed radiography and digital imaging information has been greatly expanded. As that field moves forward, the various modes of digital imaging are presented, some of which are here to stay and others which are transitional.

The intrepid contributors have, once again, presented their chapters with new images and expanded explanations of the technologies they present. It is always a pleasure to interact with colleagues who are experts in their field and to share their enthusiasm for their subjects. To that end:

Dr. Hylands has rewritten his Ultrasound chapter with new images and text.
Dr. Bonder has enlarged his chapter on Nuclear Medicine and added new images.
Horst Bruning of Animage has contributed wonderful images from technologies that are being introduced and accepted worldwide.
Stephanie Holowka has revised her chapters and added new images.

Chapters 1 and 2 once again present the science of x-ray technology.

Chapter 3 expands on how to protect your staff and the patients from the effects of radiation.

Chapters 4 to 7 present a revised and more succinct information on the modality of film/screen imaging.

Chapter 8 is the digital imaging chapter. It has been revised and expanded with a number of new sections. This field is ever evolving, and as new technology is presented, I will update the chapter on the Evolve website.

Chapter 9 presents quality control, the testing and the expected results. I have included the tests that can be completed in house if there is a problem prior to a visit from a service engineer.

Section 3 is the specialized imaging area. The experts in their fields have written their chapters, which are included to demonstrate the enhancement of anatomical parts evidenced from the use of specialized imaging.

Features of Part Two: Radiographic Positioning and Related Anatomy

This part is all about positioning and is a one-source reference for major species and procedures. Each chapter has been updated, with additional images, strategies and techniques including digital imaging. There are separate chapters on the abdomen, thorax, forelimb, pelvis and hindlimb, spine, and skull of small animals. Small animal dental radiography, special procedures, large animal, and avian and exotic radiographic imaging have also been significantly expanded.

All information required for accurate positioning is clearly indicated. Routine and ancillary views are included for each position. All chapters include an outline, learning objectives, key terms, where to measure, the location of the central ray, borders, a step-by-step approach to positioning, further comments, and tips to ensure that the perfect image is obtained both through analog and digital imaging. Technician notes scattered throughout the chapters emphasize important points.

Positioning views are accompanied by high-quality color photographs and graphic color drawings that visibly indicate ideal radiographic imaging and anatomic features. Through the integrative application of radiography and anatomy, veterinarians will receive optimized images. Further related and essential descriptive anatomy is included in the appendixes on the Evolve website.

The emphasis in these chapters is on non-manual restraint techniques required for the safety and radiation protection of the radiographer and for the benefit of our patients. It is essential that the veterinary profession understands and applies these safety principles.

Diagnostic imaging is an exciting and changing field in which the radiographer plays an important role. With the tools and information presented here, an accurate diagnosis should be ensured.

Welcome to the seventh edition. We hope that you enjoy learning from it as much as we enjoyed writing it.

Marg Brown
Lois C. Brown

Additional Learning Resources

The Evolve Student Resources include review questions, crossword puzzles, and fill-in-the-blank exercises, as well as five appendixes and a comprehensive glossary. A full complement of support materials for teaching and learning are also available and include a complete collection of all images in the text.

Acknowledgments

I express my deepest gratitude to everyone who has contributed to the production of this edition. Your dedication and constant additions keeps this resource one of the most relevant and current in the field.

A big thank you to the reviewers who gave us great input on what should be changed or continued in this edition. Your guidance has been essential to improve the content and layout. Lois, your perspective and enthusiasm continue to amaze me. It has been a pleasure to work on this with you once again.

I am forever indebted to my former colleagues of the Seneca College Veterinary Technician Program in King City, Ontario, for your constant support, generosity, enthusiasm, and dedication. Unless otherwise indicated, the positioning photographs were taken at Seneca College. Thanks to our models, Sam, Ace, and Spud, and to their owners. A big thank you to my former students. Because of your enthusiasm, curiosity and search for knowledge, I never worked a day in my life. You were a constant source of motivation and joy. Nothing gives me more pleasure than to continue learning and hearing from you.

Special thanks to Sue MacNeal, RVT, CVDT, BSc, for totally upgrading the dentistry chapter. Your knowledge and logical explanations ensure that dentistry remains a valuable chapter of this edition.

Lorelei D'Avolio, LVT, VTS (Exotics). CVPM, your expertise and years of experience significantly improved the avian and exotic medicine chapter. Shana Lemmenes, CVT, VTS-EVN, your assistance in the large-animal positioning was invaluable. Ashley Jenner, RVT, BSc, VTS-DI, your practical suggestions were indispensable for editing the small animal positioning chapters. Along with your colleague, Julia Bitan, RVT of https://handsfreexrays.com/, the images added greatly to the chapters. Jennifer White, RVT, your further images were helpful. Evelyn Kelly, RN, MRT(R), ACR, BSc, and Carolyn Bennett, AHT, your assistance with the special procedures chapter was appreciated. Heartfelt thanks to you all for your input.

I continue to express my appreciation to those who contributed to previous editions. Jeanne Robertson, your graphic images continue to be awesome.

Huge credit is extended to the editing team at Elsevier, especially Brandi Graham, Brooke Kannady and Manchu Mohan. Your inspiration, suggestions, and patience have helped make this book an essential resource.

As Albert Einstein said "once you stop learning, you start dying." May you all learn forever.

Marg Brown

I am, once again, humbled and impressed with the knowledge, experience, and enthusiasm that I received as we ventured into a seventh edition of this work.

Robert Hylands, DVM, rewrote the ultrasound chapter, adding information and new images, and sent it and responses to my questions from an island in the North country of Canada while self-isolating from the COVID pandemic. Horst Bruning, president of Animage, sent images of his FIDEX system via California as he was quarantined in Italy, unable to travel due to COVID. Stephanie Holowka, MRT(R), MRT (MR), MRSO (MRSC TM), was especially involved with the computed tomography (CT), magnetic resonance imaging (MRI) and the new positron emission tomography section, as well as reviewing the new and revised digital imaging chapter. Her thorough enjoyment of the veterinary aspect of imaging is always refreshing. Animal Health Partners, North York, Ontario invited us to visit their MRI and computed radiography departments and then contributed enthusiastically to our seventh edition. They photographed their CT and MRI units and supplied images as requested by Stephanie as she compiled the MRI and CT chapters. Darryl Bonder, DVM has contributed to all three editions with his encyclopedic knowledge of equine nuclear medicine. Raymax Medical Corporation was invaluable in reviewing the

ı Curious Tiberius—the literary—always providing assistance and voicing concerns—mainly about dinner and the lateness of the hour.

manuscripts of Section 1. Every time I called with a request, the response or the image would show up in my inbox within hours.

The many, many contributors of images and expertise would fill several pages, and to those people, veterinarians, technicians, technical educators, and other staff members, I once again offer my special thanks.

Once again, our reviewers and the suggestions they made helped immensely to guide the content of the seventh edition. The expertise of our editors, Brooke Kannady and Brandi Graham, and their staff certainly kept us on track and led to this new and very special seventh edition.

As before, Marg, great to work with you again… stay safe.

The restrictions of COVID could have made this project very difficult, but everyone worked from home, or in isolation far from home, and with the able assistance of our pets, moved the project to completion. For me, I Curious Tiberius was once again a mainstay of editing

Lois C. Brown

Contents

PART ONE

Diagnostic Imaging

In Part One, you will be introduced to the technical side of imaging. The main emphasis is on the practical applications of rules and laws guiding the principles of radiography. You will learn about the inner workings of the radiographic unit. Film, digital, and specialized imaging are also addressed. Identifying radiographic artifacts and quality control testing techniques are also included.

CHAPTER **1**

The Basics of Atoms and Electricity

Lois C. Brown, RTR (Can/USA), ACR, MSc, P.Phys

Wilhelm Roentgen's laboratory. (Photo courtesy Röntgen-Kuratorium Würzburg e. V., Röntgenring 8, 97070 Würzburg.)

Imagination is the highest form of research.
—Albert Einstein 1879–1955

OUTLINE

LEARNING OBJECTIVES

When you have finished this chapter, you will be able to:

1. Describe the events related to the discovery of x-rays.
2. List the properties of x-rays.
3. Understand the relationship between atoms and elements.
4. Describe the basics of atomic theory.
5. Understand the relationship between matter and energy.
6. Describe the basics of the table of the elements.
7. Define x-ray photons as waves and particles.

APPLICATIONS

This chapter provides basic information that will be expanded on in subsequent chapters.

KEY TERMS

Key terms are defined in the Glossary on the Evolve website.

Atomic theory	Elements	Matter	Thermal energy
Atoms	Energy	Nuclear energy	Thermionic emission
Diagnostic imaging	Fluorescence	Nucleus	Wavelength
Electricity	Frequency	Particles	X-rays
Electromagnetic spectrum	Heterogeneous	Polyenergetic	

The Discovery of X-Rays

X-rays were discovered by German scientist Wilhelm Conrad Roentgen in 1895. He was working in his laboratory and setting up experiments for the next morning when he discovered a platinocyanide plate glowing a few feet from where he was working.

The fortuitous decision by Roentgen to understand what caused the plate to glow, how to prevent it from glowing (by removing the radiation source), and how to categorize the rays that caused the glow was the beginning of the profession that we know as diagnostic imaging.

Roentgen named the rays "x-rays" because of their unknown nature ("x" in science denotes an unknown quantity). He was also the first person to patent the phenomenon at a registry office.

As Roentgen developed his experiments and identified the characteristics of the new rays that he was investigating, he listed 12 unique properties (Table 1.1). He thought that these were just the beginning of a list of properties, but such was the thoroughness of his experiments and his scientific investigation that to this day no one has added to the original list. It is important that we review the contents of the list, as we will encounter these characteristics throughout the balance of the text.

Elements and Atomic Theory

An element is the smallest particle of a substance. Elements are arranged on a table of the elements (Fig. 1.1). This table was put together to understand the nature of the atoms, which make up the elements contained within the table. Scientists realized early on that some elements were much more stable than others and some were very unstable.

Throughout the text, various elements will be described in relation to their position on this table.

The highest number of stable nonradioactive elements is #83 Bismuth, preceded by #82 Lead. We will meet Lead many times within the chapters of this text.

The smallest particle of an element is an atom (Fig. 1.2). An atom consists mainly of empty space, but the units within the atom are very small. An atom consists of a nucleus containing protons and neutrons. Protons have a positive electrical charge, and neutrons have no charge. Circling around the nucleus are negatively charged electrons. The electrons are held "in orbit" by the positive electrical charge of the protons and their own negative charge. They are arranged in very definite "rings," with specific numbers of electrons in each ring matched with specific numbers of protons within the nucleus. As the numbers of protons within an atom's nucleus increases, the number of corresponding electrons also increases. With this increase, the number of rings of electrons increases and, because of the distance from the nucleus, the electrical charge holding the electrons within the rings lessens to the point that individual electrons may leave their orbits, or they can be "boiled off" if heat is applied to the element. Boiling electrons off the filament of the cathode is the first step in creating x-rays.

◆ APPLICATION INFORMATION

When the x-ray generator is turned on and heat is applied to the cathode of the x-ray tube, electrons are "boiled off" in an effect called *thermionic emission*. When the exposure switch is closed, it is the energy of the electrons (at this point called "photons" or energy packets)—drawn across from the cathode to the anode and interacting with the anode—that produces x-rays.

TABLE 1.1	Roentgen's List of Unique Properties of X-Rays	
PROPERTIES OF X-RAYS	**NOTES**
Are invisible	One cannot hear, smell, or see x-rays.
Are electrically neutral	X-rays carry neither a positive or negative charge.
Have no mass	X-rays have no resistance or force when put into motion.
Travel at the speed of light in a vacuum	X-rays move at 186,000 miles/second in a vacuum (3×10^8 meters/second).
Cannot be focused by a lens	The beam will pass through the lens unchanged.
Form a polyenergetic (heterogeneous) beam	Multiple photon energies are contained within one exposure.
Can be produced in a range of energies (kV)	Peak kilovoltage (kVp) is the maximum energy in one exposure. One exposure equals the energy used to produce one image.
	The useful range for diagnostic imaging is 25–125 kV; 25–40 is used in specialized imaging.
Travel in straight lines	Individual photons travel in a divergent (straight line) beam from the x-ray tube.
Cause fluorescence in certain substances	Fluorescence is useful to intensify the effect of radiation on a film with the use of intensifying screens.
Can cause chemical changes to occur in radiographic and photographic film	Depending on the energy of the photons, x-rays either penetrate matter or are absorbed by it, and therefore an image can occur on film.
Can be absorbed or scattered by tissues in the body; can produce scattered and secondary radiation	Based on the energy of the x-rays and on the composition and thickness of the tissues being exposed, characteristic radiation may be produced when the photon interacts with matter.
Can cause chemical and biological damage to living tissue	Through excitation and ionization (removal of electrons) of atoms comprising cells, damage to cells may occur.

Periodic Table of Elements

Period	I A														III A	IV A	V A	VI A	VII A	VIII A
1	1 H	II A																		2 He
2	3 Li	4 Be													5 B	6 C	7 N	8 O	9 F	10 Ne
3	11 Na	12 Mg	III B	IV B	V B	VI B	VII B		VIII		I B	II B			13 Al	14 Si	15 P	16 S	17 Cl	18 Ar
4	19 K	20 Ca	21 Sc	22 Ti	23 V	24 Cr	25 Mn	26 Fe	27 Co	28 Ni	29 Cu	30 Zn	31 Ga	32 Ge	33 As	34 Se	35 Br	36 Kr
5	37 Rb	38 Sr	39 Y	40 Zr	41 Nb	42 Mo	43 Tc	44 Ru	45 Rh	46 Pd	47 Ag	48 Cd	49 In	50 Sn	51 Sb	52 Te	53 I	54 Xe
6	55 Cs	56 Ba	*	71 Lu	72 Hf	73 Ta	74 W	75 Re	76 Os	77 Ir	78 Pt	79 Au	80 Hg	81 Tl	82 Pb	83 Bi	84 Po	85 At	86 Rn
7	87 Fr	88 Ra	**	103 Lr	104 Rf	105 Db	106 Sg	107 Bh	108 Hs	109 Mt	110 Ds	111 Rg	112 Uub	113 Uut	114 Uuq	115 Uup	116 Uuh	117 Uus	118 Uuo

*Lanthanoids	*	57 La	58 Ce	59 Pr	60 Nd	61 Pm	62 Sm	63 Eu	64 Gd	65 Tb	66 Dy	67 Ho	68 Er	69 Tm	70 Yb
**Actinoids	**	89 Ac	90 Th	91 Pa	92 U	93 Np	94 Pu	95 Am	96 Cm	97 Bk	98 Cf	99 Es	100 Fm	101 Md	102 No

FIG. 1.1 A periodic table of the elements. (From Ziessman HA, O'Malley JP, Thrall JH. *Nuclear Medicine: The Requisites in Radiobiology.* 4th ed. London: Elsevier; 2014.)

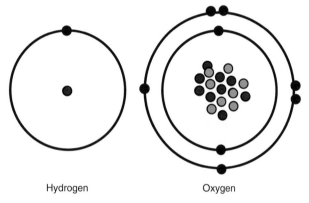

FIG. 1.2 Two examples of elements. The hydrogen element has 1 proton inside the nucleus and 1 electron orbiting the nucleus. The oxygen atom has 8 protons, 8 neutrons within the nucleus, and 8 electrons orbiting the nucleus.

FIG. 1.3 Lightning is an excellent example of electric energy. The negatively charged electrons build up in the clouds until they are attracted by the powerful force of the positively charged earth.

Matter and Energy

Every element on earth has substance, either matter (mass) or energy. It is the conversion of matter into energy that we use to create x-rays. The principal characteristic of matter is mass or weight. Weight involves gravity. The principal characteristic of energy is movement or motion (Fig. 1.3).

The combination of matter and energy in the universe is a constant. Matter can become energy. Energy can become matter. Neither can be created or destroyed. Each can only be changed in form from one to the other.

? POINTS TO PONDER

- Dr. Einstein said it best when he developed his famous formula $E = mc^2$.
- E = energy, m = mass (or matter), c^2 = the speed of light, which is a constant.
- This means that everything that has mass can be changed into energy, and energy can be converted to mass. Neither can be created or destroyed.
- This matters to the production of x-rays because the electrons that are boiled off the cathode in the x-ray tube will be absorbed into whatever they encounter.

◆ APPLICATION INFORMATION

The production of x-rays depends on the tungsten wire in the negatively charged cathode. As energy is infused into the wire, creating heat, electrons are emitted from the wire. These electrons are drawn across to the positively charged anode as "packets of energy" when the switch is closed and the circuit is complete.

The Electromagnetic Spectrum

There are several types of energy: mechanical, chemical, thermal, nuclear, electromagnetic, and electrical. Electrical energy and electromagnetism are the two major types of

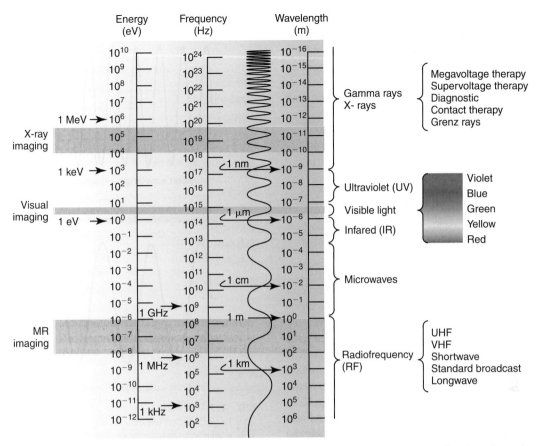

FIG. 1.4 The entire electromagnetic spectrum is much larger than just the visible light portion. This chart shows the values of energy, frequency, and wavelength for all portions and identifies the three imaging windows. (From Bushong SC. *Radiologic Science for Technologists.* 11th ed. St Louis: Elsevier; 2017.)

energy used in x-ray technology. This is evident when we turn on the power to the x-ray generator at the electrical box, and the energy (both electric and electromagnetic) is directed to the production of x-rays. The electrical spectrum covers a vast number of energies. We are concerned with the portions that involve radiation and visible light. In Fig. 1.4 the portion of the spectrum that involves radiation is near the top of the scale, whereas the visible light area is below that and divides into all the colors of the rainbow (Fig. 1.5).

The Dual Nature of X-Rays – Wave-Particle Duality

As can be seen in Fig. 1.4, visible light and x-radiation are listed on the table of the electromagnetic spectrum. They are very similar except that x-rays have a much higher frequency and a shorter wavelength.

- Visible light photons tend to react in experiments in the manner of waves.
- X-rays tend to react in the manner of particles. (An x-ray photon is a unit of pure energy).

This is known as **wave-particle duality** and is useful to know when we investigate the creation of x-rays within an

FIG. 1.5 A rainbow shows all the colors in the *visible* light portion of the electromagnetic spectrum.

electric circuit. In the electric circuit, the x-rays can be described as waves emanating from the tungsten target in the x-ray tube where they are produced. At other times during the discussion of x-radiation, the concept is changed to x-rays as particles.

An electromagnetic wave has height (amplitude) and moves at the speed of light.

◆ APPLICATION INFORMATION

Waves and particles of energy are important in the production of radiation. Setting the voltage and current on the x-ray generator controls the nature of the quantity and energy of the x-rays produced.

Energy as Wavelengths and Frequencies

Watching waves on the seashore is an excellent example of energy transformed into waves (Fig. 1.6). There are crests and troughs, and there is a measurable distance between the crests or the troughs. There is a time factor between each crest and trough. That time factor is the frequency of the waves (Fig. 1.7). One wavelength is the measurement of one crest to the peak of the following crest (or one trough to the depth of the following trough (Fig. 1.8).

A *sinusoidal (sine) wave* is the tracing of the crests and troughs that the waves describe as they travel through the ocean. Sine waves have a high point and a low point, with time being the constant that runs through the middle. This is very important when we set x-ray technical factors and choose the time over which the x-rays will be produced and the kilovoltage that is used to produce them.

Frequency is the number of waves passing a given point per given unit of time. With x-ray production, frequency is connected to the kilovoltage used to penetrate the tissue of the patient and the time that is set to produce the x-rays. Shorter wavelengths with higher frequencies penetrate the tissue more effectively than long wavelengths with low frequency.

Wavelength and frequency are inversely related so that as the frequency increases, the wavelength decreases.

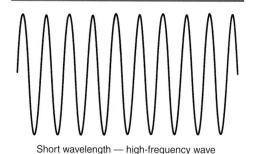

Short wavelength — high-frequency wave

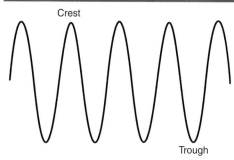

Long wavelength — low-frequency wave

FIG. 1.7 If waves have a short wavelength, they will pass a fixed point frequently (short wavelength/high frequency). If the waves have a long wavelength, they will pass that given point less frequently (long wavelength/low frequency).

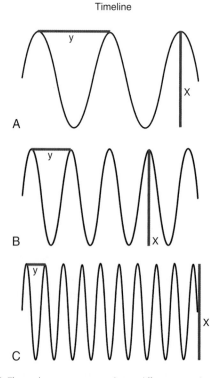

FIG. 1.8 These three sine waves have different wavelengths (y). The shorter the wavelength, the higher the frequency as measured over a constant time. The height of the wave from crest to trough is the amplitude (x). **A,** Long wavelength. **B,** Medium wavelength. **C,** Shorter wavelength.

FIG. 1.6 Energy represented by waves on the ocean. The power of the wind creates waves with frequency and wavelength. This image represents one wave with a crest and one trough. (Copyright 2015 petesphotography/Getty Images.)

◆ **APPLICATION INFORMATION**

Electrical energy can be transformed from one type of energy to another. Electrical energy applied to a hair dryer is converted to heat. Electrical energy applied to an x-ray tube is converted into heat and then, by electromagnetism, into x-rays.

Wavelength and frequency are important when setting the technical factors on the x-ray unit. The choice of increasing or decreasing each of the factors is dependent on the voltage, current, and time—all of which are directly related to wavelength and frequency.

Energy as Particles

Photons are the smallest quantity of any type of electromagnetic radiation. They have neither mass nor electrical charge but interact with matter as though they are particles (Fig. 1.9). It is this energy that has been produced within the cathode to create the potential x-ray beam. A *photon* may be pictured as a small bundle of energy. This is particularly true when using high-frequency energies such as x-rays or gamma rays. The photon particle carries a specific energy that is dependent on *frequency*. The energy and the frequency are directly proportional. If the energy is doubled, then the frequency is doubled. When described as particles, it is possible to mathematically quantify the relationship between frequency and photons and the amount of energy required to perform work.

Summary

Roentgen discovered x-rays in the late 1800s and described the nature of the phenomenon completely. The electromagnetic spectrum describes all forms of energy and categorizes it on a table depending on wavelength, with x-rays near the top of the scale and light near the middle of the scale.

The table of the elements categorizes all the elements known at this time. Throughout the text, we will describe some of these elements and show how their place on the table is important.

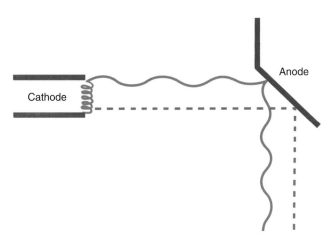

FIG. 1.9 In an x-ray tube, energy is emitted from the cathode as particles. The photons of energy are magnetically drawn to the anode when the circuit is activated.

Scientists soon realized that x-rays can act as continuous waves or as particles (photons of energy), depending on their activity. Sinusoidal (sine) waves are examples of how x-rays behave as waves. Each wave has a crest and a trough, and there is an important relationship between the crests and the troughs.

REVIEW QUESTIONS

1. X-rays are described as:
   a. Invisible, but they travel in straight lines at the speed of light
   b. Electrically neutral unless they are emitted from a charged source
   c. Visible through a lens during x-ray exposure
   d. Causing electrical changes in photographic film
2. An element is the smallest part of a substance. Which of the following statements is true?
   a. The element is combined with a proton.
   b. The smallest part of an element is an atom.
   c. The element is composed of neutrons and particles.
   d. Electrons circle the element in random order.
3. The electrons are held in place by:
   a. The neutral charge of the neutrons
   b. Their own attachment to the nucleus
   c. The ionization of the atom
   d. The positive charge of the protons
4. On the table of the elements:
   a. The elements are arranged alphabetically.
   b. The order of the elements depends on when they were discovered.
   c. The elements are arranged in specific groups.
   d. All the known substances are listed with the radioactive ones at the beginning.
5. Matter and energy are basic to every substance on earth. Which of the following statements is true?
   a. A principal characteristic of matter is mass or weight.
   b. The principal characteristics of energy are time and space.
   c. Matter represents motion and frequency.
   d. Energy cannot be created out of atoms and molecules.
6. The electromagnetic spectrum represents:
   a. The color wheel and the electrical properties of light
   b. The vast spectrum from x-rays to radio waves
   c. The intensity of light and the darkness of radiation
   d. Electricity, wavelength, and frequency
7. Energy can be represented by both:
   a. Waves and particles
   b. Waves and frequencies
   c. Mass and matter
   d. Matter and waves
8. A sinusoidal wave represents x-ray energy as waves. Which of the following statements is true?
   a. It contains the energy of the x-ray beam.
   b. It is an uneven wave, so it cannot be measured.
   c. It has frequency and amplitude in its definition.
   d. It represents the motion of the x-ray timer.

9. Energy as particles is represented as:
    a. Units of motion or as packets
    b. Individual movements of atoms within a substance
    c. Particles within the nucleus of the atom
    d. Waves with frequencies and structure
10. Photons are described as:
    a. Electromagnetic radiation that has a positive electric charge
    b. Negatively charged electrons in the nucleus or the atom
    c. Negatively charged protons within the nucleus of the atom
    d. Electromagnetic radiation that has no electrical charge

Chapter Review Question answers are located in the Instructor Resources on Evolve and can be provided to students at the discretion of the instructor.

CHAPTER 2

Diagnostic X-Ray Production

Lois C. Brown, RTR (Can/USA), ACR, MSc, P.Phys

The representation of the distribution of electricity of the world. (Courtesy US National Aeronautics and Space Administration [NASA].)

"The important thing is to not stop questioning. Curiosity has its own reason for existing."

—Albert Einstein 1879–1955

OUTLINE

LEARNING OBJECTIVES

When you have finished this chapter, you will be able to:

1. Describe the functions of each part of the x-ray tube.
2. List the four criteria necessary to produce x-rays.
3. Understand the construction of the x-ray tube.
4. Describe the anode heel effect and what causes it.
5. Discuss the line focus principle and anode heat bloom.
6. Distinguish between single-phase, three-phase, and high-frequency generators.
7. Understand potential difference.
8. Be familiar with direct and alternating current.
9. Know the difference between transformers and rectifiers.
10. Understand heat dissipation and know how to interpret the cooling charts.
11. Describe the activation of the single-stage and two-stage exposure switches.

APPLICATIONS

The application of the information in this chapter is relevant to the following areas:

1. Production of radiation using electricity
2. The use of electricity in radiography and all the other imaging modalities
3. The application of switches, circuit breakers, transformers, and rectifiers in the production of radiation
4. The use of transformers to increase and decrease the voltage of the incoming power to the x-ray unit
5. The application of electricity in all aspects of work in every area of the profession

Key terms are defined in the Glossary on the Evolve website.

Alternating current
Amperage
Anode
Anode heel effect
Bremsstrahlung radiation
Cathode
Characteristic radiation
Circuit
Circuit breaker
Current
Direct current

Exposure switch
Filament
Focal spot
Focal spot bloom
Generator
Ground
Heat bloom
Heat dissipation
Hertz
High frequency
Line focus principle

Line voltage compensator
Off-focus radiation
Photons
Potential difference
Power
Pulses (timer)
Rectifier
Resistance
Rotating anode
Rotor
Space charge effect

Stationary anode
Target
Thermionic emission
Transformer
Unsharpness
Voltage
Watt
Waveform
X-ray tube

Electricity

All x-ray units are activated by an electric source. This source may be anything from a field battery to a large, very powerful connection in a hospital setting. So to start, we will learn about electricity and the factors that generate the power to activate the x-ray tube.

The x-ray unit consists of a closed circuit with five main criteria:

1. It must have enough power to eventually produce x-rays.
2. It must have selections where the power can be increased or decreased as necessary.
3. The electric current must travel in the same direction through the x-ray tube.

4. There must be a way to produce free electrons with enough energy to produce x-rays.
5. There must be an efficient way to dissipate the heat that results in the interaction of the photons and the anode. (The production of x-rays is very inefficient and results in 99% heat and 1% x-rays).

The Wall Switch

Before the on/off switch for the x-ray unit itself is the wall switch (Fig. 2.1). It is very important—and in fact, the law in most countries—that the x-ray unit is installed with a separate wall switch mounted at eye level (about 5 feet) above the floor within reach of the x-ray generator. This is in place so that if there is an equipment malfunction and the x-ray unit

FIG. 2.1 A, The wall switch must be mounted at eye level and as close as possible to the control panel. **B,** The label on the outside notes the voltage (240V) and the current rating (100 amps) for this switch box.

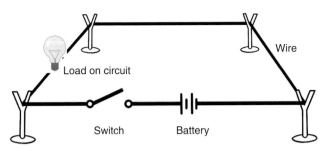

FIG. 2.2 The electric circuit. Electricity must always travel in a circle or circuit. In this drawing, the power source is a battery and the light bulb is the load on the circuit. A break in the circuit (when the switch is open) will cause the electricity to stop flowing.

FIG. 2.4 Principle of resistance. Different-sized fire hoses provide various amounts of resistance depending on their diameters. With the same amount of water flowing through the hose, the smaller-diameter hose provides greater resistance (and therefore a more forceful exit) than the larger-diameter hose.

timer does not terminate the x-ray exposure, the power can then be shut off from the disconnect switch on the wall.

The Electric Circuit

The wall switch is the main access to the electricity that will eventually generate x-rays. The electricity that is used in the production of x-rays travels in wires that have the capacity to contain the necessary amount of voltage and current. Electricity always flows in a *circuit* (Fig. 2.2). In other words, it needs to be connected in a "circle." Any interruption of the circuit will cause the electricity to stop flowing.

"Circuit breakers" are a very important part of the x-ray unit. They act as a fuse. If the voltage or current is set too high, or if a component malfunctions, the circuit breaker will cut the power to the unit. This is a very important safety feature and must never be bypassed because of inadequate service from the installer/manufacturer or the power company.

Four important factors are involved in transmitting the electricity to the x-ray tube (Fig. 2.3):

1. *Voltage* (V): Voltage is the speed with which the electrons in the electric current transfer energy along the circuit. *High voltage* (kV) produces short-wavelength/high-frequency, highly penetrating x-rays.
2. *Current* (I): Amperage is the unit used to measure the electric current that activates the x-ray tube. (In radiography, we use milliamperage.)

3. *Resistance* (R): Resistance is the factor that slows the current as it travels through a wire. A wire that is large in diameter will have low resistance. A wire that is small in diameter will have high resistance (Fig. 2.4). Very-large-diameter or long cables that are used in the x-ray unit will "leak" electric current. This is known as *line loss*.
4. *Time*: A timer controls the length of time that the x-rays are produced. This is determined by the operator selection on the control panel.

◆ **APPLICATION INFORMATION**

If the cables used to attach the x-ray generator are excessively long, the line loss will seriously affect the factors used to create the x-ray image. It is important to keep the cables as short as possible.

Two x-ray clinics owned by the same veterinarian had the same x-ray units installed: identical tubes, x-ray units, and generators, as well as identical processing. The technicians traveled between clinics and found that the technical factors in one clinic were nearly double those of the other clinic. The consultant identified "line loss" as the problem. The cables in one clinic were three times longer than those at the other clinic.

The Operating Console

Typically referred to as the "generator," the operating console displays the dials and often the digital readout of the technical factors selected by the operator: kV (kilovoltage), mA (milliamperes), and time (in seconds). On older units a line voltage compensator will be available to adjust as the incoming line voltage rises and falls depending on supply.

Voltage

The first component in the x-ray circuit is voltage. When we turn on a lamp in our homes, we make use of the incoming voltage to power the light bulb. In the x-ray circuit, we require a lot more voltage for very brief periods of time. The voltage supply in a home power supply is usually 110 volts. In the x-ray clinic, that incoming voltage of 110 is increased

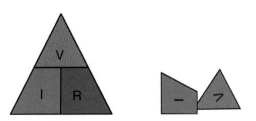

FIG. 2.3 The Ohm's law triangle. The electric circuit components are interrelated. If one component is not functioning, there is no current. Time is the shadowy fourth component as the current flows over time. *I,* Current; *R,* resistance; *V,* voltage.

to supply 220 volts. The components of the x-ray unit will increase that 220 volts to the very high voltage necessary to produce x-rays. Most veterinary x-ray units have a maximum of 125 kilovolts (125,000 volts) available to the operator. Voltage controls the penetrability of the x-ray beam. It is usually labeled on the x-ray console as kV (kilovoltage) and is the easiest selectable module.

> ◆ **APPLICATION INFORMATION**
>
> A consultant was asked to investigate a problem with intermittently very light images on x-ray films at a medical health clinic in a steel plant. When she activated the unit, she noticed that the line voltage indicator fluctuated dramatically. The exposures on the unit when the line voltage needle was at the correct point indicated that the output was calibrated perfectly. All exposures at any other point on the dial displayed very low kilovoltage readings. The cause of the problem was identified as the intermittent drop in voltage over the entire plant on the days when the plant "rolled steel." The high electricity requirement during those times resulted in lower voltages throughout the plant including the x-ray generator. The solution was to run a separate circuit from the city power line into the x-ray clinic completely independent of the steel plant.

Current (Amperage)

The current in a radiography generator is labeled as milliamperage (mA). If the current demanded by the x-ray generator is in excess of what is available, an overload light is displayed, and no exposure is possible until the technician reduces the selected factors. An exposure is still possible on a very old unit, but the unit will produce only its maximum mA and not necessarily the mA requested by the operator. It is very important that the operator is aware of the correct settings and the maximum rating of the x-ray unit.

A word of caution: The milliamperage (mA) knob on the generator panel is connected directly to the high-voltage transformer. It is very dangerous to try to service this knob if it becomes loose or is broken. A qualified service electrician must be contacted to service the generator or serious injury, or death may result.

Time

The timer on the x-ray generator is simply the time over which the radiation is produced. The operator initiates the exposure and the preset time ends the exposure. On older units, the time is graded in parts of a second starting with 1/120. On newer units, the timer is not related as closely to the local electricity supply and therefore supplies much shorter times, down as low as 1 millisecond.

On the x-ray technique chart, the time is always linked to the current and labelled mAs (mA = current, s = seconds) (see Chapter 5).

Watt (a Unit of Power)

A watt is a unit of power. It is the process of changing energy from one form to another. A single watt is equal to 1 ampere of current flowing through an electric potential of one volt.

$$\text{Power (Watt)} = \text{Voltage (V)} \times \text{Current (A)}.$$

When we discuss watts, we generally think of a light bulb. The cathode in the light bulb is an example of changing the electricity in the circuit to light.

When we discuss a technique to be used to radiograph a patient, we discuss it in terms of kV and mA and the time over which the exposure takes place. Radiography units require 20,000 to 150,000 watts to be efficient. (A household toaster requires 500 to 1500 watts.)

When a salesperson discusses the generator options, it is always in terms of kilowatts. A 37-watt generator is a 300-mA unit, whereas a 50-watt generator will produce 400 mA.

Potential Difference

Potential difference (Fig. 2.4) will cause the electrons to flow from the start of the circuit (at the generator) through the x-ray tube as part of the circuit. If we use a garden hose as an analogy, the hose is connected to a generator (the faucet). When the hose is stored, there is very little water throughout the hose itself but a great deal of potential ability to contain water from the faucet. When the faucet is turned on to allow water to flow, there is a potential difference along the length of the hose. One end has no water and the other has a lot of water, with more coming in all the time. The "potential difference" is the measurement of the full end of the hose compared with the empty end of the hose.

In radiography, the potential difference between the cathode and anode of the x-ray tube causes the electrons to flow from the cathode to the anode when the exposure switch is closed.

Line Voltage Compensator

The line voltage compensator is standard equipment on every unit. On some older units still in use today, a compensator is mounted on the control panel (Fig. 2.5). In older units and in areas of the country in which the incoming line voltage is not always as stable as it should be or the incoming power lines to a facility are limited or restricted, the compensator can stabilize the incoming power line to the x-ray unit. It is usually connected through the kilovolt (kV) meter and is a method of increasing or decreasing the incoming line voltage. The veterinary technician should always check the line voltage meter on an older unit before positioning the patient and making an exposure. If it is low or high, it must be adjusted before setting the technical factors. Newer units compensate automatically through an internal compensator.

FIG. 2.5 A, The line voltage compensator on an older-model Bennett x-ray generator circa 1985-1990. **B,** Close-up of the compensator readout on the Bennett generator. The knob on the side of the unit must be turned until the needle is centered on the black bar.

◆ APPLICATION INFORMATION

A veterinary hospital was opened in an industrial mall on the outskirts of a large city. The images were excellent, and the techniques were consistent for the first 5 years. Unexpectedly, the veterinary technician noticed that intermittent images were so underexposed as to be unreadable. He called in a consultant, who discovered an intermittent severe voltage drop on the line. After tracing the problem to the transformer on the roof of the building, it was discovered that an auto body shop specializing in trim work and welding had illegally tapped into the veterinary clinic's transformer on the roof of the building. Every time the shop used the welding and electroplating equipment and the veterinarian used the radiography unit simultaneously, the voltage dropped, and the resulting images were underexposed.

Circuit Breakers: Amperage and Ground

Amperage

When the power first arrives at the x-ray unit, it immediately encounters the circuit breaker (Fig. 2.6). This is the power supply to the x-ray unit and to the rest of the facility. It is very important that the power to the x-ray unit is connected to its own circuit breaker and not shared with other units in the facility. A circuit breaker will accept current (amperage) up to a certain point (its rating). If the maximum quantity of power exceeds the rating, the circuit breaker disconnects, and power to the electronic device is interrupted until it is manually reset.

Because the nominal voltage coming into most buildings is 110 volts, it must be doubled to 220 volts in order to provide enough power to supply the x-ray circuit. This is done by connecting two 110-volt power lines coming into the building to the x-ray unit (220 volts).

Fuses

Fuses are safety devices that will mechanically interrupt the flow of electricity if a problem arises that would overheat the circuit. In radiography, circuit breakers act as fuses (Fig. 2.6).

FIG. 2.6 An example of a circuit breaker panel. Each switch represents a circuit within the building so that power can be interrupted in one area and maintained everywhere else. A #2 wire from the electrical panel to the x-ray unit will disconnect the x-ray unit from the panel if an overload occurs.

Ground

A grounding wire provides an alternative route for the electricity to flow if the circuit is broken inappropriately. The original electrical circuit is directed to a ground wire attached to an object that will absorb excess electrons and therefore redirect the current flow. The flow of electrons will stop with the broken circuit, but the excess electrons that are still flowing will be redirected to the ground wire. In most cases the ground wire is a green wire within the switch box (Fig. 2.7).

Direct Current and Alternating Current

The electricity "flows" through wires from the main generating stations in power plants throughout the country. It is then converted into a useful power supply to be used either as *Direct* or *Alternating* Current.

FIG. 2.7 On the inside of the box, two fuses are connected to the two 110-volt lines to provide 220 volts to the radiography unit. The ground wire is green and is located to the left side of the box in this installation.

FIG. 2.8 A flashlight is an example of direct current. The batteries carry the voltage. When the switch is closed, the current flows through the batteries and the contact plate to the light bulb, which emits radiant energy in the form of light. (Modified from (c) istock.com/blueringmedia.)

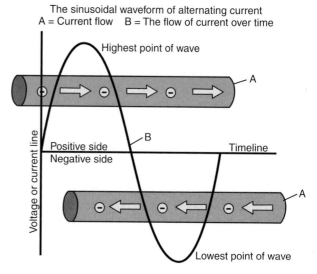

FIG. 2.9 An example of alternating current. The electrons flow through the coil (A) creating one positive portion and (B) one negative portion of one cycle.

Direct Current

A flashlight is an example of direct current (Fig. 2.8). The batteries installed in a flashlight need to be in a certain orientation so that when the switch connects the circuit, the unit produces light through the light bulb.

Direct current requires a source situated very close to the end user. If power is to be transmitted over vast distances, then a source that transmits a very low current paired with a very high voltage is less expensive and much more efficient.

Alternating Current

Alternating current produces one positive pulse and then one matching negative pulse (Fig. 2.9). In North America the pulses are paired at 120 cycles (one positive [+ve] cycle and one negative [−ve] cycle) per second.

Transformers

The power that is generated to activate x-ray units and other electronic devices originates at a power plant. The power is transmitted over vast distances, with transformer stations along the way to boost the power that is lost through transmission. What matters most to the veterinary clinic is the transformer that is mounted near the veterinary clinic and supplies power to the entire clinic. Quite often the local transformer station is within a few miles of the veterinary hospital, and an auxiliary transformer is mounted on a hydroelectric pole or within a transformer on the ground just outside the clinic (Fig. 2.10).

This transmission of power from the power station to any end point (e.g., a veterinary hospital) requires the use of transformers. Transformers step up (increase) the power at one end of the journey and then step down (decrease) the power at the destination.

For example, to send 1 million watts of power across a grid to provide electricity to a neighborhood, it is much easier and more efficient to send 1 ampere at 1,000,000 volts than 1,000,000 amperes at 1 volt (Fig. 2.11). Using transformers at each end of the journey alters the voltage as required. The shortest time on a single-phase, fully rectified generator is based on 60 full cycles per second. The 60 positive pulses and 60 rectified negative pulses provide a fastest time of 1/120 of a second. (In Europe and some Caribbean countries, 50 full cycles per second are provided and the shortest time is 1/100th of a second.)

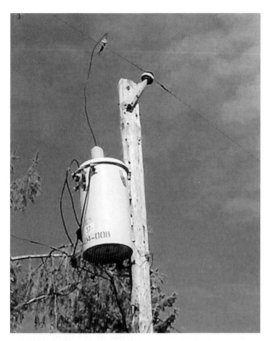

FIG. 2.10 The transformer mounted on a hydroelectric pole outside a veterinary hospital in New York State.

FIG. 2.11 An example of hydroelectric transmission lines alongside a New York highway. The sign warns potential climbers of the high voltage being transmitted through the lines.

Within the x-ray circuit, the autotransformer is used to provide the current and voltage requested by the veterinarian when they set the kV on the control panel. The high-voltage transformer increases the current and voltage to the amount requested by the operator when setting the mA on the control panel. The filament transformer reduces the current and voltage to the correct amount to heat the cathode filament and produce the electron cloud (thermionic emission) so the electrons can be drawn across to the anode and produce x-rays and heat.

APPLICATION INFORMATION

A veterinary hospital in the countryside purchased a new x-ray unit during the winter as part of a renovation project slated to be completed during the following summer. The unit was installed during the day and tested during that evening by the service engineer. All went well, and the images were consistently excellent. Everything was fine until the following August, when images were inconsistent. The images would occasionally be far too light and then would be fine. There seemed to be no pattern to the problem. The consultant was called and visited several times, testing various potential areas where a problem could occur.

Finally, it was decided to trace the electricity from the power lines. At the back of the hospital there was a power line pole with the hospital transformer mounted on the pole. A squirrel had industriously built a very large nest on the top of the transformer. There was obviously a draw on the line: when the wind blew, the wires partially disconnected then reconnected. As soon as the nest was removed, the power and the images returned to normal. The unfortunate squirrel was found at the bottom of the nest, apparently electrocuted when the nest was finally breached by the power line.

Transformers receive power from the incoming power lines and transform the power to the x-ray tube. They use the turns of a wire around a central core or around two magnetic cores in close proximity to each other to either increase or decrease the voltage in a circuit. There is a direct relationship between the windings on one side of the transformer and the windings on the other side of the transformer. In a step-up transformer, 100 turns on the primary coil and 200 turns on the secondary coil produce twice the voltage. In a step-down transformer, 100 turns on the primary coil and 50 turns on the secondary coil produce half the voltage (Fig. 2.12).

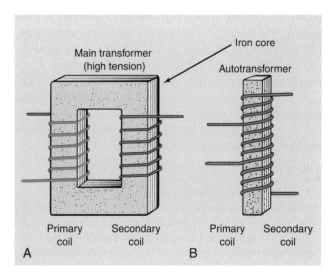

FIG. 2.12 Example of two simple types of transformer. **A,** Closed core transformer. **B,** Autotransformer. (Modified from Bushong SC. *Radiologic Science for Technologists.* 11th ed. St Louis: Elsevier; 2017.)

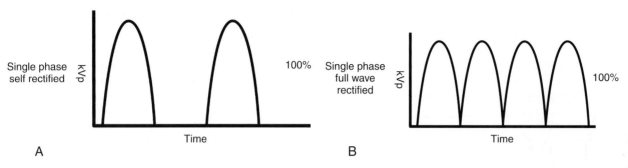

FIG. 2.13 A, A single-phase generator produces a waveform that rises and falls throughout the exposure. The negative portion of the waveform does not go through the x-ray tube, and therefore one half of the exposure is lost. B, A fully rectified single-phase generator changes the negative phase to positive. The full waveform is used during the exposure.

Rectifiers

The power supplied by the electric companies in North America and around the world is an alternating current. This means that the power fluctuates from positive to negative 120 times every second. In North America, this is called *60 hertz*; one positive and one negative pulse is one cycle—120 positive and negative fluctuations equal 60 cycles.

In Chapter 1, we discussed that electrical energy travels in pulses and waves. When the x-ray tube is producing x-rays, the available current must travel continuously in one direction (cathode to anode). However, when the power plants supplied alternating current, there was a problem. The negative pulse was blocked and only the positive pulses were allowed through to the x-ray tube (Fig. 2.13A).

In the early units, there was a problem when the electrical pulses dropped to the baseline, so the rectifier circuit was invented.

The rectifying circuit ensures that the current that travels through the x-ray tube does so in the same direction. Four diodes are paired in the circuit. In each pair, one diode allows the current to flow and one diode prevents it from flowing. The second pair repeats this when the current alternates, thereby maintaining the current flow in the same direction. The end result is that the current flows in one direction through the x-ray tube and is fully rectified (Fig. 2.13B).

If one of the rectifiers stops working, the current on that portion of the alternating current is prevented from reaching the x-ray tube, and the images will be too light by exactly one-half the density.

★ APPLICATION INFORMATION

A veterinary hospital with a simple x-ray unit called a consultant to investigate why the images started to turn out with exactly half the density that was expected. Everything seemed to be working well except that the milliampere-seconds (mAs) had to be doubled to produce a properly exposed image.

Upon investigation, the consultant discovered that half of the rectifying circuit had malfunctioned, so the film was only receiving one-half of the expected radiation.

Single-Phase Circuits

The original single-phase x-ray units were equipped with basic autotransformers, timers, and simple rectifying circuits. These units had a fastest time of 1/120 of a second, but there was a voltage drop during each pulse.

Some units had no rectifiers and were described as *self-rectified units*. The timers used the pulses of 120 cycles/second but, as there was no rectification, the radiation was produced only during the positive pulses. Therefore, the fastest time was 1/60 of a second. The problem that arose was the long exposure time due to the low power of these units and the loss of power as the voltage dropped during the exposure with the completion of each pulse (Fig. 2.13B).

Three-Phase Circuits

One solution to the dips of power in the waveform of the single-phase x-ray units was to add two more pulses of power offset from the first pulse and also from each other to make the drop in power much less significant (Fig. 2.14). This change considerably reduced the ripple effect in the power and made the output of the x-ray unit much more efficient.

These x-ray units became much more sophisticated and required a great deal more initial power when they were installed. These units are not normally used in veterinary medicine except in large veterinary hospitals, where very high milliamperes (mA) combined with short times (seconds) are necessary to image large-animal chests and abdomens.

High-Frequency

Another less expensive and better alternative to the power drop problem is to use high-frequency pulses. In this case, many phases are overlapped continuously, and the ripple stays very low (around 2% to 3%) with continuous output. High-frequency units cost a little more than the original single-phase units, but the benefit of more x-rays for each exposure allows the operator to reduce the overall exposure time, saving wear and tear on the x-ray unit and reducing the overall dose. Today virtually all new x-ray units installed in

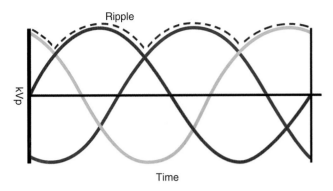

FIG. 2.14 An example of a three-phase circuit. The circuit now has three overlapping cycles and therefore very little loss of power when each cycle reaches zero. The small fluctuation at the top of the waveform is called a *ripple*.

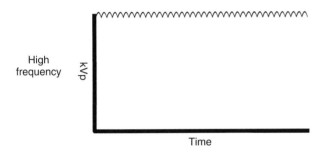

FIG. 2.15 A waveform from a high-frequency generator. There is a 3% ripple with virtually continuous output.

North American veterinary hospitals are high-frequency units (Fig. 2.15).

The Complete X-Ray Circuit

The x-ray circuit has now been explained, identifying its individual components and how they deserve their place in the circuit. Fig. 2.16 is a diagram of the x-ray circuit.

The X-Ray Unit

Components of the X-Ray Unit

Figs. 2.17 and 2.18 illustrate high frequency x-ray units installed in veterinary hospitals.

Fig. 2.19 shows an x-ray unit with the three separate components: the table, x-ray tube, and generator.

The x-ray unit consists of three component parts:
1. The high-voltage transformer
2. The x-ray generator (control panel)
3. The x-ray tube

The **high-voltage transformer** (sometimes called the high-tension transformer) is often located beneath the x-ray table (Figs. 2.17 & 2.18). It is connected to the hospital power lines and uses the power supplied to the hospital by the outside power lines.

The **x-ray generator** receives its power from the high-voltage transformer and sends it through the circuit to the rectifiers and then to the x-ray tube (Fig. 2.16).

FIG. 2.16 The complete radiography generator circuit. (From Bushong SC. *Radiologic Science for Technologists*. 11th ed. St Louis: Elsevier; 2017.)

FIG. 2.17 The Sedecal veterinary x-ray unit. The transformer is beneath the table—note that the operator controls are mounted in front of the x-ray tube. This configuration may pose a challenge with staff members who are short. In this case, the generator panel may be relocated to a stand at one end of the table.

FIG. 2.18 A, The Innovet line of high-frequency generators. Note that the cables are contained within the tube stand. B, (*Inset*) Technique selection is located on the front of the table. The x-ray generator and transformer are located beside the table.

The **x-ray tube** is the most important part of the x-ray machine because it is here that the x-rays are produced.

The x-ray generator and the high-voltage transformer are usually matched as a pair. If one of these components malfunctions, they must both be replaced. The x-ray generator is

FIG. 2.19 Typical x-ray unit with a separate generator. (Courtesy Raymax Medical Corporation, Brampton, Ontario.)

separate from the x-ray tube (Fig. 2.19). The x-ray tube can be replaced on its own but must be recalibrated to match the generator.

The x-ray unit requires a dedicated power line. It cannot share a power line or source with another piece of equipment that draws a lot of power. If another unit (such as a sterilizer or clothes dryer) is installed on the same line, the draw will reduce the power to the x-ray unit, and the transformers will not be able to compensate for the loss of power. The resulting image will be underexposed.

On some units the generator is mounted above the table on the tube stand (Figs. 2.17 & 2.18) This is fine for the staff members who are reasonably tall, but it can be awkward if the technician is short because the readouts can be difficult to see.

Fig. 2.20 illustrates a programmed x-ray generator. They are very useful, as the technical factors are programmed into the unit according to the measurement of the animal. (Chapter 5 explains technique charts.)

The X-Ray Tube

The x-ray tube (Fig. 2.21) consists of a glass enclosure that houses a cathode and an anode. The glass enclosure is a special heat-resistant glass. Pyrex is one brand of glass manufactured for x-ray tubes. The standard x-ray tube is approximately 30 cm long and approximately 20 cm in diameter. The external housing enlarges the tube to about 50 cm long and 30 cm in diameter.

Every x-ray tube is shielded with a metal covering, which restricts most off-focus (see Fig. 2.29) radiation from exiting the tube other than at the tube port.

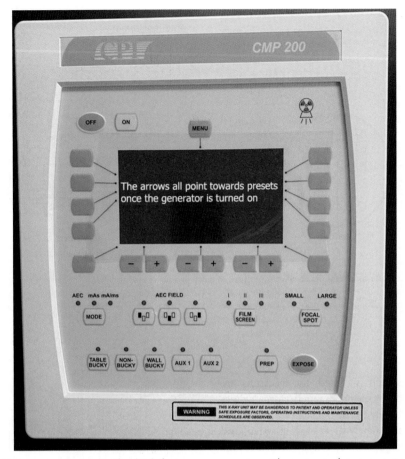

FIG. 2.20 The operator console of a high-frequency generator with anatomical programming. This unit is the size of a computer keyboard and may be mounted at the front of the x-ray tube or on a stand at the end of the table. (Courtesy Raymax Medical Corporation, Brampton, Ontario.)

FIG. 2.21 Cutaway of a typical x-ray tube to visualize the anode and the cathode. Note that the cathode is offset from the anode, so the electron beam is directed toward the outer ring of the rotating anode. The angle of the anode will deflect the beam at 90 degrees toward the patient. (From Bushong SC. *Radiologic Science for Technologists*. 11th ed. St Louis: Elsevier; 2017.)

FIG. 2.22 Cathode assembly. **A,** The two filaments are much like an incandescent light bulb filament. **B,** The wiring diagram for the filament selector and the cathode assembly. Note that the cathode is offset so the photon beam is directed toward the beveled edge of the anode. (**A** from Fauber TL. *Radiographic Imaging and Exposure.* 5th ed. St. Louis: Mosby; 2017; **B** from Fauber TL. *Radiographic Imaging and Exposure.* 4th ed. St. Louis: Mosby; 2013.)

When the exposure switch is closed, the electrons are drawn across to the anode by electromagnetic force, where they are stopped very suddenly by the density of the metal of the anode. They react immediately by (1) losing speed, and (2) converting the forward motion to energy, which results in heat and x-rays (99% heat and 1% x-rays).

The Cathode

The cathode is a thin tungsten wire that is coiled and placed in a focusing cup (Fig. 2.22A). When this coil is heated by electricity, it produces a cloud of electrons. This is called *thermionic emission* (emission due to heating).

The cathode of the x-ray tube typically has two filaments (Fig. 2.22A). The large filament (typically 1.4 mm wide and 1 cm in length) is used when large body parts are examined; the small filament (typically 0.7 mm in width and 0.75 mm in length) is used for detailed work, such as extremities and small pocket pets. These filaments are labeled on the x-ray generator as large and small focus (Fig. 2.22B). The filament used is preset on the generator panel by the milliamperage setting and selected by the operator.

The filaments of the cathode are made of thoriated tungsten, which can withstand very high temperatures without melting. The melting point of tungsten is 3410° C (6170° F). Therefore, it can withstand many x-ray exposures without melting.

The filaments are positioned opposite the outer rim of the anode in a small cup-shaped device called the *focusing cup* in such a way that they are aimed directly at the anode. The focusing cups are slightly negatively charged to focus the electrons that are boiled off the cathode filaments (Fig. 2.23). The beveled edges of the focusing cups are designed to focus on very small areas of the anode. It is here, on the focal spot of the anode, that x-rays are produced, and it is from here that the exceptional amount of heat must be dissipated.

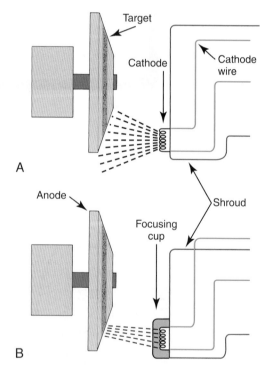

FIG. 2.23 **A,** Without a slightly negative charge on the focusing cup, the electron beam spreads beyond the anode. (Similar charges repel one another in a mutually electrostatic repulsion.) **B,** With a negatively charged focusing cup, the entire electron beam is directed toward the target. (From Bushong SC. *Radiologic Science for Technologists.* 11th ed. St Louis: Elsevier; 2017.)

When the exposure switch is closed, the circuit is activated and the filament transformer sends electricity to the cathode. The cathode temperature quickly rises, and electrons are "boiled off" the cathode filament in a reaction called *thermionic emission*. The cloud of electrons that is produced is called a *space charge,* and the whole process is called *space charge effect.*

The Anode

The anode is a tungsten plate that is beveled on the outer rim so that the x-rays produced at the anode are directed downward toward the patient (Fig. 2.24).

The anode is the partner to the cathode in the x-ray tube. It consists of a tungsten "target" upon which the electrons (now photons of energy) are focused. This very small area is called the *focal spot,* and it is this area where the x-rays are produced and sent in a downward projection to the patient.

There are two types of anode: rotating and stationary. Small-animal installed x-ray units use rotating anodes, and large-animal portable units use stationary anodes. The anode material is tungsten or a tungsten–molybdenum alloy. Tungsten has a high atomic number (74) and readily absorbs electrons and heat.

The Rotating Anode

The rotating anode is mounted on a stem that in turn is mounted on ball bearings (Fig. 2.24). The entire structure rotates very rapidly once the circuit is closed, and the anode is prepared to receive electrons. On the beveled front edge of the rotating anode is the target of the x-ray tube.

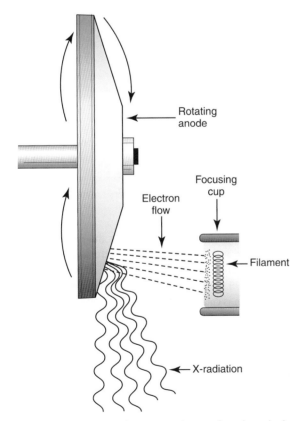

FIG. 2.24 A rotating anode receiving electrons from the cathode and converting them to x-radiation, which is directed toward the patient. The composition of the anode is a tungsten molybdenum alloy to assist in dissipating heat. (From Fauber TL. *Radiographic Imaging and Exposure.* 5th ed. St Louis: Mosby; 2017.)

The anode stem mechanically supports the electron target. It serves as a thermal dissipater by directing the heat emitted in the production of x-rays along the stem, as well as rotating so that the electrons (which are now traveling at tremendous speed across the gap toward the anode and are now called *photons*) are not always focused on the exact same spot.

The outer edge of the disk is beveled at a very specific angle in order to direct the x-rays down toward the patient being radiographed. This angle is important because it creates the deflection by which the x-rays travel toward the patient. The angle is fixed when the x-ray tube is manufactured, and it is not adjustable. The angle is usually between 11 and 15 degrees, depending on the manufacturer.

The Rotating Anode and What Can Happen When Things Go Wrong (Fig. 2.25A-D)

The rotor circuit is activated at the same time as the filament transformer starts to heat the cathode. The rotor circuit enables the rotation of the anode and will reach speeds of 3000 to 10,000 revolutions per minute. The inside of the rotor shaft contains very-high-grade stainless steel bearings that are manufactured to withstand extremely high temperatures as heat is dissipated from the rotating anode. As the x-ray tube ages, these bearings can distort and develop flat edges, as they become very hot during the exposure and then rest in one position after the exposure and termination of the motion. Because the bearings move rapidly when the rotor is turning, the noise made by the flattened sides of the bearings can become extreme. If the bearings seize and the rotor does not rotate, the heat is directed to one tiny spot on the anode, the focal spot. The accumulated heat will crack and sometimes melt the overheated anode. Usually, at this point, safety interlocks prevent further exposures.

The veterinary technician should always listen for the noise of the rotating anode before the exposure. If no noise is heard, the exposure should not be attempted, and service should be called.

The Stationary Anode (Fig. 2.26)

Equine portable x-ray units, dental x-ray units, and fluoroscopy C-arms have stationary anodes. Because a lot of heat is produced during the exposure, the stationary anode must have an efficient method of dissipating heat. The stationary anode is composed primarily of copper with a wide stem and a tungsten insert to receive and dissipate the high amount of heat produced during the exposure. The targeted end of the stationary anode is angled to direct the beam to the patient. Because the anode is not rotating to dissipate the heat, the operator must be careful to follow the warning and ready lights on the unit so the heat may dissipate between exposures.

The Anode Heel Effect

Because so few x-rays are produced per exposure, it is important that the x-ray beam is used efficiently. The bevel of the angled anode redirects the x-rays being produced at the

FIG. 2.25 Effects of overheating the anode. A, Three examples of new anodes. **B,** Effect of etching due to slow rotation of the anode due to bearing damage. **C,** Effect of repeated overload or overheating of the anode. **D,** Effect of exceeding maximum heat storage capacity. (Courtesy Philips Medical Systems.)

Cathode   Anode

FIG. 2.26 A large-animal portable x-ray tube with a stationary anode, with a tungsten target embedded in a copper shield for faster dissipation of heat. The cathode filaments enclosed in the focusing cups and are not visible on this image. They are offset within the surrounding shield, so they are aimed directly at the focal spot of the anode.

anode. The intensity of the radiation is greater on the cathode side than on the anode side (Fig. 2.27). This effect, called the *anode heel effect,* becomes important when a patient is thicker on one end of its anatomy than on the other.

The thicker end of the animal should be placed on the cathode side to take advantage of the greater amount of

radiation at that end. In Fig. 2.27, the end of the table with the higher amount of radiation would be to the right. With any new or unfamiliar installation, it is important to note the anode and cathode positions of the x-ray tube and to ascertain the correct orientation. If unsure, a call to the vendor or the installer will answer the question.

The Line Focus Principle

The line focus principle describes how the electrons interact with the anode and change direction, so the x-rays are directed toward the patient being radiographed. The angle of the bevel on the outer edge of the anode and the resulting change of direction of the radiation is called the *line focus principle* (Fig. 2.28).

If the angle of the anode is less than 15 degrees from the vertical, the resulting x-ray beam will be very narrow, and the image will have higher resolution. With an angle of less than 15 degrees, multiple exposures will heat the area around the focal spot to the point where that area will also produce x-rays, effectively enlarging the focal spot. The images will lose resolution as the focal spot enlarges *(focal spot bloom).* It would be very unusual for this to happen in a veterinary hospital, but it could be a problem in a specialty hospital in which special procedures such as fluoroscopy or angiography are practiced.

FIG. 2.27 The anode heel effect. The radiation on the anode side of the central ray is limited by the "heel" of the anode. The cathode side of the image receives more radiation. (From Bushong SC. *Radiologic Science for Technologists*. 11th ed. St Louis: Elsevier; 2017.)

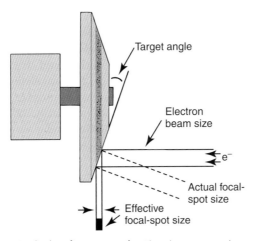

FIG. 2.28 The line focus principle. The electrons travel toward the anode and are converted into x-rays as they encounter the target. The x-rays are directed downward toward the patient. Because of the angle of the anode, the effective central ray is narrower than the primary beam, making the focal spot effectively smaller. (From Bushong SC. *Radiologic Science for Technologists*. 11th ed. St Louis: Elsevier; 2017.)

If the angle is greater than 15 degrees, the beam will be wider, resulting in less heat focused on the very small focal spot and decreasing the "bloom" effect on the focal spot. This angle also reduces resolution. The typical angle for x-ray tubes in North America is 11 degrees, which provides a very narrow x-ray beam and therefore allows for high resolution.

Off-Focus Radiation and Heat Bloom

When the exposure switch is closed, the interactions between the electrons and the anode are in effect and produce x-rays throughout the length of the exposure. The stream of electrons interacts not only with the actual target but also with the areas of the anode immediately adjacent to the target. Occasionally the electrons "bounce" off the target anode and are then attracted back to the anode but at a point beyond the focal spot (Fig. 2.29A).

It is very important to ensure that the exit area of the glass envelope of the x-ray tube is supplied with a collar of lead so that any extra focal radiation, or radiation produced outside the actual focal spot, is absorbed by the collar and does not appear on the image as an artifact (Fig. 2.29B).

Off-focus radiation effects can also occur if the kV is set higher than necessary and the collimation is inadequate. (Collimation will be discussed in Chapter 6.)

Large-Animal Portable X-Ray Units

Equine veterinarians must have the facility to travel to their patients and radiograph them on site. To do this, a small version of a full-sized x-ray unit has been developed. These units are not as powerful as the small-animal units, and they do not have the milliamperage of the larger units. However, because equine legs and feet are usually the areas of concern, the units are quite adequate.

These units can also be used in a small-animal veterinary hospital. Because the milliamperage is limited on these smaller units, longer time factors must be used to achieve the correct milliampere-seconds. Using the inverse square law, the ideal distance is 30 inches (76 cm) to compensate for the lower output of the x-ray unit (Fig. 2.30).

In a large-animal unit, the generator, transformers, and x-ray tube are all miniaturized and compressed into a very small space (Fig. 2.31A). The newest unit on the market features a completely wireless system that combines digital radiography and portable large-animal radiography (Fig. 2.31B).

X-Ray Production

The Exposure Switch

The exposure switch sets the sequence of events in motion to produce the x-ray exposure. Most small-animal x-ray units have one two-stage exposure switch (Fig. 2.32). The *first* stage activates the rotating anode and boosts the filament circuit. The *second* stage activates the exposure, and x-rays are produced.

The exposure switch should be tested on a regular basis (semiannually) to ensure that it disconnects when the foot pedal is released. This "dead man" safety factor is a legal requirement to ensure that the x-ray beam is terminated at the end of an exposure. Tube heat overload is an indication that the x-ray tube is overheated and will require time to cool before another exposure is attempted. This occurrence is very common on large-animal mobile units. Waiting for the "ready" signal is a very important part of the radiography

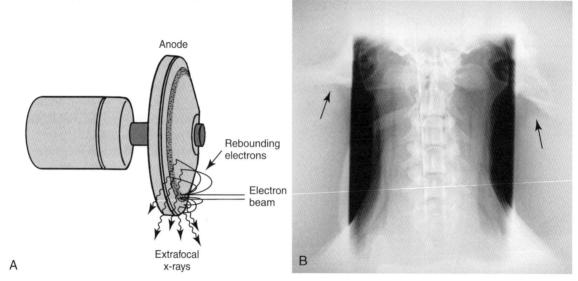

FIG. 2.29 A, The production of off-focus radiation. B, Off-focus radiation (extra focal radiation) has produced an image of the dog's ears beyond the limits of the collimator (arrows). (A from Bushong SC. *Radiologic Science for Technologists.* 11th ed. St Louis: Elsevier; 2017; B Courtesy Lois Brown, imaged at a veterinary hospital in Mississauga, Ontario.)

FIG. 2.30 Wireless digital equine imaging. The laser (*red dot*) ensures the correct distance, and the lack of electrical cords simplifies the imaging process. The assistant holding the digital plate wears a lead apron and lead gloves. If a film cassette is used, a cassette holder would be in place with the assistant standing well out of the beam. The veterinarian holding the shielded x-ray unit is also wearing a lead apron and lead gloves.

protocol and prolongs the life of the x-ray tube by not overheating it continually.

◆ **APPLICATION INFORMATION**

If the first-stage switch is activated and the sound of boiling liquid (actually oil) is heard, the exposure switch must be released immediately. It is likely that the x-ray tube has "shorted out" and the filament circuit is overheating the cooling oil in the x-ray tube housing. This situation is very unsafe because the tube could explode if the full force of the tube voltage (kV) were applied.

Exposure Switch Variations

There are several variations of exposure switches. A single-stage switch may be wired in so that the rotor begins to turn when the generator is turned on. This is not ideal because the rotor should be activated only when the exposure is about to be made. If this is the case, the unit should be turned off between exposures and activated only when the exposure is about to be made. A single-stage foot switch may also be wired in, so the rotor is initiated when the foot switch is depressed. There will be a safety delay until the rotating anode achieves the necessary speed. This installation is not efficient and should be revised as soon as possible because animals being radiographed are not necessarily cooperative and initiating the exposure depends on timing for minimal patient movement or, for certain views, full inspiration or full expiration.

Another variation is the hand switch. Most human units are activated with a hand switch, and the technologist stands behind a screen and instructs the patient. The hand switch may be replaced with a foot switch when such a unit is sold to a veterinary facility. Occasionally, the hand switch is still active on a unit with an added foot switch. This can be useful if there is a problem with the foot switch; the hand switch can be used while the service engineer is on the way.

X-Ray Production

Electrons are "boiled off" the cathode filament as it is heated up, ready for the x-ray exposure. At the same time the rotating anode reaches speeds of 3000 to 10,000 revolutions per minute (rpm). When the exposure switch is closed, the electrons are attracted to the anode at very high speeds, and their energy is transferred to the tungsten atoms in the anode to produce x-rays. Many electrons travel from the cathode to the anode, and various interactions take place

FIG. 2.31 A, The United Radiology Systems battery-operated x-ray unit paired with a Thales digital wireless plate. **B**, The image is delivered wirelessly to the computer from the digital plate.

FIG. 2.32 Two-stage exposure switch. The switch plate is depressed halfway to initiate the rotor circuit and then all the way to initiate the x-ray exposure.

during the time of the exposure. This produces an x-ray beam of a number of different energies, and this heterogeneous beam is important for diagnostic images.

Two common interactions take place. In *bremsstrahlung interactions,* the incoming electron avoids hitting a tungsten electron but travels very close to its nucleus. In doing this, it

is redirected into a different path and loses some energy, which is emitted as an x-ray photon. The name comes from the term for "braking," as in losing speed rapidly (Fig. 2.33A).

Characteristic interactions occur when an incoming electron interacts with an electron from the inner shell of the tungsten atom (the K-shell). If the incoming electron ejects the inner shell electron, it leaves a space that is rapidly filled by electrons from the next ring in a roller-coaster effect. As each electron drops into place, it emits a small amount of radiation. The K-shell electron now travels on as an x-ray photon with properties *characteristic* of tungsten. This radiation has the strongest effect on the exposure because a strong incoming electron is required to oust the K-shell electron from its orbit. Once the K-shell electron leaves its orbit, all other electrons move in to fill the vacant spaces. An L-shell electron drops into the K-shell ring, an M-shell electron drops into the L-shell ring, etc. Each time an electron drops into the next ring, it loses energy, which is also emitted as x-rays (Fig. 2.33B).

Heat Dissipation

When the x-ray beam is generated, the exposure to the image detector is only 1% x-rays and 99% heat. This heat must be dissipated quickly before the next exposure. When the target is exposed to radiation over a number of exposures in a short time, the anode can become exceptionally hot, usually 1000° to 2000° C (1832° to 3632° F). With repeated exposures the focal spot will dissipate heat into the area immediately surrounding it—this will enlarge the effective focal spot. The descriptive term for this is *heat bloom.*

Each x-ray tube is supplied with an anode cooling chart when it is installed. This chart graphically illustrates the cooling period necessary between exposures to prevent

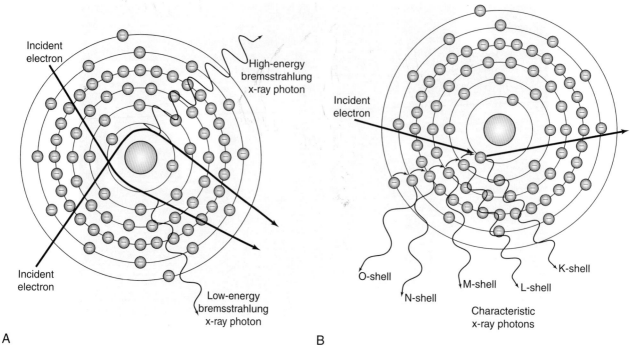

FIG. 2.33 A, Bremsstrahlung radiation. Radiation resulting from an interaction of an electron and a tungsten atom. The electron misses the nucleus but loses some energy as it swings around the nucleus and travels in a different direction. The energy lost is emitted as bremsstrahlung radiation. **B,** Characteristic radiation. The electron interacts directly with an inner orbital electron of the tungsten atom. The energy lost is emitted as a photoelectric effect characteristic of the tungsten atom. (From Fauber TL. *Radiographic Imaging and Exposure.* 5th ed. St. Louis: Mosby; 2017.)

overheating of the x-ray tube. Large-animal portable units typically have a safety shutoff that prevents overheating. In Fig. 2.34 the anode cooling chart indicates that an interval of 15 minutes should be allowed to dissipate 350,000 heat units. The maximum heat units for this x-ray tube are 350,000 units. Using this chart, if 50,000 heat units are produced, read to where the line crosses the blue curve (approx. 6 minutes) and subtract that number (6) from the maximum allowable 15 minutes (15 − 6 = 9). Therefore at 50,000 heat units, it will take 9 minutes for the tube to cool sufficiently for another exposure to be made safely.

To calculate heat units, multiply as follows (using the chart in Fig. 2.34):

kV × mA × Seconds × Number of exposures = Heat units

For example:

At 80 kV × 200 mA × 0.20 seconds × 10 exposures
= 32,000 heat units

Heat dissipation requires 15 − 9 = 6 minutes

When multiple exposures are necessary, the technician should be aware of how quickly the heat is dissipated and what the limits of exposure are for the particular unit in the facility. Each unit sold is supplied with both charts. Overheating is not likely to occur in a veterinary clinic because many concurrent exposures rarely happen rapidly during the course of the day. However, the technician should be aware that this can occur if multiple exposures are made with an older x-ray tube. It can also occur with large-animal

FIG. 2.34 An anode cooling chart. This chart shows that at maximum heating, this tube requires 15 minutes to cool between exposures. If 50,000 heat units are applied to the tube, it will take approximately 7 minutes to complete cooling (note where the cooling line crosses the 50,000 line).

portable units if many exposures are being taken rapidly, such as during prepurchase examinations.

The Tube Rating Chart

An additional chart that is useful to determine the maximum exposure on an x-ray unit is the tube rating chart. This

FIG. 2.35 A tube rating chart for the small focus on a single-phase 150-kV, 200-mA unit. (From Bushong SC. *Radiologic Science for Technologists.* 11th ed. St Louis: Elsevier; 2017.)

chart indicates the x-ray tube limits based on the equation mA × kV × time for the x-ray unit. In Fig. 2.35 the maximum exposure at 200 mA is 80 kV and 0.005 seconds. This would not be a suitable unit for a clinic whose patients included very large dogs, but it may work very well for a cat clinic.

As a guide, every technique selected above the mA rating line is not safe; every technique below the mA rating line is safe.

Each x-ray tube that is sold comes with a tube rating chart specific to it. It is important that the tube rating chart is referred to if a very large animal is to be radiographed using an old x-ray tube with a low tube rating. High technical factors may easily exceed the limits of the x-ray tube.

Focal Spot Bloom

Focal spot bloom affects the sharpness of the image. When the anode is bombarded with radiation, it becomes very hot. The heat dissipates through the surrounding metal, but if the exposures continue throughout the day and the tube is not allowed to cool, the outer edges of the focal spot become hot enough to expand the size of the focal spot, even though the heating effect of each individual exposure does not exceed the rating chart. A focal spot that started the day at 0.3 mm × 1 cm after several exposures can bloom to 0.45 or 0.5 mm. This will cause the image to lose sharpness, reducing resolution. The cause of the unsharpness is the increased area of the focal spot, as illustrated in Fig. 2.36A. The effect is demonstrated in Fig. 2.36B.

Focal spot bloom may also occur on a very old x-ray tube. The edges of the focal spot become enlarged and the images start to lose sharpness.

Minimum Power Supply Requirements

A power rating chart allows the electrician to communicate with the vendor of the x-ray unit to make sure that the power supplied by the veterinary hospital is sufficient to run the installed x-ray unit (Table 2.1).

When an x-ray unit is purchased, the veterinary hospital will receive a minimum power rating chart. This chart outlines the minimum power required to run this unit correctly using all of the stations supplied. This rating chart is usually attached to the unit itself. The salesperson must instruct the purchaser about the safest and most efficient use of the x-ray unit. If the power supply coming into the building is provided at only 80 amperes and fused at 60 amperes, then the power will not run a unit that is rated at 100 amperes and fused at 80 amperes. *It is very important to make sure that the electric circuit is equipped to handle the requirements of new x-ray equipment.*

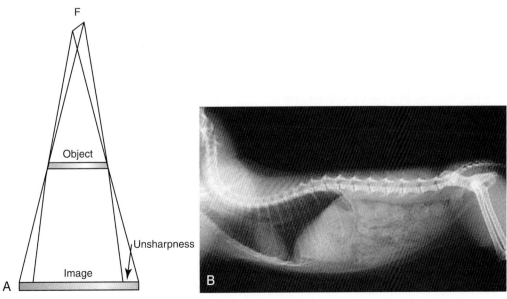

FIG. 2.36 A, The geometrical effect of an enlarged focal spot. **B,** The image loses resolution and lack of sharpness predominates. (**A** from Fauber TL. *Radiographic Imaging and Exposure.* 5th ed. St. Louis: Mosby; 2017.)

TABLE 2.1	Minimum Power Requirement Chart				
X-ray unit rating	Max kilovoltage (kV)	100	125	125	125
	Milliamperage (mA)	200	200	300	400
Power supply from wall	Power supply	60	60	100	100
	Disconnect fuse	40	50	80	80

◆ APPLICATION INFORMATION

A consultant was called in to diagnose a problem on a brand-new x-ray machine in which the images for large dogs were always light. If the technician increased the settings, the circuit breaker tripped and turned the machine off. The consultant discovered that the electrical panel was rated at 80 amperes and fused at 60 amperes. The x-ray machine required 100 amperes and fused at 80 amperes. The electrical circuit was not equipped to handle the technical factors necessary to x-ray large dogs.

Summary

In this chapter, we have reviewed the parts of the electrical circuit that are required for an x-ray unit to function. The most important parts of the unit are the x-ray tube, the generator, the rectifiers, the transformers, and the exposure switch, all of which enable the technician to select the correct technical factors to produce an image and ensure that the current travels through the x-ray tube in the correct direction.

The filament transformer, which is activated before the exposure, ensures that the cathode of the x-ray tube is heated correctly in order to produce the free electrons necessary to close the circuit and produce x-rays. The anode attracts the electrons, which are drawn across to the target area, producing 99% heat and 1% x-rays.

The main interactions that produce the photons of x-rays are bremsstrahlung and characteristic radiation. The line focus principle ensures that the x-rays are directed toward the object being radiographed. The anode heel effect uses the more powerful part of the x-ray beam at the cathode end of the x-ray tube.

REVIEW QUESTIONS

1. A transformer is used to step up or step down electricity. It receives:
   a. High voltage and low amperage
   b. High amperage and low voltage
   c. High wattage and low resistance
   d. Low wattage and high resistance
2. In x-ray technology, potential difference refers to the difference between:
   a. The charge between the cathode and the anode of the x-ray tube
   b. The technical factors used with large dogs compared with cats
   c. The voltage and the amperage in an electric circuit
   d. The power ratings of two different x-ray units
3. The purpose of a transformer is to:
   a. Transform the voltage to enable the unit to access power
   b. Maintain the voltage and decrease the current
   c. Increase the voltage in a step-up transformer
   d. Decrease the voltage in a step-up transformer
4. Rectifiers are used in the x-ray circuit to ensure that:
   a. A direct current flows in the x-ray circuit
   b. An alternating current flows through the x-ray tube
   c. The current flows through the x-ray tube in a continuous direction
   d. The voltage is maintained in the x-ray circuit
5. The high-frequency x-ray unit is _____ efficient than a/an _____ unit.
   a. less, equine mobile
   b. less, single-phase
   c. less, three-phase
   d. more, single-phase
6. The cathode in the x-ray tube is a coiled _____. It is made of _____.
   a. tube, aluminum
   b. tube, tungsten
   c. wire, copper
   d. wire, tungsten
7. The filament circuit is used to:
   a. Boost the current to the x-ray transformer
   b. Send voltage to the cathode to heat it
   c. Increase the current to the collimator light
   d. Increase the intensity of the electron beam
8. The anode rotates in order to:
   a. Dissipate the heating effect of the electrons as they hit the target
   b. Dissipate the heat emitted in the production of x-rays
   c. Decrease the size of the focal spot to form a clearer image
   d. Increase the size of the focal spot and increase contrast
9. X-rays are produced when _____ electrons are attracted to _____ by an electromagnetic force.
   a. negative, a negative cathode
   b. negative, a positive anode
   c. positive, a negative anode
   d. positive, a positive anode
10. Heat builds up on the anode and must be dissipated by:
    a. A long tungsten stem and a rhodium filter
    b. A rotating anode or a thick copper stem
    c. A rotating anode or an aluminum coil
    d. A stationary anode and a tungsten alloy target
11. The rotor circuit is responsible to activate:
    a. The rotating anode
    b. The x-ray filament
    c. The internal rectifiers
    d. The production of x-rays

12. The exposure switch must _____ and _____.
    a. activate a two-stage exposure, will not reexpose until the door is closed
    b. be depressed to activate the exposure, will continue to expose until it is released
    c. expose only when the correct factors are set, must not reexpose until the switch is released and reactivated
    d. terminate when the exposure is complete, must not reexpose until the switch is released and reactivated

13. The line voltage compensator is situated_____ and controls the _____.
    a. on the incoming line, incoming voltage
    b. on the autotransformer, incoming voltage
    c. at the on/off switch, incoming current
    d. at the filament transformer, current to the cathode

14. A ground wire is installed in every generator. Which of the following statements is correct?
    a. It prevents electric shock if there is a fault in the incoming line.
    b. It uses the excess electrons after the exposure.
    c. It always feeds the on/off switch to the generator.
    d. It provides an alternative route for the electricity.

15. Direct current is necessary to produce x-rays; the current must flow through the x-ray tube:
    a. From the cathode to the anode without interruption
    b. From the anode to the cathode without interruption
    c. From the transformer circuit directly to the x-ray tube
    d. From the filament circuit to the anode in one direction only

Chapter Review Question answers are located in the Instructor Resources on Evolve and can be provided to students at the discretion of the instructor.

Correct storage of leaded accessories.

CHAPTER **3**

Radiation Safety and Protection

Lois C. Brown, RTR (Can/USA), ACR, MSc, P.Phys

I investigated. It seemed at first a new kind of invisible light.
It was clearly something new, something unrecorded.
...There is much to do

— Wihelm Roentgen — German Physicist — 1845–1923

OUTLINE

LEARNING OBJECTIVES

When you have finished this chapter, you will be able to:

1. Understand radiation risks.
2. List the effects of excess radiation doses.
3. Define stochastic and deterministic effects.
4. Describe radiation and DNA.

5. Discuss radiation exposure and radioactivity.
6. Describe radiation-protective apparel.
7. Know the laws and regulations regarding radiation protection.

APPLICATIONS

The application of the information in this chapter is relevant to the following areas:

1. Protecting the hospital or clinic staff from primary, secondary, and scattered radiation

2. Protecting the patients and their owners from radiation dose

KEY TERMS

Key terms are defined in the Glossary on the Evolve website.

'ALARA' principle
Distance
DNA molecules
Dosimeters
Fluoroscopy
Gonadal shields
Half-life
International Commission
    on Radiological Protection
    (ICRP)

Linear energy transfer
Meiosis
Mitosis
Must/should
National Council on
    Radiation Protection and
    Measurements (NCRP)
Nonradiation worker
Nonstochastic effects
Organogenesis

RAD
Radiation dosimeter
Radiation Emitting Devices
    Act
Radiation worker
Radioactive decay
Radioactive disintegration
Radiography
Radionuclides
REM

Roentgen
Secondary radiation
Shielding
Stochastic effects
Thermoluminescent
    dosimeters
Time

This chapter discusses the various methods of radiation protection and the means by which veterinary health care workers can ensure they are protected from excess amounts of radiation. Each staff member should be encouraged to use the guidelines within this chapter and to check the specific guidelines that relate to his or her geographical area. Included throughout the chapter are quotations from both the National Council on Radiation Protection and Measurements (NCRP) in the United States and Safety Code 28 in Canada. International radiation protection is administered by the International Commission of Radiological Protection (ICRP).

Employees within a veterinary facility must be educated regarding radiation protection. All the regulations are very similar, and a copy of the appropriate regulations should be available in the veterinary hospital for employees to review when necessary. In most countries, it is the law that, during the initial interview for any prospective employee, the employer must discuss the fact that the clinic uses radiation in the diagnosis of patients. This includes all personnel and not just the employees who will work directly with radiation.

Radiation doses to workers and patients within the veterinary facility must be reduced to a level *as low as reasonably achievable* (ALARA). This is a universal principle. It is very easy to become lax in the strict standards set out in the law because radiation in the radiography room is invisible. Protecting the staff and the patients from excess amounts of radiation over the course of a career is vital.

All the handbooks on radiation protection are available online by typing in the handbook number. Hard copies may be ordered from the various organizations. (Contact information for the various organizations is listed at the end of this chapter.)

Radiobiology

Cell Biology in Brief

There are millions of cells in the bodies of the veterinary patient. Each animal stays alive by these cells dividing and subdividing in a process known as *mitosis*. This process occurs throughout the life of every living being. The exception to this are the genetic cells, which are involved in procreation and divide in a process called *meiosis*.

The energy contained in radiation will disturb the natural sequencing of these processes and can have various effects depending on what stage of cell division is occurring and which cells are affected. There are also various gradations within these effects, and it should be noted that these effects are demonstrated over many cells, not just an isolated cell.

It is also important to be aware that radiation dose is cumulative. Even though the effect of a single exposure or even multiple exposures is not felt immediately, radiation does affect the cells, and a late-effect consequence may be the result of carelessness throughout one's career if excessive exposures are not avoided. The mammalian body is roughly 80% to 95% water. It is the interaction between the fluid in the body and x-radiation that primarily affects the cells.

When a radiation disaster strikes at a nuclear plant anywhere in the world today, the many precautions that have been established since the radiation disasters at Hiroshima, Nagasaki, Chernobyl, and Fukushima are very effective in containing the fallout and preventing radiation illness and death. Although the amounts of radiation in diagnostic imaging are considerably lower than in national disasters, it is important to be aware of the potentially devastating effects of excess exposure, even in small amounts, over the course of a career.

Radiation Effects

There are two main types of radiation effects: stochastic (somatic) effects and deterministic (nonstochastic) effects.

Stochastic effects occur by chance and may occur without a threshold level of dose. The probability of this type of effect is proportional to the dose, and its severity is independent of the dose. These late-term effects usually do not appear right away but often appear many years after the initial exposure or appear as a genetic effect that causes mutations in offspring from the initial victim of the dose. The effects of such amounts of radiation are stochastic in nature because the radiation is delivered intermittently over long careers. It must be understood that exposure reactions are cumulative. Even if a person is not immediately affected by a very low dose, the cumulative result of a repeated dose over a long career in radiation can be devastating. The most common stochastic effect is cancer. Other stochastic effects are cataracts, hyperthyroidism and hypothyroidism, and sterility.

◆ APPLICATION INFORMATION

Twelve technicians in a medical radiography department were rotated through the various rooms. In the gastric examination room, the patient stood in front of the table and the technologist stood to one side of the table. Although the technologists wore leaded aprons, thyroid collars had not been manufactured at this time. Over the next many years, 10 of the 12 technologists developed thyroid problems. This was a stochastic effect.

Deterministic effects (nonstochastic effects) are noticeable in the short term. Several documented effects are noticeable immediately and are very rare in a diagnostic imaging setting. Erythema is the most common effect and will cause reddening of the skin, radiation burns, and tissue necrosis. A common nonstochastic effect is sunburn.

Radiation effects are mainly demonstrated in the DNA of the cell. This is the most vulnerable area, and the cell is particularly vulnerable during cell division. Radiation is nonselective. It affects the area of the cell upon which it arrives. DNA molecules, and particularly the nucleus of the cell, may be affected by the disintegration of the side rails of the DNA double helix. Four effects may occur when DNA is affected by radiation:

1. The radiation may pass through the cell and not affect a critical point. Mitosis may be suspended, but the cell is not damaged.
2. The cell may display no immediate effects, but damage may have occurred internally that will affect the individual

later, when mitosis (cell division) occurs. In this case, cell division may not occur successfully and the cell dies.

3. Cell damage may be obvious, with portions of the DNA compromised.
4. Cell death may occur from the "hit," severely damaging the molecule.

Diagnostic radiation workers are not as concerned about the massive cell damage that occurs with radiation therapy doses and nuclear disasters. The main concern in diagnostic imaging are the latent effects (stochastic). To produce these latent effects, the radiation dose over time must be substantial. There are currently no recorded cases of death after diagnostic x-ray exposure. The principal effects experienced by radiation personnel who do not take the necessary precautions consist of thyroid effects: radiation-induced malignancy and genetic effects.

Early radiation workers did develop malignancies from radiation exposure before implementation of the safety precautions that are in effect today. Marie Curie, one of the original researchers in radiation in the early 1900s, died of radiation-induced cancer. Her household items, even her cookbooks, are still contaminated with radiation today. This is because she lived and worked with radiation—even in her home while she was cooking.

The doses that cause severe radiation sickness are far above any that would be delivered in a veterinary hospital. These types of effects result from radiation accidents, usually at a nuclear facility. Severe radiation sickness is usually threefold, and often the person cannot recover. Death from these effects is inevitable. The effects are listed here to show how cells are devastated by severe amounts of radiation:

- Hemopoietic effect (disturbance of blood cell formation)
- Gastrointestinal effect (the effect on the gastrointestinal system)
- Central nervous system effect (the effect on the nervous system and brain)

✦ APPLICATION INFORMATION

The consultant was called in to a major hospital. The technicians were very upset, stating, "Something is wrong with our CT scanner. It is putting out major amounts of radiation, even in the control room!" The consultant asked how this information was obtained and verified.

The CT room was situated next door to the nuclear medicine department. (Chapter 14 describes nuclear medicine and the meters that are used to measure output doses from the patient.) The technicians explained that a meter was on a countertop near the wall that divides the CT unit from the nuclear medicine department. When the main contactor to start the CT exposure was activated, the nuclear medicine Geiger counter spiked with a high reading. A Geiger counter is an unshielded meter and will read radiofrequencies as well as levels of radiation.

A large patient was on the table of the CT scanner, so the consultant placed a dosimeter detector at the end of the table during a sequence. No dose was registered. Next, the consultant placed the detector on the main console of the scanner; again, no dose was registered.

It is wise to determine which type of meter—and which level on the meter—is used when measuring radiation doses.

Radioactivity

This section is particularly applicable to nuclear medicine, but the radiographer also should be aware of radioactivity in the earth and atmosphere.

Certain atoms exist in an abnormally excited state characterized by an unstable nucleus. The nucleus becomes unstable as a result of an imbalance of neutrons and protons with reference to the number of electrons encircling the atom. To reach stability, the nucleus of the atom spontaneously emits particles and energy (decays) and transforms itself into another atom with a stable and proper ratio. This process is called *radioactive disintegration* or *radioactive decay*. The atoms that emit particles and energy in order to become stable are called radionuclides. The radionuclides may be in the form of solids, liquids, or gases. These unstable atoms are used in the field of imaging called *nuclear medicine.*

Nuclear medicine technicians use radioisotopes, which are administered to patients by injection, inhalation, or oral consumption (see Chapter 14). Isotopes are variants of atoms of a particular chemical element that have differing numbers of neutrons. If the isotope is radioactive, it is called a radioisotope. Radioisotopes may be produced artificially in machines such as particle accelerators and nuclear reactors. For example, seven radioisotopes of the element barium have been artificially produced within nuclear reactors. Radioisotopes were also produced naturally during the formation of the earth, and because they are very slow to decay, they are still emitting radiation today. An example is uranium, which ultimately decays to radium, which in turn decays to radon. Other isotopes, such as carbon (C^{14}), are produced continuously in the upper atmosphere by the action of cosmic radiation.

Each radioisotope has its own pattern of decay. The energies of particles or waves emitted have unique characteristics that can be associated with that specific radionuclide. The decay rate of a radionuclide is called its *half-life.* A half-life is the amount of time it takes for half of the radioactive atoms to disintegrate or decay into a stable form.

Intensity of Radiation

All types of radiation have the ability to penetrate tissue and transfer energy. This ability is called *linear energy transfer (LET)* and describes the amount of energy imparted to the tissue. In radiography, LET is a measure of the rate at which energy is transferred from ionizing radiation into the tissue of the patient. The higher the value of the LET, the greater the amount of energy being transferred to tissue per interaction. If large amounts of energy are transferred rapidly, the ability of the particle to penetrate is reduced because the energy decreases rapidly. However, this also means that the risk of potential damage to the target material is increased because the energy is absorbed into the tissue.

Alpha and beta particles (weaker radiation) have high LET with low penetrability. These are commonly the secondary

TABLE 3.1	Tissue Compositions and Radiosensitivities		
TISSUE	**ABUNDANCE IN THE BODY**	**RADIOSENSITIVITY**	**EFFECTS OF OVERDOSE**
Lymphoid tissue	Minimal	High	Atrophy
Bone marrow	4%	High	Hypoplasia
Gonads	Minimal	High	Atrophy
Skin	3%	Intermediate	Erythema
Gastrointestinal tract	3%	Intermediate	Ulcers
Eyes (cornea)	Minimal	Intermediate	Cataracts
Growing bone	4%	Intermediate	Growth arrest
Organs	12%	Intermediate	Nephrosclerosis/ascites
Muscle	43%	Low	Fibrosis
Fat	14%	Low	Atrophy
Brain	Minimal	Low	Necrosis
Skeleton	10%	Low	Transection

FIG. 3.1 A simple radiation dosimeter. This unit is shielded to measure cumulative x-rays, beta rays, and gamma rays. It will measure both a single exposure and a fluoroscopic exposure of continuous radiation.

and scattered radiations from which the health care worker requires protection. X-rays and gamma rays have low LET with higher penetrability. This means that their ability to travel through matter is high, producing less immediate effects on the tissue through which they pass. X-rays and gamma rays are produced in the radiography department. The patient's body absorbs the photons of radiation according to the density of the tissue exposed to the x-ray beam (Table 3.1).

Bone is much denser than soft tissue or fat. Bone efficiently absorbs the radiation reaching it and therefore prevents the image receptor from being exposed. This explains why bony areas are white on the image. Fat and air, which are radiolucent, allow the radiation to penetrate through to the image receptor and show up as black or dark areas on the image monitor.

Learning how to optimize images by varying the settings on the machine is discussed in Chapter 5. It is important to note that the higher the kilovoltage (kV), the higher the energy of the x-ray beam and thus the greater the amount of scattered and secondary radiation and the potential risk to the x-ray worker. When a technique chart is developed, the kV should be optimized to penetrate the body part, and then the milliamperes/seconds (mAs) value should be set to provide the correct density on the film/monitor.

Radiation-Monitoring Equipment

Measurement of Radiation Doses

Radiation doses are measured by means of a dosimeter (Fig. 3.1). Radiation is emitted from objects over which we have no control, such as the sun and even the concrete in the pavement we walk on or the walls in our houses. The fluorescent lights in our clinics and hospitals are activated by ballasts, which ionize the gas within the light tubes and produce light.

If radiation is measured with an incorrect meter, these levels can be alarming because the meters are set to a random sensitivity level and are exceptionally sensitive. When beta, gamma, and x-ray levels are measured, it is important to use a shielded dosimeter specifically set to measure these types of radiation.

Types of Dosimeters

Handlers who are regularly required to work within the radiography room or who may be exposed to radiation during the course of their work are required to wear a personal radiation dosimeter (Fig. 3.2A). Personal radiation dosimeters capture the radiation dose from x-ray, beta, and gamma radiation and maintain it until it is read by a dosimetry service. Several companies supply personal dosimeters, with the most common types as follows:

- **Thermoluminescent dosimeters (TLDs).** A TLD demonstrates radiation exposure by measuring the intensity of light emitted from a crystal within the detector when the crystal is heated. The intensity of light emitted is dependent on the radiation exposure (thermo = heat; luminescence = light) (see Fig. 3.2D).
- **Optically stimulated luminescence (OSL).** An OSL contains sensitive elements that absorb radiation and store some of the energy in the form of excited electrons. The dosimeter is read by stimulating the sensitive elements using light-emitting diodes, which release some of the stored energy as light. The amount of released light is measured and used to determine the radiation exposure received by the dosimeter's user during the wearing period (see Fig. 3.2C) (obtained from the National Dosimetry Services website: www.hc-sc.gc.ca).

The radiation protection officer or his or her designate replaces the dosimeters at specific time intervals so they may be read by an outside independent company. They can be read monthly, quarterly, or biannually.

Spare dosimeters may be maintained for visiting personnel or for dose studies in certain areas. These dosimeters should be labeled and noted on the remittance form when they are sent in to be read.

FIG. 3.2 A, Radiation dosimeters at a veterinary clinic. These units are stored outside of the x-ray room, away from any possible extraneous radiation exposure. **B,** The control dosimeter is kept in the original packaging, well away from any possible exposure within the facility. If the dosimeter indicates a radiation exposure, this would mean that all of the dosimeters were exposed during shipping. **C,** The reverse side of the dosimeter indicating the facility and wearer's identification. This is read by the dosimetry service and prevents misidentification. **D,** Thermoluminescent dosimeters stored outside the radiography room.

Control dosimeters are kept in the container received into the facility and removed from any possible radiation exposure (see Fig. 3.2B). The dosimeters are sent back to the laboratory along with the control. If the control dosimeter registers a radiation dose, then it is likely that all of the other dosimeters in the package received the same dose during shipping.

Use of Dosimeters

The rules of use apply to all dosimeters (Box 3.1). When a health care worker is issued a dosimeter, his or her personal information is required by the facility to which the service is registered. This process enables the dosimetry service to combine reports from other employers in order to calculate total exposure for an annual reading. If the worker is employed at more than one site, he or she must wear a different dosimeter at each site. In this way, incidents can be tracked to a specific site.

Radiation Exposure

Recommended Dose Limits for Radiation Workers and Nonradiation Workers

Specified dose limits apply to both radiation workers and nonradiation workers. There is no dose discrimination between men and women of reproductive capacity. Once pregnancy has been confirmed, the woman's fetus should be protected from all types of x-ray exposure. X-ray radiation worker dose limits specifically apply only to irradiation resulting directly from their occupation and do not include radiation from medical diagnosis and background radiation.

Dose limits for nonradiation workers are considerably lower than those for radiation workers because radiation workers wear protective garments over the most sensitive areas of their anatomy.

BOX 3.1	Dosimeter Guidelines

- A dosimeter must not be taken home.
- A dosimeter must be stored in a location where it is not likely to be exposed to radiation.
- A dosimeter must not be stored where it will be exposed to heat and/or sunlight.
- A dosimeter must be worn only at the site to which it is registered.
- A dosimeter should be worn attached to the thyroid collar outside the leaded apron by any worker who is potentially exposed to radiation.
- A dosimeter must never be shared with another worker.
- A dosimeter must not be worn on a jacket or laboratory coat that might then be removed and hung in a radiation area.
- If the dosimeter is to be worn under the leaded apron during fluoroscopic examinations, a second dosimeter should be worn attached to the thyroid collar outside the apron. These dosimeters must be clearly marked and must never be exchanged.
- Visitors to a radiography room during an examination must be provided with personal dosimeters, and service personnel working on x-ray equipment must also wear personal dosimeters. These are for individual use only and must be annotated when they are submitted to the dosimetry facility.
- Each facility is responsible for posting the results of the dosimetry readings as they are received. Reports should be kept as a medical record according to the protocol of the facility.

The Radiation Emitting Devices (RED) Act in Canada, the National Council on Radiation Protection and Measurements (NCRP) in the USA, and International Commission of Radiological Protection (ICRP) clearly state the dose limits for radiation and nonradiation workers (Table 3.2 and Boxes 3.2 and 3.3). The ICRP specifies the allowable doses and should be consulted for further information (www.icrp.org).

The Occupational Health and Safety Acts (Canada, United States, and International)

The Occupational Health and Safety Acts specify that it is the employer's responsibility to ensure that the health care worker is protected against any excessive radiation exposure. Several sections refer specifically to radiation protection of the health care worker. All of the legislation is similar across international borders. The terms *must* and *should* in the Canadian Safety Code are *shall* and *should* in the American report (NCRP Report No. 148). **Shall and must are mandatory in both countries; *should* is optional.**

These sections of legislation apply to radiography and to all other modalities addressed in this text, including nuclear medicine and positron emission tomography:

1. A supervisor shall ensure that a worker is instructed in the use of the protective devices and that he or she uses or wears these devices appropriately.

TABLE 3.2	Maximum Permissible Dose Recommendations

	AMOUNT
Occupational Exposure Limits	
Annual	50 mSv
Cumulative	10 mSv × Age
Public Exposure	
Effective dose limit, continuous or frequent	1 mSv
Effective dose limit, infrequent exposure	5 mSv
Embryo or Fetus Exposures Monthly	
Equivalent dose limit for the embryo or fetus	0.5 mSv
Negligible Individual Dose (Annual)	
Effective dose	0.01 mSv

Note: All dose limits exclude medical exposures and exposures to natural sources.
For further information on this Table, refer to NCRP Report #148, Table 2.1. http://ncrponline.org/publications/reports/ncrp-reports-148/.

BOX 3.2	Employer Prerequisites Necessary to Maintain Radiation Safety

- A health and safety representative has the power to review any and all testing procedures that in any way affect the occupational, biological, chemical, or physical health and safety of any worker.
- The employer must provide information regarding any potential or existing hazards to any worker.
- A health and safety committee has the power to identify hazardous situations in the workplace and make recommendations to establish monitoring programs that will improve the present status of safety to the workers.
- The committee will designate a member representing workers who shall monitor the testing procedures to ensure the safety of the workers.
- An employer shall ensure that equipment, materials, and protective devices are provided in good condition to the workers and are used as proscribed.
- An employer must appoint a competent safety officer who will supervise the handling, storage, use, and disposal of any article, device, equipment, or biological, chemical, or physical agent. The safety officer will prepare and post a written health and safety report in a conspicuous location and review and maintain it annually.

2. The supervisor must advise the worker of any potential of actual danger of which he or she may be aware and take every precaution to protect the workers under his or her advisement, including providing written instructions regarding any unusual circumstance concerning dangers in the workplace.

BOX 3.3 Further Legislation Regarding the Employer and the X-Ray Worker

1. If a worker exceeds the allowable dose, the employer shall investigate the cause and shall communicate the process of the investigation and the outcome and corrective measures taken to ensure compliance with the legal authority in that jurisdiction.
2. In each facility the owner of the radiation-emitting equipment or source must either assume the duties of the designated competent person or assign those duties in writing to an officer designate. That individual will ensure that the directives of the appropriate government body are carried out. Further duties include the training of the staff of the facility regarding radiation protection. He or she will also ensure that appropriate measures are in place to protect the patients and members of the general public who visit the clinic.
3. It is recommended that the equipment in a veterinarian's office be tested every 2 years. This testing will include, but is not limited to, accuracy of kilovoltage, half-value layer, milliampere linearity, reproducibility, timer accuracy, and collimator accuracy (see Chapter 9).
4. In addition to the responsible user of the diagnostic facility, a radiation protection (safety) officer must be delegated to act as advisor regarding all matters directly connected to the radiation protection aspects of the facility during the initial stages of construction, during installation of equipment, and during subsequent operations.
5. The specific duties of the radiation protection officer are outlined in the relevant act. They include the provision of a determination of responsibility and monitoring of radiation doses emitted by the equipment and received by both personnel and patients.

3. The worker shall observe all the provisions of the Health and Safety Act of the country in which he or she is employed. Report to the supervisor any defect in any of the measures provided to ensure the safety of the workers.
4. No worker shall remove any protective device required by the regulations or by his or her employer without providing adequate temporary protection. No worker shall engage in any act that would render the protective devices installed to be ineffective or nonexistent.

5. Every person who supplies any equipment shall ensure that the equipment is in good condition and complies with the safety measures outlined in this act.
6. Where a biological, chemical, or physical agent is used in a workplace, the local legal authority must be notified and shall decree whether the use is prohibited, limited, or subject to the safety conditions outlined in his or her directive.
7. A distributor must provide clear written instructions as to the use of any hazardous physical agent that he or she manufactures or designs to be used in the workplace.
8. Where an employer has an item described in subsection (1) {a piece of protective apparel in the radiography department}, the employer must ensure that those workers are aware of any potential hazard and are thoroughly instructed as to the proper use and maintenance of that item.
9. The employer must post prominent notices identifying and warning of the hazardous physical properties of the item in the place in which the item is to be used or operated.
10. Notices must be written in English and whatever appropriate languages are prescribed.

Legislation Regarding Radiation Doses to the Health Care Worker

It is the responsibility of the radiation worker to read the entire act in terms of its context before making a claim against any employer or section of this text. Each country provides legal direction specific to radiation workers within their borders, and it is the responsibility of the individual worker to be familiar with these legal directions. A radiation worker is defined as an individual who "could be exposed to radiation from manmade sources *during their work*." The nonradiation worker includes the rest of the population. The doses allowed for the radiation worker assume that the individual has been supplied with and is wearing protective devices on the parts of his or her body that would be susceptible to radiation damage (e.g., leaded aprons, thyroid collar).

Radiation Units

Radiation units were named as they were discovered. Recently the names have been changed to follow an international naming code, and the quantities have also been altered. The names and quantities in Table 3.3 are the most common in a veterinary practice.

TABLE 3.3 The Most Common Units of Dose in a Veterinary Practice

Radiation units were named as they were discovered. Recently the names were changed to follow an international naming code. When this occurred, the quantities were also altered. The names and quantities that are mentioned here are the most common in a veterinary practice.

NAME	QUANTITY	SYMBOL	SI UNITS	EQUIVALENTS
Roentgen	Exposure (dose)	R	Coulomb/kg (C/kg)	$1 \text{ R} = 258 \times 10^{-4} \text{ C/kg}$
RAD	Absorbed dose	rad	Gray (Gy$_1$)	$1 \text{ rad} = 0.01 \text{ Gy}$
REM	Effective dose	rem	Sievert (Sv)	$1 \text{ rem} = 0.01 \text{ Sv}$
Curie	Radioactivity	Ci	Becquerel (Bq)	$1 \text{ Ci} = 3.73 \times 10^{10} \text{ Bq}$

The following radiation units are of most concern to veterinary personnel:

1. **Absorbed dose.** The RAD (Radiation Absorbed Dose) changed to the gray (Gy), which measures the amount of radiation absorbed per unit mass of matter. This usually concerns biological effects and is not monitored in diagnostic imaging because the effects are minimal.

2. **Dose equivalent.** The REM (Radiation Equivalent Man/Mammal) changed to the sievert (Sv). This is the unit measured by the radiation-monitoring dosimeters that are worn by personnel who regularly are exposed to minimal amounts of radiation during the course of their work.

3. **Measured radiation.** The Roentgen, the dose output of the x-ray unit, changed to the air kerma (Gy_a). This is the dose measured by service personnel calibrating the x-ray unit. Most meters still measure in roentgens and milliroentgens.

Dosimeters are usually read in REM (Sv) and usually display both units on their reports. Both the NCRP in the United States and the RED Act in Canada use the dose limits developed by the ICRP. Table 3.2 is a summary of the maximum permissible dose recommendations for ionizing radiation. **Persons under 18 years of age are not allowed to work in radiographic areas.**

Principles of Radiation Protection

Once Roentgen had discovered the potential of the "x-ray," its value to medicine was immediately recognized. Shortly thereafter, the detrimental effects of radiation were also identified.

Historical Note

Roentgen discovered and researched x-radiation. However, he was one of a very few x-ray pioneers who did not suffer radiation induced illness. He was a careful researcher who always protected himself from his "x-rays."

The science of health physics develops protocols to protect health care workers, x-ray radiation workers, patients, and the general public. The three cardinal rules for radiation protection are *time, distance,* and *shielding.* Reducing the time of exposure, increasing the distance between the source of the radiation and the subject, and placing a shield or barrier between the operator and the source are the three primary methods for reducing exposure.

Protection from radiation is important for any individual. Particular attention should be paid to males or females who have the ability to reproduce. This group includes all males of any age and all females before menopause. In all geographical areas, it is illegal to employ a radiation worker under the age of 18 years.

One consideration that must be emphasized is protection of the pregnant veterinary worker. Research indicates that the severity of the response of the fetus to radiation is related to both dose and time. The second to the tenth week of pregnancy is the period of major organogenesis and therefore is the most critical time. Because it is quite possible that a female may not yet be aware that she is pregnant, protection of any female of childbearing age is essential.

Time

Exposure refers to two different occurrences: exposure rate and exposure time.

RULE: Exposure = Exposure rate × Exposure time

The exposure rate to an operator during radiographic examinations is obtained either by holding a patient during radiography or by standing too close to the x-ray table when the exposure is produced. This is measured by a personal radiation dosimeter worn by the operator. In veterinary medicine, the dosimeter must be worn on the thyroid collar when the operator is handling the patient. This will track the dose from secondary and scattered radiation. The radiation dosimeter is not meant to track primary radiation.

Every precaution must be taken to limit exposure time, or the time that the operator is exposed to radiation. Exposure time is measured by the radiation dosimeter, which measures an immediate dose—either a per-exposure dose or a fluoroscopic (real-time) dose. There is no delay in this reading. A radiation dose measured over time results in a given amount of exposure. The dosimeter will measure a dose over time, and a monitoring company will read the dosimeter and email a report to the facility.

During fluoroscopy (real-time imaging), the veterinarian is trained to pulse the exposure rather than leaving it on continuously. Pulsing the exposure limits the time of the exposure and thus the dose to the patient and to any staff member who must restrain the patient. A 5-minute reset timer on the fluoroscopy unit notifies the veterinarian exactly how much exposure time has elapsed during each procedure. Many facilities note the time elapsed for each procedure on the patient's chart so the dose calculation may be completed easily if a question arises regarding the examination.

Distance (The Inverse Square Law)

To calculate the intensity of radiation at a particular point (distance) away from the source, one must know the following three things:

- The intensity of the radiation (I_1) at a fixed distance from the source (focal point) (e.g., 123 mR)
- The fixed distance (D_1) (e.g., 180 cm)
- The calculated distance (D_2) (or the distance at which the intensity is to be calculated) (e.g., 160 cm) to obtain a patient entrance exposure (if the patient measured 20 cm.) Calculate using the formula:

$$\frac{I_1}{I_2} = \left[\frac{D_2}{D_1}\right]^2$$

For example, if I sit 1 foot away from a lamp, the intensity of the light reaching me is 1×. If I move to 2 feet from the source (2×), the intensity of the light reaching me is now decreased to one fourth (¼) of its original value. This is the

Focal spot of X-ray beam

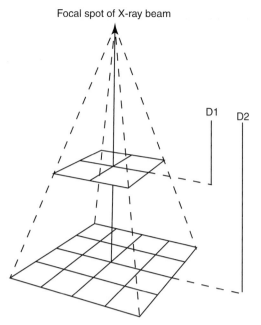

FIG. 3.3 The intensity of radiation is inversely proportional to the square of the distance (D_1 and D_2) of the object from the source.

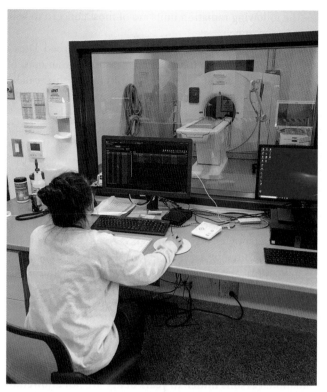

FIG. 3.4 An example of a leaded glass window between the operator of a CT unit and the CT unit. (Courtesy Toronto Animal Health Partners: Emergency and Specialty Hospital – North York, Ontario, CANADA.)

application of the *inverse square law,* and it must be observed whenever a patient is being radiographed.

The Inverse Square Law

The intensity of the radiation at a location is inversely proportional to the square of its distance from the source of radiation.

The rule of distance is also important when a new facility is planned, or renovations are contemplated (Fig. 3.3). Enlarging an x-ray room means that the technicians can stand farther away from the patient and still be able to react if the patient moves or requires repositioning.

Shielding

RULE: Positioning a shield or barrier between the health care worker and the radiation source greatly reduces the level of radiation exposure (Fig. 3.4).

Ideally the operator exposes the patient while standing behind a shield or barrier. In some cases, doing so is not possible because the veterinary patient must be restrained and cannot be sedated. Shielding material is usually defined with reference to the thickness of lead. Other construction materials may be used, but they are commonly calculated according to their comparison with lead. For example, at 100 kV, 2.20 cm of concrete is equal to 0.79 mm of lead. Large sheets of lead may be purchased for construction. The minimum thickness is usually 0.79 mm ($\frac{1}{32}$ inch). Calculations for the shielding of x-ray rooms are beyond the scope of this text. Legally, in every country, the barriers (walls, ceiling, floor, and doorways) of the radiography room must be designated radiation barriers.

The maximum amount of radiation that may affect these barriers over the course of time must be calculated to ensure that the appropriate protection is installed before the first exposure of the imaging equipment. The necessary calculations may be carried out only by radiation-trained personnel or a medical radiation physicist. The calculations for each barrier must be submitted to and approved by the appropriate legal authority (Fig. 3.5).

If the equipment in the room is changed by either upgrading or downgrading, a new set of plans must be submitted. If the adjoining areas of the facility are changed, a new set of calculations must be submitted. Any room containing an x-ray generator must be designated with the appropriate legal signage (Fig. 3.6).

Radiation-Protective Devices

Leaded Protection Materials

Shielding material used to protect the patient is usually in the form of leaded drapes and/or gonadal shields (Figs. 3.7 and 3.8). Leaded aprons are typically measured for their effectiveness at 125 kV.

In film/screen radiography the cassette may be divided, and the area to be radiated is then restricted so leaded dividers can be used to limit scattered radiation from fogging the unexposed part of the cassette (Fig. 3.9).

Leaded gloves, leaded aprons, and thyroid protectors must be worn by the health care workers present in the room

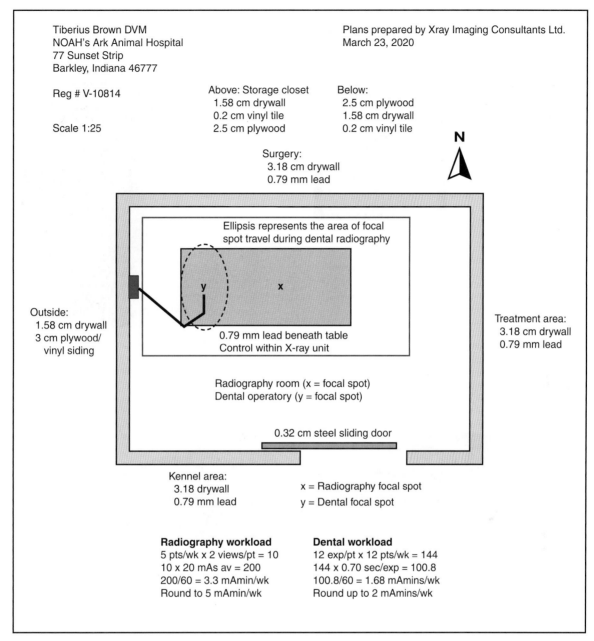

Tiberius Brown DVM
NOAH's Ark Animal Hospital
77 Sunset Strip
Barkley, Indiana 46777

Reg # V-10814

Scale 1:25

Plans prepared by Xray Imaging Consultants Ltd.
March 23, 2020

Above: Storage closet
1.58 cm drywall
0.2 cm vinyl tile
2.5 cm plywood

Below:
2.5 cm plywood
1.58 cm drywall
0.2 cm vinyl tile

Surgery:
3.18 cm drywall
0.79 mm lead

N

Ellipsis represents the area of focal
spot travel during dental radiography

y

x

Outside:
1.58 cm drywall
3 cm plywood/
vinyl siding

0.79 mm lead beneath table
Control within X-ray unit

Treatment area:
3.18 cm drywall
0.79 mm lead

Radiography room (x = focal spot)
Dental operatory (y = focal spot)

0.32 cm steel sliding door

Kennel area:
3.18 drywall
0.79 mm lead

x = Radiography focal spot
y = Dental focal spot

Radiography workload
5 pts/wk x 2 views/pt = 10
10 x 20 mAs av = 200
200/60 = 3.3 mAmin/wk
Round to 5 mAmin/wk

Dental workload
12 exp/pt x 12 pts/wk = 144
144 x 0.70 sec/exp = 100.8
100.8/60 = 1.68 mAmins/wk
Round up to 2 mAmins/wk

FIG. 3.5 A sample floor plan designating the barriers of the radiography room and the installation of lead protection in the walls.

during the radiographic examination (Fig. 3.10). Leaded glass goggles are also available to protect the lenses of the eyes from scattered and/or secondary radiation (Fig. 3.11).

Movable leaded barriers are available as added protection in imaging rooms where the workers are exposed to a higher amount of radiation than their colleagues (Fig. 3.12).

Use and Care

The lead used in aprons, leaded blockers, and drape shields is usually manufactured in thin sheets that are then layered together to achieve the correct amount of radiation protection. The sheets of leaded rubber are very thin and must be handled carefully in order to last for many years. Guidelines

for the use and care of protective devices are included in Box 3.4.

If a patient must be supported or restrained during an imaging procedure, the x-ray worker should stay as far away from the source of the radiation as possible. Whenever possible, a nonradiation worker should be asked to restrain the patient. Nonradiation workers should be rotated throughout the shift so that no one worker is continuously exposed to radiation.

Lead Specifications

Radiographic and fluoroscopic leaded aprons must provide attenuation equivalent to at least 0.5 mm of lead at 150 kV.

CAUTION X-RAYS

**ATTENTION
RAYONS X**

A   B

FIG. 3.6 A, A legal door sign in Canada warning of the potential for radiation in the room behind it. The image denotes an early x-ray tube. **B,** A legal door sign in the United States. This sign also warns of nuclear isotopes in both the United States and Canada.

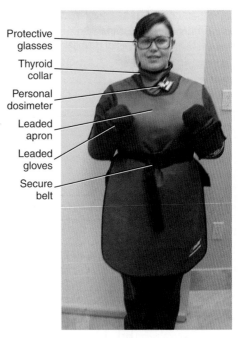

Protective glasses

Thyroid collar

Personal dosimeter

Leaded apron

Leaded gloves

Secure belt

FIG. 3.7 Radiation-protective wear. The apron is secured across the shoulders with a hook-and-loop (Velcro) band so that it will remain in place while the technician is positioning a patient.

A   B

FIG. 3.8 A, Leaded shields used to protect the patient from excess or scattered radiation, to shield the detector from excess scatter, and to be placed on the patient to act as a mild restraint. **B,** Gonadal shields to be used to protect gonadal areas, particularly with breeding animals.

The lead equivalency must be permanently marked on the apron. **NOTE:** Most leaded aprons are rated at 125 kV. To meet 150 kV standard, an extra layer of lead needs to be added to the basic apron during manufacturing.

Protective gloves must provide attenuation equivalent to at least 0.25 mm of lead at 150 kV. This protection must be provided throughout the glove, including the fingers and the wrist.

◆ APPLICATION INFORMATION

There are many different shapes and designs of protective mitts or gloves. It is important to ensure that the hands and fingers are covered during the radiation exposure if it is necessary to restrain the patient. For further information on patient restraint and safe handling practices, please review all of Part Two of this text.

Further Methods to Reduce Radiation Exposure to the Veterinary Handler

Immobilization Equipment

Equipment to restrain and/or immobilize the patient during any imaging procedure should be available in each imaging suite. Such equipment includes radiolucent foam blocks, cloth restraints, and tie-downs (Fig. 3.13). The patient must be held in place by any person who is fully clothed in protective apparel and shielded from the direct beam by accurate collimation. (See also Part Two regarding protection and positioning with nonmanual restraint.)

Veterinary Facilities Inspection Checklist

Fig. 3.14 provides a checklist for a typical facility. It is available on the Evolve website for any facility to download and post.

FIG. 3.11 Radiation glasses. These are made with leaded glass lenses and can also be ordered as prescription glasses. They are fairly heavy and should always be worn with a neck strap, as they are quite fragile.

FIG. 3.9 Various blockers that can be used to protect the image detector from scattered or secondary radiation. Collimation is vital in digital imaging.

FIG. 3.10 An example of a leaded apron. It must be tied around the waist and secured on the shoulders so that the radiation worker is protected when they are in the room during a radiation exposure.

FIG. 3.12 A leaded screen. This unit can be placed in the room so that the technician can stand behind it when the exposure is made. This does not replace a leaded apron.

Radiation Safety Websites

General sites for additional radiation safety training include:

- Occupational Health and Safety Act (www.osha.gov)
- X-Ray Safety Regulation (www.radiationsafety.ca)
- Radiation Emitting Devices Act (Safety Codes 20A and 35) (http://laws-lois.justice.gc.ca)
- Radiation Protection in Veterinary Medicine (Safety Code 28) (www.hc-sc.gc.ca)
- International Commission on Radiological Protection (www.icrp.org)
- National Council on Radiation Protection and Measurements (ncrponline.org/)

BOX 3.4 Use and Care of Protective Devices

- Aprons should be hung up by the shoulders when not in use.
- Aprons should not be folded or creased under any circumstances.
- Aprons should be cleaned regularly with warm water and a mild soap.
- The leaded apron should fit correctly. It should have a method to secure it on the wearer's shoulders so it does not fall off the shoulder during use. Simply adding a strap with a piece of hook-and-loop (Velcro) to the shoulder units of the apron will ensure that it stays in place when the handler bends forward. If the apron is worn during fluoroscopy, it should wrap around the technologist's back. In this way, protection is ensured while the technologist is in the room during continuous radiation.
- Thyroid collars should always be worn in conjunction with the leaded apron. They should be treated with the same care as the leaded aprons.

FIG. 3.13 Foam block used to assist in positioning patients.

Checklist regarding the safety of and the information provided to radiation workers.

_____ X-ray source not operated for the irradiation of a worker [section 4]

_____ Informed Workers in Writing (at time that employment begins) that worker is employed as an x-ray worker (i.e. higher dose equivalent limit), informed workers of those dose equivalent limits, and if female, limit for pregnant x-ray workers [section 9;1]

_____ Employer created and maintains a list of x-ray workers [section 9;2]

_____ Dose is ALARA and within dose equivalent annual limits [section 10;1]

_____ Employer takes every precaution reasonable to ensure mean dose equivalent received by the abdomen of a pregnant x-ray worker does not exceed 5 mSv during the pregnancy [section 10;2]

_____ X-ray warning signs or devices posted in conspicuous locations (i.e.door signs) [section 11;1]

_____ Label on X-ray control stating that the machine is a source of x-rays [section 11;2]

_____ Locks/interlocks in areas where air kerma may exceed 100 microGrays in one hour [section 11;3, i]

_____ Barriers and warning signs if the x-ray source is portable or mobile and is so used and where air kerma may exceed 100 microGrays in one hour [section 11;3, ii]

_____ Structural or other shielding shall be installed as per Ministry of Health plan approval [section 11;4, i]

_____ Diaphragms, cones and adjustable collimators used to limit size of beam [section 11;4, ii]

_____ Each x-ray worker has approved dosimeter [section 12;1]

_____ X-ray Worker using dosimeter as instructed by employer [section 12;2]

_____ Employer ensures dosimeter is read accurately [section 12;3]

_____ Employer furnishes worker the record of dosimeter results [section 12;3]

_____ Employer verifies dosimeter results as reasonable and informs MoL otherwise [section 12;4]

_____ Employer retains dosimeter results for at least 3 years [section 12;5]

_____ Copy of X-ray regulations posted and available to workers [OSHA section 22;2, i]

FIG. 3.14 Checklist for a typical facility in Canada. _ALARA,_ As low as reasonably achievable; _MOL,_ Ministry of Labour; _OSHA,_ Occupational Safety and Health Act.

- U.S. Nuclear Regulatory Commission, Radiation Information Regarding Disposal of Nuclear Waste (https://www.nrc.gov/waste.html)

Summary

In this chapter, we explored the regulations that have been put into effect to protect radiation workers, nonradiation workers, and patients undergoing radiographic examination from harmful doses. Protective apparel and its use and care have been discussed. The world of the radiation worker is much safer today than it was when the early pioneers were exploring this exciting new field.

REVIEW QUESTIONS

1. Radiation workers should always reduce radiation doses by following the:
   a. ALARA principle
   b. The least dose principle
   c. The no dose–image gently formula
   d. The principle of radiation doses
2. The radiation dose that workers are subjected to today is _____ than the _____ doses of early researchers.
   a. far higher, high
   b. far higher, low
   c. far less, high
   d. far less, low
3. When radiation strikes a cell, the most vulnerable area is the:
   a. Cell wall
   b. DNA
   c. Mitochondria
   d. Mitosis
4. If there is damage to the DNA, one of the outcomes is:
   a. Cell damage disrupting the cell walls
   b. Cell death from damage to the entire cell
   c. Cell death from other effects
   d. No change because the DNA can mend itself
5. Late-occurring effects are evident long after the damage has occurred. They are:
   a. Latent effects
   b. Nonstochastic effects
   c. Radiation effects
   d. Stochastic effects
6. Radiation exposure to veterinary workers is usually due to:
   a. Primary and secondary radiation
   b. Scattered and primary radiation
   c. Scattered and secondary radiation
   d. Secondary and stochastic radiation
7. Isotopes are variants of elements. They have differing numbers of:
   a. Electrons
   b. Neutrons
   c. Nuclei
   d. Protons

8. Linear energy transfer is defined as:
   a. The type of energy available only through radioactive disintegration
   b. The ability of radiation to affect DNA
   c. The ability of radiation to affect tissue
   d. The ability of radiation to transfer energy into tissue
9. X-rays and gamma rays have:
   a. High LET with high penetrability
   b. High LET with low penetrability
   c. Low LET with high penetrability
   d. Low LET with low penetrability
10. Bone is much denser than fat, so it absorbs more radiation than fat.
    a. True
    b. False
11. Three methods of radiation protection are:
    a. Distance, leaded aprons, and leaded gloves
    b. Time, distance, and shielding
    c. Time, inverse square law, and distance
    d. Time, LET, and shielding
12. The most susceptible tissue is tissue that is rapidly dividing. Which of the following is true?
    a. Postpubertal adolescents would be highly affected.
    b. Prepubertal children would be most affected.
    c. This includes the healing of surgical wounds.
    d. This includes the tissue in a 2- to 10-week fetus.
13. Shielding of radiography rooms is essential in all installations. Which of the following is true?
    a. Most radiation therapy suites are excused from this regulation.
    b. This applies to all imaging suites where ionizing radiation is used.
    c. This applies to only dental and nuclear medicine suites.
    d. This applies to only units that use over 90 kilovolts.
14. Leaded aprons are composed of thin sheets of leaded rubber. Which of the following is true?
    a. The rubber is flexible and not likely to split if folded.
    b. The rubber is heavy and does not react to bending or splitting.
    c. The sheets of rubber are fragile and will split apart over time.
    d. The leaded apron should be hung up when not in use.
15. Radiation dosimeters must be issued to every radiation worker. Which of the following is true?
    a. Personal dosimeters should be hung in the x-ray room when not in use.
    b. These are personal dosimeters and must not be shared with other workers.
    c. They can be shared by people who job-share.
    d. They should be taken home at the end of each shift to ensure they are safe.

16. The radiation worker is described as:
    a. A person who works in the same building where radiation is produced
    b. A worker who does not work with radiation but may be exposed to it
    c. A worker who works with radiation during his or her normal duties
    d. The employer of people who work with radiation
17. An employer is legally bound to instruct new employees that:
    a. There is equipment that produces radiation on site.
    b. There is a radiation source but they will not be exposed to it.
    c. They are in a facility where there is a radiation source for radiography.
    d. They are not allowed to work with radiation.

18. When maximum doses allowed are listed, there is no discrimination between men and women of reproductive age.
    a. True
    b. False

Chapter Review Question answers are located in the Instructor Resources on Evolve and can be provided to students at the discretion of the instructor.

CHAPTER **4**

Imaging on Film

Lois C. Brown, RTR (Can/USA), ACR, MSc, P.Phys

Sometimes you will never know the value of a moment until it becomes a memory.
—Theodor Geisel (Dr. Seuss) — American author – 1904–1991

OUTLINE

LEARNING OBJECTIVES

When you have finished this chapter, you will be able to:

1. Identify cassettes, screens, and film, and understand
   how they work together to produce an image.
2. Understand the purpose of screen and film speed and
   screen colors and how they affect the image.

3. List the characteristics of various commercial cassettes
   and screens.
4. Understand latent image formation.

APPLICATIONS

The application of the information in this chapter is relevant to the following areas:

1. Producing x-ray images (radiographs) for evaluation
   and diagnosis
2. The selection of intensifying screens that will serve the
   requirements of the animal hospital

3. Ensuring that the film selected is compatible with the
   intensifying screens
4. The selection of appropriate storage space for both
   unused film and cassettes and film in use

KEY TERMS

Key terms are defined in the Glossary on the Evolve website.

Artifacts
Calcium tungstate
Cassette
Conversion efficiency
Crossover effect

Emulsion
Film base
Film/screen contact
Generator
Halation

Image receptor
Intensification factor
Intensifying screens
Latent image
Light spectrum

Luminescence
Manifest image
Resolution
Screen characteristics
Supercoat

Preamble

As technology moves forward into new and interesting areas there are two still items of great importance in imaging:

(1) the x-ray generator, which produces the x-rays
(2) the receptor, which receives the x-rays and produces the actual image.

Chapters 1 and 2 discussed the functions of the x-ray unit and how x-rays are produced via an electrical circuit through the x-ray tube.

This chapter introduces the other side of imaging—the image receptor. Many veterinarians have made the transition to digital imaging and we will discuss the changes that are inherent in that transition in Chapter 8.

There are also many veterinarians around the world who still rely on imaging on film and processing using manual tanks or automatic processors. This chapter and the ones that follow will discuss the techniques of imaging with film and then processing the film to obtain the final image.

FIG. 4.1 Imaging Then. The first radiograph—the hand of Mrs. Roentgen. It also contains the first artifact; can you identify it?

? POINTS TO PONDER It is very important to remember the two separate components of the x-ray system. If one component is changed (e.g., the receptor), it is not always necessary to change the second component (e.g., the generator, transformer, table, or x-ray tube).

When we review various image receptors, we are immediately aware of how much imaging has changed over the years (Fig. 4.1). Since Roentgen's discovery of x-rays just over 100 years ago, the field of imaging has evolved to encompass areas that could not have been imagined in the 1800s (Fig. 4.2).

As new concepts evolve, new units are manufactured and tested in the marketplace. Such testing always leads to upgrades as each new x-ray unit is challenged by its supporters and its competitors. Every unit that is successful in the veterinary clinic has some merit. It may be smaller or larger or faster or more efficient to use, but each design is changed as the imaging community demands even more convenience and better imaging.

The age and appearance of the generator make little difference to the final image. If the technical factors are correct and the generator is calibrated correctly and produces consistent results, a very old generator will produce the same image as a brand-new generator.

X-ray film was the common receptor until a few years ago. Computers have now taken over the medical imaging world, and veterinary hospitals and clinics are rapidly following this trend. The concept of simplifying the selection of technical factors beyond the control of the operator and allowing the computer to manipulate the image reflects the

FIG. 4.2 Imaging Now. **A,** Magnetic resonance imaging evolved from radiography and **B,** ultrasound, although neither modality uses x-rays to produce images.

lack of knowledge of the commercial vendor and the operator regarding technical factors and how they unify to produce an optimized image.

The term *photography* derives from the Greek words *phos* (*photós*), meaning "light," and *gráphein*, meaning "to write." From this the term *radiographer* denotes the technician or technologist who "writes with radiation." Obtaining a superior image and maintaining good imaging practices is achievable only if the operator has a basic understanding of technical factors and a solid background in x-ray image production and radiation protection.

> **? POINTS TO PONDER**   Just as a camera must be set correctly to record the perfect image, so must the x-ray generator. A local camera store would be seriously remiss if they sold a digital camera with the concept that there is no need for operator training and support, or if the camera store told the proud new owner that there is no need to adjust the settings because every image can be optimized with postprocessing. In both photography and diagnostic imaging, the image data cannot be created with postprocessing if they are not recorded correctly.

There are three receptor components to every film-based imaging system: the cassette (the film holder), the intensifying screen (permanently installed within the cassette), and the film. Each item is an integral part of the imaging system. Each one is laterally important, so we will start from the outside and move inward.

X-Ray Cassettes

The x-ray cassette is a film holder designed to contain one pair of intensifying screens (attached to the front and back of the inside of the cassette) and one sheet of film of the appropriate size, which is placed between the screens (Fig. 4.3).

The cassette front is the "tube" side of the cassette and is located adjacent to the patient when it is in position. The cassette back is the side farthest from the object of interest. The cassette back usually contains the intensifying screen information and contains the opening device. When the cassettes are opened, they are placed on the counter with the front side down.

Early cardboard and later plastic holders were used to encase the thinner and more flexible film because, unlike photography, the radiation penetrated the film holder. These holders were vulnerable to repetitive handling, and it soon became evident that a more substantial product was necessary. However, the early film holders are still in use in some facilities that radiograph very small animal extremities and small birds (Fig. 4.4).

With the introduction of intensifying screens, the entire package needed to be protected by a holder that was sturdy and unbendable because the emulsion of the intensifying screen could be damaged if it was folded or bent. Manufacturers finally developed a cassette that met all the necessary criteria.

An x-ray film cassette must:
- Be sturdy so it does not crack under the heavy weight of a patient or several cassettes in a pile
- Not break apart in very cold conditions (equine radiography)
- Withstand considerable abuse during many years of service
- Be inflexible and not warp if the patient's weight is unevenly distributed on the front
- Have secure latches that do not come undone inappropriately, exposing the film to light
- Have a radiolucent front that will not produce artifacts on the film

Kodak always yellow on back

Konica cassette Double deck   Wolf cassette with DuPont Hi Plus screens

FIG. 4.3 A, Cassette fronts. These labels indicate the screen type within the cassette and also the placement of the mask for the film identifier. **B,** Cassette backs from three different manufacturers. Sometimes the screens of one vendor are mounted within a cassette made by a different company. The labels on the back of the cassette should always be compared with the screen stencil stamped onto the screen itself. Note that the cassette front shows where the film identifier is located; the cassette back identifies the type of intensifying screen enclosed.

Front of plastic/cardboard holder.

B

Inside film holder
with flap folded out
and single screen
installed.

FIG. 4.4 A and B, Film holders were originally made of cardboard and, later, plastic. They usually had a paper liner and can still be used for small body parts (wings and rodents' feet).

- Have a balanced weight from back to front so the cassette does not warp with age
- Contain a leaded foil or steel back to absorb scattered radiation emitted from the patient
- Contain some method of ensuring that the x-ray film is in good contact across the entire intensifying screen on both sides of the cassette (usually either foam or felt); film/screen contact is essential to high resolution (see Chapter 9)
- Have material on the outside that is washable and impervious to cleaning solutions, blood, and other effluents

Intensifying Screens

Very soon after discovering x-rays, Roentgen noticed that a paper covered with barium platinocyanide reacted quickly to the x-rays, converting them to light. Because he already knew that film is more sensitive to light than to x-rays, the logical conclusion was to convert the x-rays to light after they penetrate the patient and to record the resulting image on glass plates coated with an emulsion that maintains the image.

Barium platinocyanide was the first material used as an intensifying screen. Other physicists carried on his research, and in February 1897 the first commercial intensifying screen was developed. Thomas Edison, a fastidious inventor, applied for the first U.S. patent, but intensifying screens became widely used throughout the world within months of Roentgen's discovery of x-rays.

Screen Composition

The modern intensifying screen is composed of a base with an emulsion painted onto it. Often there is an adhesive layer that glues the emulsion to the base. Currently, the base is a plastic/polymer, which is virtually indestructible within the hospital. The screen emulsion adheres to the base with an adhesive layer.

Screen Characteristics

Film has an infinite resolution. Film that is contained in the appropriate light-tight film holder and exposed and processed under perfect conditions will produce a near-perfect, high-resolution image. Problems arise because of the exposure time necessary to acquire that image. Patients are not always cooperative, hearts beat, lungs move ribs, and abdominal contents gurgle their way through the system.

Intensifying screens provide a faster, more efficient method of image acquisition. An added benefit of intensifying screens is the enhancement of contrast. When film alone is used on body parts greater than 10 centimeters, the amount of radiation required to expose the film causes scattered/secondary radiation to reduce the contrast dramatically. Visualization of the anatomy is compromised, making diagnosis from the film virtually impossible.

When x-ray photons penetrate the front of the cassette and arrive at the intensifying screen(s), they are immediately converted to light by the phosphor in the emulsion of the screens. The intensity and color of the light depend on the components of the phosphor.

This is one of the most important areas of imaging with film/screens.

The speed (or rate) at which the x-rays are converted to light by the individual phosphors is called the *intrinsic conversion efficiency* of the phosphor. Each screen is rated by how quickly or how slowly the conversion occurs. This number determines the speed of the screen (screen speed), or how quickly that particular screen converts radiation to light. A calcium tungstate emulsion (the older technology) has a 30% to 40% conversion efficiency, whereas a rare earth emulsion (the newer technology) has a 50% to 60% conversion efficiency. This means that less exposure time is required to produce an image on film that uses rare earth intensifying screens than on film that uses calcium tungstate screens.

The concept of screen speed classifications was introduced in order to compare the screens produced by each manufacturer. A standard film and rigidly controlled processing was used to test the system speeds. The speed of the system was measured by the amount of radiation required to produce a certain specific density (1.0) on a film (Fig. 4.5). A density of 1.0 is exactly in the center of the visible density range and is the density imaged in the middle of the ilium or in the center of the cranium of a lateral skull on a correctly exposed radiograph. (See Chapter 9 for more information on uniform density.)

A measurement of the exposure needed to produce a density of 1.0 *with* intensifying screens compared with the exposure needed *without* the use of intensifying screens is called *the intensification factor (IF)*. One example of a reduction in exposure time are the technical factors required for a radiograph of a bird's wing. All other factors being equal, the time required with no intensifying screens is approximately 0.03 seconds, whereas the time required using 400-speed intensifying screens is 0.003 seconds.

$$IF = \frac{\text{Exposure without screens}}{\text{Exposure with screens}}$$

$$= \frac{.03}{.003}$$

$$IF = 10$$

This type of calculation is useful if no screen/cassette is available. Usually it is used when very high resolution is necessary to visualize very small, thin body parts.

Until the 1970s, calcium tungstate ($CaWO_4$) was the phosphor of choice for producing intensifying screens. In the 1970s a scientist at 3M in Minnesota experimented with phosphors while conducting research to collect light from distant stars, and she identified several phosphors as being very efficient at capturing light photons. These phosphors all belonged to a group of elements known as the *rare earths,* so-called because of the difficulties encountered when mining them from the earth. 3M produced system speeds of up to 1200; however, the company settled on a 400-speed system.

Rare earth phosphors produce three to four times the amount of visible light per absorbed photon than the calcium tungstate phosphors. This means that the technical factors and thus the amount of radiation necessary to produce the same image density (optical density [OD] 1.0) may be reduced by a factor of 3 or 4. An examination requiring 0.10 seconds with calcium tungstate phosphors would now be perfectly acceptable at 0.025 seconds with rare earth phosphors. The older calcium tungstate screens are still available but are not recommended for use in any medical or veterinary facility.

The Blue/Green Question

Until 1981, all radiography film was manufactured to react to blue light from the blue light–emitting intensifying screens (Fig. 4.6). In 1981, Kodak introduced the rare earth lanthanum oxide intensifying screens, which emitted green light. This event threw the imaging world into chaos. Now the competitive film companies, who were just perfecting the blue systems, had to "play catch-up" and manufacture two completely different emulsions—an intensifying screen emulsion and a companion film emulsion. In addition, Kodak introduced the 24 cm × 30 cm x-ray cassette, which replaced the standard 10 in × 12 in (25 cm × 30 cm) cassette. The added metric cassette (1 cm smaller on the short

FIG. 4.5 An example of density 1.0 + base + fog. This density on a film is exactly midway between completely black (density 3.00) and completely clear (density 0.10). For a further explanation, see Chapter 9.

Blue Systems

Screens Emit Violet Blue light

Require   receiving film

Demonstrate various speeds of conversion efficiency

Green Systems

Emit Green or Blue-Green light

Require Green receiving film

Usually demonstrate single speed of conversion efficiency

FIG. 4.6 Blue Systems vs. Green Systems.

side) was a marketing ploy that confuses people to this day. The green screen technology was definitely a superior imaging system, and the research dollars spent to improve this system have given it an advantage over the blue systems.

At the time of this writing, blue systems are being phased out and eventually will not be supported as the production of blue-receiving film slows down and eventually ceases. Research into blue systems ended in the mid to late 1980s, which means that the technology used to produce any blue-emitting screens is at least 40 years old.

It is vitally important to know which color system is in place at the veterinary facility. Ordering or accepting a delivery of incorrect film and trying to optimize imaging is a very common problem in the radiography room.

More About Color

A rainbow is the result of light traveling through the atmosphere. Each of the colors of the rainbow is refracted at a slightly different angle (Fig. 4.7), resulting in a perfect spectrum of color. Every time light is refracted, whether through a prism of glass, a sudden shower, or a perfect diamond, the colors remain in the same orientation and order. This arrangement is known as the *visible light spectrum*. Infrared light is at the far "outside" of the curve, and blue and ultraviolet light are on the "inside" of the curve. Violet morphs to blue and then to green, yellow, orange, and red. This order is important when investigating x-ray film and intensifying screens and when setting up a darkroom and using a safelight (see Chapter 7). If the film reacts to only the blue-green side of the spectrum, it will not react to the deepest red part of the spectrum. If it reacts to green, it will react to an orange-yellow color because there is a yellow component in the color green (blue + yellow = green).

FIG. 4.7 The Importance of Spectral Matching. The film must be able to "see" the light emitted from the intensifying screen. In this case, blue light is emitted and blue film overlaps the emission and therefore reacts to the light. The film would not "see" green light as it is too far removed to the right of the spectrum to be activated. It does, however, "see" a small amount of the blue light because there is a blue component in the green light. (Modified from Bushong SC. *Radiologic Science for Technologists.* 10th ed. St Louis: Elsevier; 2013.)

> **✓ CHECK IT OUT**
> 1. The easiest way to identify the color of the screen in your facility is to remove the film from each cassette in the darkroom and store it in a light-tight container.
> 2. Place the open cassette on the x-ray table under the x-ray tube and set the factors on the generator—usually 100 mA, ¼ (0.25) of a second, and 70 kV. (It is important to set a long enough time to be able to identify the color of the screen while the exposure is being made.)
> 3. Make sure the room is darkened and that the collimator light is off. Now make an exposure and watch for the phosphors to fluoresce.

The early intensifying screens were made of calcium tungstate ($CaWO_4$), which emits a very pretty blue-violet light. When the rare earth phosphors were developed, the striking difference (apart from their rapid conversion efficiency) was the bright green-yellow color of their phosphor emission. This changed the entire world of imaging. The x-ray film that had been developed to respond to blue light did not "see" the extended yellow-green portion of the spectrum. Therefore, a new film had to be developed that responded both to blue light and to yellow-green light.

> **? POINTS TO PONDER** Many facilities today still have a problem confusing the film that is ordered. Green-sensitive film must be used with green-emitting screens. Blue-sensitive film must be used with blue-emitting screens.

Green-sensitive film "sees" the blue light portion of the green screens, but blue film does not react to the green portion of the green-emitting screens. If the incorrect film is used, the technical factors will need to be revised because the imaging is not optimized. This increases patient and staff radiation dose considerably and results in a less-than-optimal image. If blue film is inserted between green screens, the images will be a dull gray, lacking contrast that does not improve even if the technical factors are raised or lowered.

> **? POINTS TO PONDER** DuPont Quanta V screens were the green-emitting answer to Kodak's Lanex Regular screens. They were never successful and were eventually abandoned.
> The replacement technology led to the introduction of DuPont UV (Ultraviolet) screens, which moved the sensitivity to the left of the spectrum and into the ultraviolet range. These screens were mostly successful with extremities and thinner body parts. They do show up in the veterinary market occasionally but are no longer produced, and the UV film is no longer sold.
> If the facility has purchased UV screens, the film that would be ordered is blue receiving film. This film is available but usually "not in stock." They do not respond well to the light of green-emitting screens. Ideally the screens should be replaced.
> We will visit this topic again when we discuss radiographic film, both blue-receiving film and green-receiving film. The concept is important and frequently confused.

400 speed
Green emitting screens
presently slowed
to ~300 speed

200 speed
Green emitting screens
presently slowed
to ~100 speed

400 speed
Green emitting screens
presently remains
at 400 speed

600 speed
Green emitting screens

FIG. 4.8 The Backs of Various Cassettes and Screen Speeds.

Screen Speed

- The conversion efficiency of the phosphor reflects the components of the x-ray screen; unfortunately, not all screens are created equal (Fig. 4.8).
- Green-screen technology has two screen speeds: fast response to radiation and slow response to radiation (Table 4.1). (A medium-speed screen was available but not in general use and is now mainly phased out.)
- The phosphor thickness is a factor in the screen speed, but so is the thickness of the emulsion. Slower-speed systems have thinner emulsions.
- Faster systems with thicker emulsions produce more photons of light per incident ray than the slower systems. Faster systems reduce the radiation dose to the patient, but they also reduce the *spatial resolution* (the ability to see very fine detail).

TABLE 4.1	The Influence of Slow Screens vs. Fast Screens on Images	
FACTOR	**SLOW SCREEN SPEED RESPONSE TO RADIATION**	**FAST SCREEN SPEED RESPONSE TO RADIATION**
Technique	Increase technical factors	Decrease technical factors
Dose	Higher dose	Lower dose
Resolution	Better resolution	Lower resolution
Contrast	No difference	No difference
Density	Lighter image if factors are not adjusted	Darker image if factors are not adjusted

- The slower the screen speed, the more detail is evident on the image (higher resolution).
  - To produce the same density on the film every time, more radiation must be used to produce an image from a slow screen than from a faster screen.
  - The screen type does not influence contrast—only film and technical factors influence contrast. Over time, many applications were developed using a variety of screen speeds and mixing and matching screens became quite common.
- This interchanging of screens was known as *asymmetrical systems,* and 3M was the company best known for this technology.

Cassette Identification vs. Screen Identification

Cassette/screen manufacturers place labels on the back of the cassettes to notify the user which screens have been installed. 3M cassettes are often labeled 2/6 or 6/12; this labeling denotes an asymmetrical system.

Screens are always labeled in very fine print on the edge, usually along the long side. The imprinting is very tiny and sometimes hard to read, but it is essential that the operator is aware of the phosphor emission color and the screen designation. Cassettes do have the screen type labeled on the back, but occasionally screens are replaced in cassettes and the labels are not changed. The positive identification is on the screen stencil (Fig. 4.9).

Luminescence and Phosphorescence

Intensifying screens react to the incoming radiation by a process called *luminescence.* The photons of the x-ray beam are converted to light when they reach the emulsion of the screen.

There are two types of luminescence: fluorescence and phosphorescence.

- Fluorescence is an instantaneous reaction that lasts exactly as long as the phosphor is stimulated.

3M Trimax 2

Kodak Lanex Regular   Kodak Lanex Fast

FIG. 4.9 Screen Stencils: 3M and Kodak. The numbers identify when the screen was manufactured and the batch number.

FIG. 4.10 An Example of *Phosphorescence.* The light from the sun causes the crystals to glow, which remains long after the excitation of the crystals. The effect that the screens must have is *fluorescence,* which means the crystals stop glowing immediately after the stimulation is removed. (Copyright myshkovsky/Getty Images.)

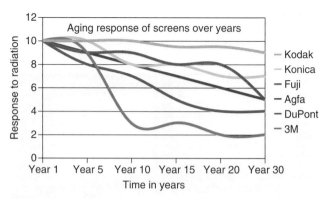

FIG. 4.11 Chart Depicting the Typical Responses of Screens Over 30 Years. The Lanex screens retain their original speed throughout their lifetime. Most other screens deteriorate in speed. This is not the result of a controlled experiment, but rather an observation over 50 years of imaging consultation.

- Phosphorescence occurs when the phosphor continues to emit light after the stimulation has ceased (Fig. 4.10). Phosphorescence is not desirable in medical imaging and is termed *screen lag or afterglow.*

Screen Aging Response

As intensifying screens age over time, the response of the phosphor reduces in brightness and speed. A screen that responded to the incoming radiation 100% when new may respond only 50% after 15 or 20 years. The response of the screen, both in brightness and over time, is called *screen speed.* Technical problems arise as the products age. The reaction time of the screens deteriorates and the techniques have to be increased to give a uniform image density (Fig. 4.11). If older screens from various manufacturers are used in one clinic, the screen speed may differ widely, and the images produced can vary in density and contrast. This is often the reason why a particular cassette is discarded because "it doesn't work properly." Actually, it may be reacting to the x-ray beam correctly according to its manufacture, original screen speed, and age. It is very important to know which screens are in use at the veterinary facility and whether they are matched for screen speed and age. (See Chapter 9 for screen speed testing procedure.)

If a facility has a mixture of various manufacturers' screens, there is most likely a wide variation in the speeds of the intensifying screens. In this case, adherence to a standard technique chart is impossible, as is the production of consistent, optimized images. Intensifying screens are often replaced in cassettes, but the change is not necessarily noted on the outside of the cassette. A cassette label on the back of the cassette may note that it contains Quanta 111 Screens installed in 1982, but the actual screens may be Fuji HR or Kodak Lanex Regular and installed very recently (see Chapter 9).

Speed Response Differences

In order to compare screen speeds, the manufacturers agreed on a numbering system that is still used today. The DuPont (E.I. DuPont de Nemours) Hi Speed Screen is used as a baseline and called 100-speed class. Table 4.2 lists the common manufacturers with the names and speeds of their systems.

It must be remembered that each manufacturer has its own concept of the speed of its particular phosphor "recipe," so the speeds are not all exactly the same; this is why we use the term *"speed class."* For example, Kodak Lanex screens are a true 400-speed, whereas DuPont Quanta 111 screens in the 400-speed class are actually closer to 350-speed. More radiation must be used with the Quanta 111 screens than with the Kodak Lanex screens to produce the same density on a film.

3M Corporation originally developed the technology to use the rare earth phosphors for intensifying screens and therefore had many more varieties and combinations than are listed in Table 4.2. Old Agfa screens, often donated by medical facilities to veterinary clinics, demonstrated phosphorescence and would fog the film in the cassette as it waited to be used. Agfa's Ortho 400s had the most frequent problems. DuPont rare earth screens were never very good, with poor resolution and very little contrast, and the emulsions tended to absorb moisture (see Chapter 9).

As screens age, their response to radiation will slow down. Screens of various companies lose their speed over time in and at various rates. Fig. 4.11 lists the average speed loss of screens from six major manufacturers over a 30-year period.

If there is a problem with imaging, the first place to investigate is always the film/screen combination. It is common for the incorrect film to be ordered or even supplied by the film vendor. Checking the film/screen combination is the easiest place to start the investigative process.

TABLE 4.2	Screen Manufacturers and Their Speed Classifications			
MANUFACTURER	**SCREEN NAME**	**SPEED CLASS**	**COLOR OF PHOSPHOR**	**RARE EARTH?**
Agfa	Ortho Fine	100	Green	Yes
	Ortho Medium	200	Green	Yes
	Ortho 400*	400	Green	Yes—no longer available
	Ortho	400	Green	Yes
DuPont	Par	50	Blue	No: These screens were produced from 1960–1980 and are now obsolete. The speed of the screens has diminished to the point that they should no longer be used, ever.
	Hi Speed	100	Blue	
	Hi Plus +	200	Blue	
	Lightning Plus	150	Blue	
	Quanta 11	300	Blue	Yes—no longer in use. These were very "noisy" screens and were either dumped onto the vet/chiropractor/osteopath market or scrapped.
	Quanta 111	400	Blue	Yes
	Quanta V	400	Green	Yes. These were manufactured only by DuPont and are no longer available; they had very poor resolution.
	Quanta UV	400	Ultraviolet	Yes. These were available only around 1985–1989. They produced good imaging for extremities but very poor imaging for abdomens. They were removed from the medical market around 1990.
Fuji	G4	200	Green	Yes
	G8	300	Green	Yes
	G12	400	Green	Yes
	HR	400	Green	Yes
Kodak	Xomat	200	Blue	No
	Fine	100	Blue	No
	Lanex Fine	100	Green	Yes
	Lanex Med	200	Green	Yes
	Lanex Regular	400	Green	Yes
	Lanex Fast	600	Green	Yes
Konica	KMC	200	Blue	Yes, with type HB film
	KMC	400	Blue	Yes, with type A film
	KF	100	Green	Yes
	KM	300	Green	Yes
	KR	400	Green	Yes
	KS	600	Green	Yes
3M Corp[†]	2 or 3	100	Green	Yes
	6	200	Green	Yes
	12	400	Green	Yes

*Old Agfa screens often donated to a veterinary clinic demonstrated phosphorescence and would fog the film in the cassette as it waited to be used. Agfa's Ortho 400s had the most frequent problems.
†3M corporation developed the technology to use the rare earth phosphors for intensifying screens and therefore had many more varieties and combinations than are listed here.
With assistance from Leo Reina, X-ray Cassette Repair Company, dba Reina Imaging, Crystal Lake, Illinois.

Radiography Film

Several companies manufacture film, and several more cut and sell the film. The one standard among all these companies is the film size (Table 4.3).

Film is sold in very specific sizes to match the sizes of the cassettes. It is important to know what size cassette is in use in the facility and then order the appropriate size film. Kodak's introduction of the 24 cm × 30cm film and cassette made the industry even more complicated. Film price is based on the square inch of the product. A box of 25 cm × 30 cm film (traditionally 10 in × 12 in, or 120 in²) is more expensive than the 24cm × 30 cm (113 square inches) film introduced by Kodak and now sold universally. Film that is 25 cm × 30 cm will fit into a 24 cm × 30 cm cassette only if it is cut down to size in the darkroom; 1 cm must be removed from the long side. This is a lengthy procedure and unnecessary if the correct size is originally ordered. It is expensive to order the incorrect film in terms of both time and money.

TABLE 4.3	Film and Cassette Sizes (Metric vs. Inch)*		
FILM SIZE (INCHES)	**FILM SIZE (CENTIMETERS)**	**TYPICAL IMAGING USE**
6 × 8	18 × 24	Extremities, pocket pets
8 × 10	20 × 25	Equine and extremities, pocket pets
	24 × 30	Equine and feline, also skull and extremities
10 × 12	25 × 30	Equine and feline, also skull and extremities
11 × 14	28 × 35	General radiography
	30 × 35	General radiography
14 × 17	35 × 43	General radiography

*Some of the inch sizes do not have an equal-sized metric partner, as is the case with the cm sizes.

Regular cow hide   X-ray film

FIG. 4.12 One use for recycled radiography film! This is a band in Cuba. Used x-ray film has many uses, including fencing and fence posts, lawn chairs, and fashion jewelry. It is very important to find a recycler for used x-ray film; it should not go to a landfill. (Courtesy James Duhaime, St Clair Veterinary Facilities, Toronto.)

★ **APPLICATION INFORMATION**

Ordering x-ray film has been made complicated by the mixture of centimeter sizes and inch sizes. Often the film supplier will send 10 in × 12 in film, which is one centimeter wider than 24 cm × 30 cm film. This means that the staff has to send the product back, which is time consuming, or they have to stand in the darkroom (in the dark) and cut 1 cm off the long edge of the film so it fits into their 24 cm × 30 cm cassettes. This happens frequently if the person ordering the film is not familiar with the correct film sizes. The correct order numbers must be very clearly understood by the purchasing staff.

The Development of Film-Based Imaging

Cellulose nitrate was introduced as a film base in 1914. The old emulsions were flammable and did not archive well.

Along with the new film bases, more efficient emulsions were investigated.

The cellulose triacetate base was used into the 1960s when E.I. DuPont de Nemours introduced the film base that is in use today.

Along the way, the company also invented nylon, Dacron, Kevlar, and many related substances, but their major achievement in imaging was the invention of Mylar. Mylar or a derivative has been used in medical imaging for about 60 years. Before the introduction of Mylar, the film would tear apart and be destroyed if it became caught in a processor. With the introduction of a film base that was nontearing and inflammable, x-ray film became virtually indestructible.

? **POINTS TO PONDER**   Recycled radiography film has been used in many applications once its life in the medical world is complete, including in gardening to prevent drainage from raised beds, as windows in Third World countries, and as the heads of bongo drums (Fig. 4.12)!

When it is time to dispose of used film, the veterinary technician should always make sure that the recycler is actually destroying the film by shredding, or the veterinary facility should remove all patient identifiers from each film before it is shipped from the veterinary hospital.

Composition of Radiography Film

The x-ray film base is translucent and flexible. Light-sensitive film emulsion coats either one side of the base (single-emulsion film) or two sides of the base (double-emulsion film) (Fig. 4.13A,B). Between the base and the emulsion is an adhesive layer that is so thin it is basically incorporated into the emulsion layer. The supercoat is a hard, protective gelatin layer on top of the emulsion that protects the image from the rigors of processing. This is only somewhat effective, so film should always be handled with respect because the emulsion on a preexposed film and the image on a postexposed film are very tenuous and easily compromised.

Halation is the effect of light reflecting off the back of the film base and affecting the image by causing a shadow effect. Double-emulsion film contains a dye layer that prevents a crossover effect, a type of halation in which the light of one intensifying screen affects the opposite emulsion (Figs. 4.14A,B and 4.15). Single-emulsion film requires an anticurl/antihalation layer on the nonemulsion side. The antihalation layer is removed during film processing. Single-emulsion film is easily identified even in the darkroom under safelight conditions. The side with the emulsion is dull, and the side with the anticurl/antihalation layer is shiny.

Double-emulsion film is used in general radiography. Single-emulsion film is used in special applications such as high-resolution imaging (extremities and equine) and in laser imaging printing for computed tomography, magnetic

FIG. 4.13 Cross-section of double-emulsion film (**A**) and single-emulsion film (**B**). (Modified from Fauber TL. *Radiographic Imaging and Exposure*. 5th ed. St. Louis: Mosby; 2017.)

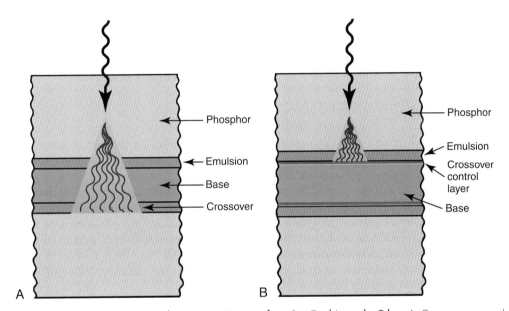

FIG. 4.14 Dye Layer *(Orange Layer)* that Prevents Crossover from One Emulsion to the Other. **A,** Crossover occurs when the film has no dye layer to prevent light from the top screen affecting the film emulsion on the opposite side. **B,** The dye layer prevents the light from the top screen affecting the light from the bottom screen. This occurs only with double-emulsion film.

FIG. 4.15 The Halation Effect. If the film has two emulsions and no antihalation layer, there will be a crossover effect.

resonance imaging, nuclear medicine, and positron emission tomography if the veterinarian needs a hard-copy image from these modalities.

✦ APPLICATION INFORMATION

Film processed to demonstrate an image is referred to with reference to its density, or the amount of darkening of the image on the film. "Light" images or "dark" images refer to the overall amount of clear or degree of blackness on the film. These densities are read using a densitometer (density-meter) and will be discussed in Chapter 9.

Please refer to Fig. 4.5, which shows an example of a density 1.0 image. This is the midrange of densities which typically start at 0.15 and rise to 3.40.

Film Base

The base material that holds the emulsion of the film:

- must be strong yet flexible.
- must bend without stretching,

- must be stable throughout changes in temperature and humidity.
- must be rigid enough to hang on an illuminator and yet flexible enough to travel through an x-ray processor.
- must be consistently and uniformly optically translucent.
- must permit the transmission of light without adding any artifacts to the final x-ray image.
- must also be thin enough so there is no crossover effect (reflection) from one side of the image to the other when the image is produced.

In the 1960s, it was discovered that the addition of a slight blue tint to the film base enabled the radiologist reading the images to work for longer periods without experiencing eyestrain and headaches from the glare of the illuminators transmitted through the lightly exposed or unexposed portions of the film (see Chapter 6).

Film Emulsion

The emulsion is the material that is coated onto the film base by means of an adhesive material that binds it to the film base. Film emulsion starts with gelatin (the same gelatin used in cooking and Jell-O). The gelatin used in this application is of very high quality and is completely translucent. The photosensitive products within the emulsion are mainly silver bromide (about 95% to 98%), silver iodide, and silver chloride. (There is very little silver chloride in film emulsion today). Collectively, the term silver *halide* is used to describe the components of the emulsion. Fig. 4.16A illustrates the old method of infiltrating the silver halide into an emulsion. As illustrated, there are large areas between the silver crystals. Fig. 16B illustrates the later "tabular grain" technology where the crystals were flattened and now overlap to cover more surface area.

The gelatin base must:
- allow the processing chemicals to infiltrate the emulsion and react with the silver halide crystals to produce the image.
- be uniform. Its thickness is usually 0.0002 to 0.0004 inch (5 to 10 μm) depending on the manufacturer.

- must be flexible enough to permit bending without stretching as the film winds its way through an automatic processor.

The Supercoat

The outside of the film is protected by a tough coating of hard protective gelatin (the supercoat) that has been treated to prevent tearing, scratching, and abrasions to the film as it is loaded into the cassettes and then processed either manually or automatically. It is not very thick, and rough handling and scratching can damage the supercoat. This supercoat also protects the film from diffusing its dye into the screens. It is important to note that once the film is wet, the gelatin absorbs moisture and the supercoat becomes vulnerable to scratches and abrasions.

Latent Image Formation

The film emulsion with the silver halide particles suspended in a gelatinous layer also contains sensitivity specks (centers), small physical imperfections within the network of the silver halide. It is these small areas that become magnets for the silver particles to adhere to one another and form an image.

If the silver halide were perfect and without any imperfections (sensitivity specks), the image would not form, and the film would exit the processor with no discernible image. Therefore, when film is first manufactured, it must remain in the warehouse for a time to allow the sensitivity specks to settle within the emulsion. This process is called *aging* or *seasoning*.

According to theory, the latent image is formed within the emulsion of the x-ray film when the x-rays and light activate the silver particles in the film emulsion. The silver particles are attracted to the sensitivity specks by electromagnetism. It is believed that there must be at least three silver atoms to each sensitivity speck in order for the image to form. The term *latent image* refers to the image that is formed but is invisible until processed either manually or in an automatic processor. This new arrangement of silver

FIG. 4.16 Magnified Portion of the Film Emulsion. **A,** Old technology silver halide crystals. **B,** New technology using tabular grain silver halide crystals. (Courtesy Carestream Health.)

FIG. 4.17 A Geodesic Dome. The pattern is similar to the lattice network that forms when an image is produced on a film. The joints are the sensitivity specks drawing the silver ions together to form the network, or lattice. (Copyright photoart23D/Getty Images.)

FIG. 4.18 Seeding of Clouds by Human Intervention. The moisture gathers on the dust until it becomes so heavy that it starts to rain. This is similar to the sensitivity specks distributed throughout the film emulsion. Once the emulsion is activated by the x-rays, the sensitivity specks form "collection points" where the latent image forms

halide particles is called the *lattice network*. It is a tenuous arrangement and may be easily destroyed.

The pattern of a lattice network is much like a geodesic dome (Fig. 4.17). The joints of the bars are the sensitivity specks. High-detail film contains more sensitivity specks than general radiography film and therefore produces a more detailed image. The silver compounds wait until they are processed to produce a manifest image.

The lattice network forms very much like the seeding of clouds to cause rain (Fig. 4.18). The water droplets require impurities in the clouds to form rain; these impurities can be added naturally by the wind raising dust clouds or mechanically by an airplane dropping dust onto the cloud. With film, the impurities (sensitivity specks) are added into the film emulsion, and the catalyst to start the process of latent image formation is the introduction of photons of light and x-rays. The actual physical process is still somewhat a mystery, but it is known that the image forms around the sensitivity specks electromagnetically and that at least three freed silver atoms must be deposited for a clump of black metallic silver to be formed by chemical development later during processing.

The latent image is fragile, and the network is very easy to break. Dropping a cassette from a table after the film inside has been exposed to radiation can destroy the network and cause an artifact of streaks radiating from the point of impact.

Time will also cause the latent image to start to fade, although it does take a fairly long time (in excess of 24 hours) to fade completely. The lattice network will form a denser (darker) image the more it is exposed to radiation, light, and heat. A continuous heavy pressure on unexposed film will prevent the lattice network from forming or will break down what has already formed, leaving a clear area outlining the area of the pressure. Therefore, film and cassettes should always be stored in an upright position in the darkroom and never flat on the counter.

Base + Fog

When the film is originally manufactured, it will be completely clear after the emulsion has been removed by processing. A very light blue dye is added as the film is manufactured in order to reduce the glare of the illuminator when the radiologist or veterinarian is viewing the image. This is called the base density.

After the film seasons, or matures, to the point that it can be sold and put into practice, it will develop a low fog level.

Freshly manufactured film will be stored for a period of time to allow the film emulsion to "season." Once it is delivered to the customer, the optical density level will increase to around 0.10–0.15. This optical density is the evidence that the sensitivity specks are active and will convert any light or radiation into metallic silver during processing. Whenever film density is discussed, the base color and the fog level are always included as part of the image (e.g., density 1.0 + base + fog). As you will recall from Fig. 4.5, density 1.0 is the mid-range density of the image.

The base + fog level is usually minimal in unexposed film. However, if the film is exposed to unsuitable storage conditions (e.g., heat, air heavy with a chemical odor) and then exposed to radiation, the base + fog will be dark enough to compromise the radiograph because the clear areas will no longer be visible, having been replaced by a fog density of 0.20 to 0.29.

> ### ◆ APPLICATION INFORMATION
> The head technologist at a large Southern veterinary hospital called the consultant with a problem. About 6 months ago, she had purchase about 50 boxes of x-ray film from a dealer who was going out of business. The veterinary technician had started using the film about 1 week ago and the images were all dark gray with very little contrast.
>
> The first indication that there was a problem was where the technologist had stored the unused boxes of film. It was very warm in the office and the boxes of film were stored on a shelf that ran along the top of two walls. Heat rises and when the consultant held a thermometer to the level of the shelf it read 90°F (32.2°C). The fog level of the film had risen remarkably, as sensitivity specks start to form a density when exposed to heat, light, and chemical fumes. The average density was Optical Density 0.40–0.50.
> There is no way to reverse the process, so after each box was tested, the film was recycled as useless.

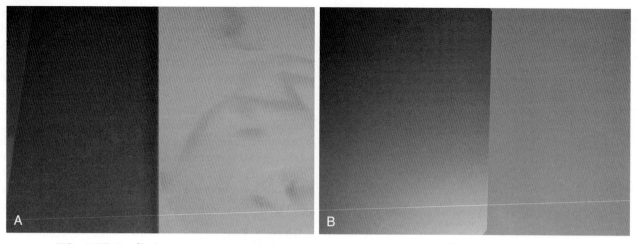

FIG. 4.19 Two film/screen systems are available on the market today. Green is the preferred color, but some facilities still use blue. Four brands of film are illustrated here, two blue and two green. **A,** Blue light–receiving film is physically green. The image is "blue" film from two different companies. **B,** Green light–receiving film is physically violet. The image is "green" film from two different companies.

The Response of Film to Light

Film Color

Modern film responds to the light emitted from the intensifying screens. This light may be either blue or green, and this can cause confusion in any veterinary facility. It is also one of the most important concepts in the practice of film/screen imaging.

Blue-emitting screens require blue-receiving film (Fig. 4.19A). Confusion arises when the blue dye used in the base "mixes" with the yellow color of the emulsion. The blue-receiving film then becomes physically green in color. Green-receiving film is physically violet. This was agreed to by the film manufacturers to differentiate between blue-receiving film and green-receiving film (Fig. 4.19B). Rather than preventing confusion, however, this step added to the confusion; to this day, green-receiving film is physically violet and blue-receiving film is physically green.

Film Speed

It is always good practice to examine every box of film delivered from the supplier to ensure that the correct film has been shipped. The type of film and the code number are clearly marked on the front and/or side of the film box.

It is common to find hospitals using a half-speed film in old blue-screened cassettes when they could decrease the dose just by changing the film they put into the cassettes (Table 4.4).

Swapping out the screens to green-emitting screens can save money (green is less expensive than blue) and improve imaging using modern technology. The imaging research on blue systems ended many years ago. If a facility is going to stay with film-screen imaging, the cassettes should be replaced with ones containing green-emitting screens or, at the very least, the screens within the cassettes should be replaced.

◆ **APPLICATION INFORMATION**

It is common to find hospitals using half-speed film and not realizing it. What can happen is that the film supplier runs out of full-speed film and, understanding that the color is important, they supply half-speed film instead. The technicians often order from the label on the box, so when the time comes to reorder, they reorder the half-speed film. Meanwhile their technical factors have all doubled in mAs, but that happens only once, so they think the x-ray machine is getting old or not as efficient, and they change the technique chart and carry on.

The problem is discovered when a new technician arrives and questions the high doses or when a consultant comes in on another matter and notices that the technical factors are very high compared with what he or she is used to seeing. The only film that should be used in a veterinary hospital is full-speed green film. (Often with green receiving film, the half-speed product is a special order.) If blue film is still being used, then it should be full-speed blue film. Half-speed and UV film is not suitable for use with any blue-emitting screens.

It is important to remember that half-speed film stored away somewhere may arrive at your facility. Because half-speed film reacts 50% slower to radiation, it will produce an image that is 50% lighter than it should be given the technical factors used for a 400-speed system.

TABLE 4.4	Common Film Types and Their Speed		
COMPANY	**FILM TYPE**	**FILM SPEED**	**FILM COLOR**
Carestream	T-mat-G/RA	Full-speed	Green
Carestream	CSB	Full-speed	Blue
Fuji	HRS	Full-speed	Green
Fuji	RX	Full-speed	Blue
3M	UD+	Full-speed	Green

The other film that may be available today in certain geographical locations is extremity film and/or single-emulsion film. Single-emulsion film has emulsion on one side and an antihalation layer on the other side. Single-emulsion film reacts to radiation and light from the screens only on the side with the emulsion, and it is far slower than double-emulsion film. Single-emulsion film is used for certain specific applications in which exceptional detail is required. It may be used in some equine practices when tiny spurs, spicules, or hairline fractures are suspected. It can also be used in wildlife practices to diagnose fractures in reptiles or on the wings of birds. Single-emulsion film requires considerably higher doses of radiation to produce an image and therefore is definitely not recommended for routine veterinary examinations. The most common use of single-emulsion film up until a few years ago was human breast imaging; thus, it is typically available only in 8 in × 10 in, 24 cm × 30 cm, and 10 in × 12 in sizes.

Other films, such as duplicating film and laser film, are not in wide practice in veterinary medicine.

Film Speed and White Box Film

Film speed is the most difficult factor to control in the production of the film itself. Mixing emulsions is a little like following a recipe from a list of dissimilar ingredients. Depending on the manufacturer, many different components are mixed in with a lot of gelatin.

If the mix is slightly "off" either way, the film may react a little too quickly or a little too slowly to exposure by radiation. Each manufacturer has a specific benchmark for the reaction time of the film, and each batch of film is tested against this benchmark. If the speed of the film is within ±10% of the perfect speed, it is accepted and boxed with the manufacturer's label. At this point the film is in huge rolls about 2 feet (0.61 m) in diameter and about 40 to 50 feet (12.2–15.24 m) in length.

If the speed of the entire roll of film is beyond the 10% parameter up to a point of nonacceptance as defined by each manufacturer (usually ±25%), it is sold as "white box" film (Fig. 4.20). This film remains unfinished—it is not given a supercoat to prevent the dye within the emulsion from leaching out onto the screens. This means that, over time, the dye will stain the screen and reduce its speed by coloring the screen emulsion.

White box film is cut to various sizes and boxed in white boxes with a film dealer's label. Because white box packagers deal only with originally rejected film, they may easily mix films of different speeds in one box. A box of 100 sheets may contain film that failed the quality control standards because it was too "slow" mixed in with film that failed because it was too "fast." It is important to remember this process when images never seem to be quite right, with some images too dark and other images too light for the same size animal under the exact same exposure and processing conditions. The easiest solution is to purchase film with the original manufacturer's label on the box. The few dollars saved by buying white box film is not necessarily a cost saving when a diagnosis is missed because of poor image quality or an uncertain speed.

FIG. 4.20 Two Examples of "White Box" Packaged Film. The film in these packages was manufactured in Belgium (Agfa film) and finished in the United States. Other film may be manufactured in the United States (Kodak film).

Typically, the original manufacturer is identifiable on the white box by the location indicated on the label. Because it is law that the country in which the film is manufactured be noted on every product, the label will state "Manufactured in USA" (Kodak film, now Carestream) or "Manufactured in Belgium" (Agfa film). This information serves only for general interest and does not reflect on the product of either manufacturer (Fig. 4.20).

If the film does not meet quality control specifications, the supercoat is not applied. It is the supercoat that prevents the dye transfering from the film surface to the intensifying screens. This uncut film is then sold to a third level film dealer. That facility cuts the film to industry standard sizes and sells it to independent dealers as "white box film".

Storage of Film, Cassettes, and Screens

Proper storage of the products used for imaging is very important. The film and chemicals must be stored on a rotating basis so that the first product in is the first product out. This is also known as *FIFO storage*.

Film

Film boxes must always be stored on edge and not flat on a counter. Film is sensitive to pressure both before and after it has been exposed to radiation. Dropping a cassette with exposed film can destroy the lattice network and ruin the image. Heavy pressure on the film can also destroy the film's capability to form a lattice network, resulting in no image in the area of the pressure. When a film is manufactured and finally presented to the market, it has aged and is ready to be used. The emulsion on the film is an unstable entity ready to react within fractions of a second to any stimulus. Heat, chemical fumes, light leaks, and aging will darken the film without any exposure to radiation. It is important to store film at room temperature and in a dry atmosphere.

FIG. 4.21 Open boxes of film should be stored in a light-tight film bin. This box should be hung on the wall so the film boxes inside remain upright.

FIG. 4.22 Cassettes should be stored upright on a counter or in a cabinet protected from radiation.

Film must be protected from light leaks in the darkroom and from scattered or direct radiation (Fig. 4.21). Film storage is important. The expiration date on the boxes is typically not a best-before date; it is the date that the film starts to gain a fog level caused by the sensitivity specks becoming active and affecting the fog level. As the fog level rises, the darkening increases dramatically, and the resulting image loses contrast because the clear areas of the film will demonstrate the increased fog density.

If the facility has several different sizes of cassettes and film, some of the film sizes may age beyond their expiration date through very intermittent use.

> **? POINTS TO PONDER** Any film that is used for imaging in a camera or imaging in a radiography room is manufactured to be instantly responsive to light. Once the film has been exposed and the lattice network has formed, the film is ten times more sensitive to fogging than it was in its unexposed state. For this reason, any exposed film that is used during a radiography examination must be placed well away from the radiation source and from any scattered radiation.

Cassettes and Screens

Cassettes should be stored upright in a cupboard or in the darkroom without the possibility of exposure to radiation (Fig. 4.22). They should not be stored on the floor, where they could be knocked over or subjected to spills and liquids. They should not be stored in a pile on a counter because the pressure of one cassette on top of another will affect the film. In addition, pulling a cassette out from under a pile of cassettes exerts extra wear and poses the risk of damage to the cassettes.

Cassettes should be loaded with film and ready to be used. It is important to ensure that the correct film is used in each cassette. The cassettes should be kept closed in the darkroom in order to protect the integrity of the screens. Humidity and dust adversely affect the screen and compromise the image.

Screens should be protected when the film is being removed from the cassette. Sliding the film in the cassette will cause wear artifacts on the screen. If the film is not readily removable, the cassette should be held on edge to allow the film to separate from the screen naturally (Fig. 4.23).

Other Equipment and Accessories

We will examine the tabletop, the grid, and the illuminators in other discussions of equipment and accessories (see Chapter 6), technical factors (see Chapter 5), and processing and processing artifacts (see Chapters 7 and 9).

Summary

An optimized system is possible only if the correct products are matched, purchased, and used correctly. This chapter discussed various x-ray cassettes and screen types along with some of the problems inherent in selecting the correct combination to produce an optimized image. Screen/film combinations and the blue versus green problems were reviewed. Latent image formation, base + fog, and general film fog were discussed, and the importance of correctly storing and handling these products was outlined.

Image Gallery

Figs. 4.24 to 4.36 illustrate what can go wrong with film, cassettes, and screens.

FIG. 4.23 Two Ways to Remove Film from a Cassette. **A,** Stand the cassette on edge and let the film fall away from the screen. Then lay the cassette on its front and remove the film from the cassette. **B,** The film may be removed by lifting it from the cassette as shown. DuPont cassettes have a small spring that lifts the film away from the bottom screen.

Magnetized rubber back   Metal foil fixed to back of screen

FIG. 4.24 Agfa cassette with the screens peeled back to demonstrate the structure of the cassette beneath the screen. The front screen has metal foil attached to the back. The back of the cassette has a magnetic rubber sheet.

FIG. 4.25 The foil-backed screen is not firmly attached to the cassette front and can be lifted up and moved forward on two strips of radiolucent polyethylene. The manufacturer's philosophy was that the front screen would be pulled forward by the magnetic rubber and provide excellent film/screen contact across the entire cassette. This did not work well and the film/screen contact was imperfect, especially on larger cassettes. See Fig. 4.29.

FIG. 4.26 **A,** DuPont cassettes are opened when the locks are released. The back of the cassette is slightly curved and is supposed to spring up so the cassette can be opened and the film removed. Over time the cassettes lose the "spring" opening and become more difficult to open. **B,** To correct this problem, open the cassette and lay the back over the edge of a flat surface. Very carefully and slowly press down on the side suspended from the table and the side still on the table. The pressure needs to be firm but not hard. Gently press and release four or five times. Now close the cassette and reopen. The back should now spring up correctly.

FIG. 4.27 Kodak cassettes have a rubber surround that is vulnerable to cracking and breaking. These cassettes have come completely apart at the hinge back and are not reparable. Even if taped with heavy tape (such as duct tape), they cannot be taped tightly enough to provide excellent screen contact. The screens can be removed from each half of the cassette and placed into an intact cassette. Using another Kodak cassette is not recommended, because opening it completely will compromise the rubber hinge. When removing the screens, be very careful to keep the screen intact and not bent or creased, because this will render an artifact on the image. Kodak screens are excellent and have a long life with little deterioration of speed, so they are worth retrieving.

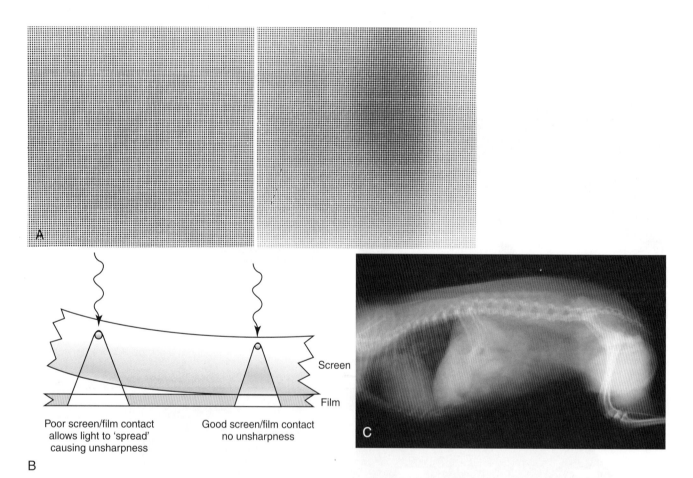

Screen

Film

Poor screen/film contact allows light to 'spread' causing unsharpness

Good screen/film contact no unsharpness

B

FIG. 4.28 **A,** Two images of a film screen contact mesh test tool. The image on the left shows a test image with excellent screen contact. The image on the right demonstrates poor screen contact *(larger darkened area)* on the upper right. **B,** Poor screen contact produces a darkened area of the film. If the film is lifted away from the screen for any reason during the exposure, there will be an area that lights up the screen but spreads very slightly around the specific area because of the lack of good contact. This area of penumbra will translate onto the image as a fuzziness or blurriness. **C,** An image taken using an Agfa screen/cassette with particularly poor screen contact. (From Fauber TL. *Radiographic Imaging and Exposure.* 4th ed. St. Louis: Mosby; 2013.)

A. Minus density artifact from fingers pressing too hard on the film emulsion

B. Minus density artifacts caused by rough handling of the film

FIG. 4.29 A Resolution Test Tool. The tool consists of two different scales, but each lists the line pairs per millimeter demonstrated on the film. A line pair consists of one white line and one black line. This tool is placed on the top of a cassette to test the resolution of the film screen system. The exposed film is processed and checked with a small magnifier. The line pairs will visually blend together when the highest resolution is reached. This tool is not used for digital systems. Typically, the highest resolution for film screen imaging is nine line pairs. The highest resolution for film/screen extremity imaging is 15 to 20 line pairs.

FIG. 4.30 Processed film demonstrating a density 1.0 + base + fog. On the film are two major artifacts: **A,** A minus-density artifact from damp fingers handling the film as it is placed in the processor. The salts from sweat will loosen the emulsion, which will float away in the processor and leave fingerprint evidence. **B,** A long, vertical minus-density artifact where the film was roughly dragged out of the film box, destroying the ability of the emulsion to form a lattice network across this trauma line. Film must be handled with care from the time the box is opened until it is processed, dried, and ready for viewing.

FIG. 4.31 A, Overuse of commercial screen cleaners builds up residue on the screen, which eventually causes artifacts on the film as they cause plus-density artifacts across the image. The artifacts are actually areas of the film that were affected by the components of the screen cleaner causing the silver in the emulsion to coagulate. **B,** Intensifying screen emulsion becomes physically worn after many years of films being drawn across its surface and is not able to uniformly convert x-rays to light to expose the film. The lighter areas on the film replicate the wear areas of the screen. The *inset* demonstrates an enlarged part of the indistinct image due to screen wear.

FIG. 4.32 Using the incorrect screen cleaner (e.g., cleaner manufactured by a company other than the screen manufacturer) can cause severe yellowing of the screen. This causes a loss of speed because the light emitted from the screen is an altered color.

FIG. 4.33 Chemical Stains on a Cassette. These may be wiped off if the screen has a cellulose supercoat. Typically, they penetrate the emulsion of the screen and are permanent. **A** and **B** are caused by drips from manual processing that have penetrated the emulsion. **C,** A small drip may look like pathology on an image until the veterinarian notices that every view is demonstrating the same "pathology" on the same place on the film whether or not there is overlying anatomy.

FIG. 4.34 A, The result of DuPont using water-based screen emulsion. The screens worked well in hospitals because the atmosphere in most hospitals is fairly dry. Once the screens were used in private clinics and particularly veterinary hospitals, the water-based emulsion absorbed moisture from the air and swelled to the point where the lattice network was destroyed as soon as the exposure was made and the film stayed in the cassette for any length of time waiting to be processed. This also occurred with films that were preloaded into cassettes waiting to be used. The pin points exerted such pressure that the ability of the film emulsion to form a lattice network was compromised. The screens are not repairable and must be replaced. New screens can be purchased and placed into the cassette. **B,** A close-up of the particularly compromised screen. The swellings are most visible on the UV screens. With Quanta 111 screens, the swellings are not always visible but usually can be felt as tiny pin points. The presence of the swellings is always evident.

FIG. 4.35 The screen emulsion has torn away from its polyester base. This was a particular problem with DuPont UV screens.

FIG. 4.36 A piece of hay in a cassette. This can be a problem with large-animal veterinarians trying to change films in a darkened room in a barn.

REVIEW QUESTIONS

1. There are two completely separate components to an imaging system; they are:
   a. X-ray generator and imaging receptor
   b. The x-ray tube and the generator
   c. The generator and the film
   d. The x-ray tube and the processing unit

2. It is very important that the x-ray generator is the latest model available.
   a. False
   b. True

3. A good technique chart and knowledge of image production is essential because:
   a. The technique chart supplied by the vendor is always correct
   b. The technique chart set up by the previous tech is always the best
   c. Setting correct technical factors is essential to good imaging
   d. Technical factors change over the years and service is not always available

4. The front of the x-ray cassette:
   a. Must absorb scattered radiation
   b. Should have a reflective coating to match the screen
   c. Should have an adhesive layer to hold the film in place
   d. Must be radiolucent and free of artifacts

5. The purpose of an intensifying screen is to:
   a. Enhance the x-ray beam to make it stronger
   b. Convert the x-ray beam to x-ray photons
   c. Convert the primary x-ray beam to light photons
   d. Change the x-ray beam to scattered radiation

6. The intensifying screen is composed of a _____ and a(n) _____.
   a. base, emulsion layer
   b. cardboard base, adhesive layer
   c. polyester base, supercoat
   d. cardboard base, emulsion layer

7. Conversion efficiency is _____ at which the x-ray photons are converted _____.
   a. the rate, to x-rays
   b. the speed, to silver
   c. the speed, to polyphotons
   d. the speed, to light

8. Screen speed is defined by the:
   a. Intrinsic nature of the photons
   b. Conversion efficiency of the phosphor
   c. Atomic mass of the phosphor
   d. Comparison of rare earth elements

9. The density chosen to represent a midline density is:
   a. −1.0
   b. 1.0
   c. 10
   d. 2.0

10. The intensification factor is the _____ necessary to produce an image _____ screens vs. the exposure necessary to produce the image _____ screens.
    a. photon number, with, without
    b. exposure, with, without
    c. speed, without, with
    d. electricity, with, without

11. Imaging relies on a sound knowledge of the colors of the rainbow; the following is true:
    a. It doesn't matter because we can't see color in the dark.
    b. Ultraviolet, on the outside of the curve, cannot be affected by infrared.
    c. Ultraviolet is in the middle of the curve; infrared is on the outside of the curve.
    d. The color of the light that film emulsion reacts to must match the screen color.

12. The green-receiving film will "see" blue light:
    a. But will not "see" the green color, so the film will be light
    b. But needs the green light to produce an optimum image

c. But it will not make use of it when it produces the image

d. But requires the full spectrum to produce an optimum image

13. Knowledge of the system speed is critical to produce the correct amount of radiation:
    a. To determine which cassette will be used to radiograph the animal
    b. To optimize imaging and produce a diagnostic radiograph
    c. To set the technical factors and calculate the weight of the animal
    d. And determine the rate of conversion efficiency of the photons

14. Luminescence is the reaction of the screen to the photons; the reaction is called:
    a. Fluorescence
    b. Phosphorescence
    c. Thermionic
    d. Light speed

15. If the screen continues to emit light after the photon source is removed, the effect is called:
    a. Phosphorescence
    b. Thermionic emission
    c. Fluorescence
    d. Photon lag

16. Intensifying screens age _____ and _____ over time.
    a. at the same rate, maintain their speed
    b. at different rates, increase the rate of reaction
    c. at the same rate, slow down
    d. at different rates, slow down

17. A knowledge of screen color assists in optimizing imaging and ensuring uniformity of images.
    a. True
    b. False

18. Two types of film are _____ emulsion and _____ emulsion film.
    a. double-, extremity
    b. triacetate, polyester
    c. polyester, general radiography
    d. double-, single-

19. Film emulsion is composed of mainly:
    a. Silver iodide crystals and gelatin
    b. Silver halide crystals and sensitivity specks
    c. Carbon halides and silver atoms
    d. Silver carbide and silver halide

20. The combination of the color of the film base and the initial aging of the film:
    a. Is not a part of the image
    b. Does not affect the overall film density
    c. Is called base + fog
    d. Only affects the image before processing

21. If a film is exposed to alternative energy, it will acquire a density before exposure. Which of these statements is true?
    a. This may be caused by heat, light, or chemical fumes.
    b. This density does not affect the overall image.

c. Film fog is a natural part of imaging.

d. Fogging a film is not important in image production.

22. The following factor distinguishes a preexposure fogged film as opposed to overexposed film.
    a. The two factors cannot be separated.
    b. The density decreases if the technique is changed.
    c. Fogged film feels "different" when it exits the processor.
    d. The density does not change if the technique is altered.

23. Blue-receiving film is physically _____; green-receiving film is physically _____.
    a. green, violet
    b. blue, green
    c. violet, green
    d. green, blue

24. The following method is used to determine the color of the screens in order to use the correct film:
    a. The cassette is opened and the stencil is read.
    b. The color is obvious when the cassette is opened.
    c. The cassette is placed open on the table and exposed to radiation.
    d. A blue or green label is attached to the back of the cassette.

25. "White box film" is so called because:
    a. It is sold off in batches; it is no different from regular film
    b. It did not meet the quality control standards of the parent company
    c. The companies that sell it are overstocked
    d. It is mainly blue film that is being phased out and so it needs to be sold

26. New, unused boxes of film should be stored:
    a. Upright in an area unaffected by radiation and heat
    b. Upright wherever there is room in the clinic
    c. Lying flat on the darkroom counter
    d. Lying flat on the darkroom shelf so it is available

27. X-ray film has an expiration date, which should be:
    a. Within 5 years of the date noted on the box
    b. Checked carefully and then noted when the box is empty
    c. Ignored as it is used by the supplier and not the facility
    d. Noted upon delivery by the facility staff

28. The standard film sizes are important to the ordering process because:
    a. The film sizes all match the cassette sizes in the facility
    b. All film sizes may be either in centimeters or inches and fit the cassettes equally
    c. The film sizes are critical to the size of the cassette
    d. 10 in × 12 in film will fit into a 24 cm × 30 cm cassette

Chapter Review Question answers are located in the Instructor Resources on Evolve and can be provided to students at the discretion of the instructor.

CHAPTER 5
Producing the Image

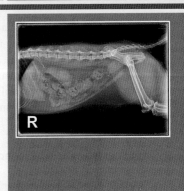

Lois C. Brown, RTR (Can/USA), ACR, MSc, P.Phys

Pleasure in the job puts perfection in the work.
Aristotle — Greek critic, philosopher, physicist, and zoologist — 384–322 BC

OUTLINE

LEARNING OBJECTIVES

When you have finished this chapter, you will be able to:

1. Recognize exposures on film.
2. Define film fog, density, and contrast.
3. Know the difference between subject contrast and radiographic contrast.
4. Understand the importance of correct patient measurement.
5. Know how to establish and develop a technique chart.
6. Record your exposures in a radiography log book.

APPLICATIONS

The application of the information in this chapter is relevant to the following area:

1. Producing optimized images (radiographs) for evaluation and diagnosis

KEY TERMS

Key terms are defined in the Glossary on the Evolve website.

Contrast	Kilovoltage	Quality/quantity	Tabletop
Density	Log book	Radiographic contrast	Technique chart
Direct Radiation	Measurement	Remnant radiation	Time
Expiration date	Milliamperage	Scattered radiation	Tissue fluence
Fog	Optimized image	Secondary radiation	
Grid tray	Positioning	Source image distance (SID)	
Inverse square law	Primary beam	Subject contrast	

The main objective of all imaging systems is to demonstrate the differences in tissue density. Air, water, fat, tendons, muscle, and bone all have different tissue densities, and it is this differentiation, this contrast, that must be optimized. In addition, optimal imaging is achieved with correct measuring, correct positioning, and correct technique.

This chapter will deal only with producing images for film/screen combinations. Digital imaging and computed radiography are to be found in Chapter 8.

The Radiography Unit

Every complete x-ray unit is composed of three individual components: an x-ray tube, a generator, and a high-tension transformer. In a small-animal facility, the other necessary component is the radiography table.

Some radiography units have add-ons for convenience, such as a cassette holder or a recessed control at the table side, but these are not necessary. The only two components that must be matched every time are the generator and the high-tension transformer.

Quite frequently, a tabletop becomes scratched, broken, or marred in some way (Fig. 5.1). Most tabletops can be removed and replaced with a new medical-grade, radiolucent tabletop. The new tabletop should be attached to the frame of the table with hook-and-loop tape to facilitate removal for cleaning or if a kitten escapes and goes exploring beneath the x-ray table.

The factors to consider when selecting an x-ray table are stability, height, ability to install a grid tray and, most important, radiolucency. The x-ray photons must be transmitted through the tabletop without superimposing an image of the grain of the tabletop onto the radiograph. Test for table lucency by placing a cassette beneath the tabletop, without the grid. Use 50 kV and 4 mAs to produce a 1.0 density image (Fig. 5.2A,B).

The cassettes exposed during an examination should be removed from the radiography room and placed well out of possible exposure by scattered radiation.

The Technique Chart

There are several ways to set up a technique chart. Every imaging department is slightly different, and all of the factors discussed in previous chapters must be taken into consideration. A technique chart that works in one clinic does not necessarily produce optimized images in a neighboring facility.

Most equipment suppliers will supply a technique chart with a new radiographic unit. Some of these charts have been set up by salespeople who have no concept of all the factors that are components of the image. Therefore, some charts are suitable and some are not. Typically, if the images are good for a 10-cm abdomen measured and positioned correctly, then the chart may be extrapolated to produce optimized images for any size animal for that particular unit and the accompanying film/screen combination.

The production of an optimized radiograph is an art and a science. The x-ray generator is the same basic unit now as it was 60 years ago. On a correctly calibrated radiography unit, 70 kilovolts is still 70 kV, and 200 milliamperes is 200 mA; all the rest is cosmetics. If the generator has the variables necessary to produce good radiography, there is no need to replace it because a newer imaging system is introduced or because it is old and not as attractive as the newer models. As long as the unit is correctly calibrated and the parts and service are available to keep it that way, there is no need to upgrade to a different unit.

A technique chart is a guide. It should be developed to work with a specific system (film and intensifying screens) in a specific radiography room. The technique charts in this chapter are suggestions only. Slight variations in power supplies, film/screen combinations, or x-ray unit setup may necessitate some adjustment but, if all the rules are followed, these charts will provide good basic imaging.

These technique charts are in use in many hospitals and clinics and have proven to produce excellent images when the radiography units are calibrated correctly and the rules for positioning and measuring are followed exactly. If the technique chart is correctly set up and the patient is measured correctly, the image should never be too light or too dark. The flow chart in Fig. 5.3 can be used to evaluate and correct any technical difficulties. A technique chart can be developed to work with any x-ray unit from a large-animal portable unit to a highly sophisticated medical model.

This chapter explores the development of these technique charts. Two charts are presented in which we have followed the rules of chart development, and these charts are arranged so the technician can choose the type of chart that matches the model of the generator in use. The third chart is a large-animal portable chart and is an example used by the owners of the Poskom veterinary unit. All large-animal units are supplied with a technique chart to be used with that specific x-ray unit. If the unit is to be used as a small-animal unit, the company usually supplies a technique chart for small-animal radiography.

Technical Factors

To produce a radiographic image, the contrast that separates the tissue densities must be optimized. The four factors of

FIG. 5.1 A Badly Damaged Tabletop. This crack will show up on any image that is exposed with the cassette in the grid tray.

FIG. 5.2 A, An example of a density 1.0 + base + fog image. It is similar to the density at the caudal aspect of the ilium. On the phantom film, if this density is matched, then the rest of the technique chart can be filled in according to the rules. **B,** An example of a pelvis image produced using the technique developed by using the water phantom. Note that the density at the caudal ilium is density 1.0 + base + fog.

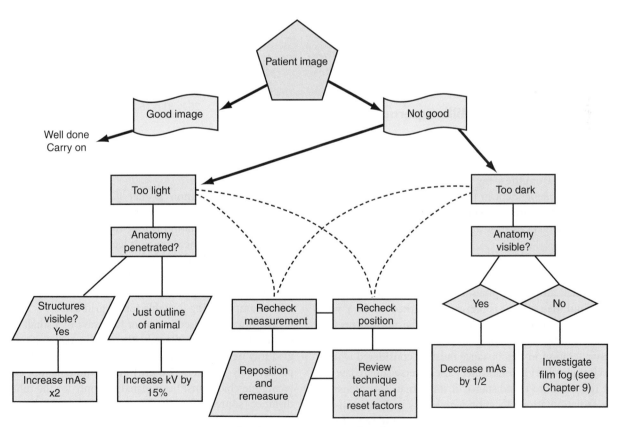

FIG. 5.3 Flowchart Demonstrating Technical Diagnostics.

TABLE 5.1	Subject and Radiographic Contrast Components	
SUBJECT CONTRAST (ALL FACTORS CONCERNING A PATIENT)	**RADIOGRAPHIC CONTRAST (ALL FACTORS CONCERNING THE EQUIPMENT)**	
Patient thickness	Kilovoltage	
Body part being examined	Milliampere-seconds	
	Distance	
Bone-to-muscle-to-fat-to-fluid ratio	Film/screen combinations	
	Processing parameters	
Use of contrast media (barium, etc.)	Grid, filters	
	Collimation	
	Anode heel effect	

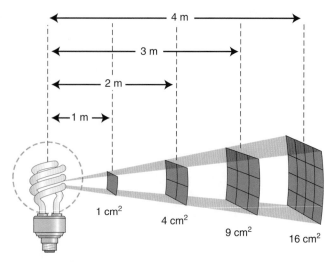

FIG. 5.4 The Inverse Square Law. The intensity of radiation at a location is inversely proportional to the square of the distance. For example, doubling the distance from 2 meters to 4 meters increases the area covered by a factor of four. At 2 meters, it is 4 squares; at 4 meters, it is 16 squares. (From Johnston J, Fauber T. *Essentials of Radiographic Physics and Imaging,* 2nd ed. St Louis: Mosby; 2016.)

exposure—kilovoltage (kV), milliamperage (mA), time (seconds), and distance (inches or centimeters)—must be manipulated in such a way that the tissue absorption of radiation is exactly correct to demonstrate anatomy and pathology and to minimize any external artifact that may obscure the desired result.

Radiographic Contrast vs. Subject Contrast

There are two main areas in which contrast may be manipulated (Table 5.1):
- The patient's thickness and shape (subject contrast)
- The mechanical variables available to enhance contrast (radiographic contrast)

Please note that the factors that manipulate radiographic contrast in a digital system are quite different than with imaging on film. See Chapter 8 for more on digital and computerized images.

Distance, Kilovoltage, Milliamperage, and Time

Three factors that are set on the x-ray unit are kilovoltage, milliamperage, and time. A fourth factor, distance, is based on the distance from the x-ray tube to the receptor. All these factors are interdependent in terms of film/screen imaging. A change in one factor dramatically affects the other three. In common practice, mA and time are combined and called *mAs.*

Distance and the Inverse Square Law

In most small-animal hospitals, the distance between the x-ray tube and the receptor is preset and marked on the x-ray tube column. Forty inches (100 cm) is the normal preset distance from the x-ray tube to the table.

Any alteration in this distance must be considered when the technique chart is established. The inverse square law is a rule that refers to this distance. It states that "the intensity of the radiation at one location is inversely proportional to the square of its distance from the source of the radiation" (Fig. 5.4). Basically, the inverse square law states:

$$\frac{\text{Original mAs}}{\text{New mAs}} = \left[\frac{\text{New source image distance (SID)}}{\text{Original source image distance (SID)}} \right]^2$$

For example: If the technique chart calls for 20 mAs at 40 inches and the x-ray tube height needs to be changed to 36 inches:

$$\frac{20 \text{ mAs}}{X} \times \left[\frac{(36 \text{ inches})}{(40 \text{ inches})} \right]^2$$

$$\frac{20 \text{ mAs}}{X} \times \frac{1296}{1600}$$

$$20 \times .81 = 16.2 \text{ or } 16 \text{ mAs}$$

The mAs would be reduced to 16 mAs, and the density on the image would be the same as one exposed at 40 inches.

Another application is that if the original distance is 40 inches (100 cm) and we halve it to 20 inches (50 cm), the intensity of the radiation is four times higher. This can be a very useful tool if the x-ray unit has low power and the body part that we need to examine is thick.

Keep in mind that the grid factor, which is discussed in Chapter 6, may negate having to use the inverse square law when compensating for table top or grid use.

The film is exposed in one of two ways in a small-animal clinic. The cassette is placed either on the tabletop or into a grid tray beneath the tabletop. The grid tray usually sits approximately 3 inches (7.6 cm) below the tabletop, and the technique chart must be adjusted not only for the tube–tray distance (source image distance, or SID) but also because of the grid (see Chapter 6). The operator is often encouraged to change the height of the x-ray tube, lowering it when the cassette is placed in the grid tray and raising it when the film is on the tabletop. This change of x-ray tube height is not necessary if the technique chart is adjusted slightly to

TABLE 5.2	Grid Factor Formula
GRID RATIO	**MULTIPLY mAs BY**
5:1	2
8:1	3
10:1	3.5

compensate for the extra 3-inch (7.6-cm) distance, because it must already be adjusted to account for the grid. The grid factor formula is detailed in Table 5.2 and discussed further in Chapter 6.

> ### ✦ APPLICATION INFORMATION
>
> Quite frequently, the small amount that the tube is raised and lowered is confused in the facility, and often the tube is mistakenly lowered for the tabletop exposures and raised for the grid tray exposures. It is far preferable to compensate for the extra SID by adjusting the technique chart for both the grid and the distance, leaving the x-ray tube stationary.

Kilovoltage, Milliamperage, and Time

Kilovoltage, milliamperage, and time are often referred to as the *factors controlling the quality of the radiation* (kV) and the *quantity of the radiation* (mAs).

In the case of kV, quality refers to an increase in the penetrating power. When the kV is increased, the beam is said to be "hardened." This means that fewer low-energy x-rays are produced and more high-energy x-rays are produced. This leaves the x-ray beam with more capability to penetrate denser tissue.

Kilovoltage mainly affects contrast in the image. It also affects density because setting the kilovoltage too high will blacken the film and so eliminate any contrast.

An ***increase in mAs, directly affects the density of the image*** because a greater quantity of photons are produced, which in turn yields an increased number of x-rays. The increase in the number of x-rays is directly proportional to the amount of the increase in mAs. For example, if we increase the mAs from 20 to 40, we are producing twice the number of x-ray photons and therefore doubling the density on the radiograph. The mAs value primarily affects density; however, this value will also eliminate contrast if set far too high or far too low, and then the overall image will be black or clear.

Billiards Analogy

The best analogy for understanding the interaction of the technical factors is represented in the game of billiards (pool). A certain number of balls are racked or positioned on a felt-covered table. A cue ball is aimed at the prepositioned balls, and the cue stick is used to hit the cue ball and scatter the racked balls to put them into play (Fig. 5.5). *The milliamperage (mA) represents the number of balls on the table.* If there are a lot of balls on the table, there will be a high number of interactions and a greater potential to have a high-density or dark film image. If there are very few balls on the table, a light film will result. ***The mAs value is responsible for density.*** It is directly proportional—doubling the mAs doubles the density on the film. There is no higher math to calculate when determining how to optimize an image using mAs.

The *kilovoltage (kV)* is the power behind the cue stick. It is how hard the balls are hit and how much energy is transferred to the balls. If the balls are hit very hard (high kV), more of the balls travel straight through and reach the end of the table. The high-energy scattered balls bounce off the sides and ends of the table, and as they do, they transfer a little energy to the table side and move off to interact with other balls or the other side of the table until they come to rest. Each interaction, whether it be with table edges or with other balls, subtracts energy from the initial moving ball until all the balls finally come to rest.

The cue ball and some of the other balls travel straight through the mass of balls to the other end of the table. This represents *primary radiation*. In the world of radiation, the primary beam is the useful beam with varying energies but enough to penetrate the patient and reach the detector (either film or detector plate). The radiation that reaches the

FIG. 5.5 The game of pool can be used as an analogy of the technical factors of radiation exposure. The kilovoltage (kV) is the power behind the cue stick; milliamperage (mA) is the number of balls on the table.

TABLE 5.3	Relationship Between Kilovoltage and Contrast
HIGH kV PRODUCES	**LOW kV PRODUCES**
Long scale (more grays)	Short scale (fewer grays)
Low contrast	High contrast
Less contrast (fewer "clear" areas)	More contrast (more "clear" areas on the film)

TABLE 5.4	Technical Factors Affecting Contrast
INCREASING THIS FACTOR	**RESULTS OF INCREASE**
Kilovoltage	Decrease in contrast (more grays)
mAs (milliampere-seconds)	Decrease in contrast (at very high mAs, image is black)
Collimation (narrowing the x-ray beam)	Increase in contrast (reduction in secondary radiation)

film or detector is called *remnant radiation.* The scattered balls move according to how much energy is transferred down the cue stick to the balls and at what angle that energy is transferred. As these balls move, they will bounce against the sides of the table and lose some of their energy. Energy is transferred when the photons bounce off one another or bounce off the atoms within the patient. This deflected energy becomes *scattered radiation,* or *secondary radiation,* and is either visualized on the image as nonuseful radiation or not visualized because it is absorbed by another interaction within the animal. Scattered radiation is not nearly as strong

as the primary radiation but because it emits the energy at an angle to the primary, it can fog the film and irradiate the animal handler. This is the reason why we wear protective aprons, thyroid collars, and gloves, and why we employ the nonmanual restraints outlined in Part Two of this text.

Nonuseful radiation contributes to either the radiation dose to the patient or technician or appears as film fog. When the technique chart is developed, the kilovoltage must be set as low as possible in order to have enough energy to penetrate the body part but keep the scattered/secondary radiation to a minimum. The kilovoltage is responsible for the penetrating power of the x-ray beam. In our analogy, it is the power behind the cue stick.

The energy (the kV) of the x-ray beam affects contrast, as illustrated in Fig. 5.6A and Tables 5.5 and 5.6. With a low kilovoltage, the x-ray beam has longer wavelength primary radiation and penetrates fewer structures, producing a shorter scale of contrast (black and white), which is demonstrated as a larger density difference between steps. It does not take long to read the image from black to white. Fig. 5.6B has long-scale contrast (black, gray, gray, white), is produced by increasing the kV, and represents a greater number of steps between black and white but less of a density difference between each step.

When the veterinarian states that he or she would like to see more contrast, this needs to be clarified.
- More contrast = higher contrast = fewer shades of gray = fewer steps from black to clear
- Less contrast = lower contrast = more shades of gray = more steps from black to clear

FIG. 5.6 An aluminum wedge with a series of graduated steps is used in this model. How contrast affects the image: **A,** Low kilovoltage = short-scale contrast. **B,** High kilovoltage = long-scale contrast; with very high kilovoltage, the entire wedge is penetrated and there is no contrast.

TABLE 5.5	Optimum Kilovoltage per Average-Sized Body Part for Film and Digital Imaging	
BODY PART	**OPTIMUM kV FOR FILM/SCREEN IMAGING**	**NOTES**
Extremities	40–55	Techniques in this range work for pocket pets.
Cervical spine/skull	60–75	
Thorax/abdomen/pelvis	64–90	For larger animals, the kV may be increased to a maximum of 95.

TABLE 5.6	Standard Factors for Average Patients Using a 400-Speed Film/Screen System (Cat at Low End of Scale, Dog at Upper End of Scale)		
BODY PART	**OPTIMUM kV RANGE**	**OPTIMUM mAs**	**NOTES**
Extremities	40–55	3–8	These are techniques for an **average** patient.
Cervical spine and skull	50–60	4–10	
Thorax	60–90	12–25	
Abdomen/pelvis	60–90	12–25	

Do keep in mind that if the energy is set so high that it penetrates every tissue evenly, there will be no contrast and the image will be black. Similarly, if it is set so low that nothing is penetrated, there will be no contrast on the image, as there will be no image. Thus, in that way the extremes of kV also affect density.

◆ **APPLICATION INFORMATION**

Contrast is the key word on any radiographic image. If the veterinarian requests more contrast, it is always wise to clarify whether he or she wants to see more shades of gray (long scale) or a shorter-scale, high-contrast, black-and-white image. Sometimes that is not clear.

A veterinary radiologist called the consultant in to discuss the x-ray images and said he wanted more contrast. The consultant changed the chart and then also changed the film/screen combination to give him more short-scale contrast (black-and-white images). The veterinary radiologist called the consultant back and explained that what he wanted was more contrast—more shades of gray! She had done everything to produce fewer shades of gray. The problem was quickly resolved by increasing the kV and reducing the mAs. It is always best to clarify what is being requested.

Optimizing Kilovoltage

The normal range of use of kilovoltages on a general radiography unit is usually between 40 and 90 kV. When the technique chart is developed for the facility, it must be fine-tuned to consider all the variables inherent in the production of the final image (Fig. 5.7). The main objective in optimizing the technique chart is to use the lowest kV value that will penetrate the region of interest within the body and enhance the tissue contrast surrounding it. Each body part or component can be penetrated by an optimum kilovoltage. Table 5.5 is provided as a starting point to develop a technique chart for an average-sized animal.

For larger animals or for pocket pets and smaller animals, the kilovoltage is adjusted on the final chart. Because kilovoltage is the energy with which the x-ray beam passes

FIG. 5.7 Optimized Kilovoltage Versus High Kilovoltage. **A,** Optimized kilovoltage. The bony structures are visible and trabecular patterns are well visualized. **B,** High kilovoltage. The bony structures are overpenetrated and now blend in with the muscle tissue. Trabecular patterns are no longer visualized.

through the body, a change in kilovoltage is not in direct proportion with the increase or decrease in tissue. This difference is due to a variation in tissue absorption (tissue fluence).

The optimum kV is the kilovoltage that penetrates the anatomy so that it is identifiable on the radiographic image. For an abdomen, for example, there is proper contrast and density if the anatomy is visible on the film after it is processed, the spine is evident, and the intervertebral spaces are clearly defined. If the whole image is slightly dark or light, the mAs must be altered to optimize the image. However, if the image is far too light or so dark that the anatomy is obscured, the 15% rule for kV may also be used.

The 15% Rule for Changing Kilovoltage

The 15% rule is used to optimize kilovoltage only when a body part has not been imaged satisfactorily. Do not use kV to increase or decrease overall *density* on an image. Density should be increased or decreased only by using mAs.

To increase penetration: multiply the original kV by 1.15 (kV + 15%).
For example, 80 × 1.15 = 92 kV
To decrease penetration: multiply the original kV by 0.85 (kV – 15%)
For example, 80 × 0.85 = 68 kV

Applying this rule will increase or decrease the penetration of the region of interest. This rule will be effective for a kilovoltage between 40 kV and 90 kV, which is the normal range of use in radiography. If the technique chart is optimized and the patient is positioned and measured correctly, the technician will never need to use this formula.

> **? POINTS TO PONDER**   The technique chart is a tool that provides suggested techniques based on anatomy and positioning. The factors presented are completely dependent on the accuracy of the technical staff. The radiography system does not discriminate between species, a prime rib roast, a bucket of water, or your Rottweiler's abdomen. It produces an image based only on accurate and precise measurements and the accompanying correct technical factors matched with the correct image receptor.

Developing Technique Charts

The three factors that may be adjusted on the generator are kV, mA, and time. The limits outlined in Table 5.6 are the standard for an average patient. Figs. 5.7 and 5.8 show the result of stepping dramatically outside those limits.

The images in Fig. 5.7 represent changes in kV while adjusting the mA to maintain density 1.0 + base + fog in the ilium of the pelvis. These images demonstrate that an increase in kilovoltage causes a substantial change in contrast as the x-ray beam becomes "harder" or more penetrating.

The images in Fig. 5.8 represent changes in mAs as the kV is adjusted to maintain density 1.0 + base + fog in the ileum of the pelvis. These images show that a decrease in mAs causes a substantial change in density but does not affect the contrast.

Use of a Phantom

Developing a technique chart for a film/screen system requires a certain amount of experimentation. A phantom

FIG. 5.8 Optimized mA Versus Low mA. **A,** The density provides a black background with the bony structures well visualized. **B,** The inadequate mAs value provides a flat image with loss of visualization in the bony structures. Note that the contrast is maintained.

FIG. 5.9 A Standard Flat-Bottomed Container. Note the standard measurements on the side. These duplicate extremity, skull, and abdomen equivalents, and the water level can be altered easily.

(a facsimile of a patient) is used instead of using a live patient in human medicine throughout the world; the phantom is always the same size and density with no variations. Using an animal as a phantom introduces problems with identical positioning and cooperation on the part of the animal. If the animal is stretched out on one view and not positioned identically for the second view, an unnecessary variable is introduced. In addition, the dose to the animal must be considered if multiple exposures are to be made. The use of a uniform density phantom eliminates the variables introduced by using an animal.

A uniform density phantom consists of water in a container that mimics the thickness of a patient. The body of a mammal is composed of 98% liquid, so a water bucket works well as a standardized patient phantom (Fig. 5.9). The uniform-density phantom creates a density 1.0 + base + fog image from which the rest of the technique chart can be extrapolated. There will be no contrast demonstrated unless soup bones are placed in the container, but they are not necessary in setting up the technique chart. Make sure the bucket is plastic; a metal bucket will act as a filter and reduce the amount of radiation reaching the film.

Procedure

1. Start with tabletop techniques. Check to establish the speed of your system (films/screens, processing temperature). The techniques listed on the charts are for a 400-speed film/screen combination using a correctly calibrated generator and processing on a recently serviced processor.
2. Refer to the technique charts (Fig. 5.10A,B) to determine which chart should be used with your x-ray unit.
3. Fill the plastic bucket with 5 cm of water.
4. Place a cassette on the tabletop and place the bucket on the cassette.
5. Collimate to the limits of the edges of the bucket; place a marker on cassette #1.
6. Choose the chart that matches your x-ray unit.
7. Set the technical factors found in the charts.
8. Make adjustments if needed, using Fig. 5.3.
9. Expose the film and process, ensuring that the processor is clean and well serviced.
10. A density of 1.0 + base + fog is the ideal density (Fig. 5.2). This density is exactly in the midrange of densities as discussed in Chapter 9 (quality control).
11. Go back to the chart and change the water level to correspond with greater or lesser thicknesses of a patient. (Once you have reached a measurement of 10 cm or greater, place the cassette in the grid tray; for any measurement below 10 cm, the cassette will be on the tabletop with the bucket placed on top of the cassette.)
12. This should now work well for any level of water in the bucket, assuming that a change in technique is accompanied by an appropriate change in water level according to the chart.
13. If the images turn out very light using these techniques, you may have a 200-speed system or the temperature in your processor may be incorrect.
14. Start over and recheck the speed of the system, the calibration of the unit, and the processing parameters. Only then should you increase the mAs.
15. To confirm the settings, position and correctly measure a patient on the table. Set the technical factors from your modified chart and process the film. The density of the soft tissue immediately cranial to the iliac crest should be density 1.0 + base + fog. The image should demonstrate good density and contrast.

Sante's Rule

Sante's rule is an alternative method of developing a variable kV technique chart. This chart is useful if the mA and time factors are limited on the radiography unit (Table 5.7). It will only be useful with a single-phase unit. It is not accurate for a three-phase, high-frequency unit. It is also not accurate for a digital system (see Chapter 8). This rule estimates kilovoltage in relation to patient thickness. Because it is based on a variable kilovoltage chart, it does not accommodate gradual changes in mAs (or density) as the patient becomes thicker and the tissue becomes less differentiated. The substantial increase in kV will produce scattered/secondary radiation, which will seriously compromise the image if the kV is allowed to exceed 80 kV. A change in mAs is also needed to minimize the kV increase above 80 kV. mAs totals used are tested for each body part and then preset (Table 5.8).

To use Sante's rule, place the patient in the correct position and measure the body part (in centimeters) where the central x-ray will penetrate. Double the measurement and add to the distance (in inches) of the x-ray tube to the tabletop (usually 40 inches).

A — Single Phase x-ray unit

		Table Top –						GRID ▶	8:1 Grid Cassette in Grid Tray														
Chest	CM.	4	5	6	7	8	9		10 11	12 13	14 15	16 17	18 19	20 21	22 23	24 25	26 27	28 29	30 31	32		
Thoracic Sp	mAs	2		3		4			12	14	16	18	20	22	24	26	28	30	32	34		
Shoulder	kV	48		50		52			60	62	64	66	68	70	72	74	76	78	80	8		

		Table Top – 100 mA						GRID ▶	8:1 grid Cassette in Grid Tray														
Abdomen	CM.	6	7	8	9	10	11		10 11	12 13	14 15	16 17	18 19	20 21	22 23	24 25	26 27	28 29	30 31	32		
Lumbar Sp	mAs	2		3		4			12	14	16	18	20	22	24	26	28	30	32	34		
Pelvis	kV	48		50		52			60	62	64	66	68	70	72	74	76	78	80	82		

		Table Top						GRID ▶	8:1 Grid Cassette in Grid Tray			
Skull	CM.	4	5	6	7	8	9		10 11	12 13		
Cerv Sp	mAs	2		4		6			12	14		
	kV	50		52		54			56	58		

		Table Top –						NO Grid ▶	NO GRID All limbs are radiographed table top		
Limbs	CM.	1	2	3	4	5	6		7 8 9		
Stifles	mAs	2		4		6			8 10		
	kV	46	48		50	52			52 54		

Read page from left to right – Measurement of the animal correctly is essential
Log all measurements and exposure factors so that any problems may be identified

B — Three-phase, high-frequency unit

		Table Top –						GRID ▶	8:1 Grid Cassette in Grid Tray														
Chest	CM.	4	5	6	7	8	9		10 11	12 13	14 15	16 17	18 19	20 21	22 23	24 25	26 27	28 29	30 31	32		
Thoracic Sp	mAs	1		2		3			6	8	10	12	14	16	18	20	22	24	26	28		
Shoulder	kV	44		46		48			54	56	58	60	62	64	66	68	70	72	74	7		

		Table Top –						GRID ▶	8:1 grid Cassette in Grid Tray														
Abdomen	CM.	4	5	6	7	8	9		10 11	12 13	14 15	16 17	18 19	20 21	22 23	24 25	26 27	28 29	30 31	32		
Lumbar Sp	mAs	1		2		3			6	8	10	12	14	16	18	20	22	24	26	28		
Pelvis	kV	44		46		48			54	56	58	60	62	64	66	68	70	72	74	76		

		Table Top						GRID ▶	8:1 Grid Cassette in Grid Tray			
Skull	CM.	4	5	6	7	8	9		10 11	12 13		
Cerv Sp	mAs	1		2		3			6	8		
	kV	46		48		50			52	56		

		Table Top –						NO Grid ▶	NO GRID All limbs are radiographed table top		
Limbs	CM.	1	2	3	4	5	6		7 8 9 10		
Stifles	mAs	0.50		1		2			3 4		
	kV	44	46		48	50			50 52 54		

Read page from left to right – Measurement of the animal correctly is essential
Log all measurements and exposure factors so that any problems may be identified

FIG. 5.10 A, The single-phase chart. The completed radiography chart for a small-animal clinic using a single-phase unit, 400-speed system, and correct processing. B, Three-phase, high-frequency chart to be used with correct processing, correct measurement, and a 400-speed film/screen system on a correctly calibrated unit.

TABLE 5.7	Sante's Rule for Grid Use	
GRID RATIO	**ADDED kV**	**OR ADDED mAs**
5 : 1	6–8	×1
8 : 1	8–10	×2
12 : 1	10–15	×3

TABLE 5.8	Sante's Rule for Variable mAs
BODY PART	**SUGGESTED BEGINNING mAs**
Extremity	5
Thorax (no grid)	7.5
Abdomen (grid)	10
Pelvis/spine	12.5

TABLE 5.9	Effect of Grid Ratio on mAs	
GRID RATIO	**LINES/MM**	**AVERAGE GRID FACTOR**
8 : 1	103	mAs × 1.5
10 : 1	103	mAs × 2.0
12 : 1	143	mAs × 3.0

Note: This table gives the information for the most common grid ratios.

Therefore, if a body part measures 4 cm:

$$4 \text{ cm} \times 2 = 8 + 40 \text{ inches} = 48 \text{ kV}$$

If a body part measures 16 cm:

$$16 \text{ cm} \times 2 = 32 + 40 \text{ inches} = 72 \text{ kV}$$

In addition, a body part of 16 cm requires a grid. The increase in factors due to grid use can be accounted for by either adding the grid factor, which for an 8 : 1 grid ratio will increase the kV by 10 to 82 kV, *or* by doubling the mAs (×2) (Table 5.9).

Tabletop vs. Grid Tray in Film/Screen Imaging

Any body part that measures less than 10 cm will be radiographed on the tabletop. Any body part that measures 10 cm or greater will be imaged with the cassette either beneath the tabletop in the grid tray (with a grid installed beneath the tabletop) or using a grid taped to the cassette.

Grids were developed to absorb scattered and secondary radiation. They also absorb a certain amount of primary radiation which is why when a grid is used, the technical factors must be increased as outlined in Table 5.9. Grids above 12:1 should not be used. Grids are positioned normally under the tabletop between the patient and the film. Digital imaging often does not use a grid, so the following paragraphs assume a film/screen system. Chapter 6 describes the manufacture of the grid and the different uses for various grids.

Producing a Working Technique Chart

The objective of any radiograph produced by any imaging system is to optimize the differences in tissue density of the anatomy being examined. A basic knowledge of veterinary anatomy is essential to setting up a technique chart. The anatomy of the animal chest is quite different from that of a human. The human heart is much narrower and takes up far less space in the chest cavity. This is mainly because of our upright stance and greater overall heart-to-lung ratio, which produces maximum contrast on a radiograph. The typical human chest is always imaged upright with the x-ray tube at 6 feet (180 cm) or more from the grid tray. Because of these differences, human technique charts do not transfer well to veterinary charts, which normally use a consistent distance of 40 inches (100 cm) with a prone (DV [dorsoventral]) or supine (VD [ventrodorsal]) animal.

The tissue density of the animal chest is very similar to the animal's abdominal density; the heart occupies a large proportion of the chest, and there is a fairly even mix of muscle tissue, air cavities, and bone. Therefore, the techniques for thorax and abdomen can be virtually the same.

The Three "Rules"

Three rules must be followed before attempting to develop a technique chart for any medical, veterinary, or research facility.

Rule #1

The x-ray unit must be calibrated by a qualified x-ray service engineer. Quality control tests must be carried out on every station that will be "within normal range of use" to ensure that what is being set exactly conforms to the output of the x-ray unit. There is no point in setting up a chart only to find that a setting of 70 kV is 76 kV on one mA station and 68 kV on a second mA station.

It is essential that every x-ray unit should be calibrated a minimum of once every 2 years. As the unit ages, it should be recalibrated annually.

◆ APPLICATION INFORMATION

When the mA stations are tested, they must be linear. Because the output of the mA station is directly proportional to the increase or decrease, 200 mA must produce double the radiation of 100 mA. In addition, each kV station must be matched so that the output of 70 kV at 100 mA is double the output of 70 kV at 50 mA, and so on.

This can be determined on the engineer's test tools and should be checked by the veterinary technician before the service person leaves the facility. If the service engineer does not calibrate the unit correctly or does not match the unit to the incoming electricity, it will be impossible to set up and follow a technique chart.

Rule #2

The technique chart is set up to reflect the thickness of the body part that is being radiographed. The animal must be placed in the correct position on the x-ray table before being measured. Fig. 5.11 demonstrates a possible difference in

FIG. 5.11 Microchip, the cat, being incorrectly measured (16 cm) **(A)** and then correctly measured (8 cm) **(B)**. The staff will immobilize Microchip and step away from the table for the exposure.

measurement of 8 cm between when Microchip (the patient) was not measured correctly and when he was in the correct position and measured accurately. This represents a huge difference in technical factors.

> **? POINTS TO PONDER** Measuring correctly cannot be stressed enough. The x-ray unit is not intuitive. It will produce the radiation that is requested for the measurement that is set.
>
> The consultant was asked to help out with constructing a technique chart. Every staff member in the hospital obtained different densities using the same chart. The difference in measurement at one clinic for one dog (a medium-sized hound) measured separately by seven people was 17 cm! Every person obtained a different measurement, depending on how the dog accepted the person with the calipers. Because the staff measured the dog standing either on the tabletop or on the floor, it could either shrink away from the technician or stand quietly. Once the dog was in VD position with legs extended, the measurement was entirely different again. Training the staff to measure uniformly with the animal in position resulted in consistently optimized radiography. The technique chart was quite correct, but the patient measurement method was at fault.

Rule #3

The measurement must be made at the area of particular interest. The central x-ray must enter the body part that was measured. If the area of interest on a greyhound or a whippet is the bladder (8 cm) and the dog is measured at the level of the kidneys (17 cm), the image will be far too dark in the area of interest.

If the area of interest is a dog with a very high thorax-to-abdomen measurement ratio, then the widest part and the narrowest part should be measured and the technique set at

the midrange (e.g., 20 cm for a thorax measurement and 10 cm for a pelvis measurement, with the technique set for 15 cm). The central ray would then enter the midrange of the abdomen (see Chapter 16). The anode heel effect can be used in this instance (see Chapter 2).

> **? POINTS TO PONDER** The x-ray generator will deliver only the amount of radiation requested by the operator, and it will not take operator error into account when the exposure is made. Measuring patients correctly is fundamental to the use of a technique chart. The amount of tissue to be penetrated is finite. It is not a guessing game and has no relation whatsoever to the weight or species of the animal.

Manipulating Technical Factors: The 15% Rule

Earlier in this chapter, we discussed the codependency of kV, mA, time, and distance. The following example helps illustrate how to manipulate a factor for a particular result.

You have produced a good image, but the veterinarian now requests that you increase the contrast to image an obscure bladder stone. All other factors taken into consideration, the optimum kV for the abdomen was 70 kV at 22 mAs.

If we like the original density of a film and we want to manipulate the kV to change the contrast, we need to also change the mAs in the opposite direction to maintain the density. 70 kV will penetrate the bladder, but what do you do with the mAs, because the density on the first film was fine?

When decreasing kV, multiply by 15% ($70 \times 15\% = 10.5$). Subtract that from your original kV (59 kV) with the .5 kV rounded off.

To maintain the same density, multiply the original mAs by 2 (44 mAs in this example)

When increasing kV, multiply by 15% ($70 \times 15 = 10.5$). Add that to your original kV (80 kV) with the .5 kV rounded off.

To maintain the same density, divide the original mAs by 2 = (11 mAs in the example).

It is important to understand that the 15% rule applies only to kV values of 40 kV to 90 kV, which is the usual range of kVs in veterinary medicine. Outside these parameters, the characteristics of the x-ray beam are completely different, and different rules apply.

Technical Rules

- **Rule 1.** When the machine is being calibrated, it is essential that the kVs *must* be verified on each mA station individually. 70 kV must be 70 kV (± 1 or 2 kV either way is not a problem; ± 5 to 10 kV is a problem).
  - The output of 100 mA *must* be 50% of the output of 200 mA. The output of 300 mA *must* be three times that of 100 mA.
- **Rule 2.** Review the three "rules" of calibration, positioning, and measuring. A technique chart cannot be optimized unless these rules are followed.
- **Rule 3.** If the technique chart is usually accurate, reposition and remeasure if the image is not diagnostic.
- **Rule 4.** When you have a radiograph of the correct region of interest that is unsatisfactory, always adjust the mAs first, but not before you have reviewed Rule #3. A change in density on the image is directly proportional to a change in mAs. 20 mAs is half as dense (lighter) as 40 mAs and two times as dense (darker) as 10 mAs. Changes in kV are semilogarithmic, and therefore the end result is not easy to predict or calculate.
- **Rule 5.** If the film is very light and it is usually satisfactory, check the temperature of the chemicals, either in the tank or in the developer of the processor (see Chapter 7).
- **Rule 6.** If the image is dull gray and does not improve with a change in technique, assume that the film has been fogged and look for light leaks in the darkroom or an opened or broken cassette (see Chapters 4 and 7).

Anatomical Considerations

Skull and Cervical Spine

Both the skull and cervical spine represent bone and tissue with high-contrast tissue densities. They do not require high kilovoltage or mAs.

Thorax, Abdomen, Lumbar Spine, and Pelvis

The thorax, abdomen, lumbar spine, and pelvis are similar in the differences in tissue density and are a mix of air, fat, tissue, muscle, and bone. These body parts will be difficult to image if very high kilovoltage is used because the potential for photons producing secondary/scattered radiation increases as the thickness of the animal increases. It is important to keep the kilovoltage as low as possible to image the area and to increase the mAs proportionally as the tissue thickness increases.

Extremities

The tissue-to-bone ratio in extremities is high, and because the body parts are thin, a low kilovoltage is indicated. This will emphasize the contrast between the bone and the small amount of soft tissue.

Pocket pets and birds should be radiographed with technical factors similar to the extremities of cats and dogs unless a special film/screen combination is used. In addition, mAs will be proportionally low.

> **? POINTS TO PONDER** The hospital has just installed a new x-ray unit. A supplied technique chart produced poor images, particularly on large dogs. The technique chart is a variable kV chart with very little change in the mAs. The kVs increase by 2 kV for every centimeter measured. The kV for 10 cm is 60. The kV for 20 cm is 82 and 30 mAs when a grid is used.
>
> Dramatic increases of kV without adjusting the mAs as the animal becomes larger produce less contrast and more scattered radiation—the tissues in a larger patient become more uniform. To summarize:
>
> Large dog = less tissue contrast + high kV
> = low contrast images.
>
> The ideal technique chart increases the mAs proportionately with the increase in centimeters as indicated in Fig. 5.10 A,B.

Completing the Technique Chart

Provided that the densities on the test images were satisfactory, each of the techniques may be extrapolated. Fill in the blanks on your chart. Increase 2 mAs for every 2-cm increase in density and increase 2 kV for every 2-cm increase.

Take careful measurements, and record the results in your clinic logbook. Always make sure that the patient is measured correctly and that the techniques are logged correctly. The only way to optimize the chart is to monitor it carefully, correctly, and consistently.

Small-Animal Technique Charts

The charts shown in Fig. 5.10 are in use in many clinics in North America. They are set up to be used on the specific units identified in the legends. These units must be correctly calibrated, and the patients must be correctly measured and correctly positioned, with obedience to the rules outlined previously.

The use of a large-animal portable unit in a small animal radiography clinic can produce acceptable images; however, the lack of technique selection and the limited mA values (usually a maximum of 30 or 50) can be frustrating.

Nonstandard Radiography Units (Alternative Charts)

If the radiography unit is limited in the number of mA stations or time stations, then adjustments need to be made within the chart to compensate for the lack of variables.

If a 200-speed system is used in the hospital/clinic, the mAs should be doubled from the suggested charts (Fig 5.10), and the kV left at the same settings. With a 200-speed system, it is important to compare system speeds to ensure that the system is actually 200 using the procedure outlined in Chapter 4. (These screens typically would be quite old and therefore may have deteriorated dramatically.)

Non-rare earth systems are not normally available for sale at this time. They can be specially ordered at a premium price.

Equine Radiography

Equine radiography is typically carried out on location using a large-animal portable radiography unit that is specially adapted to be transported from location to location.

The technique chart shown in Fig. 5.12 will work well with standard units. This chart is typical for a typical large-animal unit. The film/screen system speed is 400-speed class, and the films were processed in an automatic processor.

The unit must be calibrated correctly, and it is essential that any personnel in the vicinity wear leaded aprons, thyroid collars, and gloves while the examination is in progress. Each unit is equipped with a measuring device that must be used to ensure that a consistent distance is used for each view. The cassettes must be protected both before and after the exposure is made, and a method of separating exposed cassettes and unexposed cassettes must be used consistently so there is never a question as to whether a cassette has been used or is available for an exposure.

**All these techniques are set up for 30" distance
All views are full size horse unless otherwise noted

Body part	Size/view	kV	mAs	Grid (if used)
Navicular	**AP**	**74**	**2.5-2.8**	**4.0-5.0**
Coffin	A.P.	74	.8	
Coffin Jt/foot	Lat	74	.5	3.2
Coffin Jt./foot	Obl.	74	.5	3.2
Fetlocks and	**A.P.**	**74**	**.5**	**2.5-4.0**
splint bone	lat	74	.6	
	Obl	74	.5	
	Flexed lat	74	.5	
Knees	**A.P/Lat/Obl**	**74**	**.5**	
	Flexed lat	74	.5	
	Skyline	74	.5	
Hock	**A.P.**	**74**	**.8**	
	Lat/Obl.	74	.6	
	Flexed lat	74	.6	
	S1 talus	74	.5	
Stifle	**Lat Jt.**	**76**	**1.2**	**4.0-5.0**
	Lat patella	76	1.0	
	A.P.	80	3.2-5.0	8.0-10
Elbow	**Lat**	**74**	**.8**	
	A.P.	74	1.0-1.2	
Shoulder		**80**	**6.2-8.0**	
Thoracic sp./	**T 1-3**	**76**	**.5-.8**	
withers	**T 4-6**	**80**	**.8-1.8**	
Cerv. sp.	**Foal C1-C2**	**76**	**.6**	
	Foal C3-C4	76	.8	
	Foal C4- C6	78	.8	
Skull	**Incisors/Wolf teeth**	**74**	**.5**	
	Malaise	74	.8	
	A.P.	76	1.0-1.6	
	Jowl	74	1.2	

FIG. 5.12 The Large-Animal Portable Chart. Note that the time stations and kV stations are limited; therefore, the images will not always be optimized, but they will be diagnostic.

Date	Film #	Client	Breed	Area of body	Measure-ment Cm	kV	mA mAs	Time	Comment

FIG. 5.13 A Radiography Sample Log Book Page.

? POINTS TO PONDER The consultant was called to visit with a large-animal veterinarian who was concerned that his images were too dark. He thought there was an x-ray unit problem and that perhaps his unit required service.

The consultant assured him that any deterioration in his unit would cause lighter images, not darker images.

When the consultant arrived at the farm, the horse was positioned, and the veterinarian was in place to image a right hock. The distance from the focal spot to the cassette was 15 inches (38 cm). The distance on the technique chart he was using was 30 inches (76 cm). The amount of radiation the film was receiving was 4 times the radiation necessary to produce a correctly exposed image (calculated by the inverse square law [Fig 5.4]).

The Radiography Log Book

Legally, the clinic must keep a record of every patient radiographed (Fig. 5.13). The log book must include the patient's name, identifiers, the views taken, the measurements, and the technical factors. Leaving a space for a comment is often useful. The log book must be completed every time a patient is radiographed.

The technical factors and measurements are critical to maintaining a working technique chart. It is much easier to diagnose the cause of a problem if the technical factors are completed correctly.

Summary

The technical factors introduced and discussed in Chapters 2 and 4 have now been explored and put to use.

In this chapter, we have examined the variables of kV and mA and how each of these factors affects the overall image. It is vitally important to approach the technique chart with a scientific mind. The settings on the unit indicate the correct settings in order to produce an optimized image. If a service consultant is on site, the first place he or she will look is the log book to see if any inconsistencies of exposures have been occurring.

Each facility is unique, but the universal truth is that 70 kV is 70 kV, and the generator and the technical factors set on the generator must be accurate and reproducible.

REVIEW QUESTIONS

1. The main objective of all imaging systems is to:
   a. Produce a radiograph with a recognizable image
   b. Demonstrate differences in tissue density
   c. Demonstrate the image with no movement
   d. Show how much contrast and density are alike
2. Every radiography generator has kV, mAs, and time. The following statement is true:
   a. These may vary from unit to unit.
   b. These must be calibrated correctly so that 70 kV is 70 kV on every unit.
   c. The factors are variable and should be adjusted when the chart is set up.
   d. The factors do not matter as long as you follow the chart.
3. Film fog is a plus density artifact on an image. The following statement is true:
   a. It may be caused by light leaks in the darkroom.
   b. Film is not sensitive to light, only to x-rays.
   c. Film fog shows as a minus density after development.
   d. It may be caused by dropping a cassette after exposure.
4. Base + fog, which is an inherent part of the exposure:
   a. Does not appear on the processed film
   b. Appears only on reflected images
   c. Must always be included as part of the exposure
   d. Is a part of the manufacturing process and not important

5. The expiration date on the film box:
   a. Is not important because it has to do with the manufacturer
   b. Is important because it affects the processing of the film
   c. Is a critical piece of information when the box of film is used
   d. Has to do with the purchasing of film and not with its use
6. Radiographic contrast is part of the image controlled by:
   a. Patient thickness, density, and grid ratio
   b. The body part being examined and the bone-to-muscle ratio
   c. Grids, anode heel effect, and technical factors
   d. Collimation, distance, and patient thickness
7. Subject contrast is part of the image controlled by the patient thickness.
   a. True
   b. False
8. The inverse square law is particularly important in:
   a. Measuring the distance from the top of the patient to the grid tray
   b. Adjusting the technical factors between kV and mAs
   c. The distance between the table and the grid tray
   d. The distance measured in equine radiography
9. Kilovoltage is primarily responsible for:
   a. The hardness of the x-ray beam and its penetration
   b. The amount of density on the radiograph
   c. The intensity of the radiation and the density
   d. The blackness of the perimeter surrounding the image
10. The 15% rule is primarily used:
    a. When the image is far too dark or too light
    b. When the density on the image needs to be a little darker
    c. When the contrast on the image needs to be enhanced
    d. To reset the technical factors because of fogged film
11. If the original kV is 80 (we will increase the kV), the 15% rule calculation yields the following value:
    a. 87
    b. 92
    c. 97
    d. 79

12. Milliamperage is responsible for the intensity of the radiation, which:
    a. Translates to the density on the image
    b. Translates to the contrast on the image
    c. Relates only to the time of the exposure
    d. Does not concern the blackness of the background.
13. The rules of using a technique chart correctly include:
    a. Positioning on the table, measuring, and centering the central ray
    b. Positioning the animal on the floor and centering to the film
    c. Measuring the animal in the cage and then setting the technical factors
    d. Measuring the animal upright, setting the techniques before measuring, and then centering to the grid tray
14. If the images are consistently dull and gray, the first check should be made in the:
    a. Processing to see whether the fluids are still fresh
    b. The cassettes to make sure they have not changed
    c. The darkroom to ensure that there are no light leaks
    d. The generator to ensure that the techniques did not change
15. The radiography log book is a record of exposures. The following statement is true:
    a. It is also a legal necessity and maintains a record of technical factors.
    b. It is not necessary because we always remember the techniques.
    c. It is not necessary because the animal always measures the same.
    d. It is necessary only to write down the animal's name for accounting purposes.

Chapter Review Question answers are located in the Instructor Resources on Evolve and can be provided to students at the discretion of the instructor.

CHAPTER 6

Optimizing the Image

Lois C. Brown, RTR (Can/USA), ACR, MSc, P.Phys

A photograph is usually looked at—seldom looked into.
—Ansel Adams – American photographer – 1902–1984

Sometimes you need to "jump through hoops" to obtain a good image.

OUTLINE

LEARNING OBJECTIVES

When you have finished this chapter, you will be able to:

1. Define motion, distortion, magnification, and blur.
2. Understand the purpose of filters.
3. Define collimation.
4. Understand the purpose of illuminators.
5. Know when to use a grid.

6. Understand the grid ratio and the difference between various grids.
7. Determine the importance of line pairs in relation to the grid ratio.

APPLICATIONS

The application of the information in this chapter is relevant to the following area:

1. Optimizing the images (radiographs) to aid in diagnoses

KEY TERMS

Key terms are defined in the Glossary on the Evolve website.

Blur
Central ray
Coincidence
Collimation shutters/leaves
Collimator
Collimator indicator
Compensating filters
Diffusion
Distortion

Filtration
Grid
Grid deterioration
Grid ratio
Grid tray
Heterogeneous beam
Illuminator
Illuminator mask
Inherent filtration

Line pairs/inch (grids)
Line pairs/mm (resolution)
Magnification
Motion
Object image receptor distance (OID)
Off-focus radiation
Region of interest (ROI)
Resolution

Scattered radiation
Secondary radiation
Source image distance (SID)
Source object distance (SOD)
Umbra/penumbra

This chapter is the compilation of all the technology introduced thus far and introduces the tools necessary to optimize the image. This chapter refers to the central ray, which is the x-ray beam produced off the central point of the focal spot of the anode and directed at 90 degrees to the image receptor (Fig. 6.1). The ROI (region of interest) is the area of the patient through which the central ray must pass to obtain a correctly positioned radiograph.

It is essential to ensure that as much cooperation as possible is obtained from the patient. If an animal is so ill or terrified that it tremors continuously, obtaining an optimized radiograph will be very difficult unless the animal can be reassured or sedated to the point at which it will be cooperative and remain motionless throughout the x-ray examination. Many veterinary facilities are limited to $1/120$ of a second on their radiography units, and at times this is not fast enough to arrest involuntary motion such as tremor or panting.

Other factors, such as magnification, distortion, and blur, can be minimized by understanding the principles behind these factors. The use of collimation and grids reduces the scattered/secondary radiation. Understanding the principles of grids, the limitations of various grid ratios, and how to position the grid correctly is vitally important to obtaining a good, clean image. Filtration eliminates a certain amount of secondary radiation and prevents most of the scattered radiation. Illuminators are vitally important to film/screen radiography, and the correct placement of the illuminator and the correct lighting tubes within the illuminator will optimize viewing of the x-ray film image.

The central ray

FIG. 6.1 The central ray of the radiography unit is the point at which the x-ray beam enters the patient.

Motion, Distortion, and Magnification

Motion

Resolution is the ability to differentiate fine details within the x-ray image (Fig. 6.2A). Motion will destroy resolution. Unsharpness resulting from patient motion may be voluntary or involuntary. Reducing involuntary motion or waiting a few extra seconds until the patient settles is very important to good radiography.

Diagnosis is impossible if the patient appears to be leaving the table as the exposure is made. This is also true if a wagging tail is moving across the image. The use of sandbags and rolled towels can support body parts that are unstable and out of the ROI. Sandbags can be obtained commercially or, if someone in the facility can sew, can be made quite

FIG. 6.2 A, An example of involuntary motion (tremor); the abdominal contents are no longer distinct. B, Blur can be very subtle. Here the patient is in tremor; the image almost looks like a double exposure except for the trachea and the heart, which are clear.

easily. Be aware that sandbags are not radiolucent and should never be placed where they will obscure the ROI. For all other methods of nonmanual restraint, please review Chapter 15 and each of the views in Part Two.

> ✓ **CHECK IT OUT** A sandbag can be made out of heavy vinyl. A piece of vinyl 15 in (38 cm) long and 15 in (38 cm) wide will make a sandbag 15 in × 5.5 in (38 cm × 13 cm). The vinyl should be folded over twice on each seam, and the seams should be oversewn so that the sand does not leak out over time.

Colorful slipcovers can be sewn and secured at the top with hook-and-loop (Velcro) strips to make a standard-size sandbag. Larger or smaller sizes are also useful. If no one at the facility can sew, sandbags and foam blocks for positioning can be purchased from commercial suppliers.

Blur

Blur is another factor in patient motion, which in some cases may be useful when imaging a particular body part that is obscured by overlying anatomical structures. Blur is the principle of computerized tomography; we investigate this principle in depth in Chapter 12.

Blur can be dramatic, with the structures completely obscured and the image appearing as if the patient is leaving the table. It can also be subtle, such as in Fig. 6.2B, in which the patient is in tremor and every body part uniformly appears as if it is a double exposure. In this case, the large organs appear in focus, but resolution is lost in the extremities and spine.

Distortion

Distortion is the foreshortening or elongation of a body part due to angulation of the body part, x-ray receptor, or x-ray tube (Fig. 6.3). Distortion can be useful when one body part obscures the area of interest. For example, if the left (upper) shoulder obscures pathology of the right (lower) humerus on an upper-right lateral thorax view, the x-ray tube may be angled obliquely so the left shoulder is projected away from the right humerus. The patient may also be rotated slightly to demonstrate pathology. Useful distortion is practiced regularly in dental radiography and is discussed in Chapter 22.

> ◆ **APPLICATION INFORMATION**
> The best resolution and least magnification of the body parts occurs when the ROI is closest to the image receptor.
> It is due to these factors that when a patient's spine is radiographed, the patient is positioned in the ventrodorsal (VD) position. If the left side of the thorax is of concern, then the patient must be turned onto the left side for the lateral view.

Distortion is not useful if it results in elongation or foreshortening of the ROI. Shape distortion can occur from inaccurate positioning of the central ray. For example, if the ROI is the thorax and the central ray is directed to the abdomen, the anterior ribs will be projected cranially and the shape of the thorax will be distorted. It is important that the ROI is centered beneath the central ray of the x-ray tube.

FIG. 6.3 Distortion. A, Body part not parallel to the image receptor. B, Image receptor not parallel to the body part. (From Fauber TL. *Radiographic Imaging and Exposure.* 4th ed. St. Louis: Mosby, 2013.)

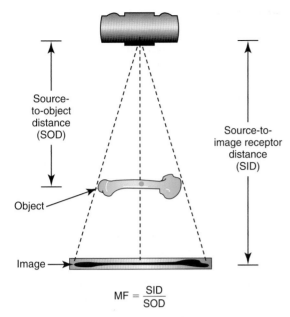

$$MF = \frac{SID}{SOD}$$

FIG. 6.4 Example of Magnification of an Image Structure. *MF, Magnification factor.* (From Fauber TL. *Radiographic Imaging and Exposure.* 5th ed. St. Louis: Mosby, 2017.)

? POINTS TO PONDER Elongation and foreshortening are eliminated by ensuring the correct alignment of the x-ray tube, body part, and image receptor and central ray.

Magnification

Magnification of a body part is reduced if the body part is placed as close as possible to the image receptor (Fig. 6.4). The source image distance (SID) on most veterinary radiography units is 40 inches (100 cm). If the object of interest is raised or anatomically positioned above the image receptor, the object will be magnified. In everyday practice, the actual measurement of an object in question is not an issue. If the radiography is used to measure cardiac enlargement, then positioning correctly becomes a major factor.

Magnification Calculation

To calculate the size of an object (e.g., a kidney stone), the source-to-object distance (SOD) first needs to be calculated by using the following formula:

$$SID - OID = SOD$$

Measure the distance of the object from the image receptor (object-to-image receptor distance; OID) by measuring on the lateral view. To do this, position the film on the illuminator and measure the distance (in cm) from the dorsal surface of the abdomen to the object in question. (For a kidney stone, this measurement is typically one-third of the measurement from the dorsal surface to the ventral surface.) The SID on most veterinary radiography units is 100 cm.

If the OID is 12 cm, then the SOD will be:

$$100 \text{ cm} - 12 \text{ cm} = 88 \text{ cm}$$

The magnification factor (MF) is calculated by using the following formula:

$$SID/SOD = MF$$

If the SID is 100 cm, then the MF will be:

$$100/88 = 1.13$$

Actual object size is calculated by using the following formula:

$$\frac{\text{Measurement on a radiograph}}{\text{Magnification factor}} = \text{Object size}$$

From our previous calculation, we know that the MF is 1.13. If the object size on the radiograph is 1.5 cm, then the actual object size will be:

$$\frac{1.5 \text{ cm}}{1.13} = 1.327 \text{ cm}$$

Geometrical Unsharpness

Every feature in the image is best viewed in its natural size unaffected by unsharpness caused by geometrical factors. Therefore, both the SID and OID are vitally important. The source of the radiation is the x-ray tube. The collimator ensures that the beam is focused directly on the ROI. Together the SID and the OID, along with the size of the focal spot, determine the sharpness of the image.

Unsharpness Due to Increased Focal Spot Size

In very rare cases, the focal spot of the x-ray tube can become enlarged due to overheating or age. In this case the bony structures appear to be double-exposed, with a second image exactly superimposed on the original image but offset by approximately $\frac{1}{8}$ of an inch (0.32 cm). There is no way to remedy this problem, and the x-ray tube must be replaced.

Filters and Filtration

? POINTS TO PONDER A quick review: Radiation produced by the x-ray tube is made up of many different wavelengths. It is described as **a heterogenous beam**. As the kilovoltage increases, the scattered photons of the beam also increase. The lower energy radiation (alpha and beta) is not useful and must be filtered out, as it only contributes to patient dose and does not have the energy to penetrate the patient and contribute to the image

Aluminum is the element of choice for filtration. It has a low atomic number and will absorb the low energy radiation without filtering much of the useful beam. It is also widely available and inexpensive. It can be milled to a very thin sheet so it can be added to the x-ray unit in gradations of 1 mm.

Once radiation became useful in general radiography, the problem of scattered/secondary radiation had to be addressed. As the body parts being examined become thicker, the technical factors need to be increased, and there is even greater scattered/secondary radiation, particularly as the kilovoltage (kV) is increased.

The standard reaction to increased body size is to increase the kV: 2 kV per centimeter is usually the norm, starting around 40 or 50 kV. A proportionate increase in kV along with an increase in patient thickness causes two factors to enter the equation:

1. There is less difference in tissue density because fat and flabby muscle tissue become more prevalent.
2. The production of scattered/secondary radiation is greater because the kilovoltage controls the penetrating power of the x-ray beam. An increase in the penetrating power of the x-ray beam (obtained by increasing the kV) will produce higher levels of secondary radiation and then more scattered radiation, which will fog the film and reduce contrast considerably.

Chapter 5 explains how to control the technical factors to reduce secondary radiation. It also explains *kilovoltage, milliamperage,* and *time* and how kV affects the image.

When radiation enters the patient, it does so as a heterogeneous (many different energies) beam. When 70 kV is set on the x-ray unit, only a portion of the actual radiation produced will be 70 kV. This is the *effective kV.* Therefore a 70 kV beam contains radiation representing 70 kV but also contains photons of varying amounts of energy (alpha, beta, gamma energies) that are both absorbed within the patient and scatter from the patient as scattered/secondary radiation. Because this radiation is not useful, it must be filtered out either before it enters the patient or after it exits the patient. The first method to filter out the soft or lower-energy radiation before it reaches the patient is through inherent filtration within the x-ray tube and collimator.

Inherent Filtration

The collimator of the radiography unit is equipped with inherent filtration when it is installed (Fig. 6.5). Before the x-ray beam exits the port of the x-ray tube, it is attenuated by the glass envelope of the tube, the oil surrounding the tube, the mirror, and an added filter made of aluminum just inside the port of the collimator (the beam restrictor located just below the x-ray tube). This is inherent filtration—the filtration that is part of the x-ray tube assembly that includes the collimator. This filtration cannot be changed in the radiography room.

Added Filtration

The beam is further attenuated by the added filtration installed by the manufacturer. Federal (legal) guidelines are very clear regarding the amount of filtration that must be installed in each radiography unit. This added filtration may be adjusted according to the typical procedure in the radiography room. Canadian and U.S. federal guidelines specify a minimum of 2.1 mm of aluminum for x-ray units operating above 70 kV (National Council on Radiation Protection & Measurements, 1988).

Most installations include a label on the back of the x-ray tube. This is a legal requirement in most countries. The label must include the date and country of manufacture, the amount of inherent filtration of the x-ray tube, model number, and serial number.

Special Filters

Other filters known as *compensating filters* may be added to the primary beam to enhance the imaging process. For example, a wedge filter may be added to the collimator, with the thicker part of the wedge over the thinner area of the abdomen if the ROI is the upper abdomen of a dog with a large discrepancy between the measurement of the pelvis and the area of the diaphragm (Fig. 6.6). The technique would be set for the caudal rib measurement, with the x-ray tube positioned over the ROI at the level of the spleen and kidneys.

FIG. 6.5 The back plate of a collimator showing the amount of inherent filtration within it.

FIG. 6.6 A wedge filter will even out the difference in tissue measurement. It is attached to the collimator with the thickest end at the thinner part of the patient. The technique set is the measurement of the thicker body part.

FIG. 6.7 A, Simple intravenous saline bags absorb scattered radiation if the region of interest is on the outer aspect of the anatomy. **B,** Special lead blockers also work well as long as they are not pushed under the patient, which would block primary radiation. Leaded rubber gloves and cut-up pieces of lead apron also serve this purpose.

Many other filters are available, both to even out the discrepancy between different areas of the body and to absorb scattered/secondary radiation.

Blockers

Filtration to eliminate scattered radiation on the image is as simple as laying a mask of leaded rubber on the tabletop along the lumbar spine for a lateral exposure (Fig. 6.7). (This is particularly useful if the suspected pathology is within the dorsal aspect of the spine.) The leaded rubber absorbs the scattered radiation and prevents it from reaching the image receptor. Other effective blockers and filters are large intravenous saline bags and plastic bags filled with flour or rice. The advantage of the saline bags and flour bags is that they are radiolucent and do not produce an artifact. Leaded blockers may also be used to reduce or eliminate the effect of scattered/secondary radiation, which will "splash" onto the image and blacken areas of interest. Leaded gloves are particularly useful, as the curve on the glove can lie along the abdomen and not encroach on the anatomy. It is important that these blockers lie beside the patient and not beneath the area of interest.

Collimators and Coincidence

The unit immediately beneath the x-ray tube is the collimator (Fig. 6.8). There are many varieties of collimators, but they all have one main function—to produce a light beam that is coincident with the x-ray beam and covers the ROI. It is very important that the light beam be centered and coincident within 0.50 inch (1 cm) of the area of the x-ray beam.

In addition, the x-ray beam and the light beam should completely match each other in position and size. If the collimator light and the x-ray beam overlap each other completely, they are said to be "in coincidence." Chapter 9 discusses quality control tests regarding collimators and collimation.

> **? POINTS TO PONDER** As the collimation increases, the area covered becomes smaller, the beam size becomes smaller, and the amount of scattered radiation is reduced. As the collimation decreases, the area radiographed becomes larger, the field size increases, and the potential for scattered radiation is increased.

Scattered/Secondary Radiation

Scattered/secondary radiation produced has much lower energy than the usable x-ray beam and does not have the capability of producing an organized image beyond the limits of the collimator (Fig. 6.9). The presence of scattered/secondary radiation is the main reason that anyone in the room at the time of exposure should never be in the field of view, should be appropriately gowned and gloved, and should stay as far from the x-ray beam as possible (see Chapter 3). Refer to Chapter 5 to learn how to evaluate technical factors on a radiograph.

Collimation and Contrast

As the collimator blades are closed, the radiation area decreases. The amount of radiation scattered from the ROI also decreases. Scattered radiation that reaches the film is not

FIG. 6.8 Two Different Collimators. **A,** Collimator for Raymax LX125 (Raymax Medical, Brampton, Ontario, CA). Note the indicators for height of the x-ray tube and film size on the front. **B,** The collimator for Sedecal APR VET (Sedecal USA, Inc., Arlington Heights, Illinois) is mounted directly below the generator control panel.

FIG. 6.9 A, An example of scattered radiation. The collimated field is visible, but the radiation is strong enough to scatter to the outer edges of the image receptor. In this case, it is caused by high exposure. The kilovoltage should be reduced so that the lung markings are visible and the spinous processes of the thoracic spine fade as the spine descends caudally to the abdomen. **B,** Evidence of extrafocal radiation *(arrows)*. Note that this is different from scattered radiation because the folds of the dog's ears are also evident along with the much thicker shoulder area.

useful radiation. Its only effect is to increase the base + fog density and reduce the contrast between the base density and the imaged structures. If collimation restricts the beam size dramatically, the technical factors may need to be increased slightly to accommodate for the restriction of some of the useful radiation (Table 6.1). To change the density on a radiograph, only the milliamperes (mAs) should be increased, not the kV.

Collimator Problems or Scatter from the Patient?

The collimator is the last filtration system of the x-ray beam before it reaches the patient. In some cases, when the beam is collimated, there is a shadow of the patient's anatomy on the image beyond the edges of the collimator (see Fig. 6.9A). This may be caused by scatter from the patient itself. If the "splash" of radiation is larger when the patient being

TABLE 6.1	Effect of Changing Collimation*
COLLIMATION	**RESULT**
Decrease field size	Patient dose decreases
	Scattered radiation decreases
	Radiographic contrast increases
	Radiographic density decreases
Increase field size	Patient dose increases
	Scattered radiation increases
	Radiographic contrast decreases
	(due to increased scattered/
	secondary radiation)
	Radiographic density increases

*Increasing the collimation narrows the field of view. Increasing the field size is the same as opening the collimator shutters.

radiographed is large and is not visible when the patient is quite small, the problem is most likely scattered/secondary radiation from the patient. Placing a lead strip along the side of the patient prevents this scatter from affecting the image.

? POINTS TO PONDER When placing any blocker alongside the patient to absorb scatter, it is very important that the blocker does not overlap the anatomy being imaged.

Extrafocal Radiation

If parts of the patient's anatomy are clearly visible, such as the outline of a leg or the spinous processes in an otherwise collimated spine, then the fault is most likely *extrafocal radiation* (see Chapter 2) or *off-focus radiation* (see Fig. 6.9B). This is radiation that is created by the photon stream outside the actual focal spot. It may be due to a defect in the design and manufacture of the x-ray tube and shielding system or the collimator filtration, or the kV may be set too high, causing excessively active photons in the thermionic cloud at the anode.

Umbra and Penumbra

The umbra is the portion of the x-ray image that is sharp and clearly collimated. The penumbra is the outside edge or shadow where the film has been imperfectly collimated. This image is not magnified or distorted. Most modern collimators are efficient enough that penumbra is eliminated.

Changing the Collimator Light Bulb

When the light bulb inside the collimator burns out, it may be replaced by veterinary staff, but a service person should be called the first time to demonstrate the correct method of changing that particular light bulb. The installing engineer of a new unit should demonstrate how to change the light bulb during the demonstration of the unit to the veterinarian.

New radiography units should be supplied with a spare collimator light bulb. The replacement bulb should be kept in a specific place and its location noted on the x-ray genera-

2 mm AL. EQ.
LAMP TYPE: FCS, 24 VAC, 150 W

FIG. 6.10 Cover plate on the back of a collimator. Note the lamp type information. This collimator label also includes the amount of filtration inherent in the components of the collimator.

tor. Whenever the light bulb is changed, a new one should be ordered right away so that there is always a spare on "hot stand-by." Collimator bulbs are usually supplied by x-ray service companies or can be ordered online (just type in the alphanumeric code of the bulb followed by the words "light bulb" in your search engine). Always make sure that the voltage of the bulb you are ordering is the same as the one you are replacing. The wattage should also be the same, but the voltage is more important. If you are not sure which bulb to order, check the back of the collimator. There is usually a label specifying voltage and wattage (Fig. 6.10). If there is no label, then carefully follow these instructions:

- Make sure the generator is turned off at the wall switch. Have a multiple-tip screwdriver handy to remove the cover of the collimator. Select the tip appropriate for the screw heads on the collimator.
- Search for a cover plate on the collimator. It is usually on the back or on the side. Remove the cover plate. Typically, the light bulb is now visible. On some collimators, the shutters must be closed to expose the bulb, and other collimators have a small black box that must be removed. Carefully note the position of the box before you remove it.
- Once the light bulb is exposed, remove it, **noting whether it requires turning or just a gentle tug to do so. This is very important.** Some light bulbs are mounted between what appears to be two steel plates. If you look very closely, you will see a slight opening for the end of the new bulb. Some light bulbs have a bayonet mount and require turning as well as pulling to remove them. **Be very gentle; these bulbs are often small and fragile!**
- Check to ensure that the bulb you are replacing is identical to the new bulb. The code numbers or letters may differ, but the wattage and, particularly, the voltage must be the same.
- The new light bulb will probably be a halogen bulb, so it is important not to touch it with bare hands or fingers. The bulb usually comes wrapped in a plastic cover from which the bottom may be cut away to reveal the insertion end of the bulb. Using the cover, gently and firmly insert the bulb in the exact spot from which you removed the old bulb, then slide the plastic cover off the bulb.
- Once the bulb is firmly in place, turn on the main power to test that the bulb is working.
- Turn off the power again and reaffix the collimator cover plate.

Illuminators

Illuminators transmit light evenly through a specially produced glass in order to visualize and interpret radiographic

FIG. 6.11 A, A typical stand-alone illuminator. This illuminator may be placed on a table, mounted on a wall, or inserted into the wall between the upright joists. **B,** This two-bank illuminator is mounted on the wall of the x-ray room. A mask would direct the intensity of the light through the image and prevent glare from the areas surrounding the radiograph. (**B** Courtesy Westbridge Veterinary Hospital, Mississauga, Ontario.)

images (Fig. 6.11). This is the means by which the veterinarian, and often the client, view and discuss the results of the radiographic examination. It is very important that the conditions under which the radiographs are interpreted are of the highest possible quality; therefore, it is vital that the illuminators be checked regularly for optimum brightness.

Illuminator Specifications

The inside of the illuminator must be painted a bright white to reflect as much light as possible toward the diffusion glass. Illuminators with the light tubes mounted in unpainted wooden or stainless-steel boxes are not suitable because they absorb the light and diminish the amount projected toward the diffusion glass. The luminance across the entire face of the illuminator should be the same. The illuminator must be equipped with a diffusing glass or Plexiglas so the corners of the illuminator are the same brightness as the central portion.

Commercially available bulbs may be purchased at a hardware store. The light tubes must be labeled "daylight" or "blue/white" light to match the color spectrum of radiographic film. Bulbs with a green, yellow, or pink tone are not suitable for viewing radiographs. If one light tube becomes faulty, all light tubes within that illuminator should be replaced so the brightness is uniform across the width of the illuminator. The face of the illuminator should be cleaned regularly using a commercial glass cleaner whenever the countertops and shelves are dusted. The switch must be a safety switch and must be checked to ensure that it is not worn, loose, or faulty. At least once per year, the glass panel should be removed so the illuminator box can

be dusted and cleaned and the bulbs checked for brightness and consistency.

✔ CHECK IT OUT

- A combination of correct color and brightness enhances the contrast of the radiographs. As a quick test to reveal whether the color of the illuminator bulbs in the facility is correct, review a correctly exposed radiograph on the clinic illuminator.
- Now go to a window on a cloudy, bright day and review the same radiograph (this light is the same color as the daylight light tube).
- If the image looks the same, then the light tubes are most likely daylight.
- Most fluorescent tubes are labeled at one end with the manufacturer and the color.
- An illuminator that is not working correctly or does not transmit the light effectively can seriously compromise the reading of a radiograph and can actually affect the technical factors used to produce the image.

Illuminator Position

An illuminator may be mounted on the wall or positioned within the wall so that the front is flush with the wall. The films are hung from holders at the top of the illuminator, and these should be checked regularly to ensure that they do not catch and hold the film so firmly that it cannot be removed without incident.

The illuminator should be positioned in the room so that the overhead light may be switched off. This way, there will

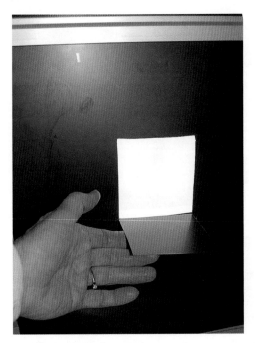

FIG. 6.12 Illuminator Mask. Keep the piece that is cut out and use it to cover that hole. Then you can cut out similar areas to fit the various sizes of film that are used in the facility. Make the cutout close to the middle of the illuminator to ensure you have the brightest light.

be no backlighting to reduce the brightness of the light transmitted from the illuminator.

Illuminator Masks

Illuminator masks (Fig. 6.12) should be available to cover any part of the illuminator panel not covered by the film so that all available light reaching the eye of the clinician is directed through the radiograph.

✔ CHECK IT OUT

To construct radiographic masks, remove a sheet of film from the film box in the darkroom. Close the box and return it to the holder. Turn on the light in the darkroom to expose the film. Process the film normally. The film will be completely black and will act as a mask for radiographs hung on an illuminator. Ensure that you have enough masks to cover any size area corresponding to the sizes of the film you use in the clinic.

For dental films, take the 14 in × 17 in (35 × 43 cm) mask and cut out a hole the size of the dental film in the middle of the mask. Cut out as many holes as necessary. Return the cutouts to the film and tape them in place. Place the tape along the bottom of the hole so that the cutout can drop down when the hole is in use by the dental radiograph and be returned to position when it is not in use.

Grids and Grid Trays

Scattered/secondary radiation is a problem as the body parts to be radiographed become larger. Any body part more than 10 cm will produce enough scattered/secondary radiation to seriously compromise the contrast on an x-ray image.

In 1913, Gustave Bucky invented the radiographic grid (Fig. 6.13). This consisted of vertical, very fine strips of metal interspaced with a radiolucent material. The strips are positioned parallel to the sides of the table, and the entire "grid" is positioned between the patient and the cassette.

The original grid was positioned with a spring that had to be set (or cocked) before each exposure; when the exposure was made, the lock released, and the grid moved across the face of the cassette to absorb scattered/secondary radiation.

This somewhat complicated contraption worked on the principle of the windshield wiper moving across the car windshield—your eyes do not focus on the windshield wiper but rather through the window to the road outside.

A couple of problems arose when this technology was transferred to the veterinary market. The grid oscillating device made a fairly loud noise as it was released. Once the spring was converted to a motor, the whirring noise of the motor was bothersome to some animals. The other problem was the timing of the original units, which needed an exposure time of at least $1/10$ of a second for the strips to move rapidly enough to blur out the image of the individual strips. Most veterinary exposures must be far less than $1/10$ of a second, so the vertical lines of the grid material are a problem. These units have occasionally been installed in veterinary hospitals, and the motorized mechanism should be removed and the ancient grids replaced by newer stationary grids.

Grid Nomenclature

Every grid manufactured throughout the world is imprinted or labeled with the grid ratio, the lines per inch, and the manufacturer.

✔ CHECK IT OUT

Remove the top of the x-ray table carefully. Most tabletops are screwed to the frame either on top of the table or beneath the table. Most medical-grade tabletops are screwed to the frame beneath the table. Remove the screws carefully. The tabletop can always be reattached with strips of adhesive-backed hook-and-loop (Velcro) tape.

(If the tabletop does not come off easily and it is necessary to change the grid, contact a service person to remove the grid from beneath the tabletop.)

The grid is seated above the grid tray. The grid lines should run parallel to the length of the x-ray table. There should be a line etched or drawn on the grid indicating the center of the grid and the direction of the lines. A label or etching on the front or top of the grid indicates the grid ratio and the line pairs per inch.

Grid Ratios and Line Pairs per Inch

A ratio is expressed as a number with a relationship to a second number; for example, the ratio of 25 apples to 5 apples is 5:1. It is always expressed with a colon (:) in between the two numbers.

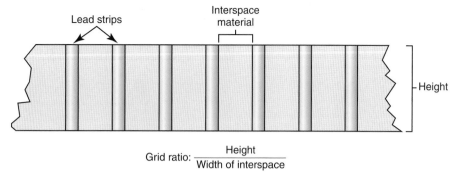

FIG. 6.13 Grid ratio is the ratio of the height of the lead strips to the distance (interspace) between them. (From Fauber TL. *Radiographic Imaging and Exposure.* 5th ed. St. Louis: Mosby; 2017.)

Grid ratio = Height of the lead strips: Distance between the lead strips.

As grids were used in various procedures, the manufacturers made them more sophisticated. The best way to identify them was by expressing a ratio of lines of the material used to "clean up" the scatter: 5:1, 6:1, 8:1, 10:1, 12:1, and 16:1. It was soon discovered that grids with lower ratios (5:1 and 6:1) did not work as well as grids with higher ratios because they did not absorb enough scattered/secondary radiation. Introducing more leaded strips and a higher ratio eliminated secondary/scattered radiation more efficiently. Also, the grids with very high ratios—16:1 and higher—were useful only for specific applications and not for general radiography. The higher ratio grids required much more radiation because they were so efficient that they absorbed much of the primary beam as well as the scattered/secondary radiation, thereby increasing patient radiation dose. (If some of the useful beam is eliminated, then technical factors would have to be increased, thereby increasing patient dose.)

The problem with expressing the grid ratio alone is that it does not specify the number of line pairs (lp) per inch. One line pair is one vertical strip and one interspace strip. A grid may have an 8:1 grid ratio, but if the lines are spread too far apart, they will show up on a radiograph.

Because the ratio numbers identify the height of lines or strips compared with the space between them, the number of line pairs is as important as the grid ratio.

In the medical and veterinary general radiography field, grids with ratios of 8:1 and 10:1 with 103 lp/inch work the best. The scatter control is good without the need to increase the radiation dose by too much to overcome the clean-up of the grid.

? **POINTS TO PONDER** When the tabletop is removed for the grid ratio check on an older radiography unit (more than 20 years old), it is common to find a 6:1 or 8:1, 70 or 85 line pair grid. The older grids not only have lower numbers of lines, but the interspace material has usually started to degrade, and the pattern is visible on a radiograph (see Fig. 6.18).

Parallel vs. Focused Grids

The original grids were manufactured with parallel lines running in the vertical direction of the table (Fig. 6.14A). A problem arose when larger cassette sizes became available and the collimators opened to a 17-inch lateral width. The parallel grid strips cut off the radiation at the edges of the image so that the edges of the films were exposed to little or no radiation.

The solution to this problem was to "focus" the grid (Fig. 6.14B). As grid manufacturing techniques became more sophisticated, newer grids were manufactured with the lines vertical strips tilted slightly to match the divergent x-rays of the primary beam (Fig. 6.15). These "focused" grids allowed more primary radiation to reach the film edges than did the older parallel grids, but they also introduced another variable that had to be addressed—focal length.

Grid Focus and Focal Length

Grid focal length is the distance from the focal spot of the x-ray tube to the grid. The focused grids assumed a 34- to 44-in (86- to 112-cm) focal length. The divergent rays of the x-ray beam exit at a prescribed distance from the grid (40 in or 100 cm). If the primary beam is changed to a shorter or longer focal length (distance from the focal spot of the x-ray tube to the grid), a grid of a different focal length is needed to correspond to the new distance. Another problem occurs with equine radiography when the x-ray unit is held too close to the grid.

Various focal lengths are now available, and the most common are listed in Table 6.2. The following factors must be included when a grid is purchased for a veterinary hospital:
- **Grid ratio**: Usually 10:1
- **Number of line pairs:** Usually 103 lp/in
- **Focal length**: Usually 34 to 44 in (86 to 111 cm)

Grid Installation

The grid is installed beneath the tabletop and above the cassette. A grid tray is usually in place below the grid, and the folded metal edges of the grid tray holder will support the grid. It is important that the grid is centered correctly and

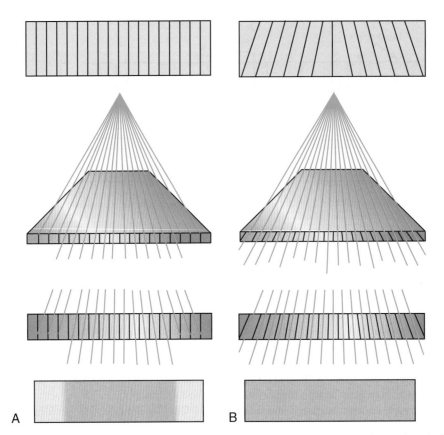

A   B

FIG. 6.14 **A,** A parallel grid absorbs the radiation at the edges of the image. **B,** A focused grid allows the x-rays to pass through to the outer edges of the image. (From Fauber TL. *Radiographic Imaging and Exposure.* 5th ed. St. Louis: Mosby; 2017.)

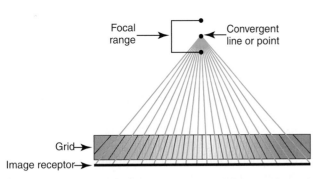

FIG. 6.15 **A Focused Grid.** The lead lines are angled coincident with the divergent primary rays. The focal length is now preset, and the focal range is slightly above and slightly below the convergent point. Typically, a 40-inch focal length grid has a focal range of 34 to 44 inches. (From Fauber TL. *Radiographic Imaging and Exposure.* 5th ed. St. Louis: Mosby; 2017.)

TABLE 6.2	Common Grid Focal Lengths	
SIZE	**INCHES**	**CENTIMETERS**
Small	26–32	66–81
Medium	34–44	86–111
Large	48–72	122–183

maintained in the correct position. An older installed grid may be screwed in place, glued in place, or held in place by hook-and-loop tape (Velcro). Strips of adhesive-backed Velcro tape work well to attach the grid to the grid tray holder. It may be necessary to cut the strips to a width of 0.5 in (1.27 cm) lengthwise so there is no chance that they will catch on the cassette as it is drawn in and out of the tray.

When replacing a grid, the size of the grid tray is important. The grid should overhang the edges of the cassette slightly to effectively absorb the scattered radiation and not be visible on the image. For example, an 18 in × 18 in (46 cm × 46 cm) grid will cover a 14 in × 17 in (35 cm × 43 cm) cassette effectively both vertically and longitudinally.

Grid Positioning

Positioning the grid is critical because it must be exactly in the center of the table or, in equine radiography, the central ray must be centered exactly on the center line of the grid. The grid must also be installed flat on the grid tray, exactly parallel to the port of the x-ray tube. If it is tilted slightly from one side to the other, it will allow the radiation on one side to pass through but will cut off the radiation prematurely on the raised side (Figs. 6.16 and 6.17).

If the grid is installed upside down, an image such as that shown in Fig. 6.20AB will result. The x-ray beam will pass

Proper position   Off-level

FIG. 6.16 A focused grid raised on one side of the table. One side of the grid acts as a parallel grid; the other side absorbs the primary and secondary radiation. (From Fauber TL. *Radiographic Imaging and Exposure.* 5th ed. St. Louis: Mosby; 2017.)

Proper position   Off-center

FIG. 6.17 A focused grid set off-center does not allow the radiation to penetrate the grid correctly, causing off-center cutoff. (From Fauber TL. *Radiographic Imaging and Exposure.* 5th ed. St. Louis: Mosby; 2017.)

through the vertical strips in the center and will be cut off on both sides evenly toward the edges.

TABLE 6.3	Grid Conversion Factors*
GRID RATIO	**CONVERSION FACTOR NUMBER**
5 : 1	1
6 : 1	2
8 : 1 and 10 : 1	3
12 : 1	4
16 : 1	5

*To calculate the grid conversion factor, multiply the mAs by the grid conversion factor number for each grid ratio.

APPLICATION INFORMATION

The consultant was called into a clinic with a problem that the hospital had finally identified as an equipment problem, but they had no idea what caused it. The images were all slightly lighter on one side than on the other. The problem worsened on the lateral edges of the film. So, on a large dog VD thorax, the right lung was considerably lighter than the left. It appeared that every dog that they x-rayed had pneumonia in the right lung, whereas the left lungs all appeared to be overinflated.

The x-ray unit had been serviced just weeks before, and the hospital hadn't had any need for grid radiographs for about 2 weeks. That was when a patient who had suspected pneumonia arrived, and the image appeared to be what the veterinarian suspected. But when the next dog came in with suspected left-side pathology and the right side was as bad as or worse than the left, they began to suspect there was a problem with the x-ray unit.

After the tabletop was removed, the consultant lifted the grid and discovered a screw had been left on the track of the grid unit. The grid was lifted about ¼ inch on the right side. This was enough to cause the left side to assume a parallel grid configuration, producing an image of overinflation in the lungs on the left. The right side of the grid with this tilt was filtering the radiation, causing a light image appearance that would look like pathology on the right.

The images showed poor aeration of the lungs on the right and overinflation on the left.

See Figs. 6.16 and 6.17 for off-level and off-center grid examples.

The Effect of a Grid on Technical Factors

The grid absorbs some of the primary beam as it impacts directly on the lead strips. The grid conversion factor is the formula that determines the increase in technical factors to compensate for this absorption. As the grid ratio increases, the radiographic density decreases, and vice versa. The mAs value changes according to Table 6.3. This table should not be necessary if the technique chart is set up correctly at the original installation.

Summary

The options discussed in this chapter are essential for producing the best images possible, no matter which radiography unit and technique chart are used. Motion, blur, distortion, and magnification have been discussed. This chapter also contains the basics of optimizing radiographic images, including the use of an optimized illuminator. The installation of a grid is necessary for reducing the scattered radiation that affects the image.

Image Gallery

Figs. 6.18 to 6.20 illustrate some of the problems that occur with grids. Because grids are located beneath the tabletop, they are out of sight and are often not included in a routine quality control protocol.

FIG. 6.18 A, The grid ratio in this image was 6:1, 85 lines. The grid lines are obvious on the radiograph, and the grid has started to deteriorate, placing a pattern on every image and obscuring a correct reading of pathology. **B,** Grid deterioration up close. The mottled pattern is the absence of the interspace material. Newsprint was frequently used as interspace material. Over time, it would disintegrate.

FIG. 6.19 A, Another example of grid deterioration. In this case a window screen was encased in plastic and used as a grid. The window screen was slowly deteriorating and leaving areas of the image produced with no grid. **B,** A close-up of a portion of **A.**

FIG. 6.20 A, A focused grid installed upside down. The divergent rays are absorbed, and only the central rays affect the film. **B,** The grid has been installed upside down and rotated 90 degrees. The grid lines should run parallel to the tabletop.

REVIEW QUESTIONS

1. The description of the central ray includes:
   a. A primary beam projected at 90 degrees to the anode
   b. A primary beam projected at 90 degrees to the photons affecting the anode
   c. The photon array projected from the cathode
   d. The number of photons affecting the anode
2. Distortion may be useful in positioning the patient:
   a. Because it is uncomfortable on the radiography table
   b. Due to anatomy that is unnecessary on the image
   c. In order to foreshorten or elongate a body part
   d. In order to project one body part away from obscuring the region of interest
3. Blur is the intentional movement of one body part to allow the underlying anatomy to be visible.
   a. True
   b. False
4. Motion degrades the image:
   a. Because it detracts from resolution
   b. Because the image becomes darker and indistinct
   c. By arresting the movement of a wagging tail
   d. By causing the density of the image to be reduced
5. Useful distortion is used to:
   a. Prevent any body parts from superimposing on any other anatomy
   b. Project one body part out of the way of the region of interest
   c. Rotate the x-ray tube to distort the final image
   d. Superimpose one foreleg on top of the other for measurement

6. Magnification is _____ if the body part is moved _____ the image receptor.
   a. decreased, closer to
   b. decreased, farther from
   c. increased, at an angle to
   d. increased, closer to
7. The source image distance (SID) is the measurement:
   a. From the patient to the image receptor
   b. From the patient to the x-ray tube
   c. From the tube to the image receptor
   d. Including the tube and the tabletop
8. The object image distance is a factor in:
   a. Blur
   b. Distortion
   c. Magnification
   d. Rotation
9. To determine the size of an object within the patient, one must measure:
   a. The area of the region of interest
   b. The distance of the object from the tabletop using the lateral view
   c. The distance from the patient to the tabletop
   d. The size of the original collimation
10. Inherent filtration includes the:
    a. Added aluminum from the installation
    b. Distance from the tube to the patient
    c. Glass envelope of the x-ray tube and the oil within the tube
    d. Thickness and weight of the patient

11. Federal law dictates that filtration must be added to equal:
    a. 2.5 mm at 70 kV
    b. 3.5 mm at 70 kV
    c. 2.5 mm at 80 kV
    d. 3.4 mm at 80 kV
12. A collimator is located beneath the x-ray tube to:
    a. Indicate that the x-ray unit is ready to be activated
    b. Outline the size and shape of the cassette in the grid tray
    c. Provide a light source so that the patient is more visible
    d. Provide a light source outlining the area of interest
13. A secondary function of the collimator is to:
    a. Change the radiation to light coincidence
    b. Demonstrate the size of the field of view and change the focus
    c. Narrow the size of the field of view and reduce scattered radiation
    d. Narrow the size of the field of view but elongate it
14. Collimation correctly applied will _____ contrast _____.
    a. degrade, by decreasing brightness
    b. degrade, by increasing brightness
    c. enhance, by decreasing scatter
    d. enhance, by increasing scatter
15. Collimation correctly applied will _____ patient dose _____.
    a. increase, by decreasing brightness
    b. increase, by increasing scatter
    c. reduce, by decreasing scatter
    d. reduce, by increasing brightness
16. Collimation correctly applied will _____ density _____.
    a. decrease, by decreasing scatter
    b. decrease, by increasing brightness
    c. increase, by increasing scatter
    d. increase, by decreasing brightness
17. Off-focus radiation is produced:
    a. By the photon stream outside of the actual focal spot
    b. Outside the area of the focal spot and has low energy
    c. Within the patient and is not harmful to staff
    d. Within the x-ray tube but outside the collimator
18. An illuminator should be mounted:
    a. In a dimly lit area so that the illuminator does not have to be so bright
    b. In a well-lit area in the treatment area so everyone can see the image
    c. In an area where the lights may be dimmed to enhance the image
    d. So that a darker image is projected in a brightly lit area
19. The fluorescent tubes within the illuminator must be:
    a. A green tone if you are using green-receiving film
    b. Daylight or a very pale blue tone
    c. Soft light or a very pale mauve tone
    d. A light pinkish tone to match the color of green-receiving film

20. The main purpose of a grid is to:
    a. Absorb scattered radiation and enhance density
    b. Reduce scattered radiation and decrease dose
    c. Reduce scattered radiation and enhance contrast
    d. Reduce scattered radiation and reduce contrast
21. Grid ratio describes:
    a. The height of the lead strips compared with how many there are to the inch
    b. The height of the lead strips compared with the distance between them
    c. The width between the lead strips and their interspace material
    d. The width of the lead strips compared with their height
22. An installed grid is positioned beneath the patient:
    a. Above the cassette and beneath the grid tray
    b. Above the cassette and beneath the tabletop
    c. Beneath the cassette in the grid tray
    d. Beneath the patient and above the tabletop
23. The focused grid is positioned _____ and at _____ distance from the tube.
    a. beneath the cassette, any
    b. above the cassette, a prescribed
    c. in the center of the table, a prescribed
    d. in the grid tray, any
24. A grid whose focal length is 34 to 44 inches will cause:
    a. Grid cutoff if the tube is set at 44 inches
    b. Grid cutoff if the tube is set at 72 inches
    c. Scattered radiation if the tube is moved to 56 inches
    d. The grid ratio to shift if the tube is not centered

Chapter Review Question answers are located in the Instructor Resources on Evolve and can be provided to students at the discretion of the instructor.

Bibliography

American Society for Testing in Medicine. ASTM E1390-90(2000), Standard Guide for Illuminators used for Viewing Industrial Radiographs. West Conshohocken, PA: ASTM; 2000. Available at: www.astm.org.

Bushong SC. *Radiological Science for Technologists*. 11th ed. St. Louis: Elsevier; 2013.

International Commission on Radiation Protection. ICRP International Conference on Recovery after Nuclear Accidents: Radiological Protection Lessions from Fukushima and Beyond. 2020. Available at: www.icrp.org.

National Council on Radiation Protection & Measurements, United States. NCRP Report No. 148. Bethesda MD: NRCP Publications; 2015.

National Council on Radiation Protection & Measurements. Quality Assurance for Diagnostic Imaging, NCRP Report No. 099. Bethesda, MD: NCRP Publications; 1988.

Radiation Emitting Devices Act, RSC: 1985, c R-1, Canada. Available at: http://canlii.ca/t/hzzs. www.hc-sc.gc.ca/ewh-semt/pubs/radiation/safety-code_20-securite/index-eng.php.

Fauber TL. *Radiographic Imaging and Exposure*. 4th ed. St. Louis: Elsevier; 2013.

A perfectly exposed and processed x-ray film demonstrates superior imaging

CHAPTER 7
Processing the Image on Film

Lois C. Brown, RTR (Can/USA), ACR, MSc, P.Phys

The more you know, the more you know you don't know
— Aristotle – Greek philosopher – 384–322 BCE

OUTLINE

LEARNING OBJECTIVES

When you have finished this chapter, you will be able to:

1. Understand darkroom specifications.
2. Understand the purpose of developer and fixer.
3. Understand processor construction.
4. Discuss the sequence of the production of the image in the processor.
5. Explain the process of washing and drying.
6. Describe the sequence of successful processing of x-ray film.
7. Discuss the causes of darkroom fog.
8. List some causes of artifacts.

APPLICATIONS

The application of the information in this chapter is relevant to the following areas:

1. Optimizing images (radiographs) to aid in diagnoses
2. Processing film images in a manual tank or in an automatic processor

KEY TERMS

Key terms are defined in the Glossary on the Evolve website.

Activator
Ammonium thiosulfate
Antifroth
Antisludge
Artifacts
Crossover rollers
Darkroom integrity
Developer

Diffusion
Electrolysis
Feed tray
Fixer
Fixing agent
Guide shoes
Hardener
Hydroquinone

Main drive
Odor masks
Phenidone
Preservative
Processing
Recirculation
Replenishment
Restrainer

Rollers
Safelight
Solvent
Stir rods
Thermostat
Wash

Introduction

Working with x-ray film and processing is slowly being phased out of the industry. Imaging with computers as receptors and monitors as the instruments of display is slowly replacing the "old-fashioned" systems. However, there are still many facilities that have retained their film and processing, automatic or manual.

The final phase of image production is processing. Film processing in the radiography department is very similar to any photographic process. It occurs either manually with the use of wet tanks and hangers or through an automatic processor. Ninety-five percent of all imaging artifacts occur during image processing. Examples of some of these artifacts are listed in the image gallery at the end of this chapter.

Darkroom Layout (Fig. 7.1)

In a new clinic, it is useful to make the radiography room light tight and to place the processor in one corner of the room. The patient can be removed during film processing or can stay on the table as long as the room is lit with two safelights so the patient can be monitored. Using the radiography suite as a darkroom makes better use of space than a very small, cramped darkroom with the risk of chemicals splashing onto the cassettes and screens during processing. In addition, many new clinics are setting up temporary darkrooms until they can afford to purchase a digital imaging system. In such cases, when the cost of square footage is an issue, many veterinarians are prompted to use the radiography suite as a temporary darkroom.

If a darkroom is set up as a stand-alone room, it must be large enough that a person can enter, open a cassette on a counter, and place it either on a hanger or in the processor without the risk of spilling chemicals on himself or herself or the cassette. The darkroom should have a countertop large enough to open a 14 in × 17 in (35 cm × 43 cm) cassette, and the processing area should be removed from the dry film area so there is no chance of chemicals being transferred to

FIG. 7.2 Chemicals spilled on the processor between the feed tray and the developer. This chemical could easily seep down onto the processing boards, causing a malfunction and an expensive repair.

the cassettes and screens. The technician must be able to walk into the darkroom, close the door, and fit inside without any possibility of bumping into the processor or wet tanks. Once the processor is in position and the tanks are filled, it is very easy to jostle the processor and cause chemicals to overflow from one tank to another or, worse still, to splash onto the control boards, destroying them completely and causing the processor to malfunction (Fig. 7.2). A minimum darkroom size of 5 feet (1.5 m) by 7 feet (2.13 m) is sufficient to position the processor or wet tanks. One extra foot (30 cm) in both directions would be an ideal minimum.

◆ APPLICATION INFORMATION

A large-animal veterinarian installed an automatic processor in a darkroom in his basement without a safelight because he felt he could work quite well in the darkened room. Every time he turned on the processor, the replenishment pumps started to run and did not stop until he turned the processor off. The consultant told him to check the switches that the film contacts when exiting the feed tray (see Fig. 7.8C); the contacts were clean.

The consultant found that chemicals had spilled out of the developer tank and onto the main circuitry board at the front of the processor (Fig. 7.2). This short-circuited the replenishment circuit, ruining the board, which had to be replaced.

The veterinarian had bumped into the processor a few times in the dark. The chemistry tanks are full when the processor is running and the racks are in place, so chemicals had spilled out of the developer and into the main circuitry. This was a large price to pay for having a small darkroom and no safelight.

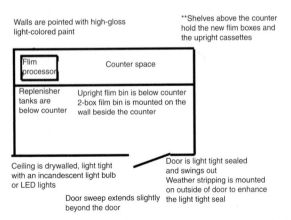

Walls are pointed with high-gloss light-colored paint

**Shelves above the counter hold the new flim boxes and the upright cassettes

| Flim processor | Counter space |

| Replenisher tanks are below counter | Upright flim bin is below counter 2-box film bin is mounted on the wall beside the counter |

Ceiling is drywalled, light tight with an incandescent light bulb or LED lights

Door sweep extends slightly beyond the door

Door is light tight sealed and swings out
Weather stripping is mounted on outside of door to enhance the light tight seal

FIG. 7.1 A Typical Ideal Darkroom Layout. The wet side is on the left and the dry side on the right. Ventilation is achieved through a door vent and a ceiling exhaust fan that is light tight.

The darkroom door should be hung to swing out from the darkroom. An inward-swinging door is not an option in a minimum-sized darkroom. Weather stripping around the entire frame of the door is essential to prevent light leaks.

Placing the weather stripping on the outside of the door prevents it from being rubbed and worn by the door opening and closing over time. Weather stripping that overlaps the edge of the door by 1 inch (2.14 cm) creates a light seal that will last as long as the room is used as a darkroom. If the floor is uneven, a light-eliminating door sweep is essential.

The temperature in the darkroom should be maintained at 68°F (20°C), and the humidity should be maintained at 40% to 60%. The door to the darkroom should be left open when not in use. This practice will maintain the temperature and humidity and will also ensure good airflow. If the darkroom is sealed too tightly, it may be difficult to close the door. A light-tight airflow pass-through is available.

The walls should be painted a light reflective color to take advantage of as much light as possible from the safelight. The countertop should be positioned between 29 inches (74 cm) and 33 inches (84 cm) above the floor.

The cassettes and film boxes must be stored upright and well away from the chemical storage (Fig. 7.3A). Ideally, a film bin will be mounted on the wall (Fig. 7.3B) to store the film out of the light and prevent accidental exposure. A metal film bin must be used if the processor and film are located in the radiography room (Fig. 7.3C). Scattered/secondary radiation will penetrate a plastic film bin unless the bin is located a minimum of 10 feet from the source of the scatter. Film should be used on a first in/first out basis so that the boxes are rotated systematically, and the film does not become stale-dated.

Ideally, the replenishment tanks are positioned beneath the tabletop processor. If this is not possible, they should be accessible both for cleaning and for "topping up" chemicals. Chemicals should be stored in their original containers until they are used. Extra chemicals should not be stored in the darkroom but rather in an appropriate storage place in the facility.

The darkroom should be cleaned regularly as part of the quality assurance program in the clinic. Dust and dirt that accumulate on the processing tray will affect the film emulsion as it is being processed. The darkroom is not a cloakroom, and coats and linens should be stored elsewhere lest the lint and dust from outdoor garments settle on the feed tray.

Darkroom Integrity

Light is very pervasive, and it is vital that all light is eliminated in the darkroom. The door of the darkroom must be light tight, and the darkroom must be completely dark. **This is nonnegotiable.** Even if the human eye does not readily see the light, the film will "see" it instantly and record it as fog.

The human eye requires about 5 to 8 minutes to adjust to darkness after being exposed to a lighted room. If the door is closed and the technician sees no visible light leaks after 5 to 8 minutes of moving about in the pitch-black dark, the integrity of the darkroom is confirmed. Complete instructions for the darkroom integrity test are included in Chapter 9.

Safelight Specifications

Film responds to color at the ultraviolet/blue-green side of the spectrum. Safelights manufactured before 1981 were Wratten series 2B red-brown. Once green light–receiving films appeared on the market, the safelight color had to change because the red-brown tint had a yellow component and the color green is made up of blue and yellow. The most common film in use today is the green-receiving film; blue-receiving film is being phased out. Therefore, when a facility purchases or replaces a safelight, the light emitted from the safelight should be dark red, with no orange or yellow (Fig. 7.4A). The safelight should be mounted on the wall a minimum of 4 feet (1.22 m) above the working surface where cassettes are loaded and unloaded.

FIG. 7.3 **A,** Cassettes are stored upright above the processor. The films are filed above the cassettes. **B,** A plastic film bin for use in the darkroom is hung on the wall. **C,** A full-sized steel bin sits on the floor and is positioned in the dual-purpose radiography/processing room.

90 seconds   60 seconds   30 seconds   Just long enough to carry to the processor

A   B

FIG. 7.4 A, A red light–emitting safelight. The filter is very important and must match the spectral sensitivity of the film. **B,** Safelight test. The film has been preexposed and placed beneath a cassette in the darkroom. The exposure time has allowed the film to fog. The safelight should be checked and altered, and then the test should be repeated.

Correctly processed film out of the box with no image will be completely clear, with only the base + fog as density. The optical density will be less than 0.10. Fig. 7.4B shows the results of a safelight test in which there was a definite problem with the positioning or wattage of the safelight. For complete instructions for performing a safelight test, see Chapter 9.

Film Identifiers

The traditional veterinary identification (ID) labels and labeling tape are slowly being phased out because they are not as efficient now that a lead replacement material is being used to produce the labeling tape (Fig. 7.5A). Individual lead lettering is certainly sharper but very time consuming because each patient's information must be set up one letter at a time (Fig. 7.5B).

An electric or battery-operated photoidentifier is preferable, and the information is much clearer on the images than those produced by the older method.

An electric or battery-operated photoidentifier works in conjunction with the cassettes (Fig. 7.5C). A light cardstock or standard typing paper is used with a template to write or type the information. Fig. 7.5D is an example of a label that has been typed. A black marker fine-point pen can also be used.

The following steps must be taken before using the labeler:

1. Choose the same corner of every cassette and put a black label on each screen in the appropriate corner inside the cassette. The label material can be black cardstock or even blackened x-ray film held in place with double-sided sticky tape. These blockers will prevent the radiation from affecting the screen in that area. Use the same label position on every cassette in the facility.
2. Label the cassettes on the outside over the blocked-off portion so that patient anatomy and identifying markers are not positioned over the blocker.

3. ID labels must be printed and include the patient's name, date, ID number, and the name and address of the veterinary facility. This is required legal information in most countries and must be visible on each film.
4. Once the film is exposed, take it to the darkroom and remove it from the cassette. Place the film in the photoidentifier and press down on the lid of the identifier. This will turn on a timed light flash, which exposes the film through the printed label and imprints the label information onto the film.
5. Process the film normally.

With this method, each film is identified before processing. This is by far the most efficient method of identifying individual films.

Secondary film identifiers such as right and left markers, positioning markers (VD, DV, upright), and time of day must all be positioned within the radiation area and must be clearly identifiable (Fig. 7.5E).

A Word About Chemicals

As human hospitals and veterinary clinics convert to digital radiography and cancel their chemical contracts, chemical suppliers have been challenged to support their business by switching to the sale of other products. As a result, the production of processing chemicals has reduced considerably. In addition, the developer and fixer components have been altered to remove any product that does not directly involve actually processing the films.

Along with the antisludge and antifrothing components, some manufacturers have removed most of the odor masks. As a result, the smell of the chemicals has emerged to a point at which it is objectionable to stay in the darkroom for any length of time. One way to address this problem is to search for a brand of chemicals that has not removed the odor mask; such brands are quite easy to find. The fixer is the

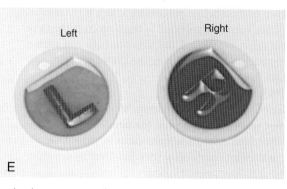

Eastern Veterinary Hospital

1234 Pet Hospital Way, Akron, Ohio, 46777

Name:	Weasily Whiskas Brown	
Views:	VD Chest, Lateral Chest	
Date:	December 21, 2017	DVM: Dr McHappy

Printed ID Label with two different labels
used for two different patients

Eastern Veterinary Hospital

1234 Pet Hospital Way, Akron, Ohio 46777

Name:	I Curious Tiberius Brown	
Views:	VD Abdomen, Lateral Abdomen	
Date:	December 21, 2017	DVM: DR McNice

Left   Right

FIG. 7.5 A, A leaded tape labeler. After the identification details are written on the tape. It is attached to a small plastic and aluminum filter that is color graded according to the kilovoltage that is used. It is then placed on the table within the collimated area. **B,** A metal marker. The metal is usually aluminum, and the individual letters are lead. The identifying letters are loaded into the guide for each individual patient. The marker is then placed on the tabletop within the collimated area. **C,** An electric ID labeler ready to be used. An ID card is written up and placed in the unit. The film is placed in the unit and the top is pressed down, which turns on a light. The image of the marker is imprinted onto the film. The film is then processed normally. **D,** An example of an ID label to be cut apart and used with the ID labeler in C. **E,** Left and right markers. The shape is less important than the thickness of the lead. They must be visible on every image.

worst culprit, and sampling various brands of fixer is quite straightforward as long as the chemicals from two different companies are never mixed together in one tank.

Another solution to the odor problem is to increase the ventilation in the darkroom. Adding a fan and keeping the darkroom door open when it is not in use is helpful. A light-tight air vent window is also available. This mesh window, which is installed in the darkroom door at eye level, allows air but not light to pass through. Known as *darkroom light-tight airflow pass-throughs*, these windows are available from any supplier of photography equipment or radiography accessories.

✎ TECHNICIAN NOTE

Safety Alert!
The Workplace Hazardous Materials Information System (WHMIS) and the Occupational Safety and Health Administration (OSHA) require that safety glasses and gloves be used whenever chemicals are handled.

The developer is highly alkaline, and the fixer is highly acidic (Table 7.1). Both chemicals must be treated with great respect. A drop of fixer concentrate can melt the lens of the eye in seconds. An eyewash station must be positioned close to the processing area and must be checked regularly by the clinic's quality assurance officer. When handling chemicals, it is essential that personnel are equipped with protective safety goggles and rubber gloves. These are inexpensive are available for purchase at any hardware or department store.

Automatic processing also helps reduce the odor to a degree because the chemical containers remain covered during processing.

One other problem that has resulted from the changes in chemistry concerns the mixing of the chemicals. In manual processing, it is very important to stir the chemicals with an up-and-down motion before processing a film. If the chemicals stratify, the hardener will sink to the bottom of the tank and will not affect the film. A stainless-steel stir rod with a flat bottom plate is ideal for stirring the chemistry.

Developer Components

The developer is an alkaline solution with a pH of 9.8 to 11.0. The two main components in the developer are phenidone and hydroquinone. Their function is to reduce the silver halide in the film emulsion to metallic silver by donating

TABLE 7.1	Acidity/Alkalinity of Processing Solutions	
COMPONENT	**ACID/ALKALINE**	**pH**
Developer	Alkaline	9.8–11.4
Fixer	Acidic	4.0–4.5
Water	Neutral	6.5–7.5*

*Ideally, the pH of water is 7.0. Most tap water is either slightly acidic or slightly alkaline.

additional electrons to the sensitivity specks in the latent image center. This is what creates the blacks and grays in the image. The other, and equally important, function is to amplify the amount of metallic silver on the film by increasing the number of silver atoms deposited in each latent image center. Unexposed silver halide in the film emulsion does not react to the developer chemicals because it has not been ionized and therefore will not accept electrons from the solution. Table 7.2 lists the developer components and their functions.

❓ POINTS TO PONDER

The components of the developer and fixer have changed dramatically over the years. The chemical manufacturers have developed products that mix together and meet most municipal hazardous waste standards. Therefore, in most communities, it is safe to dispose of the chemicals down the drain in small effluent quantities with the other waste products from the facility.

Each facility should review the chemical waste guidelines with its municipality and must always have the component sheets from the chemical manufacturer on hand. The hazardous materials sheets for most chemicals are available online and are always available from the manufacturer.

It is important to note that clear water makes up 98% to 99% of the liquid in the chemical bottles that are then diluted again when mixed for use.

Fixer Components

The main ingredient in the fixer is ammonium thiosulfate. Sulfur is another component, and if the fixer breaks down for any reason, the sulfur precipitates and a rotten egg smell pervades the area (a process known as *sulfiding*).

Another important ingredient is the hardener, which can be one of three types (Table 7.3) The function of the hardener is to ensure that the emulsion stays attached to the base. The chemicals in a manual tank must be stirred with an up-and-down motion or the hardener will remain at the bottom of the tank. If the film is then left in the wash for an extended period, the emulsion will slide off the base.

◆ APPLICATION INFORMATION

A veterinarian had an overnight emergency in which radiographs were required and accidentally left in the wash tank until the next morning. The films were completely clear with no emulsion left on the film base. The consultant who was called in reminded the veterinarian that the chemistry must be stirred thoroughly before processing the film. In her haste the night before, she had processed the films without previously stirring the chemistry. The hardener had stratified out to the bottom of the tank and so had not affected the films she processed. During the balance of the night, the unhardened emulsion had slipped to the bottom of the tank, leaving the clear film base on the hangers.

TABLE 7.2 Developer Components and Their Functions

AGENT	CHEMICAL	FUNCTION	KEY TO REMEMBERING
Developing agent	Phenidone	Fast—produces the gray densities, stable, and long lived	**Ph**enidone—**ph**ast—mainly grays
Developing agent	Hydroquinone	Slow—produces blacks; increases contrast on the image; sensitive to temperature, oxygen, and aging	**Longer** name—**longer** time—mainly blacks The sensitive one; reacts to time, temperature, gases, and air, and will be the first to become exhausted
Activator	Sodium carbonate	Produces the alkaline pH and swells the gelatin	**Bi**carbonate of soda (alkaline) reduces the acidity in your stomach if you have eaten rich food
Restrainer	Potassium bromide	Decreases the reduction of the unexposed silver halide	This is the stopper—**POT**A**S**Sium (read it backward)
Preservative	Sodium sulfite	Decreases sensitivity to oxidation	
Hardener		"Glues" the emulsion to the base to reduce scratches from the processor	
Solvent	Water	Makes up about 98%–99% of the solution	

TABLE 7.3 Fixer Components and Their Functions

AGENT	CHEMICAL	FUNCTION	KEY TO REMEMBERING
Fixing agent	Sodium thiosulfate	Clears away unexposed silver halide	This causes the rotten egg smell
Acidifier	Acetic acid	Stops development	Vinegar
Preservative	Sodium sulfite	Prevents a reaction between fixing agent and acidifier	Same as developer
Hardener	Chrome alum, potassium aluminum sulfate, or aluminum chloride	Hardens the emulsion	Similar to what is in your deodorant—a drying agent
Solvent	Water	Makes up about 98%–99% of the solution	

Manual (Nonautomatic) Processing

Some low-volume sites still process film manually. The chemicals used in manual processing are the same as for automatic processing, except that the temperature and time are very different (Fig. 7.6A and Table 7.4).

Safety and Protocols

Cleanliness is essential during film processing because it is very easy to splash chemicals onto the cassettes and screens. In the manual processing area, the cassettes must never be left open on the counter.

Chemical fumes can be irritating, and the chemicals are dangerous to ingest or splash into one's eyes. Safety glasses must be worn by anyone processing film or replenishing chemicals (see WHMIS/OSHA guidelines). A 14 in × 17 in (35 cm × 43 cm) film is lifted almost parallel with the eyes when the hangers are moved from tank to tank. It is very important that the technician is careful not to splash chemicals during this procedure.

The wet tanks are always checked for the correct temperature (68°F [20°C]), and the chemicals are agitated immediately before processing the films. This is the only time the chemicals are agitated. Agitating the chemicals before radiography is premature, and the chemicals will have settled by the time the film is introduced into the tanks.

Equipment for Manual Processing
Wet Tanks
The welds on a stainless-steel tank must be stainless steel welds. If the tanks are not welded correctly, the welding material will corrode in the first few weeks. The chemistry will be contaminated, and the wash water will always be cloudy and rust colored. After that, the tank will start to leak through pinpoint holes in the welding material.

An alternative tank construction is heavy plastic. After about 10 to 15 years, the plastic will absorb chemicals and leach out into fresh developer. This eventually will contaminate the fresh chemicals within days or even hours.

FIG. 7.6 A, Manual processing tank. Lids cover the developer tank *(left)* and the fixer tank *(right)*. The common wash tank is in the middle. Temperature is maintained by circulating water in the wash at the correct temperature. **B,** A stainless steel stir rod. Note the flat plate at the bottom with holes *(see inset)*. The stir rod is used in an up-and-down motion to bring the chemicals up from the bottom of the tank.

TABLE 7.4	Development/Fixer/Washing Guidelines*	
PROCESS	**TIME**	**TEMPERATURE**
Developer	4 minutes with agitation	68°F (20°C)
Rinse*	15–30 seconds with agitation	68°F (20°C)
Fixing	8 minutes with agitation	68°F (20°C)
Washing	12 minutes with agitation	68°F (20°C)

*Applies to manual processing only.

★ **APPLICATION INFORMATION**

A consultant received a frantic call from a veterinarian who had changed the chemicals in the developer before radiographing a dog that had swallowed a peach pit. The dog had not eaten for several days and was in distress; the veterinarian needed to know the location of the peach pit. When he took the films out of the plastic developer tank, there was a very faint image—not nearly diagnostic. Overlying the image was a "watercolor" artifact of every color of the rainbow. Reds, yellows, blues, purples, and blacks were running down the film. He took several more films and then searched for help.

The consultant was driving near the hospital when she received the call and by total coincidence had a stainless steel, 5-gallon processing tank in her car. She drove to the hospital and, together with the veterinary staff, mixed new chemistry in the darkroom. The images were perfect, the peach pit was located, and the surgery went well.

The developer drained out of the old tank was severely contaminated. They switched out the stainless-steel tank and placed it in the plastic main tank, and the next day they did the same thing with the fixer tank. The hospital never again had a problem with contaminated chemistry.

Stir Rods

One stir rod is all that is necessary, provided that it is used in the correct order: developer first, then fixer, then wash (Fig. 7.6B). The stir stick may be rinsed between the developer and the fixer, but it is not essential. The stir stick must move sequentially through the developer → fixer → wash—not the other way around—otherwise fixer will be brought back into the developer on the stir rod. This can cause an artifact called *dichroic fog*.

The stir stick must be made of stainless steel. Wooden paddles, stir rods, and broom handles will all absorb chemicals that will be leached out when used to stir fresh chemicals. The end of the stir rod is a flat plate with holes punched through it. The technician stirs the chemicals using an up-and-down motion. This up-and-down motion reduces the tendency for the chemicals to overflow the tanks, but it also brings the stratified liquids up from the bottom of the tank to mix thoroughly. Ten to fifteen vertical motions are all that is necessary to completely mix the chemicals.

★ **APPLICATION INFORMATION**

In this time of environmentally friendly chemicals, the components of the chemicals tend to stratify when they are left to sit. The "new" hardener components settle to the bottom of the tank, below the level of the hangers. This is a problem if the chemicals are not stirred immediately before processing.

If the films are left in the water too long (say, overnight), the emulsion will slide off the film base onto the bottom of the tank. This is due to the revised components in the chemicals. The environmentally friendly hardener is not as effective in "gluing" the emulsion to the base until the film is washed and then dried.

Film Hangers

Once the film is removed from the cassette and identified (if a photo ID labeler is used), it is then hung on a film hanger (Fig. 7.7) in preparation for processing. Film hangers have flexible clips at the top and stationary clips at the bottom. The film is hung on the stationary clips first and then on the

FIG. 7.7 The film is placed in a hanger for manual processing. The bottom clips are loaded first and then the spring clips are attached.

flexible (spring-equipped) clips at the top. Some hangers have channels into which the film is slid. These are rare, however, and are also difficult to keep clean.

Processing

Timing the exposure of the films to the chemicals and maintaining the temperature of the chemicals is very important, particularly in manual (nonautomatic) processing. If the developer solution is overheated or the film is left in the solution for an extended time, the unexposed crystals start to react to the solution and "developer fog" occurs.

Chemical manufacturers produce a solution that is optimized for manual processing at 68°F (20°C). It is not a coincidence that this is also the average room temperature in a veterinary clinic. The chemicals do not need to be heated or cooled before use.

The technique chart should be optimized so the film is processed at 4 minutes in the manual developer at 68°F (20°C). If the image appears too quickly or too slowly, the technical factors should be adjusted, not the temperature of the chemicals. The hydroquinone works slowly to build up the blacks and therefore enhance the contrast of the image. If the solution is either too hot or too cold, the hydroquinone does not function correctly and the image is compromised.

Developing the Image

Developing the image is the first step in processing the film. The purpose of the developer is to cause the latent image to become a manifest image. This change is achieved by immersing the film in a chemical solution. The developer has two main components and several other auxiliary components (see Table 7.2).

The unexposed areas of the film are not affected unless the film is left in the developer for too long. If this occurs, the unexposed areas will start to react to the developer, and the film will increase in overall density (developer fog).

The hanger is held by the top (handle), and the film is introduced into the chemicals slowly and steadily. Once the film is completely immersed, it is agitated slowly in an up-and-down motion several times to ensure that any air bubbles that have entered with the film are removed. The timer is set for *4 minutes*. At 2 minutes, the film is agitated up and down once again. This moves away the used chemicals directly next to the film and places fresher chemicals against the film.

◆ APPLICATION INFORMATION

With manual processing, it is very important that the technical factors used to produce the image are correct. The film must take the correct length of time to process because the hydroquinone takes longer to start affecting the emulsion than does the phenidone. Therefore, if the film is removed too early, the full effect of blackening the image will not occur. "Overexposing and underdeveloping" is not a good practice; safe exposure factors must be practiced in all facilities.

Rinsing the Film

At 4 minutes, the film is agitated up and down two to four times and then moved to the intermediary wash tank. It is agitated two to four times in the wash tank to arrest the development and remove some of the developer, and then it is placed in the fixer tank.

Fixing the Image

Fixing the image to the film is the third step in manual processing. Here the image is made visible by removing all of the emulsion that has not been affected by radiation and subsequent developing.

The film is placed into the fixer tank using the same method: introduced slowly and steadily and then agitated up and down. This agitation will remove air bubbles that have been carried into the fixer and remain on the film.

The timer is set for *8 minutes*. At 2 minutes, the light may be turned on and the film may be checked. If there is still unexposed emulsion on the film, the fixer is no longer fresh and should be changed once the films are processed. At 4 minutes, the film should have cleared completely and may be viewed momentarily on an illuminator by the staff.

Once the film is reviewed, it must be put back into the fixer to complete the fixing process. It is essential that the fixing process be completed to ensure the archival quality of the image.

Washing the Film

The film is removed from the fixer and lowered into the wash tank. It is preferable for the wash tank to have flowing water. Ideally, the water should enter from the bottom of the tank and exit from the top through a standpipe placed in the drain.

The entire film, including the hangers, must be immersed in each solution. The fixer cleans the developer out of the clips of the hangers, and the wash removes the fixer from the hangers and leaves them clean for the next film.

As the clean water flows over the film, it is washed by a diffusion process. The chemicals in the fixer are diffused into the wash water. The water must move around the film so that a concentration of fixer does not remain within the emulsion of the film.

Hanging the films in static clean water will work only if the films are agitated frequently during the wash time. The wash time is *12 minutes* with flowing water. Once again, it is important to wash the films to ensure archival quality. If the used fixer is not removed, the films will turn yellow-brown within weeks (see Fig. 7.26 in the image gallery at the end of the chapter).

Running a hose over the films for 2 to 3 minutes in a bathtub is not sufficient to wash the films thoroughly. This problem is evident on a film reviewed several weeks after it has been dried and stored. Sulfiding and staining are the result of poor washing.

It is vitally important to remove the films from the wash water and place them on the drying rack within a maximum 2 to 3 hours of washing (see the Application Information box).

◆ APPLICATION INFORMATION

A veterinarian looked at 4-week previous films of a patient with a fractured leg, only to discover that the films had changed color to a brown-yellow. Washing the films was regularly done very carefully by running the hose in the bathtub over the films for a "couple of minutes." The hose washing method cannot replace washing the films in a tank with running water for 12 minutes.

Drying the Film

If the processing is completed correctly, there are no artifacts on the films. The drying process takes several hours because even though the films feel dry to the touch, the emulsion takes longer to dry completely. If the films are placed in the envelopes too soon, they will stick together and will be impossible to separate without damaging, and in extreme cases, actually tearing the film.

The film must be dried either by hanging the films in a dryer cabinet or by allowing them to dry naturally in the air of the clinic. Drying removes 85% to 90% of the moisture in the film emulsion. If too much moisture is removed, the emulsion will crack, compromising the quality of the image.

The film is now ready to be reviewed and stored permanently.

Automatic Processing

Equipment

The automatic processor facilitates the routine of producing a manifest image on the film. It must do so quickly, efficiently, and without imprinting an artifact or scratching the emulsion off the film during the process. Most automatic processors now are sold as "90-second" processors, which means that the film enters the processor and exits within 90 seconds (Fig. 7.8A).

Because processors are smaller and fit nicely on a table or countertop, this arrangement works very well for veterinary hospitals.

Feed Tray

The feed tray is situated at the entrance of the processor (Fig. 7.8B). The film is placed either horizontally or vertically on this tray, and then accepted into the processor by means of the motor drive. It is essential that the film is placed squarely on the tray. When a film enters the feed tray, it is within 1 to 2 inches (2.5 to 5 cm) of the developer.

Once the film enters the processor, it *must not, under any circumstances,* be drawn back onto the tray, as at least three things can happen if the film is drawn back:

- Developer will be deposited onto the replenishment switches, which are situated just at the edge of the entrance to the processor (Fig. 7.8C). Developer becomes very sticky when it dries. If even one of the replenishment switches sticks open, it will pump the replenishment chemicals continuously through the processor until the tanks are empty. If this problem is not noticed in time, the pump will burn out because there are no chemicals flowing through it.
- The rack may be lifted off the gears and not only damage the gears but also compromise the position of the rack for the next film.
- The developer solution is smeared on the tray, where it will adversely affect the next film that is placed on the feed tray.

The feed tray may be stainless steel or plastic. Either way, if the air in the darkroom is dry, static may build up on the tray and discharge when a film is placed on it. The feed tray should be wiped with a fabric softener cloth at the beginning of the day to prevent static buildup (see Fig. 7.27 in the image gallery at the end of the chapter).

The processor is essentially an assembly line in which the film is drawn across a series of rollers through the developer, fixer, and wash tanks. The rollers in series from a typical processor are shown in Fig. 7.8D.

The film is affected by several systems once it enters the processor. Each system is vital to the production of the final image (Table 7.5).

Film Transport

The processor must be built so all rollers move at the same speed and are positioned to transport the film evenly and continuously with no hesitation through the developer, fixer, wash, and the dryer (Fig. 7.9). The rollers that transport the film must be close enough together to move the film but far enough apart that they transport the film without imprinting a pressure artifact or otherwise scratching the emulsion. The rollers must be firm enough to transport the film without absorbing chemicals and imprinting the stale chemicals onto films processed later in the day. In

Wash water inlet
Wash water drain
Inlet for fresh chemistry
Drain
Drain for used developer
Inlet for fresh chemistry
Dryer behind shield
Main drive shaft
Feed tray to developer

FIG. 7.8 A, Tabletop automatic processor. The round knobs on the side drain the developer, fixer, and wash tanks. The feed tray is to the right. The processed film will drop out of the dryer slot on the left onto the top of the processor. **B,** Automatic processor feed tray. The film to be processed is placed on the tray and the lid is closed, providing a light-tight seal. **C,** On this processor, four small fingers *(arrows point to two of them)* are pressed down when the film slides through the feed tray into the developer. The replenishment pumps stay activated while these fingers are depressed. **D,** The Konica SRX-101A Processor *(top view)* with the lid and racks removed.

TABLE 7.5	Automatic Processor Systems
SYSTEM	**FUNCTION**
Transport system	Chain or gear mechanism moves the rollers by a process of gears and drive shaft in order to transport the film through the processor (see Fig. 7.9).
Replenishment	Two pumps are set to replenish the chemicals (developer and fixer) so that they maintain consistent pH and solution concentration throughout the day.
Recirculation	Mixes the fresh chemicals with the working solutions so that the films are processed evenly.
Thermostats	Two—maintain a consistent temperature in the working solution and in the dryer.
Silver recovery	Not part of the processor, but an essential unit placed in the outgoing fixer line.

addition, they must be soft enough that they do not damage the fragile wet emulsion.

Every time a roller touches the film, there is the possibility of an artifact or damage to the fragile emulsion. The main drive motor must be high quality to ensure that it runs evenly and consistently for many years. The Teflon gears must be solid and resist cracking or breaking (see Fig. 7.9B).

There are several varieties of film processor on the market. The unit used to demonstrate the internal workings in this text is a Konica model SRX 101A. The film is guided by the rollers, and the curves and turns it must make are guided mostly by sheets of high-grade stainless steel or high-grade smooth plastic. These "guide shoes" have raised ridges that hold the film away from the turnarounds as it is transported through the processor (see Fig. 7.9A). This particular method of travel is called *undulating* because the film is guided in a wavelike path (Fig. 7.10).

Larger processors use a system of offset rollers and a vertical transport system. The film enters the processor and is transported by means of the entrance roller assembly into the developer tank (Fig. 7.11). At the bottom and top of each turn, a large roller (called a *sun roller*) turns the film 180 degrees and sends it back up the assembly to meet a guide shoe at the top, which then turns it back down through

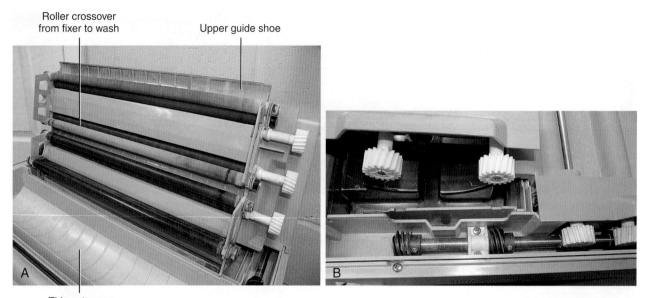

FIG. 7.9 A, The transport system. This figure shows the developer fixer rack tilted out of the processor to show the gears—which will mesh with the drive shaft when it is put in place—and the rollers. **B,** A closeup of the main drive shaft. The gears will mesh with the windings on the shaft, allowing each roller to move steadily and consistently without hesitation. The gears are lifted on the left and are in place on the right.

FIG. 7.10 A tabletop processor showing undulating film travel. The line drawing is of an Agfa tabletop processor. The large jugs behind the processor are the replenishment tanks.

the fixer. A unit of this size is most efficient when it is processing 150 films per hour. A typical veterinary clinic, even a busy clinic, does not handle that volume of films, and so a tabletop processor is quite adequate.

The most efficient and easiest processor to maintain is one with very few rollers and an efficient and reliable transport system. The Konica SRX model (see Fig. 7.8D) is an example of this type of processor. There are few rollers, and each one is easy to see and access if there is a problem. The roller assembly is fairly easy to take apart and service

because each rack assembly is easily lifted out of the processor and washed. Daily maintenance is quite simple.

The main drive motor on a tabletop processor is connected to a simple geared shaft that fits to the gears on the roller assembly (see Fig. 7.9). This arrangement ensures that all rollers turn at exactly the same speed. A broken or worn gear may cause an inconsistency in the rotation of the gears. This problem is easily identified by lifting the lid of the processor and watching for a hesitation or "bumping" of the rack assembly.

Feed tray Developing Fixing Washing

Drying chamber

Receiving bin

FIG. 7.11 A large floor-model processor demonstrating film traveling through the three tanks and into a long dryer on the right. The film exits into a bin almost at floor level. (From Fauber TL. *Radiographic Imaging and Exposure.* 5th ed. St. Louis: Mosby; 2017.)

? POINTS TO PONDER   Every time a roller comes into contact with the film, it has the potential to damage the emulsion and imprint an artifact on the film. The more rollers there are, the easier it is for them to damage films. Cleanliness and quality control of the processor are vital, especially if the processor has many rollers. In most veterinary facilities, tabletop processors work well. It is best to purchase a processor with as few rollers as possible.

Chemical Replenishment

The chemicals in the working tanks become exhausted as the chemicals interact with the silver halides in the emulsion of the film. The developer also interacts with air, which reduces its effectiveness. The fixer is weakened from the silver halides that it removes from the film base and by the introduction of developer carried over in the film emulsion.

The film is processed by the chemicals in the individual tanks. It is important that fresh chemicals are introduced as the old, used chemicals are removed. The dimensions of the film and the method by which they are fed into the feed tray

determine the amount of replenishment. The switches for replenishment are situated at the back end of the processor, immediately below the feed tray (Fig. 7.12A). Every processor built after 2000 will have a method of monitoring the replenishment, whether it is inside the processor itself or outside, as is the case with the Konica 101A.

The tanks that hold the fresh chemicals are situated close to the processor and are joined by tubing and a pump within the processor that supplies the fresh chemicals when needed (Fig. 7.12B). There are two replenishment pumps. One pump for the developer is set to deliver approximately 60 mL of chemicals for every 14 inches (35 cm) of film. The second pump for the fixer is set to deliver approximately 110 mL of chemicals for every 14 inches (35 cm) of film. The amounts of chemicals are different because the film entering the developer is dry and is affected only by the developer. The film then carries contaminant (developer) into the fixer and also removes fixer when it leaves. Therefore, the fixer requires more replenishment to keep it fresh and to replenish what is removed.

A quick check on the levels in the replenisher tanks will show that the fixer level drops almost twice as fast as the developer level. If this is not occurring, the lines and pumps should be checked for kinks or bends that are preventing the chemicals from flowing correctly.

A second form of replenishment is called *"flood replenishing"* in which the chemicals are replenished at timed intervals independent of the amount of film used. This arrangement works well if a low amount of film is being processed through a large processor. Because the volume of chemicals is great and the film volume is low, it is much more difficult to maintain stability and concentration of the chemicals. This system is not available on many tabletop processors but it is available on most free-standing large processors.

The replenishment tanks are normally positioned beneath the counter that holds the processor (see Fig. 7.12B). The developer and fixer tanks must be monitored continually so the chemicals do not reach abnormally low levels or empty completely.

Chemical Recirculation

When fresh chemicals are delivered to the working tank, they must be introduced gradually and in a portion of the

Replenishment and run light

A

B

FIG. 7.12 A, The replenishment and run lights on this processor are at the front and easily accessed. **B,** The developer *(left)* and fixer *(right)* replenishment tanks are stored beneath the processor.

processor separate from where the film is traveling. The fresh chemicals are much more active and will react quickly with the emulsion on the film. This can cause a plus-density artifact on the film—a pattern of the spray of the new chemicals across the film (see Fig. 7.25 in the image gallery at the end of the chapter).

In some tabletop processors, the working chemicals in the processing tanks are directed into an auxiliary tank within the processor. It is here that the fresh chemicals are introduced to the working chemicals, and together they enter the working tank. Some processors have a baffle system so the chemicals are introduced and immediately directed away from the film being processed.

Thermostat

There are two main thermostats in the processor. One maintains the temperature of the chemicals, and the other maintains the temperature of the dryer:

- The typical temperature of the developer and fixer solutions is 93°F (34°C).
- The typical dryer temperature is 131°F (55°C).

It must be noted that the thermostat does not have a cooling function. If the temperature in the darkroom is very hot, the thermostat will not cool the chemicals.

Heating coils may be placed in the bottom of the developer and fixer tanks, or the heaters may be placed in the recirculation system. It is essential to maintain a constant temperature in the developer and fixer tanks because the activity of the processing solutions depends directly on the temperature.

The dryer temperature is important to ensure that the films exiting the dryer are dry and not sticky to the touch. They must not be overheated or the emulsion may crack and split.

Dryer System

The rollers in the dryer must be suitable to transport the film while it dries, and the temperature must be hot enough to eliminate about 80% of the moisture. If the film is dried too much, the emulsion will crack and degrade the image. If the film is not dried sufficiently, it will be sticky to the touch, and if several films are laid on top of each other, they will stick together and be impossible to break apart.

The ideal dryer temperature depends very much on how long the film will be traveling through the dryer. The temperature will be noted in the instruction manual of each processor or can be found online by searching for the make and model of the processor.

Developing the Image

The chemistry used in the automatic processor is the same as the chemistry used in manual processing. The typical temperature is 34°C (93°F). The length of time that the film is in the developer solution is set up for every individual processor and programmed so the chemicals have time to react sufficiently to optimize the image. As noted in the replenishment section, the rates of replenishment are preset to preserve the correct concentrations of developer and fixer.

The image is in the formation stage while in the developer, and many problems can occur during this process. In fact, approximately 80% of processing artifacts occur during the development stage. The image may be deleted in places where the latent image undergoes pressure from a swollen roller, or it may acquire density from other factors. The image gallery at the end of this chapter illustrates developer artifacts.

Fixing the Image

The main purpose of the fixer (see Table 7.3) is to remove the unexposed silver halide from the film base and ensure that the image that has been developed remains intact and permanent. The fixer also stops the development of any unexposed crystals of silver halide (by removing them from the film base) and it hardens the image to the base. The image is "fixed" onto the base by a two-stage process:

- Clearing—the unexposed emulsion is cleared from the film base.
- Fixing—the remaining emulsion is stabilized onto the base.

Fixing occurs after developing and stabilizes the emulsion to the base. The emulsion before this stage is very thin and easily marked or scratched off the base. If the film is not fixed correctly, it exits the processor with a milky or even pink appearance (see Fig. 7.23 and other fixer artifacts in the image gallery at the end of the chapter).

Washing the Film

The film travels through the fixer and into the wash tank. It must be thoroughly washed to preserve its archival quality. Staining or sulfiding results if the film is not washed with flowing water (see Fig. 7.26 in the image gallery at the end of this chapter).

The wash should provide clean water that flows through the processor as the films are being washed. Washing takes place by a process called *diffusion*. The wash water contains less thiosulfate than the fixer, and so the chemicals in the fixer are diffused into the wash water. The water must move about the film so a concentration of fixer does not build up next to the film. This is achieved by the action of the rollers and fresh water running through the processor.

If the wash water is not turned on, the film will appear "dirty" in reflected light. It may be "sticky" when touched. Sulfiding and staining are the result of poor washing and are also evident on a film that is reviewed several weeks after it has been dried and stored. To review artifacts connected with washing the film, please review the image gallery at the end of this chapter.

Drying the Film

As noted, earlier, the dryer temperature should be set to ensure that the films are not tacky or sticky. Approximately 85% to 95% of the moisture should be removed from the films as they travel through the dryer. If they are too hot when they emerge, the film base may become fragile and crack.

FIG. 7.13 A Silver Recovery Unit Is Attached to the Outflow of the Fixer Tank.

FIG. 7.14 These films are stored alphabetically in a solid wood cabinet in the darkroom.

If the dryer temperature is optimized and the films are still slightly damp, adjusting the replenishment rates in the processor may solve the issue.

Silver Recovery

It is the function of the fixer to remove the unexposed silver halides from the film base (Fig. 7.13), resulting in a high concentration of silver halides floating in the fixer. If this silver is not removed from the fixer and the fixer is not correctly replenished, the silver may plate out onto the film. (See Fig. 7.22 in the image gallery at the end of the chapter.) A silver recovery unit removes the silver from the effluent of the processor as it exits the fixer tank.

> ### ◆ APPLICATION INFORMATION
>
> A good method to test whether the silver recovery unit needs to be replaced is to place a copper penny or a piece of copper pipe in its outflow. The copper penny is electrolytic and attracts the silver ions, which plate onto the copper. If the copper turns silver, it is time to replace the cartridge.

Metallic Replacement

The silver recovery unit typically used in veterinary clinics consists of a glass jar containing steel wool. The effluent from the fixer tank enters the jar on one side and is directed through the steel wool. The acidic fixer breaks down the iron in steel wool and replaces it with silver. The iron oxides are replaced by silver as it precipitates onto the remaining steel wool.

Electrolysis

A second method of silver recovery is an electrolytic process that is used mainly for large-volume units. A very low current flows through a unit equipped with metal plates, and the negatively charged silver ions bind to the plates. This method is the easiest way to collect the metallic silver, but if the current is flowing and there is no silver, the fixer may start to break down. Because the main component of fixer is sulfur, a terrible odor may result as it starts to break down. This process is called *sulfiding,* and the smell is exactly the same as rotten eggs.

Film Storage

After processing, the finished image is now available for viewing and storage. Films should be stored in individual envelopes specific to each patient. They should be stored upright in slotted shelves (Fig. 7.14).

Film should be stored in a temperature-controlled area (68° F [20° C]). Ideal humidity in the storage room is 40% to 60%. If the humidity is too high, the emulsion absorbs the moisture and the films stick together. They are virtually impossible to separate unless they are soaked in water. However, if there was insufficient hardener in the processing chemicals, soaking the films in water will only serve to lift the emulsion off the base.

Image Artifacts

Artifacts may be categorized into three groups: equipment artifacts, processing artifacts, and handling artifacts.

Processing is the single greatest cause of artifacts on the films. As already stated, 98% of all film artifacts are due to problems with processing. With automatic processing, the emulsion is softened and the rollers must touch the film as they transport it from tank to tank. The distance between the rollers is very narrow, and if a roller should swell, it will place a plus-density or minus-density mark on the film.

Artifacts are categorized as visible by reflected light (looking at the film as a page out of a book) or by transmitted light (reviewing a film hung on an illuminator). Most artifacts are visible by transmitted light. Artifacts that are visible by reflected light are very difficult to illustrate in a textbook and consist mainly of the following:

- Smear artifacts from water drips after the film is processed
- Dichroic fog from fixer that has leaked into the developer; the fixer will eventually contaminate the developer but, initially, the films will come out of the automatic processor with an array of colors visible by reflected light

FIG. 7.15 An Example of an Equipment Artifact. A collimator screw on the Plexiglas cover appears superimposed on a radiograph. The small screw fell out of the collimator shutter onto the collimator window. It was not noticed until the image was processed. Because of the distance to the patient, it is also magnified.

◆ APPLICATION INFORMATION

The darkroom of a brand-new veterinary hospital was equipped with an automatic processor, cassettes, and film. Business was slow at first, and even though the processor had been set up correctly, it was 6 weeks before a patient that needed radiographs arrived.

The films turned out gray and washed out, and subsequent films showed only a brief outline. A consultant checked the x-ray unit and found that exposures were producing x-rays and the calibration was in order.

Next, she checked the chemistry. The developer was dark brown, almost black. The processor had been used on the day the hospital opened to confirm the settings on the technique chart. The chemistry was heated and produced excellent images the first day but then sat and oxidized slowly over the next 6 weeks. As a result, the developer in the processor was completely contaminated and had to be cleared out from both the working tank and the replenishment tank.

New, fresh chemistry was installed, and the resulting images were excellent.

Summary

This chapter has discussed image processing and all of the protocols and problems associated with chemicals, films, screens, and cassettes. We also discussed artifacts and the situations that cause them. The artifacts are well represented by the quotation at the very beginning of this chapter.

Image Gallery

Figs. 7.15 to 7.30 have been collected over many years but are all possible with today's technology.

Equipment Artifacts

The following equipment malfunctions create artifacts:
- Collimator parts on the window (Fig. 7.15)
- Grid artifacts (see Chapter 6)
- Spilled chemicals (Fig. 7.16)

Processing Artifacts

Artifacts are possible throughout the entire processing cycle. Occasionally several overlapping artifacts make a diagnosis impossible. Fig. 7.17 displays handling, pickoff, and darkroom fog artifacts along with incorrect technical factors.

Transport Artifacts
- *Plus density.* These marks are darker than the surrounding emulsion.

FIG. 7.16 Spilled barium seeped beneath the front screen, and its shape was superimposed on the image. This artifact was visible on every image taken using this cassette.

- *Minus density.* These marks are lighter than the surrounding emulsion but still maintain emulsion (Fig. 7.18).
- *Scratch marks.* The emulsion is removed from the base either before processing or within the processor.
- *Pick-off.* The emulsion is picked off (removed from) the film base and redeposited on another area of the film, leaving a tiny hole in the emulsion and therefore in the image. This problem is not as evident on double-emulsion film as on single-emulsion film (Fig. 7.19).
- *Chatter.* This artifact occurs when two or more gears need to be replaced. The plus-density or minus-density marks are not deposited in a specific pattern. They may be similar to pi lines but are randomly spaced.

FIG. 7.17 A Radiograph of a Goat Abdomen. This image has many artifacts: technique, handling, and processing.

FIG. 7.19 Pickoff (visible as very small, clear "dots" on the film) occurs when the processor rollers are not clean. The emulsion is picked off by the dirt on the rollers and usually deposited somewhere else on the film.

FIG. 7.18 Pi lines are caused by a swelling of the processor roller. They may be either plus-density or minus-density lines. The roller is easily identified from the measurement of the circumference of the roller, hence the name "pi."

FIG. 7.20 Pi lines caused by wet entrance rollers, which were washed but not dried and therefore imprinted their dampness onto this image.

- *Pi lines.* These plus-density marks are specific to the circumference of the roller that caused the artifact (hence the term *pi*, the mathematical constant related to a circle's circumference) (Fig. 7.18). Pi lines are not a diagnosis of the problem but are rather the result of a problem that must be identified, such as the following:
- *Hesitation marks.* These can occur when the rollers move unevenly and the film hesitates slightly. These marks can be mild (plus-density or minus-density lines) or severe (the emulsion is removed from the base).
- *Wet entrance rollers.* Pi lines can occur when the entrance rollers are not dried after cleaning and before a film is processed (Fig. 7.20). The image of the wet roller is imprinted on the film.
- *Guide shoe marks.* These artifacts appear as fine lines on either the leading edge or trailing edge of the film and are caused by the "snapping" of the film against the film guides as it travels from one tank to the next. They can be matched against the guide shoe ridges in the processor.

Chemical Artifacts

- *Dichroic fog.* The film appears to have an oily pattern of color in reflected light. This is caused by fixer leaking or

FIG. 7.21 Film Processed with Exhausted Developer. The overall image lacks correct density and contrast; it has a washed-out appearance and is nondiagnostic.

FIG. 7.23 Film Processed with Exhausted Fixer. The film has a milky appearance and may even appear to be pink from the dye used in the green-receiving film.

FIG. 7.22 Silver has plated out onto the film as the fixer lines were crimped and replenishment had ceased.

FIG. 7.24 An example of incorrect mixing of developer in a manual tank. The image of the anatomy is completely overshadowed by the uneven chemistry.

dripping back into the developer (a reflected light artifact).

- *Underreplenishment (exhausted developer).* The films are often damp when they exit the processor, and the image has very poor contrast and is medium gray (Fig. 7.21).
- *Temperature too cool.* The hydroquinone is too cool to function correctly, and the images are dull and lack contrast.
- *Temperature too warm.* The developer will exhaust quickly and turn dark brown, and images are dark, dull, and lacks contrast.
- *Fixer not replenishing correctly.* Silver plating appears on the images (Fig. 7.22).
- *Fixer overconcentrated.* Fixer precipitates as a white, grainy material on the rollers and in the gears, causing scratches.
- *Fixer exhausted.* Films are milky white or pinkish and feel grainy and rough (Fig. 7.23).

- *Fixer tank empty.* Films are either green (blue-receiving film) or mauve/pink (green-receiving film). There is an image, but it blackens quickly.
- *Incorrect mixing (manual).* The film has a blur pattern of minus densities and plus densities (Fig. 7.24).
- *Incorrect mixing (automatic).* A treelike spray pattern appears across the film when the recirculation tank has not mixed the old chemicals with the new chemicals. The fresh chemistry is more active, darkening the image as it travels across the film. The image in Fig. 7.25 was caused

FIG. 7.25 A treelike shadow overlays the entire film. This occurred because the developer replenisher was introduced into the developing tank, bypassing the recirculation tank. The fresh developer affected the film and activated the developing process, but the older chemicals took longer to accomplish development. The solution to this problem was to install a diversion baffle for the new chemicals so they mixed with the old chemicals before reaching the film.

FIG. 7.26 Sulfiding from the residual thiosulfate is very evident on this image as the result of inadequate washing.

because a service person forgot to replace the diversion baffle in the recirculation tank, which prevented the chemicals from mixing correctly before entering the working tank.

- *Wash water tank empty*. The films are milky and look streaky in reflected light.
- *Wash water tank not circulating*. The films appear dirty and streaky. Archival quality is compromised, and the films turn yellow within 2 or 3 weeks (Fig. 7.26).

Handling Artifacts

Determining the causes of artifacts on film may turn into a Sherlock Holmes–type adventure. This is where good recordkeeping and good darkroom practices pay off. The following are some of the causes of handling artifacts:

- Foreign objects in the cassette
- Dust on the feed tray (particularly common with large-animal radiography in a barn)
- Double exposure caused by not keeping track of which cassettes are already exposed and which are unexposed
- Film fog from heat, age, or other factors
- Scattered radiation fog
- Secondary radiation fog
- Extrafocal radiation
- Static—smudge, spot, or tree static (Fig. 7.27)
- Sweaty fingerprints
- Identical to the fingerprints of whoever processed the film
- Particularly common with single-emulsion film
- Salts in sweat dissolve the emulsion so it does not develop when processed
- Film creases
- Caused by bending the film when it is taken out of the film box, roughly placed in the cassette, or roughly removed from the cassette before processing
- May be dark (caused by concentrating the ions in the silver lattice) (Fig. 7.28A) or light (caused by destroying that portion of the silver lattice so there is no longer an image beneath the crease) (Fig. 7.28B)
- Incorrect darkroom conditions:
- Safelight filter (Fig. 7.29)
- Safelight wattage
- Safelight color
- Safelight distance from countertop
- Chemical odor (a highly concentrated odor can cause film fog)
- Darkroom integrity (Fig. 7.30).

FIG. 7.27 Static from a Feed Tray. Note the flat lines produced when the film was placed onto the feed tray.

FIG. 7.28 A, Fingerprint creases are caused by flexing the film roughly; they may be plus density or minus density. **B,** *(1)* Minus-density artifact from fingers pressing too hard on film emulsion. *(2)* Minus-density artifact from rough handling of film.

FIG. 7.29 An incorrect safelight filter fogged this film from a large-animal darkroom. Film fog usually lays a gray film over the image. In this case, it caused total lack of contrast, rendering the image nondiagnostic.

FIG. 7.30 Film fog on an image caused by a light leak around the door of a darkroom. The fingers holding the film at the top protect the film from the light, and the balance of the image has a fog overlay.

REVIEW QUESTIONS

1. The temperature of the darkroom should be _____; the humidity should be _____.
   a. 40° F (4°C), 40% to 60%
   b. 60° F (15.5°C), 50% to 70%
   c. 68° F (20°C), 40% to 60%
   d. 75° F (24°C), 50% to 70%

2. If the radiography room doubles as a darkroom, cassettes and film should be stored:
   a. In a metal film bin out of the way of scattered radiation
   b. In the darkroom, on shelves, and lying flat
   c. In the x-ray room in a plastic film bin in a far corner
   d. In the x-ray room on shelves, in an upright position

3. The darkroom should be painted using _____. The safelight should be mounted _____ feet (_____ meters) above the counter.
   a. black-absorbing paint, 6, 1.82
   b. dark, light-absorbing paint, 4, 1.22
   c. light-reflective paint, 4, 1.22
   d. light-reflective paint, 6, 1.82

4. The information on the ID label must include which of the following?
   a. Clinic address, date, and time of examination
   b. Patient's name, ID number, clinic address, and date
   c. Patient's name, clinic name, and location of the clinic
   d. Patient's name, clinic name, and right or left view

5. Automatic processing a film requires four separate steps. Which of the following lists the correct order?
   a. Develop, fix, wash, dry
   b. Develop, wash, fix, dry
   c. Fix, develop, wash, dry
   d. Wash, develop, fix, dry

6. The two main components of the developer are:
   a. Hydroquinone and phenidone
   b. Hydroquinone and sodium carbonate
   c. Phenidone and potassium bromide
   d. Sodium sulfite and sodium carbonate

7. The purpose of the developer is to:
   a. Alter the chemical makeup of the film to accept the fixer
   b. Reduce the potassium bromide in the film to metallic bromide
   c. Reduce the silver halide in the film base to metallic silver
   d. Reduce the silver halide in the film emulsion to metallic silver

8. A second purpose of the developer is to:
   a. Amplify the amount of metallic silver on the film
   b. Decrease the amount of silver left on the base
   c. Increase the number of silver atoms in each sensitivity speck
   d. Reduce the number of silver halide atoms to enhance the image

9. One of the components of the developer is to reduce its activity; this is:
   a. Potassium bromide
   b. Sodium carbonate
   c. Sodium sulfite
   d. Water

10. The main function of the hydroquinone is to:
    a. Build up the blacks and enhance the contrast
    b. Slowly build up grays to enhance contrast
    c. Start to work immediately to build up the blacks in the image
    d. Steadily enhance the gray tones of the image

11. The main function of the fixer is to:
    a. Fix the contrast problems left by the developer
    b. Harden the image and fix it to the base
    c. Remove unexposed silver halide from the film base
    d. Solidify the image to the base

12. The main component of the fixer is:
    a. Acetic acid
    b. Aluminum sulfate
    c. Ammonium thiosulfate
    d. Chrome alum

13. Developer is chemically _____; fixer is highly _____.
    a. acidic, alkaline
    b. alkaline, acidic
    c. alkaline, neutral
    d. neutral, acidic

14. The main purpose of the wash water is to:
    a. Remove the leftover chemicals from the film to preserve archival quality
    b. Remove the soapy residue of the precipitate from the fixer
    c. Stop the developer from developing the unexposed silver halides
    d. Stop the fixer from removing the image from the film

15. Drying should remove about _____ of the moisture from the film.
    a. 60% to 70%
    b. 70% to 80%
    c. 85% to 90%
    d. 90% to 100%

16. Two of the systems of the automatic processor are _____ and _____.
    a. cooling anode, replenishment
    b. replenishment, recirculation
    c. thermostat, heating coils
    d. transport, cooling system

17. Every time a roller comes into contact with the film emulsion:
    a. It has the potential to imprint an artifact on the image
    b. It has the potential to stop the film from developing
    c. It is started and stopped by the action of the film
    d. The roller assists the fixer to fix the image on the film

18. Once the film is placed on the feed tray and enters the rollers:
    a. It is affecting the replenishment, so it must not be drawn back
    b. It must not be drawn back onto the feed tray
    c. It will enter the fixer and must not be pulled back
    d. The developer will arrest the motion of the film so it will be fixed

19. The transport system of the processor:
    a. Carries the films through the tanks by a series of rollers and gears
    b. Slides the film along the rollers using the guide shoes to bend it
    c. Transports the chemicals to the developer tanks by means of pumps
    d. Transports the replenisher into the processor without any air gaps

20. The developer chemicals are replenished with _____ chemicals in comparison with the fixer.
    a. less
    b. less (but diluted)
    c. more
    d. the same amount of (but diluted)

21. The fixer requires _____ replenisher because _____ is carried in with the film.
    a. less, bromines
    b. less, water
    c. more, developer
    d. more, water

22. The most typical silver recovery unit in a veterinary clinic is the:
    a. Copper replacement model
    b. Electrolytic model
    c. Ionic attachment model
    d. Metallic replacement model

23. A test to determine whether the silver recovery unit needs to be replaced is:
    a. Checking the inside of the unit for fixer precipitate and smelling the outflow
    b. Checking the inside of the unit for metallic silver and absence of steel wool
    c. Placing a 5-cent piece in the outflow, which will polish the nickel
    d. Placing copper in the outflow; silver will plate out on the copper

24. A large percentage of image artifacts are caused by which of the following reasons?
    a. Most of them are caused within the darkroom.
    b. Most of them are caused in the developer tank.
    c. Mostly they arise in the darkroom before processing.
    d. The majority are caused by incorrect concentration of chemicals.

25. Dichroic fog is caused by:
    a. Developer contaminating the fixer
    b. Fixer leaking back into the developer
    c. Fixer leaking into the wash water
    d. Wash water staining the films after drying

26. Pi lines are caused in the processor by a swelling of a roller. They are:
    a. Called this because the separation of the artifact is the circumference of the rollers
    b. Named after the Art of Pi; they compromise the image in reflected light
    c. Usually minus-density lines at random intervals along the film
    d. Usually plus-density artifacts along the edges of the film

27. Developer underreplenishment causes the film:
    a. To appear as if it had been smeared with chemicals after it was processed
    b. To have a gray, washed-out appearance due to exhaustion of hydroquinone
    c. To have a gray, washed-out appearance due to exhaustion of phenidone
    d. To look very colorful under reflected light with green and blue colors

28. Overheating the developer will cause it to _____ and turn _____.
    a. exhaust quickly, dark brown
    b. exhaust quickly, light yellow
    c. remain stable, dull gold
    d. remain stable, light yellow

29. If the fixer is overconcentrated, it will:
    a. Precipitate onto the tank and cause grainy images
    b. Precipitate out onto the gears and rollers
    c. Remain in solution and enhance the contrast
    d. Remain in solution and fix faster

30. Crease artifacts on the film are the result of:
    a. Incorrect handling before or after exposure
    b. Incorrect placement of the film on the feed tray
    c. Not maintaining good darkroom cleanliness
    d. Static electricity affecting the film transport

Chapter Review Question answers are located in the Instructor Resources on Evolve and can be provided to students at the discretion of the instructor.

CHAPTER **8**

Computerized Radiography and Digital Imaging

Lois C. Brown, RTR (Can/USA), ACR, MSc, P.Phys

There are no boundaries or borders in the digital age.
—Karim Rashid, industrial designer, b. 1960

(Image courtesy of Animage, LLC and the Animage FIDEX-FS advanced imaging system, with permission.)

OUTLINE

LEARNING OBJECTIVES

When you have finished this chapter, you will be able to:

1. Know the difference between computed radiography and digital imaging.
2. Understand the fundamentals of computed radiography.
3. List the basics of direct digital imaging.
4. Understand the purpose of the charge-coupled device camera.
5. Understand digital technique charts.
6. Know the difference between windowing and leveling and between contrast and density.
7. Know the rules to follow when purchasing a digital system.
8. Understand the software variables.
9. Understand picture archiving and communications systems.
10. Know how to look for artifacts in the images.

APPLICATIONS

The application of the information in this chapter is relevant to the following area:

1. Producing digitized x-ray images (radiographs) for evaluation and diagnosis.

KEY TERMS

Key terms are defined in the Glossary on the Evolve website.

Absorbed radiation
Ambient lighting
Automatic rescaling
Bit
Bit depth
Brightness

Byte
Charge-coupled device
Cloud storage
Contrast resolution
Contrast to noise
    ratio

Detective Quantum
   Efficiency (DQE)
Digital Imaging and
   Communications in
   Medicine (DICOM)
Dynamic range

Electronic masking
Field of view (FOV)
Fill factor
Flat panel detector
Grayscale
Histogram analysis

Continued

Caveat Emptor: Let the Buyer Beware

Please refer to the Appendix **E** to find notes and pointers regarding the purchase of a digital imaging system

---

? POINTS TO PONDER An associate veterinarian purchased a clinic with a 3-year-old digital imaging system. The amount due on the payment plan was $68,000. When the system malfunctioned, she was given the choice to repair the digital plate for $50,000 or replace the plate for $68,000. If she chose to repair the plate, it was no longer under warranty because it was a used plate.

For further information on what can go wrong (and right), refer to the Evolve website.

Introduction to Computed Radiography and Digital Imaging

Technical Terminology

Acronyms – Throughout this chapter we have used "short forms" for the names of the various components that make up the digital image and for the parts of the images themselves.

Here are the common acronyms:

ADC = Analog to digital converter
CCD = Charge-Coupled Device
CR = Computed Radiography
DI = Digital Image
DR = Digital Radiography
FOV = Field of View
HIS = Hospital Information System
IP = Imaging Plate
IR = Image Receiver
Lp/mm = Line pairs per millimeter
PSP = Photostimulable Phosphor
RIS = Radiology Information System

ROI = Region of Interest
TFT = Thin-Film Transistor

Table 8.1 and the accompanying figure outline the steps that are involved in radiographing a patient using film and cassette/screens compared to computed radiography using a cassette and computer processor and finally compared with indirect and direct digital imaging with a computer and monitor.

The major advantage with direct digital imaging is the ability to receive the image immediately, manipulate it if necessary, and then store it in an archive that does not require real estate. So, the old darkroom can now be added storage space and the radiography images can be stored in the Cloud.

This chapter will now discuss the ways in which the remnant radiation can be received, an image can be created, and the image can then be stored and viewed on various devices.

With technology, the future of imaging is limitless. One thing that remains consistent with any system is the x-ray unit itself. Any correctly calibrated x-ray generator can be joined with any digital imaging system. The two systems are completely separate. As long as the x-ray unit is calibrated and is consistent, the year of its manufacture is immaterial. "70 kV is 70kV and all the rest is cosmetics."

Digital Imaging Characteristics

When a patient is radiographed (x-rayed) the remnant radiation (that radiation which is transmitted through the patient to reach the detector) is made up of a range of densities that reflect the various tissues through which it has passed. Bones absorb much more radiation than muscle cells, and fat absorbs very little radiation (Fig. 8.1).

In digital imaging the latent image is stored as digital data. In computed radiography or direct digital imaging, the process by which the image is obtained and processed is different than screen/film imaging, but the end result is the same: an image is displayed on a computer monitor.

TABLE 8.1	Comparison of Protocols*		
TRADITIONAL FILM/ SCREEN IMAGING	**COMPUTED RADIOGRAPHY (CR)**	**DIRECT DIGITAL IMAGING (DDI)**	
Load cassette	Prepare the cassette	**This step is eliminated**	
Prepare photoidentifier	**Enter patient's data (this is completed at reception)**	**Enter patient's data (this is completed at reception)**	
Position patient	**Position patient**	**Position patient**	
Measure patient	**Measure patient**	**Measure patient**	
Place cassette in tray	Place cassette in tray	**This step is eliminated**	
Set technique/ make exposure	**Set technique/ make exposure**	**Set technique/ make exposure**	
Process film	Process the image in the reader	**This step is performed by computer**	
Reload cassette	**This step is eliminated in some units**	**This step is performed by computer**	
Hang the film	Post the image	**This step is performed by computer**	
Read the film	**Read the image**	**Read the image**	
Postprocessing not available	Postprocess the image	Postprocess the image	
Archive the film	**Archive the image**	**Archive the image**	

*__Bold__ type indicates similar processes across imaging types; red type indicates differences across imaging types.

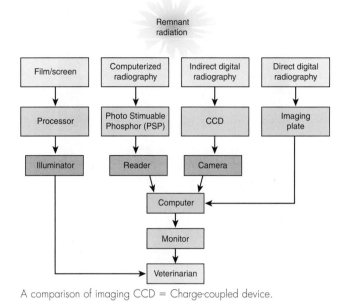

A comparison of imaging CCD = Charge-coupled device.

Defining Recorded Detail

The Image in Pixels

Digital images are composed of numerical data that can be easily manipulated by a computer. The computer overlays all graphics with a grid composed of rows and columns (Fig. 8.2).

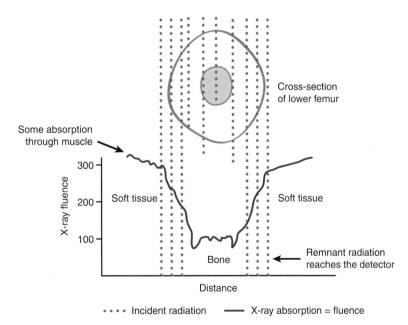

FIG. 8.1 Basic Digitization. Matrix – The image is displayed as a combination of rows and columns (array). Pixel – The smallest component of the matrix: the greater the number of pixels, the greater the resolution of the image. Pixel Bit Depth – This is the precision with which the remnant radiation is recorded, and it controls the number of bits that determines precision. It controls the exact pixel brightness that is displayed. The end goal of any imaging system is a highly diagnostic radiograph that enhances all the differences in tissue density while achieving the lowest radiation dose possible. (Adapted from Fauber TL. *Radiographic Imaging and Exposure.* 5th ed. St. Louis: Mosby; 2017.)

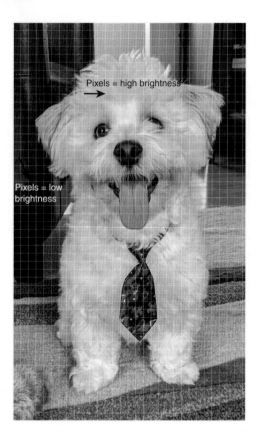

FIG. 8.2 Basic Digitization—a Grid Overlays the Image. The pixels in this image are 1400 pixels wide and 2300 vertically. The image is now a matrix of light, medium, and dark. Each pixel is assigned a brightness value.

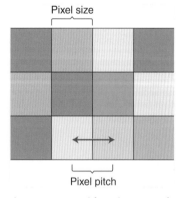

FIG. 8.3 The distance measured from the center of a pixel to an adjacent pixel determines the pixel pitch or spacing between densities. (Courtesy of Fauber TL. *Radiographic Imaging and Exposure.* 5th ed. St. Louis: Mosby; 2017.)

Pixel Pitch – This is measurement of the distance from the center of one pixel to the center of the adjacent pixel. This determines the spacing of the pixels. It is also an indicator of the relation of one pixel to an adjacent pixel (Fig. 8.3).

When displayed on a computer monitor, there is tremendous flexibility in terms of altering the brightness and contrast of a digital image by altering the brightness and contrast of any or all of the pixels. The practical advantage of such capability is that any anatomic structure can be independently well visualized.

Technique charts still play a very important role in the imaging process. The closer the technique is set to the measured thickness/density of the patient, the better the resulting image, which will reflect the appropriate contrast and brightness. Computers can then perform various postprocessing image manipulations to further improve the visibility of the anatomic region of interest.

To apply what was stated previously, a digital radiographic or photographic image is recorded as a **matrix** or combination of rows and columns (*array*) of small, usually square, "picture elements" called **pixels**. The size of a pixel is measured in microns (100 microns = 0.1 mm). Each pixel is recorded as a single numerical value, which is represented as a single brightness level on a display monitor. The location of the pixel within the image matrix corresponds to an area or volume of tissue within the patient. Given the dimensions of an anatomic area, or field of view (FOV), a matrix size of 1024 × 1024 pixels has 1,048,576 individual pixels; a matrix size of 2048 × 2048 pixels has 4,194,304 pixels. Digital image quality is improved with a larger matrix size that includes a greater number of smaller pixels.

Argo agreed to demonstrate the impact that pixel size has on the spatial resolution visualized in an image (Fig. 8.4). Although image quality is improved for a larger matrix size and smaller pixels, computer processing time, network transmission time, and digital storage space increase as the matrix size increases.

Spatial Frequency

Spatial frequency (Fig. 8.5) is defined by the unit of line pairs per millimeter (lp/mm). A resolution test pattern is a device used to record and measure line pairs. An imaging system that can resolve a greater number of line pairs per millimeter (higher spatial frequency) has increased spatial resolution. In digital imaging systems, the ability to resolve or demonstrate a specific spatial frequency is directly impacted by the size of the pixel.

Spatial Resolution and Contrast Detail

We have learned that the resolution of an image depends mainly on the size of the pixels and the number of pixels/millimeter (Table 8.2). Anatomic details are displayed as various densities, from white/clear to black, on the monitor. This is commonly called **recorded detail** and it determines, for example, how well we can visualize the minute fractures in a Great Dane's toe (Fig. 8.6).

The greater the spatial resolution, the better the visualized detail.

Every image is a combination of spatial resolution (the image in space) and contrast resolution. *Spatial resolution* is expressed in line pairs per millimeter. *Contrast resolution* is expressed as the values of black and white. The highest contrast available is an image that is completely black and white with no intervening shades of gray. The descriptor for contrast resolution is *dynamic range*.

FIG. 8.4 For a given field of view (FOV), the larger the matrix size, the greater the number of smaller individual pixels. Increasing the number of pixels improves the quality of the image. **A,** Matrix size is 531 × 863. **B,** Matrix size is 1350 × 2214. **C,** Matrix size is 1593 × 2619. Image C contains 4,172,067 pixels and demonstrates high resolution.

FIG. 8.5 This resolution test pattern measures the line pairs/mm. (Courtesy of Fauber TL. *Radiographic Imaging and Exposure.* 5th ed. St. Louis: Mosby; 2017.)

TABLE 8.2	Approximate Spatial Resolution for Various Medical Imaging Systems
IMAGING SYSTEM	**SPATIAL RESOLUTION (LINE PAIRS/MM)**
Magnetic resonance imaging	1.5
Computed tomography	1.5
Digital imaging	4–5
Computed radiography	5–6
Film/screen radiography	8–9

From Bushong SC. *Radiologic Science for Technologists.* 11th ed. St Louis: Elsevier; 2017.

The end result of digital imaging should logically be a high-resolution image. However, it is important to note that the limitations of pixel size and monitor output always result in an image that does not yet have the spatial resolution of film/screen technology.

Dynamic Range and What the Viewer Sees

The question remains: Why do digital images look so much better than film images?

Digital images take advantage of the ability of the digital process to create a greater number of shades of gray in the image. It remains a fact that no digital image can resolve an object smaller than the pixel size of the image receptor.

Film/screen imaging has a limited dynamic range. The dynamic range of film/screen technology is three orders of

FIG. 8.6 **A,** One line pair is one dark line and one (interspace) clear line. The system resolution in a digital system is also affected by the resolution of the monitor (display). **B,** The paw of the Great Dane shows up very nicely in this high-resolution image. (Courtesy of Fauber TL. *Radiographic Imaging and Exposure.* 5th ed. St. Louis: Mosby; 2017.)

FIG. 8.7 **A** and **B,** An example of a digital technique chart from a unit installed, with no grid, in 2017. This example uses very low doses and the images are excellent. Older digital plates use much higher doses, and the images may still not have the resolution of the newer digital plates.

magnitude because the optical density of the image is read from 0 to 3. This represents a dynamic range of 1000; that is, 1000 density variations, or shades of white through gray to black. The viewer can visualize only 30 shades of gray because of the limitations of the human eye.

The dynamic range of digital imaging systems is defined by the bit capacity of each pixel. Typical DR systems have a 14-bit dynamic range ($2^{14} = 16,384$ shades of gray). Digital mammography systems and some later digital systems have a 16-bit capacity and therefore image 2^{16} (65,536) shades of gray. The human eye is not equipped to visualize and appreciate all these features; it is limited to 30 shades of gray. The advantage of the digital systems is that with edge enhancement (a sophisticated computer technique that outlines each edge within the image) and the ability to manipulate the image (which is not available in a film/screen system), the

radiograph may be enhanced by the algorithms and computer processing to optimize the contrast and brightness.

Digital Detectors and Dynamic Range

The dynamic range of any imaging system is the area of the image that allows interpretation. It is the midportion of densities. In digital imaging it is the range of exposure intensities that the image receptor can accurately detect. Because the digital plate can detect a very wide range of exposure intensities, an optimum image can be produced using a very wide range of intensities.

In order to prevent ***dose creep,*** where the operator increases the technical factors beyond what is necessary, it is very important to measure each patient in position and use the technique chart to optimize exposures (Fig. 8.7). A basic digital technique chart is similar to the chart displayed in

FIG. 8.8 Digital imaging enables the viewer to fill in the clear areas of the image with a black background, which eliminates glare from the monitor. Although this image is not ideal from a positioning point of view, the surrounding black background eliminates transmitted glare from the monitor.

Fig. 8.7A. Each digital plate and computerized radiography unit will have its own sensitivity, and a chart for each separate examination can be extrapolated from this chart.

Digital Imaging Monitors

The conditions under which the images are viewed must be controlled to take advantage of the optimized image.

When the images are viewed on a monitor, the viewer's eyes must ignore the clear areas and concentrate on the image. The clear areas are still there and can cause eye strain and eye fatigue if the images are viewed for any length of time. A feature of the radiology software will darken the areas surrounding the image in order to reduce glare and viewer fatigue (Fig. 8.8).

Once the digital capture of the remnant radiation is complete, the end result to the veterinarian is the image display on the monitor. One must remember that the image has now had a further transformation from the computer/photostimulable phosphor (PSP) to the monitor. Limiting the number of steps between the remnant radiation and the monitor display is critical to the resolution of the image.

The resolution of an image is the fine detail that is, or is not, visible on the image when viewed on a computer monitor or on film. With digital imaging, the resolution of the computer display monitor is critical.

The monitor and the imaging system to which it is linked, is not as detailed as the anatomy itself. Every step in the imaging process degrades the line pair image of the patient's anatomy. Once the image has been recorded by the imaging plate (IP), it must then be displayed on a monitor. This image will not be the high resolution of the x-ray film; however, imaging systems are very competitive and therefore they will improve constantly over time.

The image will be only as good as the resolution of the monitor itself. Also, some monitors have a background color that is incompatible with the radiographic image (Fig. 9).

Soft copy viewing refers to viewing the image on a monitor as opposed to a *hard copy* such as film. This soft copy image is affected by the features of the monitor itself, the luminance, resolution, and viewing conditions such as background or ambient lighting and placement of the monitor.

It is vitally important that the monitor (Fig. 8.10A,B):
- is located in a darkened area to obtain the optimum viewing condition.
- display is situated in a space where the background lighting is eliminated.
- is positioned so that everyone viewing the image is directly in front of the monitor.

FIG. 8.9 **A,** The monitor may have built-in background lighting that is unacceptable when it is used for imaging. **B,** The yellowish tone can mask diagnostic details.

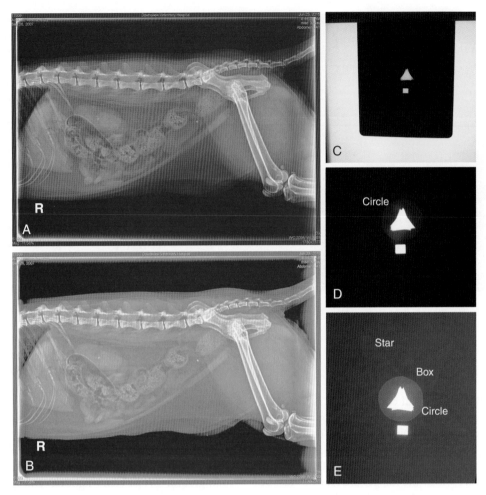

FIG. 8.10 **A,** The image as viewed in a darkened room with no reflected light. **B,** The image as viewed in a brightly lit room with reflected light. Anatomic details fade and the image loses contrast. **C,** An illustration of the enhancement of the image when ambient light is eliminated from the area surrounding the image and within the viewing room. On the illuminator with ambient light and no masking, the image is clearly seen as a triangle and a square. **D,** With the elimination of the room light, a small circle is seen surrounding the triangles. The three triangles are enhanced. **E,** Masking the image and extinguishing ambient light from the room, a circle surrounds the triangles and a five-pointed star is seen surrounding the image.

- displays the highest resolution that the vendor can supply and that the facility can afford.

The factors to be considered when purchasing a monitor and then positioning it to the best advantage are:

Luminous flux – The total intensity of light from a source

Illuminance – The intensity of light incident on a surface

Luminance intensity – The property of the source of the light. This is the luminous flux that is delivered to the total viewing area.

Luminance – Another measure of the brightness of the source

All of these factors are important when purchasing the monitor and when deciding which area will be the chief viewing area in the facility. A reading area monitor within the radiography room would not require the high definition/detail that the monitor in the veterinarian's office would display. There, the highest number of pixels and the highest resolution within a darkened area would display the highest resolution available on the system.

◆ APPLICATION INFORMATION

The client at the veterinary hospital was unhappy with the images that he was seeing:

- The images had a definite yellow tinge where the screen had aged and turned slightly yellow.
- The resolution was very poor.
- On chest x-rays, all the patients appeared to have congestion in both lungs even though upon auscultation, those symptoms were absent.
- The lights in the room were left on when the images were viewed.
- The images were "noisy" where the monitor had lost pixels, so the computer was filling in densities that were either clear or black causing the "noise."
- The digital system was ten years old. The monitor had been purchased at that time and it had a resolution of 1080p = 2 megapixels (MP) monitor.

The consultant brought a new 5MP medical monitor and set it up. The images immediately improved dramatically. Lesson learned: it is the monitor which displays the images. Quite often the reason for poor images is the ambient light or the display monitor.

The location of the monitor and the ambient light are very important. It is vital that the monitor is located in a room that can be darkened when the images are viewed. The images in Fig. 8.10C–E show the dramatic effect that eliminating all background and transmitted light can have on the image.

Histograms and Algorithms

The digital IP requires a radiation dose. It will accept scattered/secondary radiation to add density to the image. Some systems are now sold with a removable grid that will be used only on very large dogs (which produce an excessive amount of secondary/scattered radiation). The old system of decreasing kilovolts (kV) to enhance contrast is no longer an issue. The digital plate looks for dose, and the computer takes care of the rest using two very important systems: histograms and algorithms.

Histograms

A histogram (Fig. 8.11) is a graphic display of an image and is displayed on the software of virtually every digital system. Every pixel is plotted on a graph from lightest to darkest, taking into account the number of all pixels that represent the same dark/light value. Images of extremities are high on the light values and dark values, with very low levels in between. Images of an abdomen peak in the gray areas and are low on both very light and very dark values.

In some cases, the operator can manipulate the histogram slightly to enhance some of the features of the image. The histogram is then evaluated on the basis of a known algorithm to enhance the contrast and brightness of the image.

Algorithms

An algorithm is a formula or set of rules specific to a particular question used in calculations or data processing. In imaging, it is the commands given to the computer with reference to the histogram that is selected by the operator.

The computer software used in digital imaging contains a series of algorithms that provide a baseline for each type of examination. Each algorithm is based on the histograms obtained from many trials and much research. For example, a dog's foreleg typically consists of bone, muscle, and a little fat, with no internal organs. An algorithm describes what the computer will "see" when a foreleg is radiographed, and it enhances the contrast and brightness of the image accordingly. This is true for every body part on every animal. A thoracic image is enhanced as a high-contrast image. An image of an abdomen will be low contrast with many shades of gray.

When a digital unit is purchased and installed, the service engineer who sets up the computers will establish the veterinarian's preferences, such as what level of contrast is acceptable in a thoracic image and what density is preferred for abdomens and spines. Once the algorithms for that hospital are established, the service engineer can access the computer from any physical location (the office, on the road, or in a foreign country) and correct any problems. The service engineer is usually the only person who has access to the program at the algorithm level, but he or she cannot change anything within the basic programming of the software. He/she may apply filters to adjust the histogram but cannot change the manufacturer's preset algorithms.

> ### ◆ APPLICATION INFORMATION
>
> On a digital system the algorithm can be "fooled" with or worked around. For example, a client had a problem with the algorithm programmed for abdominal radiography. The images had low contrast, and the veterinarian was looking for a bladder stone on a large dog. Until the service person could change the algorithm, the consultant suggested that he request chest imaging when he was radiographing an abdomen. The higher-contrast algorithm worked just fine, and the images were diagnostic with just the right amount of contrast.

Digital Imaging Options = Image Receptors

Digital imaging came to general radiography a bit late in the game. Nuclear medicine, ultrasound, and fluoroscopy were all using digitizers to produce and save their images to computer many years before radiography finally arrived at the new frontier.

The transformer, the generator, and the x-ray tube are all involved in producing the radiation that will affect whatever image receptor is in place. It is very important to be aware that the x-ray tube and generator are completely separate from the image receptor. The generator may be quite old but as long as it is calibrated correctly, it will support a new installed digital system.

The three receptors that are universally used at this time are:

- Computed radiography using cassettes and an imaging plate
- Indirect digital imaging charge-coupled device (CCD)
- Direct digital imaging

FIG. 8.11 A histogram showing the number of each of the gray values from left to right (the horizontal axis). The total number (count) of each pixel value is added up vertically. *VOI*, Volume-of-interest. (Courtesy of Fauber TL. *Radiographic Imaging and Exposure.* 5th ed. St. Louis: Mosby; 2017.)

FIG. 8.12 A, This Agfa model has the cassette entering from the side and sits easily on a countertop. The imaging plate (IP) is removed from the cassette and drawn into the unit, wrapped around a drum, and ejected after the image is read and the IP is flashed with bright white light to erase the image. The operator will then replace it into the cassette. **B,** The Konica system is a stand-alone model. The cassette is placed in the top, and the IP is drawn straight out, read and flashed, and inserted back into the cassette, which is then lifted out of the unit by the operator.

Computed Radiography

Computed radiography (CR) (Fig. 8.12) was the first step toward digital imaging in veterinary medicine There are many similarities between CR and traditional screen/film imaging (see Table 8.1). Both use a cassette that must be processed in a separate unit. Both have IPs coated with PSPs, and the cassettes protect the PSPs from light and abuse. Both modalities require processing to archive the images.

The only step that CR eliminates from the traditional imaging protocol is reloading film into the cassette. This is done by the CR reader if that option is supplied. In some cases, the operator will remove the screen from the cassette, place it in a "reader," wait for it to be "read" and erased, and then replace it in the cassette.

A single IP in the CR cassette acquires and stores the image (ready for processing), thereby eliminating the need for film. The function is the same as in film/screen imaging except that the screen retains the image instead of the film.

The similarities between traditional imaging and CR end when we compare how the images are processed and viewed. In addition, postprocessing is available with CR but not with traditional imaging.

The Imaging Plate and Identifiers

Inside the CR cassette the single screen is referred to as an *imaging plate (IP)*. This is a distinct advantage with CR. If the facility purchases a dental ScanX (Air Techniques)(see Fig. 8.12A) unit or similar product, the cassettes can be easily substituted from film/screen imaging: the standard intensifying screens are removed, and the PSP plate is installed. The cassette is then used as holder/protective covering for the IP when it is being used to radiograph patients.

With other CR systems (Konica and Fuji), specialized cassettes must be purchased specific to the type of CR unit as the cassette is handled by a reader unit (see Fig. 8.12B). Tabletop exposures are possible and lead blockers may be used to split the cassette so that multiple images may be made on one cassette. The back of the cassette contains a small identifier that contains the patient data. It must be read by the CR unit before the IP enters the reader (Fig. 8.13). Each cassette is imprinted with the patient data as it enters the processor.

FIG. 8.13 A computed radiography cassette looks similar to a traditional radiography cassette. Each cassette has an acquisition label which links the patient information to the image produced in the reader. This is an example of the bar code read by the reader and linked to the patient acquisition numbers in the Radiology Identifier System (RIS).

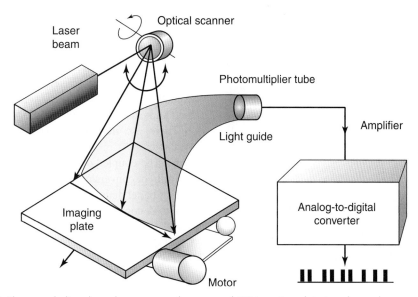

FIG. 8.14 The neon-helium laser beam scans the exposed CR imaging plate to release the stored energy as visible light. The photomultiplier tube "sees" the light, amplifies it, and converts it to an electrical signal. The electrical signal is picked up by the analog-to-digital converter, which converts the analog data to digital data and displays it on the hospital monitor. (Courtesy Fujifilm Medical Systems Inc, USA, Stamford, Connecticut.)

That way the patient data will be joined to the images as they are displayed on the monitor.

The front of the IP is coated with a PSP, usually barium fluorohalide, which reacts instantly to the x-ray beam and to light (Fig. 8.14). When the IP is placed in a reader unit, the laser (which is 50 to 100 nanometers wide and covers the plate side to side) passes over the plate as it is drawn through the reader. The laser causes the remaining unstable electrons to return to their original state with the emission of a shorter wavelength light in the blue area of the spectrum. At this point, the latent image becomes visible on the computer monitor.

The spatial resolution on the image depends entirely on the cross-sectional diameter of the laser. The laser beam tends to spread as it leaves the source, so it is collimated by a lens system that keeps it to a 100-μm diameter (μm = micrometer).

Once the image has been read, the IP is flashed with an intense white light. This light returns all the unstable electrons to their ground state, preparing the IP to be used again immediately. IPs work best if they are used immediately after processing.

If the IP is not placed in a reader unit, the image will fade within 6 to 8 hours as the electrons return to their original state.

IPs should always be "flashed" (sent through the reader) every morning because they may retain a previous image or may be "fogged" by background radiation from the ballasts of fluorescent lights or low-level radiation emitted from concrete walls. Fogging of the PSP is possible from direct or scattered radiation, heat stimulation of the IP, or light leaks within the cassette.

Sources of "Noise" in CR imaging

The term noise refers to unwanted and usually irregular densities overlying the image.

Noise is greatest in CR at the lower level of exposure as a result of background fog and scattered radiation. Table 8.3 lists sources of noise in the CR system.

The principal source of noise on the image is scattered radiation. The dose curve in CR radiography is directly linked to technique. This means that as the IP is stimulated, the response of the plate is immediate. The output of the CR image is constant throughout the diagnostic imaging range of technical factors. This may easily lead to overexposure, because technique charts are supplied by vendors who are unfamiliar with the ALARA (as low as reasonably achievable) principle. It is very important to maintain a technique chart that sets the technical factors, and therefore the dose, to an ALARA level. Typically, traditional technique charts at a 400-speed system are acceptable for CR.

TABLE 8.3	Sources of Noise Within the Computed Radiography System
SOURCES OF NOISE	**CAUSES**
Mechanical defects	Slow scan driver
	Fast scan driver
Optical defects	Laser intensity control
	Scatter of stimulating laser
	Light quanta emitted by the screen
	Light quanta collected by the optics
Computer defects	Electronic noise
	Inadequate sampling
	Inadequate quantization

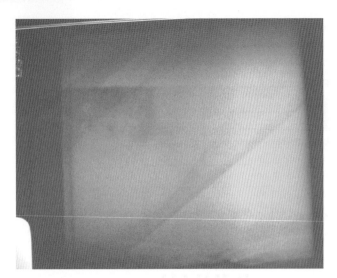

FIG. 8.15 A CR cassette that had not been used for days showed a level of exposure to background radiation. (Courtesy Bushong SC. *Radiologic Science for Technologists*. 11th ed. St Louis: Elsevier; 2017.)

Advantages of Computed Radiography

The elimination of the wet processor and the chemicals associated with traditional film processing is a distinct environmental advantage with any type of digitized imaging. Two further advantages are the wide latitude regarding technical factors and the short wait for the image display. The IPs are replaceable at a reasonable cost.

Disadvantages of Computed Radiography

IPs are consumables and therefore need to be serviced and replaced when they become worn or when the "ghosting" of previous images cannot be erased. They are prone to the effects of scattered radiation and should be flashed before each use if radiography in the clinic or hospital is infrequent (Fig. 8.15). Noise at low levels of radiation is bothersome, but newer technology promises to reduce this factor.

The readers can be a source of artifacts as the IP is drawn out of the cassette, especially in veterinary clinics, where animal hair and fur are drawn into the reader by fans or a vacuum. *Horizontal plus-density or minus-density artifacts* can be a problem as the IP is drawn out of the cassette if there is hesitation or uneven motion. *Vertical plus-density or minus-density artifacts* can be caused by dust or dirt on the rollers of the unit. These marks appear as long scratches down the length or across the width of the image.

Another disadvantage is the intermediate step of needing to process the image in a laser reader. This step delays the viewing process and requires one more piece of (expensive) equipment that must be maintained and serviced.

Direct and Indirect Digital Imaging

The acquisition of the image is variable as technology moves forward. Image acquisition is important to manufacturers because it is here that the remnant radiation meets the digital plate and the resulting image is formed and transferred to the computer. Every vendor is always anxious to have the sharpest resolution and the brightest optimum contrast image. It is the sophistication of the software and the efficiency of the monitor that allows this to happen.

I have included each of the steps along the way towards the most direct and efficient method of digital conversion available today. Each of these versions will have units in the field and each will produce diagnostic images.

There are now four forms of direct digital imaging available:

- Charge-coupled device (CCD)
- Indirect conversion detectors
- Flat panel detectors
- Direct conversion detectors

Charge-Coupled Device (CCD)

This was the very first digital imaging system that grew out of the computerized radiography research. The philosophy was that if the remnant radiation could be captured and focused to a regular single-lens reflex camera, the resulting image could then be transferred to a computer.

This technology was very popular until the price of the direct digital imaging systems gradually arrived at a level where veterinary hospitals could justify the cost and could then enjoy the direct instant imaging of the direct digital system.

Indirect digital systems use a charge-coupled device (CCD) with an IP that contains a thin-film transistor (TFT). The TFT converts the radiation to an image that is imprinted on a single-lens reflex camera that is preset and collects the image off the back of the IP. After the image is collected, it is handled in the same way as direct digital imaging.

The response of the CCD is completely linear and therefore can detect far more stimulus than the phosphor in the film/screen combination: this allows for a much greater range of sensitivity. Another advantage of CCD imaging is that the IP is considerably less expensive than that used for direct digital imaging and the CCD unit is made up of component parts that can be serviced and replaced if necessary.

A disadvantage of CCD imaging is that the image undergoes one extra step in moving from original image to computer image, so there is a chance of data loss. Research into this area has been intense, and the images from CCD units are exceptionally good. One critical aspect is the focus of the camera situated at the back of the CCD unit. The entire unit is mounted beneath the tabletop directly under the central ray. The CCD is not movable, so either the tabletop must move or the animals must be positioned in such a way that the region of interest (ROI) is centered on the CCD.

The *sensitivity* of the CCD is its ability to detect very low levels of visible light. This feature makes it valuable in radiography using its sensitivity to detect low patient remnant radiation dose. The *dynamic range* of the CCD is the ability of the detectors to respond to a wide range of light intensity. This system replicates the dynamic range of the 400-speed film/screen system.

FIG. 8.16 A photomicrograph of an active matrix array showing a thin-film transistor digital imaging image receptor with a single pixel highlighted. Electrical charges are read out from each detector element and the resulting image is instantly translated to the monitor. (Courtesy Fauber TL. *Radiographic Imaging and Exposure.* 5th ed. St. Louis: Mosby; 2017.)

Indirect Conversion Detectors

This method of translating the radiation to an image involves a two-step process. The radiation is converted to light using a scintillator (cesium iodide or gadolinium oxysulfide). The light captured is in proportion to the x-ray exposure, which is then converted to electrical charges and eventually digitized and processed in the computer to produce a raw digital image. This image is then displayed on the monitor

Flat Panel Detector Array—Direct Digital

When the radiation reaches the digital plate, it is captured by the flat panel detector that is made up in layers (Fig. 8.16). The top layer is a scintillation phosphor and the second layer contains the TFT. The third layer is a glass substrate.

The TFT array is divided up into square detector elements (DELs), and each DEL has a capacitor to store electrical charges and a switching transistor for read out.

Within the array of thousands of DELs, each element is 80% efficient in capturing radiation. Electrical charges are separately read out from each detector element. The electronic signal is then sent to the analog-to- digital converter (ADC). The DEL has an x-ray sensitive area representing each pixel in the image matrix.

Direct Conversion Detectors

This method is the most efficient and uses only one step from remnant radiation to the ADC and thus to the computer monitor (Fig. 8.17). The *direct conversion detector* uses an amorphous selenium (a-Se)–coated detector to interact directly with the incoming radiation—there is no intervening scintillation phosphor. The a-Se plate is sandwiched between two charged electrodes. X-rays that reach the a-Se plate are collected by a storage capacitor and remain there until the signal is read by the switching action of the TFTs,

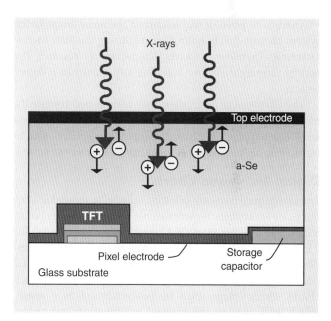

FIG. 8.17 Direct Digital Conversion. An amorphous selenium (a-Se)-coated detector directly converts the exit radiation to an electric charge. (Courtesy Fauber TL. *Radiographic Imaging and Exposure.* 5th ed. St. Louis: Mosby; 2017.)

which directly converts the remnant radiation to electrical charges that are then transferred to the ADC. Each pixel represented on the monitor has a brightness level representing the attenuation characteristics of the anatomy that was penetrated.

All of this happens very quickly and results in an image within seconds of radiographic exposure to the digital imaging plate, where it becomes an image displayed by thousands of pixels.

Digital Pixel Bundling

Our consultant had a busy day visiting two animal hospitals with a single problem. When the images on the monitor presented life size, the anatomic image was so pixilated that it was unreadable, actually, unidentifiable. The only way the data was identified was if the image was reduced to a very, very small image (by measurement 2.54 cm × 4.90 cm or 1 inch × 2 inches). Naturally at this size, there was no possibility of diagnosis.

Although the number of pixels in the digital plate is important, of greater importance is how these pixels are "wired together." In some systems the advertised pixel number is enormous, but the images are not ideal. When the image is magnified, it "pixilates" and becomes unclear. This is because these two units' pixels are bundled and read as an average. For example, the 16 squares in Fig. 8.18 represent pixels on a digital IP. Each square has a value that represents a percentage of exposure. Bundling these values together and averaging them results in a unique value of 50%. In the digital system, this bundle would give a density of 50% even though none of the squares has a 50% density. This bundling gives a noisy (grainy) image because the individual densities in the image are not represented correctly.

There is no possible way to correct the noisy image in the system because this bundling occurs during the plate manufacturing. Therefore, it is very important to research the system thoroughly before investing any money in a digital system.

The clients were told, when they complained repeatedly, that they had purchased an inexpensive system, so that was what was supplied. For these clients the only "fix" was to replace the digital plates with ones from a different company.

Digital Technique Charts

The technique charts supplied by otherwise reputable vendors can sometimes be worrisome. Setting a technique of 85 kV, 300 milliamperes (mA), and $1/120$ sec (2.50 mAs) for a kitten's paw or a cat's 10-cm abdomen illustrates the vendors' lack of knowledge in creating such charts and the problems encountered by the staff when they trust such charts. Every image must be postprocessed as a result, which adds time to the original examination and causes losses in data. Adjusting windowing and leveling (brightness and contrast) for every image compromises the information on the image. In addition, some of the images will be displayed as totally nondiagnostic. In such cases, the

high kV has penetrated every tissue evenly, eliminating any chance of enhancing contrast. The scattered radiation produced by a 110-kV exposure for a 16-cm abdomen is enough to add to the radiation dose on the technician's dosimeter if the technician is holding the patient and definitely adds unnecessary wear to the x-ray tube.

If the information has not been provided to the image receptor, either because the image is overexposed or underexposed, then no amount of postprocess manipulation will correct it. There is no "do-over," and the images are unreadable. Does the veterinarian order images that he or she knows cannot be read because the digital unit must be paid for? Does he or she have the image postprocessed as best as possible and then revert to the old system of diagnosing clinically because the images are so poor? What about the technicians who have worked at the clinic for 10 to 20 years and are now seeing dose readings on their radiation dosimeters for the very first time because of excess amounts of scattered/secondary radiation? All of these problems are experienced both in the veterinary world and in human medicine.

Technical Factors

Doses, dose creep, and poor technique charts can be a major problem in the radiography department. A technique chart must be developed that is similar to the chart used with the 400-speed film/screen combination in place when the digital unit was purchased. The chart supplied in this chapter is a guide only and can be adjusted to optimize the images after viewing the images produced using this chart (see Fig. 8.7). The best way to adapt a chart that was used before digital imaging is to measure accurately, set the generator to the measurement, and expose the receptor with a patient in place. The computer manipulates the data, but if the image is not perfect, reduce the **mAs** by a percentage. This will likely follow through for most of the chart.

For example:

16-cm abdomen, 400-speed chart, 62 kV @ 12 mAs = image dark by about 50%

Decrease technique by 50% to 62 kV, 6 mAs = image perfect, no postprocessing required

The best diagnostic images in digital imaging are acquired with a technique that is as close as possible to the parameters of the animal being radiographed. The computer will do the rest. Typically, smaller body parts will have a slightly higher technique because the digital plate requires a certain level of radiation to acquire the image. This accommodation will decrease as technology progresses.

kV, mAs, and Distance

Distance is typically not a factor in small-animal imaging because the distance is usually preset, but it is definitely a factor in large-animal imaging. An example of a technique chart is presented in Chapter 5. However, this chart may not work well with every unit. The kV and mAs combine in digital imaging to produce dose, and every system handles the dose slightly differently.

20	60	60	20
40	80	80	40
40	80	80	40
20	60	60	20

FIG. 8.18 An example of bundled pixels. Each square represents one pixel. The computer program will read all 16 pixels as an average of each value. In this example, average density on the image would appear to be 50%, even though none of these values equals 50%.

Digital Image Postprocessing

The image is now displayed on the monitor. It has excellent resolution and displays very good contrast. Now the software options become important. There are surgical tools in the software. There are filters to change the algorithms. The tools that are most commonly used and are available in every software package are **Windowing** and **Leveling**.

These are the tools that will alter the contrast and brightness of the image.

Windowing (Fig. 8.19) refers to the contrast range of densities. Window width controls the range of grayscale images to adjust the contrast on a digital image.

Leveling (Fig. 8.20) refers to density or brightness. Window level establishes the midpoint of the densities visible on the digital image. This use of windowing and leveling alters the image on the monitor.

Postprocessing and the Service Engineer

If an incorrect exposure is used and the image is compromised because of very low contrast, the operator may alter the contrast and brightness by postprocessing. However, postprocessing is not a substitute for correctly exposing the image using a correct technique chart. It is time consuming, and some information may be inadvertently lost when the image is manipulated. It is also an example of lack of regard

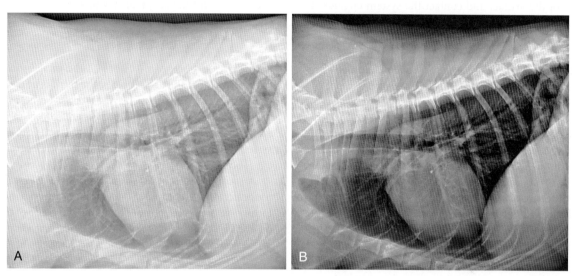

FIG. 8.19 Examples of Postprocessing an Image with the use of Windowing. As the window is reduced, the contrast flattens out so the differences in tissue density become less obvious. **A,** The image lacks contrast in the areas of the lungs and heart. **B,** Windowing the image provides better contrast and demonstrates the vascular areas of the lung tissue.

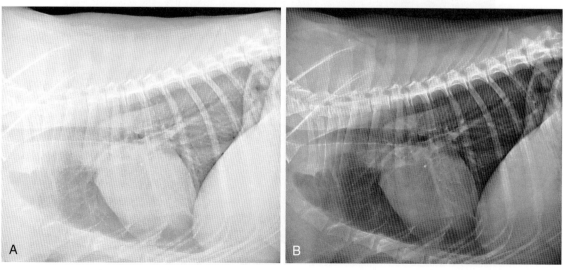

FIG. 8.20 A Change in Leveling. As the level increases, the overall density of the image becomes greater although the contrast remains the same. **A,** This image has good contrast but is overall too light. **B,** Leveling the image maintains the contrast and enhances the visualization of the anatomy by increasing the density.

for the ALARA principle, which recommends the lowest radiographic technique in order to reduce the dose to both the patient and the operator.

If the correct technical factors are used and the images are still consistently problematic, the system engineer can apply filters to enhance the overall images. However, this is not true for every system. If the software sold by the vendor is faulty or lacking in features and does not manipulate the data correctly, the image cannot be enhanced even by the experts. These are the programs that will not last in the marketplace.

Digital Imaging Artifacts

Digital imaging artifacts may be produced by the IP, grid, mechanical system, or software. It is important to identify the cause of the artifact and contact the system engineer to correct it. There are few artifacts in digital imaging, mainly because of the way the systems are installed.

Fig. 8.21A,B is an example of the anode heel effect exposure to an unoccupied plate. The subsequent automatic processing that occurred evened out the exposure without human interference. Most systems today will sort out imaging problems of this nature.

Fig. 8.22A–C illustrate human error in collimation and positioning. These are errors that the digital system cannot correct automatically. If an extremity is positioned on the plate with no collimation, the digital sensor will try to even out the exposure over the entire plate. As the entire plate is exposed and without collimation, it perceives that the exposure on the entire plate should be read and calibrated. If the extremity covers 20% of the plate and the rest is uncovered,

then the 80% density will be prioritized and the image will be very dark.

Typically, artifacts are caused by human error and can be resolved. A hardware or software problem must be addressed right away. The system engineer can usually resolve most software problems online. Hardware problems may be more difficult to resolve.

Picture Archiving and Communications Systems

Once the image is produced, it must be archived. It is very important to research the archiving of the images carefully. The archive is stored on a computer, and computers fail. All systems must therefore have redundancy, and the data must be stored in more than one place. The intricacies of data storage are beyond the scope of this text and could fill another chapter or even a book.

The simplest means of data storage is the use of interchangeable external hard drives. Most hospitals use three hard drives if they plan to store all the images onsite. Two hard drives store the day's images; the third is traded in at the end of the day, with hard drive #1 taken home by a designated person. The next day's images are stored on drives #2 and #3, and drive #2 is taken home at the end of the day. This system is complicated but inexpensive and secures the images locally.

A second means of data storage is offsite. Several companies offer offsite computer data storage and may be located locally, on the same continent, on the other side of the world, or even in cloud storage, which is becoming very popular. These companies are efficient and store masses of data from

FIG. 8.21 **A,** An image receptor exposed to an x-ray beam may show an anode heel effect response. **B,** Flat field reprocessing will make the response uniform. This must be programmed into the algorithm. (Courtesy Bushong SC. *Radiologic Science for Technologists.* 11th ed. St Louis: Elsevier; 2017.)

FIG. 8.22 Three examples of technologist error in positioning and collimation causing histogram and algorithm errors. (Courtesy Bushong SC. *Radiologic Science for Technologists.* 11th ed. St Louis: Elsevier; 2017.)

many different modalities. A word of caution: if the company is local, do not assume that the data will be stored locally. Many companies act as intermediaries and store the actual images on the other side of the world. It is wise to know where the data is stored and who controls the storage

facility. This is especially true if local politics or turbulent weather damage or destroy storage facilities.

Summary

Digital imaging either by means of CR or direct DR is a definite leap forward in radiographic imaging. The future is limitless as research continues to provide imaging applications that use technology to limit radiation exposure and provide high-quality images. Monitor technology has improved dramatically and is ever evolving. Data storage is an ever-expanding area of research, and the sophisticated methods of storage become even smaller and more convenient.

REVIEW QUESTIONS

1. Computed radiography eliminates one step in the film imaging process. This is:
   a. Archiving the images
   b. Entering patient data
   c. Processing the image
   d. Reloading the cassette
2. Digital imaging eliminates several steps in the imaging protocol. This is because:
   a. Everything to do with the image is complete when the exposure is made
   b. The technician is not required to enter patient data at the computer
   c. The technician is not required to track the image after the exposure is made
   d. The technician is responsible only for the patient, not the radiography unit
3. Computed radiography is similar to traditional radiography in that:
   a. The cassettes are identical in composition
   b. The methods of processing are similar
   c. They both use cassettes of similar sizes
   d. They both require the technician to open the cassette after the exposure
4. The imaging plate within the CR cassette:
   a. Must be processed soon because the image will degrade
   b. Can be delayed for processing for 6 to 8 hours
   c. Will hold the image for about 6 to 8 hours after exposure
   d. Will hold the image indefinitely after exposure
5. In CR, in order to read the image, a laser passes across:
   a. The IP after it is removed from the cassette
   b. The cassette after it is put into the reader
   c. The phosphor on the digital plate
   d. The IP after the exposure before it is in the reader
6. The IP should be "flashed" every morning or after a period of nonuse because:
   a. The chemicals start to develop on the plate
   b. It is sensitive to background radiation
   c. The plate is left in the reader
   d. The IP is always fogging after it has been used

7. The speed of the CR system is similar to that of 400-speed film/screen imaging.
   a. True
   b. False

8. Digital imaging is more efficient than computed radiography because:
   a. It eliminates the entire cassette reloading and processing and hanging steps
   b. It is a complete process and does not require separate image processing
   c. It is fast because the cassettes are already under the table
   d. It encourages technicians to use only one technique for every examination

9. Dynamic range is defined as:
   a. The ability to window and level the images
   b. The ability of the detectors to respond to a wide range of light intensity
   c. The latitude of the images once they are postprocessed
   d. The contrast of the images once they are postprocessed

10. A thin-film transistor (TFT) is used to:
    a. Transfer the light intensity to the computer components
    b. Convert the signal to sound and then to the electrical system
    c. Transfer the radiation signal to a circuit board within the computer
    d. Transfer a radiation signal directly to the digital receptor

11. Direct digital systems use:
    a. Cesium iodide and an intervening plate
    b. Thin-film transistors and cesium iodide
    c. Amorphous selenium to transmit the signal
    d. Amorphous silicon to transmit the signal

12. Windowing is a technique to improve images; it affects the _____.
    a. algorithm
    b. contrast
    c. density
    d. resolution

13. Leveling may enhance the radiographs, but it mainly affects _____.
    a. density
    b. frequency
    c. resolution
    d. spatial contrast

14. Picture archiving and communications systems store the images:
    a. Locally on hard drives or via the Internet anywhere in the world
    b. Locally on several hard drives that must remain in the computer
    c. On several hard drives but only within the facility for safekeeping
    d. Never on the hard drive of the computer because it may fail

Chapter Review Question answers are located in the Instructor Resources on Evolve and can be provided to students at the discretion of the instructor.

CHAPTER 9

Quality Control, Testing, and Artifacts

Lois C. Brown, RTR (Can/USA), ACR, MSc, P.Phys

*If you can't explain it **simply**, you don't understand it well enough.*
— Albert Einstein, American theoretical physicist, 1879–1955

A quality control program ensures that all equipment is functioning correctly.

LEARNING OBJECTIVES

When you have finished this chapter, you will be able to:

1. Describe the tests necessary to determine the calibration of an x-ray generator and the various problems associated with x-ray generator failure.
2. Test an x-ray unit for compliance.
3. Discuss the various methods to ensure that the collimator is installed and working correctly.
4. Describe the test tools that are used to determine resolution in fluoroscopy and radiography.
5. Identify artifacts caused by films, intensifying screens, and processing.
6. Distinguish between film artifacts and x-ray unit artifacts.
7. Identify artifacts associated with digital imaging, being able to recognize problems with a digital plate and a computerized screen.

KEY TERMS

Key terms are defined in the Glossary on the Evolve website.

Dosimeter
Generator
Half-value layer
Kilovoltage

Milliamperes
Milliampere seconds (mAs)
Patient dose

Reproducibility
Timer
Transformer
Quality assurance

Quality control

Introduction

Throughout the previous chapters, we have learned the basic workings of the imaging systems. We have also learned how to protect ourselves from overexposure to radiation. We have reviewed various methods of producing an image and then recording the image to either film or a digital medium.

This chapter identifies problems and their solutions. It is divided into sections that reflect the chapters in the text. This chapter will serve to outline quality control tests that may be incorporated into:

- Ensuring the generator is functioning correctly
- Ensuring the film/screen combination is correct and optimized
- Identifying the cause of artifacts on films caused by imperfections in intensifying screens, incorrect cleaning of the processor, or incorrect functioning of the processor
- Conducting virtually all the tests relevant for confirming the correct functioning of the generator

Quality control testing procedures are described in this chapter, though images relevant to quality control are either located in this chapter or in the specific chapters where the particular modalities are described.

Quality assurance in a digital world was addressed in Chapter 8.

FIG. 9.1 An Example of a Density 1 + Base + Fog Image. This image will be referred to throughout the chapter and throughout the text.

APPLICATION INFORMATION

- As long as the radiography unit is calibrated and functioning correctly, the generator make, model, and age have nothing to do with the digital receptor.
- The image galleries within each earlier chapter demonstrate what can go wrong and, for the most part, how to correct deficiencies.
- The most important density in the testing of films, screens, cassettes, generators, and processing is density 1 + base + fog. Thus, we have positioned an image of this density here, at the beginning of the chapter, where it will be easily found during the testing of any equipment (Fig. 9.1). Not all facilities have densitometers, and because the human eye is fairly accurate when measuring comparable densities, this figure will be of value.

Quality Control and Quality Assurance

Quality control is the identification of actions that are necessary to ensure, and then verify, the performance of equipment. It is part of quality assurance, which is the documentation of all factors relating to a certain policy or protocol within a field of study.

Quality assurance documents quality control and ensures that a facility, system, or administrative component performs safely and satisfactorily in service to a patient. Quality assurance includes scheduling, preparation, and efficiency during an examination or treatment; reporting the results; and conducting quality control.

In short, quality assurance involves the entire hospital or facility—front door to back exit—whereas quality control is the testing of each of the factors (usually the equipment) within the facility or hospital.

Radiography Equipment Testing

This section discusses quality control as it relates to Chapter 2, Diagnostic X-Ray Production.

Recall the concept that the x-ray generator produces the alpha, beta, and gamma rays (x-rays) that are produced to radiograph a patient. It is necessary to know when the exposure switch is closed and that what has been set on the generator is actually what is produced, ensuring that the exposure is correct.

The generator, x-ray tube, and main transformer are separate components in the imaging system and are not attached specifically to the image detector. They do not need to be. Frequently, an older generator is paired successfully with a new digital x-ray or computer imaging system.

X-Ray Generator Testing

X-ray generators come in all shapes, sizes, and ages; however, certain characteristics are consistent. Every x-ray generator connects to a power supply. The larger units are wired into facility power sources. The smaller portable units plug into wall outlets or have capacitors (batteries) that hold a charge and provide power when necessary.

Line Voltage

When the x-ray generator is activated, the current and the voltage of the power lines supplying the electricity to the x-ray unit must be stable and consistent. On older x-ray generators, there is a needle indicator that must be set to a certain level. The operator can adjust a setting to ensure that the needle falls within the correct boundary (see Fig. 2.5A,B).

Identify a Problem with the Line Voltage

If the images are intermittently light or dark when they are normally the correct density and all other factors are consistent, the first place to check is the line voltage meter. Newer models of x-ray generators do not have line voltage compensators, as the correction occurs automatically when the generator is activated.

Fig. 9.2 is a flow chart that indicates what procedures should be taken to ensure that the line voltage is correct. A technician/operator may use this chart to determine if the problem lies with the line voltage on older units.

If the technique is adjusted and the images do not change in density, there is a problem with the line voltage. It is very rare for the line voltage to "drift" upward. It will only do so if there is a "load" on the line for one image and that load is switched off during the next procedure.

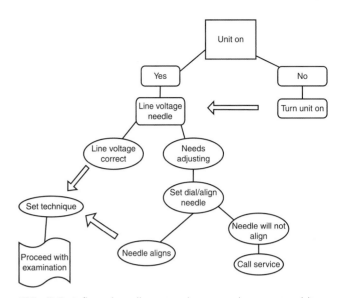

FIG. 9.2 A flow chart illustrating the steps when a manual line voltage compensator is installed.

◆ APPLICATION INFORMATION

An x-ray consultant was called into a veterinary clinic that was located in a neighborhood industrial mall. X-ray images were intermittently turning out too light to have any diagnostic value. The x-ray unit was only 5 years old, and the problem had begun about 2 months earlier. The veterinarian had assumed that the technicians were not holding the exposure foot switch down for the entire exposure, but when they insisted there was a problem, he called the consultant. This problem frequently occurred during the afternoon, but then everything was fine by the next morning. The consultant tested the x-ray generator and noticed that occasionally the voltage dropped from 70 kV to 40 kV and then half an hour later it was back up to the correct voltage.

The x-ray consultant discovered that a new business had moved in and illegally attached their power lines to the veterinary clinic's mains transformer on the roof of the building. At certain times, extra power was needed. This meant that every time they used power, it reduced the power available to the veterinary hospital—hence the inconsistencies in exposures. The solution: The business had to purchase their own transformer to boost their power when necessary.

X-Ray Unit Calibration Testing

The easiest method to identify a problem is to perform external testing using a kV meter, a dosimeter, and a timer test tool (Fig. 9.3). An alternative meter includes all three functions. Because most schools do not include this type of testing, we will simply explain the tests and familiarize the reader with the basic logic of the results.

Generator Compliance Testing

The next few paragraphs will explain how to test for x-ray equipment compliance (Fig. 9.4), will address each test individually, and will explain the procedures. The tests described here are not what is considered "invasive testing," which involves opening the x-ray unit and attaching meters to various components. The main purpose of outlining these

FIG. 9.3 **A,** Simple component x-ray test meters. A Radcal kV meter, a Radcheck dosimeter, a Nuclear Associates Timer Test Tool. **B,** Fluke/Victoreen Non-Invasive All-in-One Test Meter M-4000. **C,** Rear view of Fluke/Victoreen Non-Invasive All-in-One Test Meter M-4000.

Radiography Technical Services
X-Ray Generator Compliance Testing

Facility Name: _____

Contact Person: _____ Phone # _____

Address: _____

Control Model: _____ Serial # _____ (_Tube)

Kilovoltage (must be accurate to within +/− 8%)   Time Set _____

MA Set	KV Set			
	60	70	80	100
60 or				
120 or				
240 or				
300 or				
360 or				
			Comment	

mA	mAS	Output	mR/mAs
60 or	6	100 mR	16.6
120 or	12	200 mR	16.6
240 or	24	300 mR	16.6
300 or	30	500 mR	16.6
360 or	36	600 mR	16.6

mA Linearity (+/− 10%) __80_ kV _.10_ Time
An example of a perfectly calibrated generator

Timer (+/− 8%) _____ kV _____ mA

Time Set/ Pulses		Output
1/120 or	1	
1/60	2	
1/30	4	
7/120	7	
1/10	12	
3/20	15	

Reproducibility 80kV 10 mAs - +/− 20%
Or___ kV @ ___ mAs

	Output
1st	
2nd	
3rd	
4th	
5th	

Filtration 80kV, 10 mAs
or ___ kV @ ___ mAs

0 mm Al	
2.3 mm Al	
3.3 mm Al	
HVL= @80kV	

Survey Date _____ Completed by _____ Notes _____

FIG. 9.4 An Example of a Generator Test Page for a Veterinary Clinic. Tests include kV, mA linearity, half-value layer, timer test, and reproducibility.

tests is to explain what is involved if a service engineer is called to a facility and uses test meters to determine the calibration of the unit.

Kilovoltage
Testing Techniques
Kilovoltage is tested using a kV meter. The kV stations that are tested are within the normal range of use in graduations of 10 kV. Each station must be tested at every milliampere (mA) setting within the normal range of use.

The kV meter is positioned on the tabletop with the collimator open to the size of the detector. The typical allowance of ±8% is legal in most countries. These parameters are listed in Fig. 9.5. When 70 kV is set on the unit, one expects to receive 70 kV at every mA station in the normal range of use. It is important that the kV does not drift higher or lower than 8% of this total. mA stations and/or kV stations not in the normal range of use should be disconnected and labeled as such on the generator by the service engineer.

Takeaway Tips
Accurate calibration is vital for every kV station at every mA setting. When a service person is in the x-ray room calibrating the x-ray unit, the veterinarian or technician should request a copy of the report to ensure that all the stations within normal range of use are calibrated correctly. A unit may be installed in an area where the higher stations are not available due to insufficient power coming into the building. These stations must be marked as unavailable, and the technique chart must not include them.

Half-Value Layer
The **half-value layer** (HVL) indicates the thickness of an absorber necessary to reduce the intensity of the x-ray beam to half its original value. In radiography, that absorber is aluminum. HVL is a measurement of the amount of filtration between the x-ray tube and the patient.

As the x-ray beam leaves the tube, it goes through three different filters:
1. The glass envelope of the x-ray tube
2. The inherent filtration of the tube port, mirrors, and collimator
3. Added filtration to meet legal requirements

Legally, there must be enough filtration to eliminate non-useful x-rays (which will add to patient dose) and scattered radiation (which is not part of the useful beam).

Testing Techniques
The HVL is tested using a **dosimeter**. The kV may have to be adjusted to deliver the specific amount if the x-ray unit is not calibrated correctly. A technique is set (usually 80 kV and 10 mAs), an exposure is completed, and the dose is recorded. Filtration, in the form of aluminum plates, is added to the collimator until the dosimetry reading is half the original value. The plates of aluminum are measured in increments of 1 millimeter. This final reading is the HVL (Fig. 9.6).

Takeaway Tips
Legal filtration is typically 3.4 mm of aluminum at 80 kV. As the kV changes, the penetration value changes, so the HVL

KILOVOLTAGE ACCURACY TEST

Default kVp	Allowable Range +/− 8% Limits	Actual KvP Allowable Range (Leave blank if default values used)	Small Focus Time ___ mA ___ mAs ___			Large Focus Time ___ mA ___ mAs ___		
			25	50	100	100	200	300
50	46.0–54.0							
60	55.2–64.8							
70	64.4–75.6							
80	73.6–86.4							
90	82.2–97.2							
100	92.0–108.0							

On some units the default kV is not available. Use the middle column for closest values available.

FIG. 9.5 Chart for Testing Kilovoltage at Various mA Stations on both Large and Small Focal Spots.

HALF-VALUE LAYER TEST

Setup:

1. kVp set at ___**___ to deliver 80 or _____ kVp.

2. mA _____ Time _____ (or) mAs _____

3. Focal/meter distance _____ cm Focus _____

4. Filtration: Fixed _____ Variable set at _____

> **The kV must be calibrated correctly or the HVL total will be incorrect.**
> **As kV increases, the x-rays emitted by the x-ray tube become progressively harder (i.e., more penetrating). The HVL at 80 kV will be different than the HVL at 90 kV since the beam at 90 kV is "harder" than the beam at 80 kV.**

Readings	
0 ____ mm Al added	_____ mR
3 ____ mm Al added	_____ mR
____ mm Al added	_____ mR
____ mm Al added	_____ mR

Actual kVp	HVL
@ 80 kVp	_____ mm Al
@ kVp	_____ mm Al

FIG. 9.6 Chart for Testing Half-Value Layer. The half-value layer is a measurement of the amount of filtration necessary to reduce the x-ray beam to half its original intensity at preset factors.

mA	Output
60 or	
120 or	
240 or	
300 or	
360 or	

A   mA linearity (+/– 10%) _____kV _____Time

mA	mAs	Output	mR/mAs
60 or	6	100 mR	16.6
120 or	12	200 mR	16.6
240 or	24	300 mR	16.6
300 or	30	500 mR	16.6
360 or	36	600 mR	16.6

B   mA linearity (+/– 10%) __80__ kV __.10__ Time
An example of a perfectly calibrated generator

FIG. 9.7 A, Chart for testing mA linearity. **B,** mA linearity chart filled in. As the mA increases, the dose (output) increases proportionally. This is a 1:1 ratio. Increase the mAs by two times the amount, and the dose will double.

will change with an increase or decrease in kV. For example, a higher kV will produce a more penetrating beam, so more aluminum is required to reduce the intensity of the radiation to half its value. The equipment manufacturers arbitrarily set the standard for testing at 80 kV. This way the HVL can be compared uniformly across various x-ray units. The kV reading may need to be adjusted so that the actual kV output is 80 kV. If the HVL is too low, the "softer" radiation will not be filtered out, adding to the dose to the patient. If the HVL is too high, parts of the useful beam will be filtered out. This puts extra wear on the x-ray tube and decreases contrast in the image ("flattens" the contrast).

mA Linearity Test

The mA linearity test is a measure of the output from each of the mA stations and is done to ensure that the output is consistent from one station to the next.

Testing Techniques

The instrument used for testing is a dosimeter. This test measures the radiation dose to the dosimeter. (kV and time are not changed between exposures.)
- 60 mA must have an output of one-half of 120 mA.
- 120 mA must have an output double that of 60 mA and half that of 240, etc.
- The legal variable is ±10%.

Takeaway Tips

The kV and time are always constant for each exposure and must be accurately calibrated (Fig. 9.7). The source-image distance (SID) must also remain the same. The output will be unique for each x-ray unit, but it must be linear. In an ideal generator, dividing the milliroentgens (mR) dose value as read on the meter by the mA value will give the same number for each station. Many meters

Timer (+/– 8%) _____kV _____mA

Time Set/ Pulses		Output
1/120 or	1	
1/60	2	
1/30	4	
7/120	7	
1/10	12	
3/20	15	

A

Timer (+/– 8%) __80__ kV __100__ mA

Time Set/ Pulses		Output
1/120 or	1	**1 or .0083**
1/60	2	**2 or .016**
1/30	4	**4 or .033**
7/120	7	**7 or .058**
1/10	12	**12 or .100**
3/20	15	**15 or .150**

B

FIG. 9.8 A, Chart for testing time stations. **B,** Timer test chart filled in. Note that the time is read in pulses for a single-phase unit and as decimal time for high-frequency and three-phase units.

still read out in the older dose nomenclature and not the SI units.

Timer Testing

The timer on an x-ray generator is set to control the length of time that radiation is produced.

Testing Techniques

A timer test tool is placed on the tabletop. The x-ray beam is collimated to the size of the detector. An exposure is made, and the readout will indicate the time of the exposure as measured by the radiation dose read by the timer test tool. The timer test should include all the stations that are in the normal range of use. Fig. 9.8 shows a selection of stations. Note that even though fractions are set on the generator, the meter reads in decimals only.

Takeaway Tips

Single-phase generators select time by fractions of 120 pulses in North America (100 pulses in other countries). Three-phase generators read actual time, which is in decimals. High-frequency generators read the same as three-phase generators. Three-phase and high-frequency generators have much shorter times available, as they are not limited by pulses per second.

Reproducibility

Reproducibility is a measurement of the generator's ability to produce the same output at the same settings throughout several exposures when the factors have been changed and reset between each recorded exposure (Fig. 9.9).

Testing Techniques

The instrument used is the dosimeter. The dosimeter is placed on the table, and the x-ray beam is limited by the collimator to the size of the detector. The generator is set at 80 kV and 10 mAs. After the exposure is made, the factors on the generator are changed and then reset to 80 kV and 10 mAs. This is repeated a minimum of 5 times but no more than 10 times.

The actual reproducibility mathematics are beyond the scope of this text. It is sufficient to average the output doses and determine whether any individual number is ±15% above or below the average. If any number is beyond the parameter, the service engineer must recalibrate the unit.

Reproducibility 80 kV 10 mAs - +/– 20%
Or _____kV @ _____mAs

	Output
1st	
2nd	
3rd	
4th	
5th	

A

Reproducibility 80 kV 10 mAs - +/– 20%
Or _____kV @ _____mAs

	Output
1st	**243 mR**
2nd	**246 mR**
3rd	**244 mR**
4th	**235 mR**
5th	**241 mR**

B

FIG. 9.9 A, Reproducibility chart. The test is carried out by setting a technique (usually 80 kV and 10 mAs). A dose reading is taken and noted. The dials or light-emitting diode (LED) settings are changed and then changed back to the original, and an exposure is taken. This is done 5 to 10 times. The test ensures that the exposures are reproducible. **B,** Reproducibility chart filled in. Note that the output will vary slightly between exposures. If it varies by more than 15%, the generator should be recalibrated.

FIG. 9.10 **A,** Typical collimator without an angulation scale. This particular tube stand has a preset height (100 cm); therefore, the dial indicates cassette sizes at that height. **B,** Another collimator that has a variety of SID (source-image distance) settings available. This would be mounted on a variable-height tube stand.

Takeaway Tips

Reproducibility is very important in order to produce consistent radiographs. The actual calculations for this test are quite complicated, but it is enough to take 5 to 10 exposures and ensure that they are well within ±15%. The selectors should be changed between each exposure, just as they would be if the x-ray unit was in constant use. If this test demonstrates a greater or lesser than 15% flux, it may explain why some images turn out considerably darker or lighter than others at the same setting.

In-Clinic Collimator Tests

The collimator is the final exit point for the radiation from the x-ray tube. It is composed of a metallic outer shield with plates (leaves) installed to widen or narrow the x-ray beam to control the radiation affecting the target (Fig. 9.10). The following tests demonstrate how to ensure the integrity of the collimator and its requirements are met.

The collimator must be tested (Fig. 9.11) to ensure that:
- It produces a light field that is perpendicular to the tabletop
- The alignment of the visual field (the light field on the table) is not greater or less than 2% of the actual film size when the axis of the x-ray beam is perpendicular to the table
- The minimum collimation does not exceed 5 cm × 5 cm
- The indicated collimation is accurate, if present
- There is a stepless adjustment of the field size
- The dimensions of the field can be adjusted smaller than the field size

Test 1. Collimator Alignment
Objective
To test the alignment of the visual (light) field to the x-ray field.

Equipment
- One cassette loaded with film or a digital imaging plate

Procedure
1. Ensure that the focus film distance (FFD) is 100 cm or 40 inches from the tabletop.
2. Use 50 kV, 100 mA, and a minimum of .03 ($^1/_{30}$ second).
3. Place the cassette on the tabletop so that the central ray will pass through the exact center of the cassette.
4. Place coins on the cassette so that their edges are within the light field but right at the edge of the light field (Fig. 9.12).
5. Place a larger coin on one corner so that you can identify the position of the cassette or plate after processing.
6. Process the exposed film and place it on the front of the cassette in the exact position it was in before the exposure.
7. Turn on the collimator light.
8. Measure the amount of "shift," or lack of coincidence, between the light field and the radiation field.

Digital Systems
Follow the same procedure but leave the coins in place while you view the image. Any offset of the x-ray field will be demonstrated on the monitor, which you will compare with the light field on the tabletop.

Conclusion
- The coins mark the edge of the light field.
- If there is a "shift," or lack of coincidence, greater than 2 cm, then an adjustment is necessary.
- Sometimes this adjustment may be made in-house with an adjustable lever mounted above the x-ray tube. More often, a service person will have to make the adjustment.

Collimator, Table, and Tube Stand Tests See following procedure charts	Yes	No	Not Available
1. Alignment of the visual field (with the light on) to the x-ray field meets the 2% guideline when the axis of the beam is perpendicular to the plane of the image			These tests are all available with every collimator
2. Minimum collimation does not exceed 5 cm by 5 cm at a target to image receptor distance of 100 cm			
3. Dimensions of light field can be adjusted smaller than the image receptor			
4. Stepless adjustment of field size			
5. Collimator light is visible with room lights on			
6. Perpendicularity of light beam @ 90 degrees to table top			
7. Focus Film Distrance is accurate to +/− 3%			
8. Indicated collimation accurate			
9. Angulation indicator correct			
10. Tube, table, and tube stand stability			

FIG. 9.11 A Chart to be Completed when Testing the Collimator.

FIG. 9.12 Testing Collimator Alignment. The coins are placed at the edges (corners) of the light field. An image is generated. In this case the light field and the x-ray field are not coincident. The x-ray field is 1 cm to the left of the coin edges. This is due to a very slight angulation of the x-ray tube.

- Occasionally, on older x-ray tubes the weight of the tube will bend the tube arm and cause a horizontal shift due to the weight of the tube and the length of the tube arm. This is quite common and must be adjusted by an x-ray engineer unless the tube stand is equipped with an adjustment handle.

Test 2. Minimum Collimation
Objective
To ensure the minimum collimation does not exceed 5 cm × 5 cm (2 inches × 2 inches) at a target to the image receptor distance of 100 cm (40 inches).

Equipment
- Ruler with centimeter and/or inch markings

Procedure
1. Position the x-ray tube over the center of the table at 100 cm (40 inches) above the tabletop.
2. Turn on the collimator light
3. Minimize the collimated field (Fig. 9.13).
4. Measure the lighted area on the tabletop.

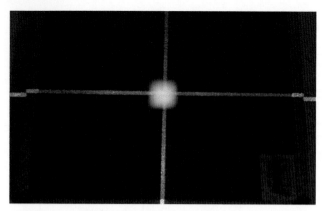

FIG. 9.13 Minimum Collimation. This collimator is equipped with a laser light source to assist in viewing. The collimator leaves are closed to less than 5 cm × 5 cm (2 inches × 2 inches).

FIG. 9.14 The light field can be adjusted to cover an area smaller than the smallest image receptor.

Conclusion

The lighted area should be closed to allow a minimum light field/x-ray field of 5 cm × 5 cm (2 inches × 2 inches).

Test 3. Dimensions of Light Field Can Be Adjusted Smaller Than the Image Receptor
Objective

To ensure that the leaves of the collimator can be adjusted to an area smaller than the smallest image receptor. This will ensure that each image demonstrates collimation.

Equipment
- One cassette (the smallest cassette in the normal range of use in the facility)

Procedure
- Position the x-ray tube on the center of the table.
- Position the cassette on the tabletop beneath the collimator.
- Turn on the collimator light (Fig. 9.14).
- Collimate to smaller than the outer edges of the cassette.

Conclusion

The collimator should close so that the lighted area is smaller (both horizontally and vertically) than the smallest cassette in the facility.

Test 4. Stepless Adjustment of Field Size

This test ensures that the field size can be made larger or smaller by turning the collimator knobs without hesitation or "notching."

Equipment
- Collimator

Procedure
1. Position the x-ray tube over the tabletop (Fig. 9.15).
2. Open and close the collimator to make sure that it opens and closes smoothly with no hesitation or "notching."

Conclusion
- This test is essential to ensure that the collimator leaves are not being obstructed by the internal components.
- Collimators are difficult to service in-house, but any difficulties with their movement must be addressed.

Test 5. Collimator Light Visibility
Objective

To ensure that the collimator light is visible with the room lights on.

Equipment
- One x-ray cassette
- One piece of black paper or cardstock with a textured design

Procedure
1. Position the x-ray tube over the center of the table at 100 cm (40 inches) above the tabletop.
2. Turn on the collimator light and open the leaves to 10 cm × 10 cm (4 inches × 4 inches).
3. Slide the piece of black paper into the light field, and observe whether the light is still visible (Fig. 9.16).

Conclusion
- The light should be clearly visible on the black paper.
- The Plexiglas plate covering the collimator light can become stained or burned with age. If the light is a standard (nonhalogen) bulb, it may not be bright enough to penetrate the discolored Plexiglas plate.
- If the light is not visible on the black paper, it will not show up on the black coat of a patient.

Test 6. Perpendicularity of Light Beam at 90 Degrees to Tabletop
Objective

To ensure that the light beam of the collimator is perpendicular to the tabletop.

FIG. 9.15 A, Stepless adjustment of field size. A sliding bar at the front of the collimator adjusts the horizontal collimation (front to back of the table). **B,** The sliding bar at the side of the collimator adjusts the vertical collimation caudal-cranial.

FIG. 9.16 Collimator Light Visibility. The laser light is visible, but the collimator light is also visible on this textured surface.

FIG. 9.17 Perpendicularity of Light Beam at 90 Degrees to the Tabletop. The bubble in the level on top of the collimator indicates that the tube is not angled and the central ray will be perpendicular to the tabletop. It corresponds to the reading of the level mounted within the collimator.

Equipment
- One carpenter's level

Procedure
1. Position the x-ray tube over the tabletop.
2. Place the level on the x-ray tube (or the front edge of the collimator if possible) so that it rests evenly on both ends.
3. Observe the bubble in the level, and adjust the angle of the x-ray tube if necessary so the bubble is centered and that the central ray from the x-ray tube is perpendicular to the tabletop (Fig. 9.17).
   1. If the x-ray tube has an angulation feature, it may slowly rotate to a slight angle when the tube is moved along the table during routine radiography.

Test 7. Focus Film Distance Is Accurate to ±2%
Objective
To ensure that the FFD is correctly marked on the x-ray tube column.

Equipment
- Measuring tape
- Yardstick ruler or meter stick that is at least 1 yard (meter) long

Procedure
1. Position the x-ray tube column in the center of the table longitudinally.

FIG. 9.18 The level of the focal spot is marked on the tube. The measurement is taken at 100 cm (40 inches). This is then compared with the marking on the tube stand.

2. Locate the position of the focal spot on the x-ray tube which should be one-third of the diameter of the tube starting from the bottom of the x-ray tube. The focal spot position is usually marked on the x-ray tube. If it is not marked, then mark this spot.
3. Tape the meter (yard) stick to the table so that it extends over the edge of the table and rests against the tube column.
4. Raise the x-ray tube until it is positioned at the 100-cm (40-inch) mark on the tube column (Fig. 9.18).
5. Measure the distance from the meter stick to the focal spot mark on the x-ray tube.

Conclusion
- The focal spot must be within ±2% of 100 cm (40 inches).
- If the focal spot is beyond these parameters, then the measuring point on the tube stand must be corrected.

Test 8. Collimation Indications Are Accurate
Objective
To ensure that the measurements on the collimator indicating the cassette size are accurate both horizontally and vertically.

Note: Keep in mind that not all collimators are equipped with field size indicators (Fig. 9.19). However, the law states that if they are part of the collimator apparatus, they must be correct.

Equipment
- One cassette of each size in the normal range of use in the facility

FIG. 9.19 Collimator Size Indicator. The outside partial ring is for 180 cm (72 inches). The inside ring is for 100-cm (40-inch) measurements.

Procedure
1. Ensure that the focal spot is 100 cm (40 inches) above the tabletop.
2. Place a cassette on the tabletop under the collimator.
3. Adjust the indicators on the collimator to coincide with the set size of the cassette both horizontally and vertically.
4. Turn on the collimator light and observe whether the light is coincident with the size of the cassette.
5. Repeat this for each size of cassette in the normal range of use in the facility.

Conclusion
- The indicators must be accurate for the size of the cassette.
- Correcting the indicators in the field by a service engineer can be difficult and expensive.
- Sometimes it is easier and less expensive to mark the correct measurements on the collimator in black marker for the size of cassette in the facility.

Test 9. Angulation Indicator Is Correct
Objective
To ensure that the angulation indicator is accurate.

Equipment
- Carpenter's level
- Protractor with angles clearly marked

Procedure
1. Position the x-ray tube over the center of the table.
2. Ensure that the central ray is perpendicular to the tabletop (see Test 6).
3. Angle the x-ray tube so that the angle indicator is at 45 degrees (Fig. 9.20).
4. Position the protractor so that the angle indicated is 45 degrees. The collimator angle and the protractor angle should be coincident.
5. Repeat this procedure for 60 degrees and 90 degrees.

FIG. 9.20 This Tube is Angled to 45 Degrees as Evidenced on the Protractor.

Conclusion
- The angle indicator must be completely accurate.
- If x-ray tubes do not have angle indicators, keep the protractor in the x-ray room if angled views are required.

Test 10. Tube, Table, and Tube Stand Stability
Objective
To ensure that the x-ray table, the x-ray tube, and the tube stand do not move during an exposure (Fig. 9.21).

Equipment
- X-ray tube, table, and tube stand
- Carpenter's level

Procedure
Note: Some x-ray tubes are mounted directly to the wall and do not move along the table. Some tube stands are mounted to the ceiling or the floor. Some x-ray tables are not mounted to the floor.
- Position the tube stand at the center of the table.
- Turn on the collimator light and position exactly over the center of the table. It is vital that the table does not move at all, particularly if a grid is to be used. If the table is not bolted to the floor, mark on the floor where the table legs must be before each exposure.
- Move the tube steadily and quickly along the table and then release the tube. It should remain stationary.
- Stand at either end of the x-ray table, and move slightly toward the tube-stand side of the table.
- The tube stand should be vertical and not be angled slightly toward the table.
- The collimator base should not be even slightly angled across the table (from table front to table back).

Conclusion
- The tube stand must be stable and must not move once it is placed in position. The x-ray table must be bolted to the floor directly in line with the center of the central ray.

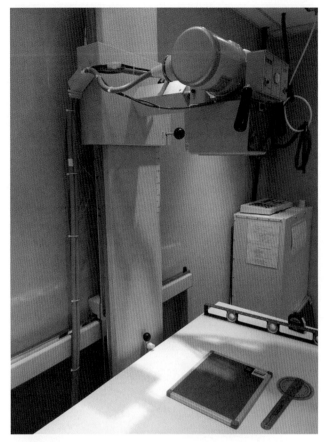

FIG. 9.21 X-ray Tube and Tube Stand Stability. The x-ray tube stand is moved to the end of the table and stopped. It must be mounted correctly so that it does not sway or move when the operator's hand is lifted from the handles. Standing at the end of the table, the operator should also note whether the tube is slightly angled front to back from the operator moving the tube while pulling downward on the handles.

- The tube stand must not lean in toward the table.
- The tube hanger must be parallel to the floor and must not allow the tube to "sag" so that the bottom of the collimator is not absolutely parallel with the table front and back and side to side.
- The table and the bottom of the collimator must be parallel to one another both vertically and horizontally.

Radiobiology and Radiation Protection for the Patient and the Worker

This section discusses quality control as it relates to Chapter 3, Radiation Safety and Protection.

The leaded products that are purchased for the x-ray room will deteriorate over time. Lead-impregnated rubber will harden and crack. Leaded protective garments should be tested annually and logged on a chart (Fig. 9.22). Each apron, thyroid collar, and pair of gloves should be identified and dated when they are purchased and marked with an indelible marker.

Date	Apron #1	Apron #2	T. Collar #1	T. Collar #2	Leaded Gloves / Masks Visual Inspection

FIG. 9.22 Leaded Products Integrity Test.

FIG. 9.23 A, Lead apron testing. The apron is spread over the cassette, which is placed horizontally on the tabletop. Two images are generated: one for the bottom of the apron and one for the top of the apron. **B,** Leaded apron radiograph showing the even stitch lines on the edge of the apron and two simulated apron cracks to demonstrate the difference between the stitch line and actual cracks (no one would agree to having their apron slashed, even for the textbook!).

Leaded Aprons

Equipment

- X-ray unit set at 60 kV and 6 mAs or whatever setting gives a density 1 + base + fog on the image through the leaded apron.
- Two 35- × 43-cm (14- × 17-inch) cassettes or a digital detector
- Method of marking

Procedure

- Place a 35- × 43-cm (14- × 17-inch) cassette crosswise on the tabletop. Place a leaded apron on the cassette so that the bottom of the apron is aligned with the lower edge of the cassette (Fig. 9.23A).
- Select the exposure as indicated above
- Open the collimator to include the entire detector.
- Expose and process the film OR check the digital image.
- The density on the film should be 1 + base + fog.

- Repeat the exposures, exchanging the cassette with each exposure and moving it up toward the neck with each repositioning until the entire apron has been tested.
- Remember to mark each section with the same identifier so that there is a referenced image for each section.

Takeaway Tips

Leaded products are not designed to be penetrated by primary radiation. They are designed for protection against secondary radiation. Therefore, high technical factors are not required to penetrate them with direct radiation. If the film image is too dark, any cracks will not appear. If the film is too light, the cracks will still appear as dark gray lines. Stitching on the sides of the apron will show up as a line of black dots and is normal. Any cracks or holes will show up as black lines or black holes. Areas of lighter density demonstrate overlaps or stretching of the lead sheets within the apron. To prevent cracks, aprons should be stored on a hanger or specially made rack and not be folded or permanently bent over a wire hanger.

Thyroid Protectors

Procedure

These can be tested using the same technique as with the leaded aprons. They can be logged on the same chart. If the thyroid protector is attached to the apron, it should still be labeled individually.

Gloves/Leaded Rubber Masks/Blockers

Because gloves are double-sided, it is impossible to test them individually using radiation, as one side will mask the other. Gloves must be pliable and easily folded when used. Old leather gloves and mitts can become stiff and unbendable. They should be replaced with new pliable mitts/gloves. The old gloves may be repurposed as leaded masks for absorbing scattered radiation. They should be labeled as masks with indelible marker.

Gloves should be examined manually by inserting a hand into the glove and palpating to identify any cracks or splits in the leaded rubber. Leaded masks should be examined regularly and should be stored lying flat.

Imaging on Film

This section discusses quality control as it relates to Chapter 4, Imaging on Film.

The image gallery in Chapter 4 demonstrates many different problems associated with film-based imaging. These problems are usually identified by their effects on the image after processing. The following are a few additional tests that may be necessary if film artifacts are noted.

Testing Film/Screen Resolution

In radiography, recorded detail is measured and expressed as resolution. Resolution is the ability of the viewer to distinguish separate line pairs. A line pair is described as one black line and one white line in an image. Line pairs are expressed as lp/mm. The test tool that is used is a resolution test pattern (see Fig. 4.29).

Very-high-resolution images are 30 to 35 lp/mm (for extremity and mammography images in medical imaging). Standard full-speed x-ray film with appropriate 400-speed screens is typically 8 to 9 lp/mm. Advertised line pairs in digital imaging are typically 4 to 5 lp/mm.

X-ray film alone has virtually infinite resolution but is only one part of the imaging system. When a veterinarian looks at an image and attempts to diagnose a hairline fracture, he or she is looking at the combination of the technical factors used to produce the image: the cassette front, the film, the intensifying screens, any tabletop artifacts, the grid, processing artifacts, the patient's anatomy, and, finally, the illuminator. Each of these factors can degrade the image and yield a far-less-than-perfect result.

Resolution becomes even more important when digital imaging is considered. The comparison between digital imaging and film/screen imaging is always, primarily, about resolution.

Equipment

- Resolution test tool
- Cassette with film
- X-ray unit

Procedure

1. Place the resolution test tool on one side of the cassette with a leaded blocker on the other side.
2. Set the x-ray unit factors to 55 kV and 3 mAs or whatever factors are required to expose the film to a density of 1 + base + fog outside of the resolution test tool.
3. Now move the leaded strip across to the unexposed side of the cassette.
4. Turn the resolution test tool 90 degrees and place it on the cassette.
5. Expose this side of the cassette and process the film.
6. Use the guide on the resolution test tool to determine the resolution of the film/screen system by counting the line pairs until they appear to run together and cannot be differentiated.

X-Ray Cassettes

Uniform Speed of Intensifying Screens

Objective

To identify the uniformity of the intensifying screens in your facility. (First, ensure that the generator is correctly calibrated and has good reproducibility.)

Equipment

- Every film cassette in use in the facility
- Leaded numbers to identify each cassette (Cassettes may also be identified permanently by writing small numbers on the screen with a fine black felt-tip marker. The same number should then be marked on the outside of the cassette.)
- X-ray generator that has been tested for reproducibility as indicated above. Each exposure must be the same as the one before and the one after.

Procedure

- Place the cassettes on a table outside the x-ray room ready to test in ascending order of size.
- Bring in one cassette at a time and remove it from the room once it has been exposed. (This will eliminate the possibility of scattered radiation affecting the cassette.)
- Place one cassette containing film on the tabletop and center it beneath the central ray.
- Collimate to the size of the cassette. Use 50 kV, 100 mA, $\frac{1}{30}$ second (3.3 mAs). (This is a typical technique for a 400-speed system. If your system speed is different, then adjust the mAs according to the chart in Fig. 5.3.)
- Process your film and record the density. (If you do not have a densitometer, record the value that is different from or similar to the reference image (see Fig. 9.1).

- Adjust the technique if necessary, until the image is density 1 + base + fog.
- Expose the film in all the cassettes using the same technique. (If you had to adjust the technique, then retest the original cassette.)
- Check the speed of the intensifying screens, and compare the images using the same illuminator with the room lights turned off.
- Slower screens produce a lighter image; faster screens produce a darker image. Ideally, all images should be the same density. Replace any screens that produce a vastly different density so that every cassette in the hospital produces uniform densities.

The Blue/Green Question
Objective
To identify the color emission of a blue or green screen.

Make sure that the correct type of film corresponds to the correct screens. Remove one sheet of film from the box, close the box tightly, and turn on the light. Recall that blue-receiving film is green and green-receiving film is mauve or very light purple.

Before "new" cassettes are put into use, always follow this procedure.

Equipment
- Cassettes to be tested, which were identified earlier
- X-ray generator

Procedure
1. Use 70 kV, 100 mA, and 0.25 (¼) second.
2. Turn off the lights in the room and ensure that it is completely dark.
3. Place an open cassette beneath the central ray.
4. Open the collimator to cover the open cassette and turn off if required.
5. Make an exposure and record the color of the light.
6. Mark a large G for green or B for blue on the back of each cassette as it is tested.

Conclusion
Screens that are not the same emission as the ones already in use must be disposed of. If they are kept in the hospital because the cassettes may be used later, then they must be clearly labeled with the color of the screens.

Film/Screen Contact Testing
The intensifying screens must be held in the cassette in close overall proximity to the film. Any air gaps between the screen and the film will result in a fuzzy image (Fig. 9.24A–D). Most companies use foam rubber, which is glued to the back of the cassette, holds the screen evenly and permanently with the correct amount of pressure against the front screen, and maintains the film in good film/screen contact.

Equipment
- Screen contact test tool
- Cassettes to be tested containing film

- X-ray unit
- Leaded numbers or black markers to identify each cassette

Procedure
- Place a cassette on the tabletop centered beneath the central ray.
- Open the collimator light to cover the cassette.
- Place the screen contact test tool on top of the cassette.
- Set the technique at 55 kV, 5 mAs. (This is a suggestion only and may have to be altered depending on the generator and film/screen combination.)
- The density of the overall image should be 1 + base + fog (see Fig. 9.1).
- Some technicians drill a small hole with a diameter of 0.635 cm (¼ inch) in the center of the test tool. This enables a density reading to ensure that the technical factors are correct and that the screen speed is consistent with every cassette.
- Once the correct density has been verified, test all the other cassettes in use within the facility.
- Check the density in the center hole for every cassette to ensure that the screens in use are functioning correctly and have not lost speed.

Conclusion
Every film image should demonstrate a clear mesh pattern with no darkened areas. Dark areas within the pattern indicate areas of poor screen contact, which will degrade the image and make it fuzzy.

◆ APPLICATION INFORMATION

All cassettes are vulnerable to problems and should be reviewed once per year. The films should be removed in the darkroom (or the cassette should be left unloaded after use). The cassette should be examined under room light to ensure that the foam rubber has maintained its integrity and that the hinges and latches are in good working order. The screens should then be cleaned with gauze dampened with distilled water to remove any dust or fingerprints. The cassettes should be stood open and upright on the tabletop for a minimum of 10 minutes until the screens are completely dry. A record should be kept to note any problems observed during the inspection.

Inspecting Cassettes for Stability and Integrity
If the latches break or cassette rubber hinges break apart, the intensifying screens can be removed with caution and placed into a new cassette with no screens or a used cassette whose screens have deteriorated.

Equipment
- Double-sided tape
- Replacement cassette with old screens removed
- Sturdy table or floor space

FIG. 9.24 **A,** This screen shows the perfect screen contact image. **B,** A problem with screen contact caused by the light being allowed to diffuse between the screen and the film. There is an area of "fuzziness" in the caudal thoracic and cephalic lumbar area of the spine. This corresponded with poor film screen contact when the cassette was tested. **C,** Poor screen contact across the entire image. The Kodak cassette had a split back, which the staff tried to correct using duct tape. The overall poor screen contact demonstrates that this method is not a solution. The screens must be changed into a new cassette. **D,** A small piece of dirt was discovered on the screen, causing a minus density artifact in the image. This artifact was in a different place each time. As the films were drawn out of the cassette, it would be moved around—but never out of—the image. (**A** from Fauber TL. *Radiographic Imaging and Exposure.* 5th ed. St. Louis: Mosby; 2017.)

- Distilled water
- 4- × 4-inch (10- × 10-cm) gauze pads

Procedure

- Place the cassette on a sturdy table and peel a corner of the screen away from the back of the cassette.

- Very carefully, pull the screen back away from the corner, making sure that the screen does not crease or bend in any way. The emulsion of the screen can be "rolled" away, but it must not crease. Kodak screens are difficult to remove because they are glued over the entire back surface. Other companies just use double-sided tape to attach the screens.

- Make sure that the tabletop is clean and dust free.
- If the foam starts to rip away, just pull the screen out carefully and place it face down on the tabletop.
- Now peel away the foam from the screen. It will probably rip away in sections; this is fine as long as all of it comes away. This can be a messy job, as some of the older screens had a very thin rubber backing that deteriorated into a rubbery glue.
- Once the screen is free of the backing, place double-sided tape on all four sides and place it in the cassette on the same side as it was in the original cassette. For example, if the screen you are working with was on the back of the cassette, then place this screen on the back.
- The easiest method for replacing the screen is to place the front screen into the front of the cassette and then place the back screen on top of the front screen and close the cassette.
- Now open the cassette and clean the screens with distilled water and gauze.
- Stand your cleaned cassette upright on the tabletop to dry for at least 10 minutes before reloading it with film.

Takeaway Tips

This is a worthwhile exercise if you have Kodak screens. They are excellent screens and maintain their speed virtually indefinitely. Make sure that you do not crease the screen when you remove it from the cassette. If you need smaller screens and you have smaller cassettes, you can cut the screens with regular scissors.

Reinstating the Curve on Curved-Back Cassettes

DuPont and a few other cassette companies bent the back of the cassette slightly to enhance the film/screen contact (see Fig. 4.26A). Over time, the bend decreases as the cassette opens and closes.

Equipment
- Cassette to be adjusted
- Firm, stable tabletop

Procedure

Place the cassette over the edge of a table and carefully press gently but firmly and evenly on the back of the cassette (see Fig. 4.26B). The pressure does not have to bend the cassette very much, so gentle pressure and then a check to ensure that the back has been recurved is sufficient.

Takeaway Tips

These cassettes also have a very tiny "handle" that was added to assist the operator in opening the cassette (Fig. 9.25). This worked well if the cassette back popped up when the cassette was opened, but if the bend was eliminated and the cassette was opened without the back rising slightly, it became difficult to open the cassette once it was unlocked. Carefully rebending the cassette solves this problem.

FIG. 9.25 These cassettes have a tiny handle that is useful for opening the cassette if the curved back is curved correctly.

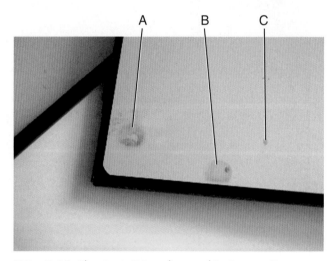

FIG. 9.26 Chemistry Dripped onto this Screen. The screen emulsion is porous and will absorb chemicals of any variety that are dripped onto it. It is important to remove the film and close the cassette when manually processing.

Miscellaneous Screen Artifacts

The emulsion of the intensifying screens can be compromised in various ways. A few of these problems are demonstrated in the following images. There is no particular test protocol to identify these problems because they are obvious once the cassette is opened in the light. The cause of the artifact that was clearly displayed on the image is now visible (Figs. 9.26 and 9.27; see also Figs. 4.33 and 4.34A,B).

Cassettes must be handled with care to ensure that the front remains undamaged and radiolucent. Any foreign material introduced into the cassette shell may show up superimposed on the image. Patient effluent, barium, or contrast material can leak between the front of the cassette and the back of the screen. If seepage occurs, the screen and backing must be removed and cleaned thoroughly (Fig. 9.28).

FIG. 9.27 A, A particular problem with DuPont Quanta 111 and later screens. In a humid environment, the screen emulsion absorbed moisture from the air and swelled into tiny raised points. These points broke up the lattice network of the image, causing small minus density artifacts. These artifacts started at the screen edge and migrated across the entire screen as the process continued. **B,** An enlarged view of a portion of part A. The screen is destroyed and must be replaced. There is no "fix" to this problem.

FIG. 9.28 An Example of Overuse of Screen Cleaner. Overuse of commercial screen cleaners builds up residue on the screen, which eventually causes artifacts on the film as they cause plus-density artifacts across the image. The artifacts are actually areas of the film that were affected by the components of the screen cleaner that caused the silver in the emulsion to coagulate.

Cleaning Intensifying Screens
Equipment
- Cassettes to be cleaned that are open and have the film removed
- Distilled water
- 1 package 10- × 10-cm (4- × 4-inch) gauze pads

Procedure
This procedure is best carried out on the x-ray table, as it is a wide surface for cleaning the cassettes and standing them upright to dry after cleaning. Make sure there is no pet hair or debris.
1. Open the cassette and remove the film in the darkroom.
2. Lay the open cassette on the x-ray table.
3. Dampen a 10- × 10-cm (4- × 4-inch) gauze wipe with distilled water. The gauze should be damp, not wet.
4. Wipe the screen lightly in one direction; then wipe again at a 90-degree angle. The screen should be very slightly damp with no visible water marks. Any surface dirt or dust is removed with this technique.
5. Stand the cassette upright on the table and leave it to dry for at least 15 minutes. The cassettes should be placed upright so that dust in the room does not settle and adhere to the screens.
6. Check that the screen is dry and that it is adhering to the cassette front and back. If the screen is loose (as might be the case with Agfa cassettes and some generic brands), make sure there is no dirt or dust beneath the screen. (Use a flashlight if necessary.)

Takeaway Tips
Commercial screen cleaning agents are often specific to the manufacturer and can stain screens that are manufactured by other companies. Screen cleaners that are not matched to

FIG. 9.29 Screen Wear. The emulsion of the screen becomes worn over many years. The thinning emulsion is not as effective at converting x-rays to light. The lighter areas on the film replicate the wear areas on the screen. The insert demonstrates an enlarged part of the indistinct image.

FIG. 9.30 Collimator Splash. The image is overexposed. The boundaries of the collimator are clearly visible, yet the film has been exposed by secondary/scattered radiation beyond the collimator limits.

the manufacturer can discolor the screens, reducing their x-ray–to–light conversion (see Fig. 4.32). Screen cleaners often build up a residue, which eventually becomes visible on the images. Home remedies such as alcohol and other cleaning agents should never be used on screens because they can dissolve the protective layer and damage the emulsion.

Distilled water and lint-free gauze are the best combination to use to clean screens. It is very important that a screen is completely dry before reinserting the film. Film emulsion is manufactured to absorb moisture rapidly, and any remaining moisture on the screen would be absorbed into the film emulsion and would adhere to the screen, ruining the film as well as the screen. Stains and scratches that have penetrated the emulsion of the screen are not removed by the technique just described. If the emulsion from the screen is missing, there is no way to repair the screen.

Intensifying Screen Wear: Emulsion Loss
Older intensifying screens exhibit wear artifacts (Fig. 9.29). Over many years of use, the emulsion of the screens thins and then disappears completely as thousands of films are inserted into and removed from the cassette. There is no solution to this problem other than replacing the screen with one of similar speed.

Producing the Image

This section discusses quality control as it relates to Chapter 5, Producing the Image.

Testing for Extrafocal Radiation

This test is used to determine that the scatter/secondary radiation as seen in Fig. 9.30 is actually from the patient and not from extrafocal radiation, as is seen in Fig. 9.31.

Equipment
- Aluminum foil folded so that there are 8 to 10 layers in a strip about 4 inches wide and 15 inches long (10 cm × 40 cm)

FIG. 9.31 An Example of Extrafocal Radiation. This imprints the image of the dog's ears beyond the edges of the collimator *(arrows)*.

- A market chicken about 5 pounds*
- X-ray unit

Procedure
1. Wrap the aluminum strip around the x-ray tube hanger just at the attachment of the collimator to the bottom of the x-ray tube (Fig. 9.32).

---

* This experiment can also be carried out in the veterinary hospital using live patients. It does not increase the dose to the patients, but rather solves a mystery as to why the extrafocal images are occurring.

FIG. 9.32 A, Aluminum foil will reduce the effect of the extrafocal radiation if it is radiating from the front and sides above the collimator. The foil should be at least 8 to 10 layers thick and wedged tightly against the mounting brackets. **B,** The aluminum foil surrounds the collar of the x-ray tube. In this case the staff has rotated the collimator so that it is easy to turn on the light if it is necessary to hold the patient.

2. Place the patient (or phantom) on the tabletop, and set the technical factors according to the technique chart.
3. Collimate to the edges of the patient's anatomy.
4. Process the film and view the image.

Conclusion
If the images previous to this one demonstrated extrafocal radiation, the aluminum foil will absorb the soft radiation and the regions beyond the collimator will be clear. If the densities are caused by secondary/scattered radiation, it will remain the same, with or without the aluminum filter.

Optimizing the Image

This section discusses quality control as it relates to Chapter 6, Optimizing the Image.

Grids, Grid Lines, and Grid Artifacts
Grid Quality Test (Fig 9.33)
Equipment
- Cassette with film
- X-ray unit containing a grid

Procedure
- Place the cassette with film enclosed into the grid tray, and close the grid tray.
- Do not put any object on the tabletop, and make sure the tabletop is clean.

FIG. 9.33 This grid was an old metal door screen from about 50 years ago. A new veterinarian was puzzled by the artifacts that affected every image taken in the grid tray.

- Set the technical factors to 55 kV and 8 to 10 mAs (or whatever technique is necessary to expose the film to a density of 1 + base + fog).
- Process the film and examine the resulting image closely.

Takeaway Tips
Any grid artifact will be immediately visible (Fig. 9.34). The image should be a gray film at density 1 + base + fog. Faint

FIG. 9.34 A, Grid deterioration places an overall indistinct pattern of vertical lines on this image. **B,** Magnified view of part A. The vertical lines are more obvious. The film was positioned on the illuminator vertically to mask the lower portion of the illuminator, causing the artifact to become more visible.

vertical lines may be visible, but they will be uniform, will be very faint, and will not affect the images.

Grid Artifact Images

These images are taken to demonstrate incorrect grid position. The grid artifact problems are easy to identify as shown in Figs. 9.34 to 9.36.

Illuminators: Characteristics and Test Tables

Once the film is processed and ready for viewing, the next piece of equipment in use will be the illuminator (Fig. 9.37). The illuminator is a vital link in the imaging chain. It is important to be aware that the illuminator provides light by ionizing the gas within the illuminator tubes. It does this by means of a ballast and an electric current. If the illuminator is mounted in the x-ray room and the room is also used as a darkroom, the gas will continue to ionize for up to 30 minutes after the illuminator is switched off. This situation will definitely fog any x-ray film within the room even though the light is not visible to the human eye. With older illuminators and fluorescent lights, the shape of the light is actually visible after the light is switched off. This is the reason why fluorescent lights should never be mounted in a darkroom.

The illuminators should be on the list of cleaning and maintenance protocols within the veterinary hospital. Each

FIG. 9.35 This grid is placed in the holder upside down and horizontally. The grid lines should run vertically; that way if the tube is angled, there will be no grid cut-off.

illuminator should be checked at least once per year or if any discrepancy is noticed between any of the light tubes in the facility (Fig. 9.38). Fluorescent tubes are sold in many different colors. The tubes for the veterinary hospital are standard tubes and can be purchased at any hardware store. It is essential that the light tubes are matched and are a blue-white light. They must not be any other color. X-ray film is tinted blue to reduce the glare of the illuminator when the

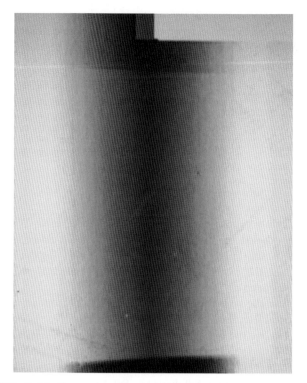

FIG. 9.36 This grid is placed in the holder vertically but upside down. Because it is a focused grid, the grid lines absorb the lateral radiation and only the center of the image shows the exposure.

FIG. 9.37 The light from the illuminator with no mask is glaring to the eye of the viewer and decreases the brightness of the image so that small details are lost.

Illuminator Position	Color	Brightness	Both bulbs bright	Flicker?	Clean screen Y/N
X-ray room					
Examination room 1					
Examination room 2					

FIG. 9.38 Test Table for Illuminator Condition.

veterinarian is viewing the images. The illuminator light tubes must be blue-white to match the blue tone of the film base. The front of the illuminator is a specially treated glass that will diffuse the light from the light tubes. This glass is expensive and not readily available except from a radiography illuminator supply company. The back of the illuminator behind the light tubes must be a shiny white in order to reflect the light through the front of the illuminator.

An Illuminator Mask

A mask can be easily made from a 35-cm × 43-cm (14- × 17-inch) sheet of film (Fig. 9.39).

- Remove the film from the film box.
- Seal the box and then expose the film to the light.
- Process the film and cut small or large holes in it to mask only the areas with no image.

- Keep the portion of the film that was cut away and use it if a second hole is cut in the film to view a second image.
- The mask will eliminate light from around the image, causing small details to be seen more easily.

Processing the Image on Film

This section discusses quality control as it relates to Chapter 7, Processing the Image.

Protecting the unexposed film from any kind of exposure to heat, light, and chemicals is vitally important to the production of an optimized image. Containers for storing unexposed film are available, and they must be positioned in the darkroom with no possibility of light seeping in (Fig. 9.40).

FIG. 9.39 A Simple Illuminator Mask Cut from a 35- × 43-cm (14- × 17-inch) Film. A hole is cut in the mask and then taped onto the film. The "window" allows the light to illuminate the image but masks the brightness of the surrounding light.

Darkroom Integrity

Testing safelight integrity must always be completed using a film that has been exposed to radiation. The film is now 8 to 10 times more sensitive to any form of film fog or artifact.

Equipment
- Cassette with film
- Stopwatch preset to 2 minutes (to be turned on by pressing a switch)

Procedure
1. Position a cassette on the tabletop.
2. Collimate to the edges of the cassette.
3. Lightly expose the film using 50 kV and 2 mAs. When processed, the lightest section of the film should be considerably lighter than the density 1 + base + fog density.
4. Take the cassette to the darkroom and place it on the counter.
5. Turn the safelight off, secure the darkroom from any noticeable visible light, and open the cassette.
6. Remove the film from the cassette, and place half of the film beneath the cassette, leaving half of the film exposed to any light leaks within the area.
7. Press the stopwatch to start counting down from the 5-minute preset.

FIG. 9.40 A, An example of a standalone metal film bin. The metal bin is essential if the film is stored in the x-ray room. This one doubles as a counter. B, A plastic wall mount bin in the darkroom. This model holds two sizes of film.

FIG. 9.41 The safelight test film will quickly demonstrate that there is a problem with the positioning and brightness of the safelight.

8. While the stopwatch is counting down, slowly and carefully move around in the darkroom as your eyes acclimate to the dark (only after 5 minutes will you start to see light leaks). Look around to see if there is any visible light.
9. Once the stopwatch counts down to zero, place the film on the feed tray and process the film. If there is a problem with the darkroom integrity, the half of the film that was exposed to the light will show a density that is not present on the half of the film that was beneath the cassette.

Safelight Testing

Testing safelight integrity must always be completed using a film that has been exposed to radiation (Fig. 9.41). The film is now 8 to 10 times more sensitive to any form of film fog or artifact.

Equipment
- Film in a cassette

Procedure
1. Expose a film in a cassette on the tabletop using 50 kV and 2.0 mAs or just enough radiation to cause a low density on the film. It does not have to be as high as density 1 + base + fog.
2. In the darkroom, place the cassette on the counter.
3. Turn the safelight on, secure the darkroom, and open the cassette.
4. Remove the film from the cassette, and place three-quarters of the film beneath the cassette, leaving one-quarter exposed to the safelight. Count to 30 seconds.
5. Slide the next quarter of the film out from under the cassette, and count to 30 again. (Now half of the film has been exposed to the safelight.)
6. Repeat this once again so that three-quarters of the film has been exposed to the safelight.
7. Immediately remove the rest of the film from under the cassette, and process it.

The last quarter of the film was exposed to the safelight for just the length of time it took to take the film to the processor. If there is a problem with the safelight, the areas exposed will be darkened in proportion to the length of time that they were exposed to the light plus the amount of the original exposure. The total length of exposure time is 1.5 minutes (90 seconds).

Ideally, the processed film will be completely clear with no fog on it. Fig. 9.41 shows the results of a safelight test where there was definitely a problem with the positioning or wattage of the safelight.

Processor Tests

Developing, Fixing, Washing, and Drying

Problems with artifacts in automatic processors can be a challenge to diagnose. Some problems, such as the ones in the image gallery in Chapter 7, are easy to diagnose. Occasionally there is a problem that is more difficult, or the veterinarian would like to evaluate two different films and the way they react to light from the intensifying screens.

As the film is placed on the entrance tray and is moved forward toward the entrance rollers, it is affected by the solutions in the developer, fixer, and wash. The dryer rollers can also cause artifacts, but this is rare.

Automatic Processors vs. X-Ray Equipment

The majority of processor problems occur in the developer. First, it must be determined that the problems occurred in the processor and are not a result of a problem with the x-ray equipment. A simple test for this follows.

Equipment
- Two cassettes loaded with film
- X-ray unit
- Processor at the correct temperature and ready to process film
- Leaded pencil

Procedure
1. Place the first cassette on the tabletop.
2. Set the technical factors at 50 kV and 5 mAs (or whatever factors are necessary to give a density of 1 + base + fog).
3. Press the exposure switch.
4. Remove the cassette from the x-ray room.
5. Place and expose the second cassette using the same technical factors.
6. Take the cassettes to the darkroom and open them both.
7. With the leaded pencil, mark the direction of travel of each film on the film itself.
8. Film #1 will be processed horizontally (long side in first).
9. Film #2 will be processed vertically (short side in first).
10. Process each film individually, one film after the other, through the center of the feed tray
11. Review Fig. 9.42.
12. If the artifact lines are horizontal on the one image and vertical on the next image that was rotated 90 degrees, then the artifact is caused by the x-ray unit and not the processor.

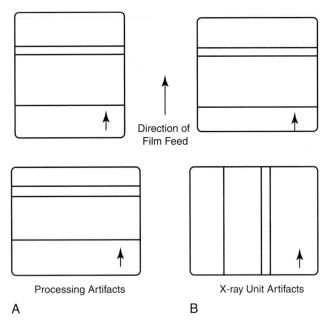

Direction of Film Feed

Processing Artifacts

X-ray Unit Artifacts

A

B

FIG. 9.42 A Processor Test Film. **A,** The two films are processed individually at 90 degrees to one another. The artifacts do not rotate with the orientation of the film. This indicates that the artifact problem is in the x-ray equipment. **B,** The two different films are processed individually, and the artifacts change with the rotation of the film. This indicates the problem occurs within the processor.

13. If the artifact lines stay in the same direction even if the film is rotated, then the artifact is caused by the processor.

Sensitometry/Densitometry

Sensitometry/densitometry is a method of tracking processing parameters. It has nothing to do with the x-ray equipment, as the x-ray equipment is not involved in this procedure. Sensitometry makes use of a device called a *sensitometer* (Fig. 9.43A). This unit has a stepped table on the bottom with a light beneath it. The table has 21 steps, or small strips of graded densities, that increase from base + fog level to the maximum blackness that the film will attain. It is manufactured so that when the light exposes a film, the middle step (Step 10) will be density 1 + base + fog (Fig. 9.43B). The top step will be base + fog only (D_{min}), and the bottom step will be the maximum density of the film (D_{max}).

The density will be read on a companion unit called a *densitometer* (Fig. 9.44). The densitometer contains a "platform" where the film is positioned for each of the 21 steps. These steps are then plotted on graph paper to produce a sensitometry curve (Fig. 9.45).

Every radiograph is made up of densities, from the clear areas on the film to the very black areas. It is the combination

1	Density Base + Fog
10	Density 1.0 + B + F
21	Density 3.25 + B + F

Time: Date: ID No:

B

FIG. 9.43 **A,** The sensitometer is a highly calibrated light source that exposes the film to a stepped wedge. The 21 steps on the wedge are used to plot contrast and consistency of the processor. **B,** A sensitometry strip produced by the sensitometer and processed. The top step is base + fog only. The bottom step is the maximum density of the film. Step 10 is density 1 + base + fog.

FIG. 9.44 A Companion Densitometer. The inset shows the small area that the light shines through to read the film. The readout is a digital screen at the top of the unit.

FIG. 9.46 It is possible to read all of the various densities in a radiograph using the densitometer. Sensitometry provides a way of arranging the densities in sequence from the lightest to the darkest density provided by that particular film.

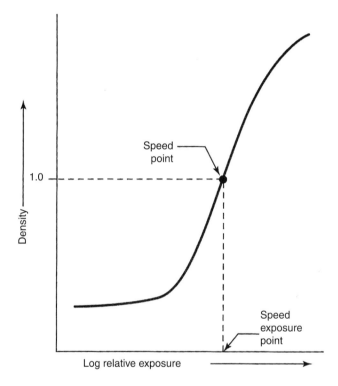

FIG. 9.45 A Typical Sensitometry Curve. At the x-y axis, there is virtually no density other than base + fog. As the steps increase, the density increases to step 21, which gives the maximum density.

of these densities that demonstrates the anatomy/pathology of the patient (Fig. 9.46). Sensitometry is one easy method to sequentially arrange the densities on the radiographs to ensure that the processing parameters are stable day to day. A chart is filled in that measures two steps above density 1.0 (Step 12) and two steps below density 1.0 (Step 8) (Fig. 9.47). When the total of Step 12 minus Step 8 is filled in on the bottom line, the number should be virtually identical every day, only varying by 2 to 3 points.

If the processing varies from day to day as the chemistry in the processor becomes older and more contaminated, this would demonstrate that the replenishment is not working

well and does not maintain fresh chemistry. The resulting films will become flat and lack contrast. This will show up quickly on the images, but the sensitometry strip will also confirm there is a problem, even if no images are taken that day.

Another use of sensitometry is to compare the contrast and speed of two different films. If a sales representative convinces the veterinarian that his or her film is better than the present film in use in the hospital, the first thing that must be done is to determine the contrast and speed of the new film. Is it more black and white (higher contrast), and does it react faster to radiation (speed) than the present film? Both films should be tested in the darkroom before any exposures on patients. Speed will affect the technique chart, and contrast may enhance or degrade the image.

Fig. 9.48 demonstrates three films, and it is easy to read that the stepped wedge on the left is very low contrast and the film on the right is very high contrast. Fig. 9.49 demonstrates the curves plotted for two different films. The speed point should always be read at density 1 + base + fog. In these curves, Film A is considerably faster (reacts to the radiation) than Film B. However, the contrast of both films is virtually identical. In this same figure, the bottom row shows that in order to achieve density 1 + base + fog on Film A, you need to reduce your exposure from 2.0 to 1.5. This can be translated to a 25% speed advantage for Film A over Film B. Another film may be manufactured to show several different gray steps and never get to solid black.

Month _____

Day	Mon	Tues	Wed	Thur	Fri	Mon	Tues	Wed	Thur	Fri	Mon	Tues	Wed	Thur	Fri	Mon	Tues	Wed	Thur	Fri
Date	3	4	5	6	7	10	11	12	13	14	17	18	19	20	21	24	25	26	27	28
Step 12																				
Step 8																				
Con-trast																				

FIG. 9.47 Monthly chart plotting the sensitometry contrast levels every operational day.

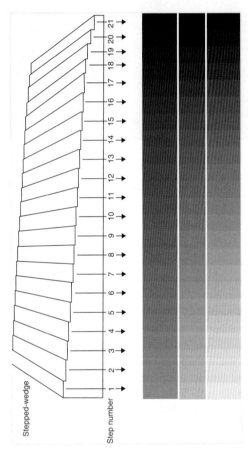

FIG. 9.48 Comparing Three Different Sensitometry Strips from Three Different Films. The film to the left is very low contrast with many steps of gray. The middle film is a standard general radiography film with more contrast than film number 1. The film on the right is a specialty high-contrast film with few gray steps.

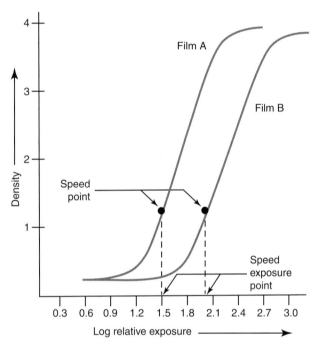

FIG. 9.49 Comparing Two General Radiography Films from Two Different Manufacturers. Film A reacts more quickly to the radiation than does Film B. The comparable densities are measured at density 1 + base + fog, which is known as the *speed point*. The bottom of the graph indicates the relative exposure levels.

Fluoroscopy

This section discusses quality control as it relates to Chapter 11, Fluoroscopy.

As veterinary hospitals become more sophisticated, fluoroscopy and real-time imaging become necessary. The equipment is more sophisticated, but a few simple tests can be easily carried out before any examinations. One is the fluoroscopy resolution test procedure.

Fluoroscopy/Image Intensifier Resolution

Objective
To identify the resolution of the fluoroscopy monitor and to log image lag or fade to identify if the image is severely distorted at the edges of the monitor screen.

Equipment
- Fluoroscopy unit with the monitor turned on
- Fluoroscopy resolution test tool (usually the lower-resolution test tool [16 to 60 mesh] is sufficient for most hospitals)

Procedure
1. Position the fluoroscopy unit over the tabletop so the image intensifier is as close to the table as possible.

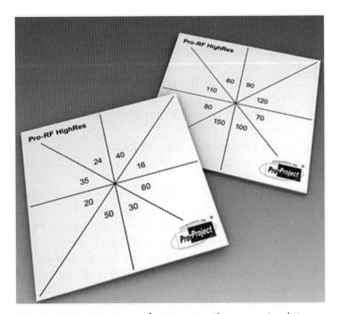

FIG. 9.50 Two Test Patterns for Measuring Fluoroscopy Resolution on the Monitor. Mesh (corresponding to the number on the front covers) is embedded between the two covers. The lower test tool measures a resolution of 16 to 60 mesh. The other measures a high-resolution screen from 60 to 150 mesh. These test tools can also be used to view edge distortion and lag.

2. Place the resolution test tool on the tabletop (Fig. 9.50). Position the central ray of the x-ray unit over the center of the resolution test tool.
3. All personnel in the room must wear leaded protection.
4. Stand close to the table and the resolution test tool so that a view of the image intensifier is unobstructed.
5. Depress the foot switch so the test tool appears on the monitor with the center of the test tool in the exact center of the monitor.
6. Identify the finest mesh that is visible on the monitor.
7. Release the foot switch and rotate the mesh 90 degrees. Depress the foot switch and verify your first reading.
8. Step 7 will identify if the mesh was correct or if it was enhanced by the raster lines of the monitor.
9. Record the finest mesh that was identified. This is a subjective test, so if you are wearing eyeglasses, ensure that they are clean and unmarked with fingerprints or dust.
10. Now move the image intensifier from side to side and watch the image. It should move and stop with no lag or "drag" of the image.
11. The mesh should now be located in the exact center of the monitor. If there is any distortion of the image at the edges of the monitor, it should be noted, as this may increase with the age of the monitor.

Takeaway Tips
As stated, this is a subjective test, so the observer must make sure that his or her eyes are unobscured by fogged or marred eyeglasses. The minimum mesh should be 30 or higher. A mesh reading of 16 indicates that the unit should be recalibrated. This test should be repeated at least once every

6 months for every monitor in the facility. The distortion is a natural result of the curvature of the lens in the monitor. It can deteriorate as the monitor ages.

REVIEW QUESTIONS

1. Quality control and quality assurance are defined as follows:
   a. Quality control is concerned with performance of equipment; quality assurance is documentation of all factors.
   b. Quality control is concerned with performance of people; quality assurance is the assurance that people are working.
   c. Quality assurance is the performance of equipment; quality control is the documentation of assurance.
   d. Quality assurance is identification of the actions necessary to assure performance; quality control is the performance.
2. Correct line voltage is confirmed by reading the dial on the front of the generator. Which of the following statements is true?
   a. There is always a dial on the front of every generator.
   b. Modern generators do not have a dial; calibration is internal.
   c. There is no particular importance to reading the dial.
   d. Once the machine is turned on, every generator will recalibrate.
3. kV testing is carried out with a kilovolt meter. Which of the following statements is true?
   a. The typical allowance is ±8% of the station tested.
   b. Accurate kV is not important, as the unit will compensate.
   c. Testing of every mA station is unnecessary, as the unit is always consistent.
   d. The typical allowance is ±15% of the station tested.
4. Half-value layer is defined as:
   a. The amount of filtration that reduces the intensity of the x-ray beam by 50%
   b. The amount of aluminum that reduces the penetration of the beam by 50%
   c. The amount of filtration needed to calibrate the generator to 50%
   d. The amount of aluminum that reduces the output of the generator by 50%
5. mA linearity is described as follows:
   a. The mA stations are mathematically linked.
   b. The output of each station must be exactly the same or within 50% of each other.
   c. The output of each station must be linear; the output at 50 mA is 50% of the output at 100 mA.
   d. The output of a generator is dependent on its linearity; all the stations should be the same.
6. Collimator testing is essential to ensure that the area to be radiographed is exactly delineated. Which of the following statements is true?
   a. The minimum collimation is the same size as the smallest cassette.

b. The indicated collimation must be in place and be accurate.

c. The x-ray tube can be misaligned up to 5%.

d. The alignment of the visual field and the x-ray field is coincident.

7. Testing leaded aprons with film involves:
   a. Placing the apron under the fluoroscope and scanning it
   b. Just testing the areas of concern on each apron
   c. Placing the apron on a cassette and radiographing it
   d. Setting a very high technique because it is made of lead

8. When an image consistently appears to be out of focus across the entire surface, one problem may be:
   a. The film/screen contact has been compromised
   b. The patients all move when this cassette is used
   c. The manufacturer built in a soft focus to this screen type
   d. The processing parameters are not functioning correctly

9. One cassette always appears to give lighter-than-normal images. Which of the following statements is true?
   a. The technician should mark this cassette and not use it.
   b. The technician should examine the screens to see if they are the same manufacturer and type.
   c. The veterinarian should throw out the screens and cassette and buy new ones.
   d. The staff should mark the cassette and always increase the technique when they have to use it.

10. One cassette always produces very gray films with little to poor contrast. A cause could be:
    a. The source-image distance is too great
    b. The screens emit blue light and the film is green receiving
    c. The screens emit green light and the film is blue receiving
    d. The processing chemistry is contaminated

11. One cassette always produces images with reasonable contrast but requires twice the radiation. A cause could be:
    a. The screens emit blue light and the film is green receiving
    b. The screens emit green light and the film is blue receiving
    c. The patient is very large with little contrast in its anatomy
    d. The source to patient distance is too great

12. The service person has just left, and the veterinarian brings you an image with an outline of the patient's ears on it. You diagnose this as:
    a. Scattered radiation and nothing can be done about it
    b. The service person left the collimator plates out of the collimator
    c. The problem is extrafocal radiation because the collar was left off the collimator
    d. The image is too dark and this is the result

13. The test for grid quality includes:
    a. The film in the grid tray and keys and syringes on top of the table for contrast
    b. The cassette on the tabletop and a very light exposure
    c. The cassette in the grid tray with nothing on the tabletop
    d. The film is exposed on the tabletop, and the grid lines should not be visible

14. The test for darkroom integrity includes:
    a. Turn out all the lights except the safelight, then look for light leaks
    b. Turn out the light and wait 5 minutes for your eyes to adapt before looking for light leaks
    c. Turn out the light and immediately look for light leaks, then process a film out of the film bin
    d. Expose a film, place it on the counter halfway beneath the cassette, turn all the lights off, and process after 5 minutes

15. The test for safelight integrity includes:
    a. Expose a film, place it on the counter three-quarters beneath the cassette, draw it out a quarter at a time, and then process
    b. Turn out the light except the safelight, look for housing cracks, and process a film from the bin
    c. Safelight is on; stand for 5 minutes, look for light leaks, and process a film
    d. Safelight is on; expose a film and process it, then look for cracks in the housing

16. Sensitometry is defined as:
    a. A method of testing processing parameters
    b. A method of testing the integrity of the x-ray equipment
    c. A testing device using a densitometer on exposed films
    d. A density measure for films exposed by the sensitometer

17. One type of artifact is the appearance of clear minus density "dots." Which of the following statements is true?
    a. The cause of this is unknown.
    b. The screen must be cleaned and dried before reuse.
    c. This is a rare occurrence with new screens.
    d. This is caused by minute areas of swollen emulsion.

18. Chemical spills and darkroom accidents:
    a. Damage screens and film and are preventable with good darkroom protocols
    b. Are easily wiped up with no further consequences
    c. Damage cassettes but are easily wiped off screens
    d. Cause fixer and developer to settle on film, prematurely developing it

19. Commercial screen cleaners:
    a. Are the best method for cleaning screens
    b. Should not be used without adequate ventilation
    c. Can build up layers and produce artifacts on the image
    d. Must be matched to the screens or they will not work

20. Heat and chemical fumes will fog the film and cause:
    a. The films in the box to stick together and be difficult to remove
    b. An increase in activity of the emulsion, which will produce a density on the film
    c. An image on the film that can be processed
    d. Artifacts that are identifiable on the film
21. One method of ensuring good resolution is to test each cassette:
    a. For good film/screen contact
    b. To ensure that they all have the same exposure response

c. To ensure that they all require the same technical factors
d. For its ability to mask artifacts and shadowing

Chapter Review Question answers are located in the Instructor Resources on Evolve and can be provided to students at the discretion of the instructor.

Ultrasound technology is becoming an invaluable diagnostic modality.

CHAPTER **10**

Ultrasonography

Robert F. Hylands, DVM

A mind that is stretched by a new experience can never go back to its old dimensions.

— Oliver Wendell Holmes, Jr., American author, 1841–1935

OUTLINE

LEARNING OBJECTIVES

When you have finished this chapter, you will be able to:

1. Understand the principles of real-time ultrasound imaging.
2. Recognize the artifacts and limitations of ultrasonography.
3. Identify the various transducer types and functions.
4. Describe the various image modes and discuss their applications.
5. Discuss clinical applications with regard to body systems.

APPLICATION

The application of the information in this chapter is relevant to the following areas:

1. Producing ultrasonographic images when alternative diagnostic imaging is required.

KEY TERMS

Key terms are defined in the Glossary on the Evolve website.

Acoustic impedance	Continuous wave Doppler	Microconvex	Sector transducer
B-mode	Convex	Phased array	Spatial resolution
Brightness	Depth control	Phased array transducer	Transducer
Cine loop	Gain control	Presets	
Color flow Doppler	M-mode	Pulsed Doppler	

In the years since the first introduction of ultrasound to veterinary medicine, the use of this indispensable imaging tool has grown exponentially to include a vast number of applications. Ultrasound advances our diagnostic abilities in a safe and reasonably economical manner. In almost 30 years of rigorous studies focusing particularly on prenatally exposed children, ultrasound has been found to have no associated health risks. Studies in 1982 and 1987 by the Bioeffects Committee of the American Institute of Ultrasound in Medicine (AIUM) first demonstrated that there were no biological effects on the patient or instrument operators at intensities typical of diagnostic ultrasonography. In 1998, the World Health Organization stated that ultrasound imaging was both a safe and effective modality. This chapter will discuss basic principles in order to familiarize the technician with the goals of an ultrasound examination.

Throughout the chapter there are certain unfamiliar terms of which the reader should be aware. They are presented here so that the student may refer to them as they arise within the chapter.

Echogenicity: The appearance of the tissues on ultrasound, based on the ability of the tissues to reflect sound waves. This refers to the brightness of tissues that are being projected on a B-mode display.

Anechoic: A structure that is lacking in internal echoes or is echo free. Appears very dark to almost black on ultrasound.

Hyperechoic: The tissue of interest reflects back more intense sound waves and appears brighter than the tissues surrounding it. This is a subjective evaluation of adjoining structures.

Hypoechoic: The tissue of interest reflects fewer sound waves and with less intensity, making it appear darker than the tissues surrounding it. This is a subjective evaluation of adjoining structures.

Isoechoic: This a term used to describe two structures that have relatively similar echogenicity toward each other.

Attenuation: This is the loss of sound wave energy as it traverses the tissue or the medium due to absorption, reflection, or scattering.

Reverberation: The sound wave is repeatedly reflected between two highly reflective surfaces—for example, air and the ultrasound probe.

Near Field: The area of a structure of interest that is closest to the probe.

Far Field: The area of a structure of interest that is farthest from the probe.

Ultrasonography and Plain Radiology: A Comparison

One of the defining characteristics of ultrasound is the benefit of real-time imaging. During a scan, a continuous stream of live, digitized data is obtained. From this data, video recordings can be saved, which then can be transferred into a "cine loop." A cine loop is a continuous feed that allows the area of interest to be visualized over a prolonged period. In comparison, plain radiography catches the area of interest in a still frame during a split second of time when the exposure is taken.

The advantage of real-time imaging is seen when we use ultrasound for cardiac studies. We can watch the movement and function of the heart and internal structures over the course of a cardiac contraction. Newer matrix probes can even take this a step further by instantly projecting the acquired data in multiple planes. These planes are then reconstructed by computer and can allow visualization of the heart in a three-dimensional format. This is called *multiplanar reconstruction,* or MPR, and it allows the ultrasound equipment to project an image that is similar to that of more advanced technologies such as magnetic resonance imaging (MRI) and computed tomography (CT).

A second benefit to ultrasound is the ability to move the diagnostic probe in any direction that is required. In comparison, radiography usually requires standardized positioning and orientation. The ability to move the ultrasound probe over the area of interest gives us a much greater amount of information about the subject.

When we use high-quality ultrasound machines in this way, we are able to show fine anatomical detail through the use of multiple sensitive receptors in the ultrasound transducer (probe) (Fig. 10.1A,B).

And finally, as mentioned in the introduction, the safety precautions required when using ionizing radiation (x-rays) are *not* required when an ultrasound is in use. There are no protective gowns and gloves, and multiple people may be in the room during the ultrasound study.

FIG. 10.1 **A,** The white arrow represents the outline of the stomach wall on a lateral radiograph of a canine abdomen. Very little information about the wall thickness or health can be extrapolated through this image. **B,** The photograph to the right is a high-resolution image of the stomach wall acquired in a near-field ultrasound examination. In the ultrasound study, we can observe gastric motility and can visualize the detail of each anatomical layer of the stomach wall. (Images courtesy RF Hylands.)

There are many other benefits to this modality, which we will explore as we continue through this chapter, including the ability to visualize detailed pathology through tissues and fluid, which could be difficult or impossible with conventional radiographic imaging.

The Ultrasound Machine

Principles

The basic principle of the ultrasound machine is the production of sound waves by an ultrasound probe (also known as the *transducer*) and the return of that reflected sound wave. Sound waves enter the tissues and are reflected back to the probe; the intensity and speed of the reflections are influenced by the tissue densities. The probe receives the reflected sound waves and then translates the information to the computer so that it can be read on the video screen by the operator.

The most important components of an ultrasound machine are the elements in the transducer. These elements are predominantly made of piezoelectric ceramics. These materials have unique properties that allow them to change shape in the presence of an electric current. When the ultrasound machine emits a desired frequency, strong but very short electrical pulses make the ceramics vibrate. This causes the crystals within the ceramics to emit a mechanical vibration at a preset frequency. The sound frequency emitted is usually set anywhere between 2 and 18 megahertz (MHz), but can reach as high as 50 MHz in probes used for ophthalmic studies. The resulting sound wave pulses can then be directed, steered, or focused to the desired depth as set by the ultrasonographer. Each of the crystals is connected to an individual circuit known as an *element*, which allows them to be directed independently. This individual control allows the operator to steer and focus the image through timing delays.

When the sound waves are reflected back to the transducer from the various tissues, they again make contact with the transducer elements, distorting the shape of the individual ceramics and creating electrical energy that is now sent back to the machine to analyze. It is this electric current that is digitized to create a diagnostic image.

Practicality

Modern ultrasound machines come in a variety of formats, including larger cart models, laptop units, and even handheld portable devices. Each unique system offers different levels of image quality and software options. There are many considerations when selecting an ultrasound machine for use in a veterinary practice. For example, machines may vary based on their selection of available types and frequencies of their transducers, the computer processor speed, the quality of the viewing monitors, and many optional software applications. Some machines also vary by whether they will support either a cardiac or general imaging platform. Ideally, for small-animal veterinary practices, a machine with dual-function capability would be the most beneficial (both cardiac and general imaging).

Patient Preparation

Small animals are generally imaged in ventral recumbency on a padded trough, standing, or in lateral recumbency. In actuality, an animal can be examined in just about any position that achieves the desired imaging. Animals undergoing a cardiac study are often placed on a specialized cardiac table that is customized so that the transducer may be directed through the small cut-out opening of the table top on the "down" side of the patient's thorax.

Large animals are usually examined in a standing position.

It is important that the patient remain still in order to achieve an accurate ultrasound examination. Panting, struggling, and

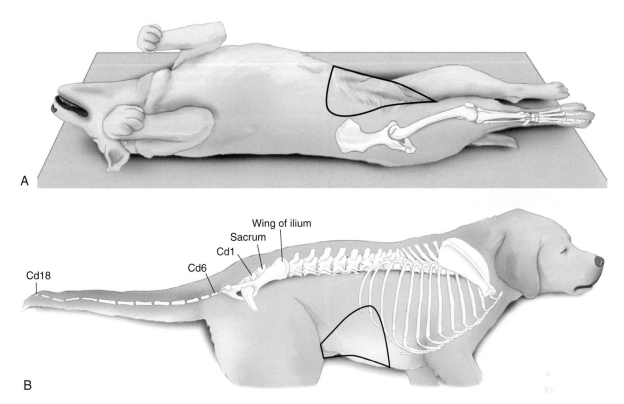

FIG. 10.2 **A,** Generally, when preparing a patient for an abdominal ultrasound, the abdomen should be shaved from the sternum to the distal border of the pubis. In deep-chested breeds the right ventral side of the thorax should also be included from the 11th to the 13th rib. This is to help visualize the gallbladder, common bile duct, and pylorus of the stomach. **B,** In preparing for cardiac studies a rectangle is shaved caudal to the axilla on both sides. To find this location, bend the elbow and find the spot where the point of the elbow touches the ribs.

tensing up will all decrease the diagnostic capabilities of the sonographer by reducing image resolution and clarity. In these instances, a diagnostic study will require sedation.

Sound waves do not travel through air; therefore, the probe must have direct contact with the skin surface. Ideally, fur is clipped away, and alcohol should be sprayed on the skin to remove superficial fats (Fig. 10.2). Next, an acoustic coupling gel is applied to the skin surface and to the surface of the probe to improve contact.

Grayscale

Ultrasonography visualizes a much wider range of tissue densities because the computer sees a larger "grayscale" than can be seen in plain radiographs (Fig. 10.3A–F). Typically, at least 256 shades of gray are incorporated into the display of an image obtained through ultrasound. This creates a much superior level of contrast compared with plain radiographs. For comparison, the human eye can only distinguish about 30 to 60 shades of gray (Fig. 10.4A–C).

Modes in Ultrasound Imaging

In ultrasound imaging, the echo data collected can be formatted into specific images that represent different interpretations of the characteristics of the tissues being evaluated.

The following list contains an abbreviated outline of the individual characteristics of each mode.

B Mode

In B mode, the "B" represents brightness. The intensity and speed of the returning echo are sent to the transducer, interpreted, and then transformed into a digitized pixel within a two-dimensional image on screen. The pixel is either classified as hyperechoic (bright) or hypoechoic (dark) (Figs. 10.5 and 10.6).

The full spectrum of 256 shades of gray is used to create each pixel comprising an image. The spatial resolution (or distance) between pixels can be as low as 0.3 mm, depending on the type of transducer and frequency used to perform the scan.

M Mode

"M" is interpreted as motion. In this mode, a cursor line is set over an area of interest as imaged in B mode. M mode simultaneously creates a B-mode image (light and dark) while displaying the motion of the tissues over a two-dimensional scale. This creates a continuous wave form and plots where each pixel intersects the cursor line.

M mode is particularly useful when evaluating the heart. Using this mode and plotting the movement of each light

FIG. 10.3 **A** and **B,** Ultrasound image showing a segment of the canine jejunum and its structural components. Acoustic impedance gives contrast to the anatomical layering of the intestines, allowing them to be visualized on ultrasound as the sound wave traverses different tissue densities at variable velocities. These variables lead to different shades of gray representing each density. This can be useful in identifying different types of intestinal pathology, as each may be associated with changes in different individual layers. **C,** The second row of images illustrate a normal section of jejunum *(left)* and a hyperechoic inner mucosa layering that is imaged as irregular segments *(right).* This represents mucosal sloughing. **D,** The ultrasound image in the middle depicts a plicated section of small intestines caused by the presence of a lineal foreign body within it. The image to the right clearly shows the same pattern of obstruction as seen at the time of surgery. Compare the detail obtained on ultrasound as compared to the radiograph to the left-hand side. **E** and **F,** The bottom set of images show a radiograph *(below left)* where there is a fluidlike radiopaque density filling the cranial aspect of the thoracic cavity *(white arrow).* This radiograph cannot differentiate between the heart, fluid in the thorax, and the outline of a mass. The ultrasound *(lower right),* because of enhanced grayscale, clearly identifies the density as a large cystic mass. This was diagnosed as a thymoma. (Images **A, C–F** courtesy RF Hylands.)

FIG. 10.4 A, The area outlined by the white box in the abdominal radiograph *(top left)* delineates the space that is usually occupied by the urinary bladder. Note that the tissue grayscale limitations in plain radiographs do not allow visualization of bladder contents other than fluid. **B,** Compare this to the significant difference in visualization of a urinary bladder polyp on ultrasound. This was previously undetected. Diagnosis of this polyp was only possible due to the increased contrast achieved through a wider dynamic range or grayscale. The fine detail is so sensitive that if you look closely, you can visualize a thin stalk **(C)** attached to the bladder wall *(white arrows)*. (Images courtesy RF Hylands.)

FIG. 10.5 B-mode image of a kidney illustrating the strong anatomical correlation between a transverse picture of a sectioned organ **(A)** and the accompanying ultrasound study **(B)**. (Images courtesy RF Hylands.)

FIG. 10.6 High resolution images from two separate kidneys demonstrate unparalleled detail of the organ's anatomy. Image to the left illustrates a fluid build-up in the renal pelvis (pyelectasia), whereas that on the right-hand side images infiltrative lines of tumor invasion into the cortex of the kidney. (Images courtesy RF Hylands.)

and dark pixel, we can determine the thickness and diameter of the ventricular wall through different stages of the cardiac cycle. We can measure cardiac dimensions and evaluate movement of the valvular leaflets within the ventricles.

Doppler

This modality is used to image the flow of blood and other liquids while measuring their velocity. There are four different Doppler techniques.

Color Doppler

In color Doppler, the information collected is presented as a color overlay above a B-mode image. This application was first introduced in the mid-1980s. There are different gradients of superimposed color, depending on the color map selected. In standard imaging, for instance, we track blood flow by using the color blue to show blood flow away from the transducer and the color red for blood flowing toward the transducer. This is best remembered through the acronym BART (blue away/red toward) (Fig. 10.7).

The addition of another type of more sensitive color mapping may add variances that detect abnormal turbulence within the normal laminar flow of blood.

Power Color Doppler

This is yet another form of color imaging that is highly sensitive to the flow of blood but does not identify its direction. It is used predominantly to detect lower velocities in tissues where the directional flow is less important than detecting the flow itself. An example of this would be in evaluating the vascularity (blood vessel pattern) of a neoplastic mass.

Pulsed Wave Doppler

As the name implies, pulsed wave Doppler (PW) is produced by a transducer that alternates between sending and receiving sound signals. This allows the area being analyzed to be set to within a very small sample volume, or "gate." The sampling or listening area can be set anywhere along a cursor line that transects the concurrent B-mode image. PW can

FIG. 10.7 A Color Flow Image of a Kidney Demonstrating the Blood Flow Within It. (Image courtesy RF Hylands.)

read blood flow velocities in the 0.4 to 0.6 m/s range, making it quite useful for small peripheral vessels. PW can detect blood flow velocities up to a maximum of 1.4 m/s. At these velocities, the probe reaches what is called a *Nyquist point*. Above this point, the transducer inaccurately displays as an inverse or flow reversal, making their true measurement impossible to quantify with any accuracy. At these velocities, continuous wave (CW) measurements should be taken instead of PW (Fig. 10.8).

Continuous Wave Doppler

This type of Doppler imaging requires that the scanner have two different sets of crystals built within it that work together simultaneously. One set of crystals is continually sending out signals and the other set receives. This allows accurate measurements during studies of very-high-velocity blood flow found in many congenital heart conditions. It is, however, less accurate when it comes to selectively measuring flow at a certain depth, and it cannot be gated as with PW studies.

Harmonic Mode

The use of tissue harmonics helps decrease ultrasound artifacts (see the section on artifacts later) in very large or obese patients. In this mode, either a single or multiple deep, penetrating frequencies are emitted into the body along with a harmonic overtone. The overall objective is to achieve deeper homogeneous penetration with fewer artifacts, as this mode utilizes software to filter the returning sound wave, which removes echoes that may interfere with a clearer image (considered "noise"). Other applications used to improve image quality include speckle reduction and compound imaging.

Multiplanar Reconstruction

MPR studies involve reconstructing images from various planes to allow simultaneous visualization on the monitor. Although MPR has been the norm in both CT and MRI studies for some time, it is a relatively new imaging format for the field of ultrasonography. Volume transducers are needed to acquire this image.

Three-Dimensional and Four-Dimensional Modes

Although currently of limited practicality in veterinary medicine, both stationary three-dimensional and time-lapsed four-dimensional reconstructions are available in human ultrasonography. This is currently used primarily for human fetal, obstetrical, and cardiac valve imaging. As newer applications arise, these technologies will likely migrate to veterinary use.

Postimaging Processing and Measurements

With the advent of digital technology, studies can be stored in their raw format for later review. This allows for a vast multitude of calculations to be made after a study is completed. The veterinary technician can be involved in reformatting the data to help complete the case study.

FIG. 10.8 Echocardiograms. The ultrasound study may also include Doppler evaluations, which can include color directional flow to detect abnormalities such as mitral regurgitation jets *(large white arrow)* and/or velocities and wave patterns of the flow of blood within the heart chambers *(smaller white arrow)*. (Images courtesy RF Hylands.)

"Knobology"

Every ultrasound machine, regardless of manufacturer, shares a common set of instrument adjustments that can modify both the performance of the machine and its image quality. These adjustments are made either mechanically (manipulating knobs and boards) or by contact on a software-driven touch screen (Fig. 10.9).

Gain

The gain adjustment affects the brightness of the image. It affects what range of the grayscale is used to format the image for that particular study. Most machines will have a

FIG. 10.9 Ultrasound Machine Panel Displaying Image Control Options. (Image courtesy RF Hylands.)

choice of preformatted grayscale and colored maps to start as the base image for the gain. These are chosen depending on the ultrasound study required. As an example, cardiac studies do not require the full grayscale range, but instead use a high-contrast image in order to better define the edges of the cardiac musculature. Abdominal studies, on the other hand, will benefit from a wide range of grayscale to better detect minor anatomical changes within an organ or tissue.

Depth

Every type and size of transducer has a set maximum and minimum depth at which it can send and receive sound waves. A common mistake when imaging an area of interest is to set the depth of the scan too deep. Although it may appear to give a better perspective of the tissue relative to the surrounding structures, it inevitably wastes valuable pixels that could give finer organ detail. As a rule of thumb, one should limit the depth of the scan so that the area of interest fills the full monitor screen for closer analysis.

Time Gain Compensation

This feature allows the operator to selectively adjust the gain at various depths. Echoes that return from deeper structures are more attenuated as they travel back through more tissues. This makes part of the far-field image appear to be darker. Time gain compensation (TGC) adjustments allow for one to compensate the gain to obtain a smooth grayscale image throughout the full depth of the scan view. This adjustment is often done through manipulating a series of sliding tabs that affect the level of brightness at various depths.

Presets

These are preinstalled settings programmed by the manufacturer. The settings included with the machine's software are meant to facilitate and maximize the performance of a transducer, depending on the type of study required. Selecting a preset for a cardiac study may affect such parameters as the sensitivity and range of the Doppler reading for either adults or neonates. Presets will affect the dynamic range, gain settings, gray map selection, frequency of the transducer, number of focal zones, and scan depth. Some machines may also allow the operator to modify these presets or create and save their own, because personal preferences can vary.

Focal Zones

Adjustments to the focal zones will allow the ultrasound beam to converge more at a particular depth during the study. This will maximize the axial and lateral spatial resolution at the area of interest (see definitions). This focal setting works best if selected within the near-field imaging parameter of a transducer. A maximum of only two focal zones should be used at a time, even though some machines will allow the operator to select up to five.

Frequency Selection

Individual transducers generate sound waves with a set range of frequencies based on the properties of the piezoelectric ceramic crystals used within the ultrasound probe. The frequency selection "knob" allows the operator to change the frequency within the range allowed by that probe. This will affect the maximum penetration depth of the sound waves in the tissues. It is important to be aware that the depth of penetration is inversely related to the level of frequency used. The advantage of using higher frequencies is that they provide better optimization of the resolution of the area.

Optimization

Another option found on many newer machines is a single-step adjustment that automatically optimizes the settings in order to obtain the best image. Choosing this setting will affect the gain settings and the tissue harmonics in order to obtain the ideal image as the sound beam travels through a particular part of the body. Ultrasound manufacturers will have different names for this option, but the end result is relatively similar. It is meant to assist operators who have limited knowledge of individual settings and adjustments to quickly obtain the best possible image.

Transducers

As we have discussed earlier, the purpose of the ultrasound transducer (or probe) is to change electrical energy into mechanical energy (sound waves), which penetrate into the tissues, and then to receive the reflected sound waves, converting them back into electrical impulses which are read by the computer. This is accomplished by piezoelectric crystal elements, which can change shape and vibrate in response to electrical or mechanical stimulation.

The greatest advancement in ultrasound imaging came in the early 1990s, when there was an explosion in the development of high-speed digital electronics and the development of powerful computer platforms. With the advent of the digitization of the systems, many fine adjustments to the processing software could be implemented, resulting in a dramatic reduction in signal noise and artifacts. The numbers of elements on individual transducers can range from as low as 64 to over 500 elements per transducer head. At the same time, improvements in the speed and quality of the receiving and processing can directly affect the image quality and resolution of the scan images for advanced studies.

Transducer Frequency

There is an inverse relationship between increasing the frequency output of a probe and the maximum depth that it can scan. This means that the higher the frequency of the transducer, the less it will penetrate. Second, there is a direct relationship between increasing the frequency of a transducer and the lateral spatial resolution (Fig. 10.10).

Lateral spatial resolution is the ability to distinguish between two objects or echoes that are adjacent to each other yet perpendicular to the sound wave. This is influenced by the sound beam's width. The lateral resolution is best when studied in the near field, where the sound beam is narrowest.

Transducer Frequencies			
Increasing frequency			
• Decreases penetration capability			
• Increases fine detail. Provides better spatial resolution			
	Depth	Wavelengths	Max spatial resolution
3 MHz	20 cm	0.44 mm	0.76 mm
5 MHz	15 cm	0.31 mm	0.62 mm
7.5 MHz	10 cm	0.21 mm	0.42 mm
10 MHz	7 cm	0.15 mm	0.33 mm

FIG. 10.10 Comparison of Transducer Frequency with Depth of Penetration and Spatial Resolution. (Images courtesy RF Hylands.)

Choosing a Transducer

A typical small-animal practice may require up to three or four different types of transducers, depending on the type of ultrasound studies that are being performed. For instance, a clinic that does both cardiac and abdominal scans will need more transducers than a clinic performing only general abdominal ultrasonography. In comparison, an equine practice devoted exclusively to lameness studies may require only a single high-frequency, linear transducer to perform most tendon studies.

Because the frequency or wavelength at which the ceramics are vibrating will affect the spatial resolution within an image, higher-frequency transducers will be required for detailed studies (Fig. 10.11). Many higher-end ultrasound machines can reach frequencies of up to 22 MHz.

Transducers have single-frequency or multiple-frequency ranges on a single probe. In veterinary medicine, the wide range in both the sizes and weights of patients makes the use of single-frequency transducers difficult.

Markers

Each ultrasound probe is tagged with a marker that may be in the form of an indentation, a raised surface, or an illuminated "in use" light. This marker will be associated with a similar identification tag on the upper-left corner of the ultrasound screen. Orienting the marker on the transducer toward the marker on the screen will assist in performing a standardized ultrasound (Fig. 10.12).

In keeping with standardized convention, in a sagittal scan plane, the cranial aspect of the patient's body should be displayed on the left side of the monitor, and when viewing transverse planes, the right side of the patient should be presented to the left of the screen as well. It is the marker icon that is represented on the screen, along with the reference point etched over the transducer, that assists the sonographer to properly orient and record the scan.

Transducer Types

A wide variety of different types of transducer probes are available to veterinarians (Fig. 10.13A–F). The most commonly used in veterinary medicine are listed next. Other types of probes include those used within endoscopes, esophageal probes, and endocavity probes used for obstetrics. The size, frequency range, and conformation of the actual footprint shape (the part of the probe that makes contact with the patient) will vary between probes and between vendors as well.

Linear Transducer

The linear transducer design was one of the first probes to appear on the ultrasound scene. It has a flat contact surface, or footprint. The earlier designs would only scan in a limited

FIG. 10.11 One of the advantages of performing ultrasound studies is that it can image in multiple planes through the simple rotation of the transducer. The set of images above represent a section of jejunum in both a short axis and long axis view. This ability adds an unprecedented amount of information with minimal effort. Another advantage, as it is imaged in real time, is that one can monitor any type of motility, including intestinal contractility and blood perfusion. (Images courtesy RF Hylands.)

FIG. 10.12 A and B, Each transducer has an identifying mark that helps align the direction of the probe with that displayed on the monitor screen *(arrows)*. (Images courtesy RF Hylands.)

FIG. 10.13 This Set of Images Represent Transducer Types and Their Individual Directional Sound Beam Shape. Please note the differences in the shape of their footprints. **A,** An example of a high-resolution linear transducer and the rectangular sound beam that it emits. **B,** A similar linear transducer demonstrating a variation of the sound beam into a trapezoid shape. This in part mimics the convex shape without losing significant resolution. **C,** A microconvex probe with a small footprint and a wide beam pattern. **D,** A larger convex probe with a similar beam pattern. Note the larger footprint. **E,** A phased array transducer designed specifically for cardiac studies. Note the conical shape. **F,** A 3D/4D transducer illustrating a volume-rendered image of a fetus. These larger probes are not yet commonly used in veterinary medicine. (Images courtesy of RF Hylands)

rectangular view of tissues directly beneath the probe. This resulted in many artifacts, such as "side lobes," forming (see the Ultrasound Artifacts section later in this chapter). With the advent of digital technology and the ability to focus the sound beam, the linear probe now has the added option of trapezoid imaging. This keeps the high resolution of the linear probe and gives some of the broader advantages of the curvilinear probe. Software changes also have resulted in a dramatic reduction of artifacts, and the faster processing time has improved the linear probe's capability. Recently, because of these adaptive changes, linear probes have reemerged in popularity as an ideal diagnostic tool for fine-detail imaging (see Fig. 10.13A).

Convex Transducer

The convex transducer (see Fig. 10.13D) is also known as a *sector or curvilinear probe* and was first introduced in the late 1970s and early 1980s. At the time, they exceeded the popularity of the linear probe because of their curvilinear shape, which offered a wider field of view at the sacrifice of spatial resolution (especially in human obstetrical studies). In some cases, the wide footprint was excessive for small-animal use. As the trapezoid imaging of the linear probe has improved and increased the detail available in the scans, the convex and the linear probes have become almost equally popular. Many ultrasonographers will use the convex probe for a general scan and then switch to the linear probes for higher-resolution inspections.

Microconvex Transducer

Although similar to convex probes because of the curvilinear shape, the microconvex transducer has a much smaller footprint size (see Fig. 10.13C). This difference makes them more practical for smaller animal patients. This is especially true for intercostal studies where the distance between the ribs limits the probe's view and contact with the patient. The disadvantage of this size change is the reduced number of elements and the spread of the wide-angle view, which ends up sacrificing some degree of image quality. Microconvex probes are particularly useful in smaller canines, felines, and exotic patients.

Phased Array Sector Transducer

Phased array transducers contain piezoelectric elements that are stimulated in complex timing sequences and controlled by circuitry to provide focus and sound beam steering at different depths simultaneously. In these types of transducers, the crystals are electronically steered through firing time delays. They are most often used in cardiac studies, as they have the unique ability to offer a CW mode (see Fig. 10.13E).

Matrix Transducer

The matrix transducer is the newest class of transducers and at the time of writing is only offered by a select number of vendors. This type of probe will likely replace many of the other probes as technology continues to improve and the size of the transducer becomes slightly more manageable. The probe offers the ability to scan in different planes at the same time due to the high density of elements installed within it. The two-dimensional matrix allows the operator to create three-dimensional images of an area in question, for example, heart valves. Unfortunately, due to costs, it has limited use in veterinary medicine at the present time.

Volume Transducer

The use of volume transducers is quite limited in veterinary medicine, mainly due to their high individual cost and the need to use optimum machines with their extended processing power. These probes are necessary for four-dimensional reconstructions, and five-dimensional models are now being released. It is just a matter of time before they will be in common use within the veterinary profession (see Fig. 10.13F).

Transducer Care and Cleaning Guides

Each ultrasound transducer can be worth thousands of dollars when new ($3000 to $16,000). When handling probes, care must be taken to avoid dropping or jarring them, as the piezoelectric crystals can become damaged.

After each use, the technician should wipe off any remaining acoustic gel found on the probe with either a dry or water-moistened *soft* cloth. Contaminated fluids on the transducer may be gently cleansed with a 10% bleach solution, a glutaraldehyde-based disinfectant, or 70% isopropyl alcohol. Check with your manufacturer's service manual, as not all companies recommend this. Follow required cleaning practices carefully to avoid warranty disruption.

Alcohol should *never* be used beyond 2 cm from the tip of the transducer, as it can damage the housing joint seals. Never use alcohol on the transducer cables (Fig. 10.14).

For probes that are used in endocavity procedures, a spray of mild disinfectant solution may be used. Although the rubber of the transducer's footprint can be immersed in fluids for very short periods, it is still not recommended. The connectors and distal cables should never be immersed. At no point should a transducer be autoclaved or gas sterilized with ethylene oxide. Care should be taken also to avoid contact with gels that contain lotions, mineral oil, or lanolin.

Safe to clean

Do not use 70% isopropyl alcohol beyond this line

FIG. 10.14 Ultrasound Transducer Probe. (Image courtesy RF Hylands.)

Applications for Ultrasound

Bovine and Ruminants

In these species, an ultrasound examination is predominantly used for reproductive work, such as follicle detection, pregnancy examination, reproductive difficulties, and so on. Ultrasound-guided biopsies and follow-up monitoring also employ ultrasound.

Equine

Two distinct imaging services exist in the equine world: sports medicine and reproduction. Ultrasound is invaluable in identifying both tendon and ligamentous strain and injuries. It is also particularly useful for monitoring progress as the horse improves and returns to normal with the prescribed therapeutics.

Fertility is also an important consideration in equine medicine, and the use of ultrasound is the standard of care when following up on the early stages of gestation and fetal development.

Porcine

The main use for ultrasonography here is for the measurement of back[fat] levels found within animals destined for meat production.

Small Animals

The list of possible applications seems to be almost endless for small-animal studies because the size of the patient is ideal for the types of frequency ranges available to the practitioner. The scope of studies is only limited by the imagination of the ultrasonographer.

Abdominal studies include all of the gastrointestinal (GI) system, from the esophagus as it transverses the diaphragm to the distal end of the colon, including the rectum, which is imaged through the perineal area. Abdominal ultrasound studies also include the imaging of the liver, gallbladder, and biliary tree. The pancreas, spleen, kidneys, adrenals, and regional lymph nodes are routinely imaged and evaluated. As an example, abdominal lymph nodes can be assessed for their level of inflammation and reactivity. The urinary bladder and excretory system (up to the bony interference from the pelvic rim) is also part of any examination, as are all of the components of both sexes' reproductive organs. The more distal structures can also be reached with more superficial scanning methods. The only major limiting factor is the obstruction from either bony structures or gas-filled organs.

Thoracic studies usually include full cardiac examinations with M-mode interpretations and Doppler vascular velocity assessments. In emergency medicine, ultrasonography is the diagnostic modality of choice when assessing trauma and suspected abdominal bleeding.

Ultrasound Artifacts

Ultrasound waves do not travel through air or bone. Because of this, there are situations where a reflected sound wave may occur that interferes with the diagnostic scan. One of the most common examples is the reflection of sound waves when the beam comes into contact with air. The resultant artifact reflection is called *reverberation*. A number of common ultrasonographic artifacts are presented next.

Comet Tail

The comet tail artifact (Fig. 10.15) appears as a series of closely interspaced and intense reverberations or reflections that appear to look like the tail of a comet. They can occur when there is reflection of the sound wave off small reflector targets, such as air pockets in the GI tract or metallic objects, a foreign body, or the tip of a biopsy needle. Fig. 10.15 shows typical illustrations of a comet tail artifact as noted in three different gastric images.

Edge Shadowing Artifact

Edge shadowing is a form of refraction, or redirection of the sound wave, as it passes through a fluid–tissue interface. It is associated with curved, fluid-filled structures such as the gallbladder, urinary bladder, cysts, and even sometimes the kidneys. The phenomenon occurs in the far field of the object (away from the entrance of the beam). It appears like a hypoechoic linear shadow that diverges from the surface of the curved structure.

Edge shadowing can occur when the incident angle of the sound beam hits the leading edge of a circular object (the near edge). The objects in question must be composed of different attenuation material, such as a liquid and solid side by side, as in a cystic structure. The images in Fig. 10.16 show such an artifact (arrows) off the surface of the gallbladder.

FIG. 10.15 Comet Tail Artifacts in Three Different Images. (Images courtesy RF Hylands.)

FIG. 10.16 Refractive edge shadowing artifacts *(arrows)* seen forming off the surface edge of the kidneys and gallbladder. (Images courtesy RF Hylands.)

FIG. 10.17 Acoustic enhancement artifact seen as hyperechoic tissue imaging deeper to the fluid-filled structures. Examples of this artifact are seen with cystic ovaries, gall bladder, and cystic spleen, as imaged above. (Images courtesy RF Hylands.)

Acoustic Enhancement

Acoustic enhancement occurs when the sound beam travels through a weakly attenuating structure such as a bladder filled with fluid. The sound beams traveling through tissues *around* the bladder will be slowed or attenuated, whereas the sound beams passing *through* the liquid will not have lost as much energy or intensity. When the sound beams hit the tissue at the far side of the bladder, the reflection will appear brighter (hyperechoic) compared with the surrounding tissues on the same plane. The resulting artifact appears as a distal enhancement (brighter on the far side of the structure) on the B mode.

This predictable artifact is quite useful in differentiating certain hypoechoic masses from cystic or fluid-filled structures (Fig. 10.17).

Mirror Image Artifact

The strong reflective surface between the diaphragm and the air-filled lungs is a common place to observe a distinct mirror image of tissues in the abdomen (Fig. 10.18). The sound beams reflected back from this interface are misinterpreted by the ultrasound machine, which then places a second image of the liver, for example, on the opposite side of the diaphragm. This artifact is important to recognize because an inexperienced ultrasonographer may interpret the artifact as a diaphragmatic hernia, a thoracic mass, or even lung pathology.

Reverberation

Reverberation is due to repeated back-and-forth reflection of echoes trapped between two strong reflectors. The resulting effect appears like a bright veil, similar to northern lights in the sky (Fig. 10.19). It is principally seen in a superficially positioned, gas-filled loop of bowel within the stomach. The bright echo display makes it difficult to see anything distal to the artifact. The result is that one cannot properly visualize the image of the opposing wall of the digestive tract.

Acoustic Shadowing

Acoustic shadowing is the simplest of all of the artifacts to understand (Fig. 10.20). When the sound beam contacts a highly attenuating surface such as a urolith (bladder stone) or bone, most of the sound beam is either reflected away or absorbed. This creates a lack of echo information distal to the dense object. The absence of data is displayed as a dark

FIG. 10.18 A mirror image artifact of the liver *(black arrows)* is seen on the opposite side to where the diaphragm is located *(curved white band)*. (Images courtesy RF Hylands.)

FIG. 10.19 Reverberation due to repeated reflection of sound waves off gas in the gastrointestinal tract. (Images courtesy RF Hylands.)

FIG. 10.20 Acoustic Shadowing Artifact as Seen in 3 Different Images. To the left, multiple struvite calculi in the bladder; in the middle, a foreign body in a fluid-filled stomach; and to the right, a dense intestinal foreign body. (Images courtesy RF Hylands.)

FIG. 10.21 Side lobe artifacts are usually seen in fluid-filled anechoic structures where there is a divergent adjacent density present (colon). These are secondary refractions that create the illusion of echo's representing real tissue. (Image courtesy RF Hylands)

streak or shadow below the object where the ultrasound beam has not penetrated. The shadow is lined up parallel to the direction of the emission of the sound beam from the transducer.

Side Lobe Artifacts

When a transducer is emitting sound beams, the majority of them are directed in a primary direction, but secondary lateral minor emissions are simultaneously created. These become more pronounced as a transducer is set at its upper threshold. These side lobe echoes can be displayed on the monitor even if they did not originate from the principal or main sound beam (Fig. 10.21). This artifact can be reduced by changing the position of the focal zone or by reducing the frequency of the transducer.

REVIEW QUESTIONS

1. One purpose of the gain control setting is:
   a. To adjust the color intensity
   b. To select for continuous Doppler
   c. To control the brightness level of an image
   d. To set the frequency of a probe

2. The piezoelectric materials within a probe can:
   a. Convert electrical energy into mechanical energy
   b. Convert mechanical energy into electrical energy
   c. Convert electrical energy into mechanical energy and vice versa
   d. All of the above

2. When recording an abdominal ultrasound, on which side of the monitor should the cranial quadrant be displayed on a sagittal view?
   a. The far field of the image screen
   b. The near field of the image screen
   c. The left side of the screen
   d. The right side of the screen

3. When performing a cardiac examination, what would be the ideal transducer to choose?
   a. A convex probe
   b. A linear transducer
   c. A phased sector array probe
   d. A sector transducer

Chapter Review Question answers are located in the Instructor Resources on Evolve and can be provided to students at the discretion of the instructor.

Fluoroscopy is real-time imaging.

CHAPTER 11
Fluoroscopy

Lois C. Brown, RTR (Can/USA), ACR, MSc, P.Phys

As we work to create light for others, we naturally light our own way.
—Mary Anne Em Radmacher, artist, poet, motivational speaker, Born 1957—still alive

OUTLINE

LEARNING OBJECTIVES

When you have finished this chapter, you will be able to:

1. Discuss the equipment necessary for fluoroscopy.
2. Describe the functions of the fluoroscopic unit.

3. Explain the difference between radiographic and fluoroscopic images.
4. List the applications for fluoroscopy in veterinary medicine.

APPLICATIONS

The application of the information in this chapter is relevant to the following areas:

1. Fluoroscopic real-time scanning and imaging in small and large animals.

KEY TERMS

Key terms are defined in the Glossary on the Evolve website.

Fluoroscopy
Image intensifier

Input phosphor
Output phosphor

Photocathode
Photoemission

Pulsed radiation exposure

Introduction

Fluoroscopy (Fig. 11.1) is an emerging field in veterinary medicine, and because of its real-time imaging, it is an invaluable tool in veterinary surgery and in interventional imaging. The primary function of fluoroscopy is to provide dynamic real-time imaging of anatomical structures. Static images are useful, but the imaging of certain activities within the body such as the insertions of catheters, lines, and manipulation of structures is enhanced if the veterinarian is able to view the activities as they happen. This is also true of fluoroscopically guided orthopedic surgery. In large-animal orthopedic surgery, fluoroscopy is vital for the positioning of plates, pins, and screws. Obtaining static images and processing them as the surgery progresses is time consuming, whereas anatomy may be imaged quickly in real time with fluoroscopy. Today the fluoroscope is connected to a digital plate, and a corresponding static image can be obtained and recorded for later viewing or for the prearchives and postarchives without interrupting the dynamic examination.

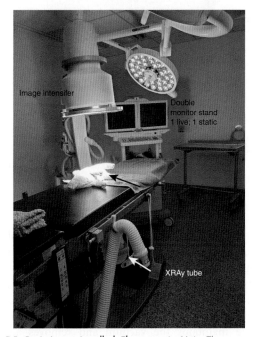

FIG. 11.1 A Large Installed Fluoroscopic Unit. The operator will stand beside the table. Handlers will also stand beside the table assisting the patient and/or the veterinarian. All personnel in the room will wear protective aprons and accessories. (Courtesy Animal Health Partners, Emergency and Specialty Hospital, Toronto, Ontario.)

Fluoroscopic Equipment

The fluoroscopic generator is virtually identical to a radiography unit. Many veterinary radiography units that are purchased from human hospitals have a fluoroscopy panel on the right side of the control panel.

The kilovoltage (kV), milliamperage (mA), and time values are the same as on a radiography unit. The difference is an added panel that allows the operator to select the "fluoro" mode, which switches the unit to a low mA (2–5) and a high kilovoltage (100–125) (Fig. 11.2). The time is not independently selected because the image is created in real time, and thus time is controlled by the operator as he or she watches the screen and obtains the imaging sequence necessary for diagnosis.

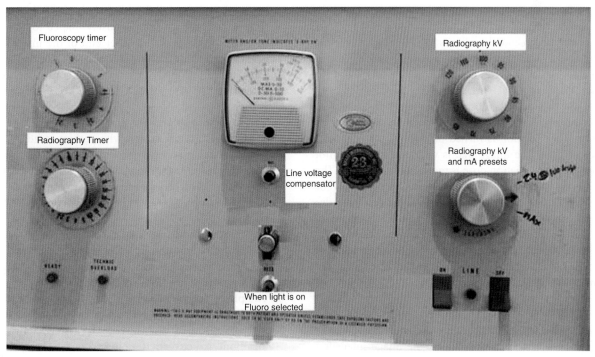

FIG. 11.2 An Older-Generation Radiography/Fluoroscopy Unit. The switch to alternate between radiography and fluoroscopy is on the side of the generator.

FIG. 11.3 The foot switch (exposure switch) has two options. One side is a single-exposure switch, and the pedal on the right is used for continuous exposure (fluoroscopy).

FIG. 11.4 The image intensifier converts the remnant radiation from the patient into a bright visible image on the output phosphor. It is then converted into a digital image to be viewed on the monitor or stored in a picture archiving system for later review and diagnosis. (Redrawn from Bushong SC. *Radiologic Science for Technologists.* 11th ed. St Louis: Elsevier; 2017.)

A foot switch (Fig. 11.3) operates as the exposure switch, and x-rays are generated continuously if the switch is depressed. A timer on the unit alerts the operator at a preset time limit (1, 2, or 5 minutes). The image intensifier monitor looks very much like a television monitor and is the display for the dynamic images.

Fluoroscopic Doses to the Patient

It is important to remember that the milliampere-seconds (mAs) is a function of mA × time. If the mA value is 3 and the operator extends the exposure time to 1 minute, the resulting mAs to the patient is 3 × 60s, or 180 mAs. Patients can receive radiation burns from a fluoroscopy unit if it is too close to the skin and remains in exposure mode for too long.

There are no specific dose limits in veterinary medicine, but the operator should always be aware of the "as low as reasonably achievable" (ALARA) principle discussed in Chapter 3 and try to keep the dose as low as possible.

One way to reduce the dose to the patient considerably is to use the pulse function on the machine. With pulsed radiation, the radiation is turned on and off for very brief periods of time. The image that is visible to the eye is not affected, but the radiation dose is reduced considerably. The radiation is pulsed, but the image on the screen is held for the brief period of time that there is no radiation. The pulse function can reduce the dose by one-half. Each manufacturer builds this function into the unit, so there is no specific time for each pulse. If the pulses are every one-tenth of a second, for example, the image is not affected, and the patient dose is reduced considerably.

The Image Intensifier

The image detector on a fluoroscopy unit is an image intensifier (Fig. 11.4). As with x-ray tubes, the image intensifier contains a cathode and an anode but in a very different design. This electronic device receives the remnant radiation exiting from the patient and converts it into a visible light image of high intensity. Modern image intensifiers consist of 11 components, each of which is uniquely important:

1. **The glass envelope.** This is the vacuum housing for the unit and must be specifically designed to withstand the outside air pressure without collapsing. An ion pump device maintains the vacuum and removes any ions produced when the intensifier is operating.
2. **The input screen.** This is the vacuum window of the intensifier. It receives the x-rays emitted from the patient. It consists of the support layer, the input phosphor, and the photocathode.
3. **The support layer.** This serves as a backing for the input phosphor and the photocathode. It is usually a thin piece of aluminum purposely shaped to help focus the electrons toward the other end of the intensifier. It is very important that the electrons are not distorted as they are intensified and projected onto the output screen. If they are distorted, then the resulting image will be distorted.
4. **The input phosphor.** The concave surface of the input phosphor is usually coated with cesium iodide. Cesium iodide crystals grow in long columns that function as pipes directing the remnant radiation toward the photocathode. This system is highly efficient, typically converting a single 60-kiloelectron volt (KeV) photon to more than 3000 light photons.
5. **The photocathode.** As light exits the input phosphor, it strikes the photocathode, which absorbs light and emits electrons. These two units are situated very close together to prevent the light from spreading.
6. **The photoelectrons.** These electrons are released by the photocathode in direct proportion to the amount of light that was absorbed. The conversion efficiency of the photocathode is between 10% and 20%. For every 60-KeV x-ray photon that is absorbed by the input phosphor, the photocathode releases about 400 photoelectrons.

25-cm
focal point

17-cm
focal point

12-cm
focal point

| 12 cm |
← 17 cm →
← 25 cm →

FIG. 11.5 The focal point of the electrons is in front of the photoanode and can be moved slightly to allow magnification of the image. (From Bushong SC. *Radiologic Science for Technologists.* 11th ed. St Louis: Elsevier; 2017.)

7. **The electrostatic focusing lens.** These lenses line the sides of the image intensifier and direct the electrons to the positively charged anode. These lenses are highly positively charged and draw the electrons with considerable force toward the anode, which has a positive charge of about 25,000 to 30,000 volts of electricity.

8. **The focal point.** The electrons are drawn rapidly toward the photoanode. As they travel, they cross each other at a spot known as the *focal point* (Fig. 11.5). This point enables the operator to control the magnification or minification of the image.

9. **The anode and the output screen.** The positively charged anode is immediately in front of the output screen. Once again, this prevents any image spread. The output screen displays the image and is read by the monitor and by any other storage devices attached to the unit.

   The anode of the image intensifier is very different from the anode in the x-ray tube. This anode merely attracts electrons as they travel past the electrostatic lenses towards the output phosphor.

   The anode merely attracts the electrons, which pass through a hole in the center of the anode. This does not interrupt the flow of electrons or distort the image as it arrives at the output phosphor.

10. **Output phosphor.** As the photoelectrons strike the output phosphor, they are converted back into light photons. Each single photoelectron that strikes the output phosphor is converted into 1000 light photons.

11. **Output window.** This is the final viewing point on the image intensifier and is usually quite thick—around 14 mm. The sides of the window are coated with a black pigment to absorb any stray light reflected in the window.

There can be modifications to these basic components depending on the manufacturer. In addition, upgrades are available to eliminate artifacts associated with a moving image.

Originally, units were supplied with a cassette holder, and individual exposures were possible. Today, with the advent of digital imaging, there is no longer a need for these holders. Now, if a single exposure is required, it can be retrieved from the bank of dynamic images and stored in a separate folder. This improvement reduces the radiation exposure for the patient because individual static images are unnecessary.

C-Arm Configuration of the Fluoroscopy Unit

The two-part C-arm where the x-ray tube and image intensifier are mounted in a "C" configuration, and the monitors and recording devices are located in a separate cabinet (Fig. 11.6), is the most common veterinary fluoroscopy unit. Many units in veterinary hospitals are purchased from human hospitals, and because their use is limited to surgical procedures in human hospitals, they are usually in excellent condition (if somewhat cosmetically compromised). They are mounted on wheels and are portable, although a little awkward to move about. Such a unit can be stored in a separate room and brought into the radiography room or surgery when required. The components are fairly rugged and withstand the bumps and shocks of uneven flooring and elevator loading and unloading.

In recent years, fluoroscopic units have been manufactured specifically for veterinary hospitals. They are virtually identical to human medical units and are operated in exactly the same manner.

The Fluoroscopy Table

One factor that is often overlooked is the table on which the patient will lie for the fluoroscopic procedure. The tabletop must be free of obstruction above and below and must be radiolucent. The radiation will travel through the patient and the tabletop, and the configuration must be accessible so that either the x-ray tube or the image intensifier can be placed beneath the table (Fig. 11.7).

An important consideration is the radiation absorption of the tabletop. The best table is custom-made of 1-inch (2.54-cm) squared tubular steel, with a tabletop made of a composite material that is completely radiolucent. The pattern for building such a table may be extrapolated from the images in the text or from the diagram provided on the Evolve website.

The tabletop may be ordered through an imaging supplier or a machine shop that has access to the composite material for the tabletop.

The table frame can be constructed by any welding shop. The outside dimensions are 56 in × 26 in (142 cm × 66 cm). The bracing of the legs can be at a 45-degree angle to each leg, or it can be in the form of rails, as shown in Fig. 11.7. The length of the image intensifier should be considered when the rails are mounted because it must be convenient to move the C-arm during surgery from the vertical position to the horizontal position. The table in

FIG. 11.6 A, The typical configuration of a veterinary fluoroscopy unit. In this case, the image intensifier is positioned below the x-ray tube. The flexibility of the unit means that the arm can be rotated so that the tube is above the intensifier or positioned for a lateral view. **B,** The two monitors are mounted on a cabinet with the recording units below. The monitor on the left shows the image in real time. The monitor on the right provides a static last image held for comparison.

FIG. 11.7 The C-arm Positioned Horizontally. The table is a sturdy construction with the support rails situated so that the x-ray tube can move beneath it unobstructed. This x-ray tube is a stationary anode tube.

Fig. 11.7 was manufactured so that the x-ray tube fits below it and the image intensifier is positioned above the patient. A surgical drape was custom made to completely encase the image intensifier. (The radiation penetrates the cloth drape.)

Radiation Dose and Service Considerations

On a standard medical unit, the x-ray tube is a high-end rotating anode tube. It must have a high heat capacity to withstand the long exposure times common in fluoroscopy. One method used to reduce the radiation dose to the patient is to pulse the exposures so that the radiation switches on and off at a predetermined rate. The image on the monitor is not affected because it is preprogrammed to react to a continuous stream and to ignore the pulses.

The x-ray tubes on a C-arm have a stationary anode, and particular care should be taken to limit the exposure times so that the tube does not overheat. Each unit is supplied with an anode cooling chart manual and x-ray tube specifications.

If a used unit is purchased from a medical hospital, all equipment manuals and service manuals must be supplied. These will give a history of any problems, as well as a wiring diagram for any future service. Each C-arm is upgraded and changed year to year, with major changes occurring at regular intervals depending on the manufacturer. The wiring diagrams from 1 year ago are not necessarily relevant the following year, even if they are produced by the same manufacturer.

If no information is available from the C-arm manufacturer, it may sometimes be obtained from the Internet.

The Monitor Tower

Two monitors are mounted on a cart and are usually positioned at about eye level (5 feet, 5 inches [165 cm]) (see Fig. 11.6B). Older models of C-arms had only one monitor; however, the double monitor serves a useful purpose. One monitor presents the static image, and the second monitor shows the real-time dynamic image. During a surgical procedure, a prosthetic device or a catheter may not be correctly positioned. The surgeon may then hold the image on the left monitor, move the device under real-time imaging, and compare the two images.

A computer keyboard and picture archiving and communications system (PACS) are mounted beneath the monitors (Fig. 11.8). These are linked to the hospital radiology

FIG. 11.8 The Computer Keyboard Mounted Beneath the Two Monitors.

information system (RIS). The patient's information may be keyed in at the monitors or may be available through the RIS. The system may also allow measurements to be calculated or positioning angles to be determined on the monitor.

The Procedure

The patient is placed on the table and wheeled into position between the x-ray tube and the image intensifier. The configuration is movable around the patient, so the tube can move from the dorsoventral or ventrodorsal position to the lateral configuration easily without repositioning the patient.

In the surgery, the unit is positioned after the animal is on the surgery table and has been draped appropriately. If the C-arm is to be moved during surgery, the unit must be thoroughly wiped down with antiseptic wipes. It can be cleaned with the same solutions used on all other operating room equipment.

Dark Adaptation

The images on the fluoroscopic screen are not in color and may be dim in comparison with the routine images read on the illuminator. The veterinarian must allow his or her eyes to become accustomed to the dim light of the room (known as *dark adaptation*) before starting the procedure. The easiest method of dark adaptation is the use of dark sunglasses.

Archiving the Images

Once the image is configured at the output phosphor, it may be viewed in several different modes.

Just as an image detector in radiography displays an image, fluoroscopic images can be digitized and sent to various recording units. Typically, the dynamic image is stored on a hard drive attached to the unit. Because the image is actually a series of still images, just like those in a movie camera, individual "spot films" may be extracted from the "movie." If a particular pathology is demonstrated, the images may be started, fast-forwarded, reversed, and then stopped and captured. If the pathology is of sufficient interest, the images may be posted to a website and discussed by many veterinarians from anywhere in the world.

Individual images may also be printed on a laser printer, such as the one illustrated in Chapter 8.

Applications in Veterinary Medicine

Real-time imaging is useful as a surgical tool in equine radiography for a review of the equine extremities. The real-time imaging does not have the resolution of the film/screen or digital imaging, so it is used mainly for fracture reductions and as a screening tool for placement of catheters, stents, and endotracheal tubes.

Contrast media studies commonly use fluoroscopy to image the function of the gastrointestinal system, as well as narrowing or blockage of blood vessels in angiography studies. The form and function of the blood vessels can be studied with the use of a contrast medium that is injected into the veins and then concentrated and excreted by the kidneys.

Miniaturizing the C-Arm

The miniature C-arm was developed in the early 1980s. This unit was originally intended to be used in the emergency department of human hospitals to image the reduction of fractures and dislocations. It is light and very portable, and even though the image is of comparatively low resolution, it is very useful for the purpose for which it was developed (Figs. 11.9 and 11.10).

Shortly after it was introduced, the miniature C-arm became a valuable tool in scanning equine legs and the joints of the extremities. It is not very powerful, but it images the equine leg very well and can demonstrate an area of trauma or pathology that should be examined further by radiography, computed tomography, or magnetic resonance imaging.

FIG. 11.9 Dan McMaster, DVM, holds the XiTec Mini C-Arm (XiTec LLC, Connecticut, USA) to demonstrate its small size and portability. The x-ray tube port is beside his left thumb, and the image intensifier is in front of his right hand. The monitor cart is behind him.

FIG. 11.10 The Monitor Cart for Two Miniature C-arms. This hospital uses one unit and stores the other for backup. The video recorder is mounted on top of the cart. A small thermal printer is mounted beside the monitor on the right.

Summary

This chapter has reviewed the evolution of real-time imaging from the original plates to the sophisticated image intensifiers now used with digital imaging. It also explored the possibilities of the mini C-arm and its application in the equine hospital.

REVIEW QUESTIONS

1. The fluoroscope is an adaptation of a radiography unit used to:
   a. Check the function of the brain
   b. Provide dynamic real-time imaging
   c. Scope the internal structures of the gastrointestinal system
   d. View the radiographic images after they are processed

2. The value of fluoroscopy during surgery:
   a. Saves money by providing real-time imaging
   b. Saves time by providing on-the-spot images
   c. Provides a functional view of the internal organs
   d. Is useful because the patient is awake

3. Because the image on the fluoroscopy unit is produced as a series of individual images:
   a. Static images cannot be taken from it
   b. Static images may be extracted without disrupting the flow of the examination
   c. All of the images show movement, and static images are useless
   d. The images removed from the program do not have contrast

4. The technical factors for fluoroscopy are:
   a. High kV and low mAs
   b. Low kV and low mA
   c. A function of the time; the kV does not matter
   d. High kV and a low mA; time is not preset

5. The mAs on a fluoroscopy examination could be as high as:
   a. 50
   b. 75
   c. 150
   d. 180

6. The exposure time is controlled by the operator:
   a. Using a timer
   b. Using a hand switch
   c. Presetting the exposure time on the unit
   d. Depressing a foot switch; there is no preset limit

7. High doses of radiation are possible during fluoroscopy if:
   a. The x-ray tube is off and the patient is not wearing a lead shield
   b. The patient is protected and the tube is too close
   c. The operator does not pay attention to the timer
   d. The image intensifier is not turned on

8. Patient positioning during the examination:
   a. Is difficult because the patient must be rotated
   b. Takes place at the start of the procedure
   c. Is difficult if the patient is large and uncooperative
   d. Is complicated because the tube arm rotates around the patient

9. The image on the intensifier screens:
   a. Is immediately visible and clear to the human eye
   b. Is dull and flat in a grainy black and white
   c. Is enhanced when the human eye is correctly dark adapted
   d. Is clear when the image intensifier is warmed up correctly

10. The fluoroscopic system functions the same way as:
    a. A film/screen combination in radiography
    b. A detector in digital imaging
    c. The x-ray tube and detector in radiography
    d. A light bulb and an x-ray tube

11. The image intensifier consists of:
    a. A photocathode and an anode
    b. A light beam and an output phosphor
    c. The input phosphor and an output phosphor
    d. Input and output phosphors, which are the same

12. The process of converting x-rays to light is called:
    a. Phototransmission
    b. Phototropic
    c. Photoemission
    d. Thermionic emission

13. A method to ensure that the electrons accelerate to the output phosphor:
    a. Uses negative photons to guide them to the phosphor
    b. Uses positive electrons and a negative charge
    c. Uses an electrostatic focusing lenses across the intensifier
    d. Uses a magnetic field within the tube

14. Each photoelectron that arrives at the output phosphor:
    a. Is intensified 50 to 75 times
    b. Is converted into 1000 light photons
    c. Produces more x-ray photons to radiate the patient
    d. Is absorbed by the input phosphor
15. The end result of the image on the fluoroscopy unit may be:
    a. Retained within the unit and reviewed on the image intensifier
    b. Converted into a WAV file and stored in a jukebox
    c. Stored on a hard drive and reviewed for diagnosis
    d. Stored on a hard drive and saved as a JPEG image

16. Applications for fluoroscopy are:
    a. Static extremity and pelvic images with contrast during surgery
    b. Contrast images of internal organs in real time converted from ultrasound
    c. Real-time images of archived radiographs converted from the films
    d. Real-time imaging of orthopedic surgery and function of the gastrointestinal system

Chapter Review Question answers are located in the Instructor Resources on Evolve and can be provided to students at the discretion of the instructor.

Sagittal cut plane. Volume-rendered CT scan of a dog showing placement of the endotracheal tube. (Courtesy Animage Imaging.)

CHAPTER 12
Computerized Tomography

Lois C. Brown, RTR (Can/USA), ACR, MSc, P.Phys; and
Stephanie Holowka, MRT(R), MRT(MR), MRSO(MRSC™)

Part of the inhumanity of the computer is that, once it is competently programmed and working smoothly, it is completely honest.

—Isaac Asimov, science fiction writer and biochemistry professor, 1920–1992

OUTLINE

LEARNING OBJECTIVES

When you have finished this chapter, you will be able to:

1. Understand the basic principles of tomography.
2. Discuss the basics of computerized tomography.
3. Understand the apparatus of the CT scanner.
4. Correlate radiographic tomography with computerized tomography.

KEY TERMS

Key terms are defined in the Glossary on the Evolve website.

Algorithm
Analog
Archive
Attenuation coefficient

Computerized tomography
CT number
Detector

Digital
Gantry
Hounsfield unit

Image data
Pitch
Raw data

Introduction

In the very early days of radiography, researchers were frustrated by the lack of resolution on the images they produced (Fig. 12.1A). In the early 1900s, several researchers worked independently in different countries with a common goal: to separate the superimposed shadows that necessarily result when complex structures of differing density are exposed to radiation and the exposure is recorded on a two-dimensional image receptor. How could the unwanted shadows be eliminated, and the structures of interest left clear and unobstructed?

The first tomography unit was established in June 1921 when Andre Bocage filed a patent for an "apparatus for radiography on a moving plate." All refinements to this original patent have left Bocage's original concept untouched.

Tomography, from the Greek word *tomos,* meaning "cut" or "section," has been defined as a special technique to show, in detail, images of structures lying in a predetermined plane of tissue while blurring or eliminating detail in images or structures in other planes. A further clarification describes the original two-dimensional radiographic image as layers of images piled on top of one another. Pathology or contrast-enhanced anatomy in one layer may be obscured by dense anatomy in an area lying on top of or below the region of interest. However, if the layers of tissue can be separated and the areas above and below the region of interest are blurred sufficiently, the anatomy in the plane of interest stands out in sharp focus against the blurred background (Fig. 12.1B).

The best way to demonstrate this concept is by visualizing the playground seesaw (teeter-totter in some countries). A child sits on either end of a board that is placed on a midway support (Fig. 12.2). The distance of the arc the children travel as they ride on the ends of the board is determined by the length of the board and by the angle at the central support. If the children sit still, there is no travel and thus no angle. As the children start to travel through the arc, the angle at the ends of the board becomes larger and larger, whereas the midpoint becomes narrower and narrower. This narrow fulcrum is called the *region of interest (ROI)* or *focal plane* (Fig. 12.3).

Principle of Rotation About a Fixed Point

The Focal Plane

The focal plane is the section, or layer, at which minimal blurring occurs (Fig. 12.4). The ROI is a fixed point in the anatomy of the patient. The structures above and below that point must be blurred out in order for the ROI to stand out in focus. If the x-ray tube and image receptor stay perfectly still, all the structures will be in focus and the layers of anatomy will be superimposed. However, if the x-ray tube moves through an arc and the image receptor follows that arc exactly, then the structures at the fixed point will remain in focus and the structures above and below that point will be blurred (see Fig. 12.4).

In Fig. 12.5, the objects at levels A and C are projected onto different areas of the image receptor and are therefore seen as blur. The objects at level B are projected onto exactly the same place on the receptor and are in sharp focus.

FIG. 12.1 A radiograph of an abdomen **(A)** next to a coronal reconstruction of an abdominal CT scan **(B)**. The benefit of the scan slice demonstrating each organ as the series is constructed is very obvious.

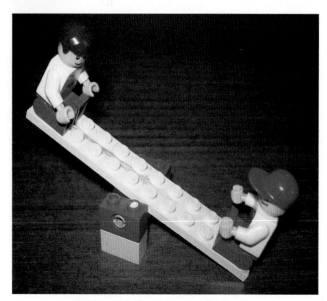

FIG. 12.2 The Concept of the Seesaw.

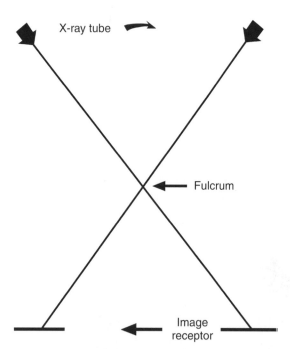

FIG. 12.3 Rotation About a Fixed Point. (Courtesy Lois Brown. From Dowdell LC. *The Joy of Sectioning: Achieving Maximum Results in Tomography.* Scarborough, Ontario: Railfare Enterprises; 1984.)

Fulcrum

The fulcrum is the central support in the playground seesaw. It is also described as the central point about which a lever rotates. In tomography, the x-ray tube sits at one end of the seesaw, and the image receptor sits at the other end. The length of the lever does not change, but the point about which the lever rotates—the pivot point (fulcrum)—can be moved up and down. This then changes the level at which the anatomy is blurred.

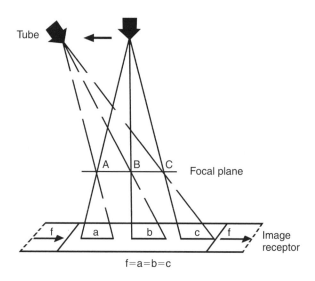

FIG. 12.4 Blurring of Points Outside the Focal Plane. The objects at levels *A* and *C* are projected onto different areas of the image receptor and are therefore blurred. The objects at level *B* are projected onto exactly the same place on the receptor and are in sharp focus. (Courtesy Lois Brown. From Dowdell LC. *The Joy of Sectioning: Achieving Maximum Results in Tomography.* Scarborough, Ontario: Railfare Enterprises; 1984.)

◆ APPLICATION INFORMATION

Hold a yardstick (meter stick) vertically in one hand. Grasp it at a midway point, say, 18 inches (45 cm). Your hand has now become a fulcrum about which either end of the stick may be rotated evenly. Now move your hand down to the 9-inch (23-cm) mark. The length of the stick has not changed, but the fulcrum has moved significantly, and the area of interest is now at the 9-inch (23-cm) mark.

Blur

Blur is the distortion or blurring of the anatomy above and below the ROI.

Computerized Tomography

The introduction of computers in the mid-1970s transformed standard tomography. The images could now be received and displayed on a computer, and the wealth of information far surpassed routine imaging on film. Invented in 1971 by Sir Godfrey Hounsfield, computerized tomography (CT), also known as *CT scanning* or *CAT (computerized axial tomography) scanning,* was the first imaging modality that enabled surgeons to noninvasively see the brain. CT took the standard analog images on film from conventional tomography and used computers to transform them into digital images. CT technology has evolved significantly over its nearly 50-year history, but the basic working principles have remained the same.

When we image structures on a radiograph, we produce a two-dimensional image (length and width of the

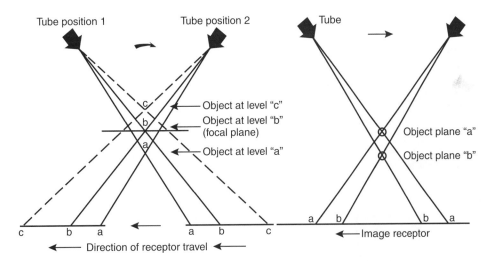

FIG. 12.5 As the x-ray tube moves coincident with the image receptor, the anatomy on the focal plane is projected onto the same place on the receptor. All other anatomy is blurred. This figure illustrates the fact that during the exposure and consequent tube and receptor movement, there is a "plane" or slice of tissue in focus, and not merely a point within the object. (Courtesy Lois Brown. From Dowdell LC. *The Joy of Sectioning: Achieving Maximum Results in Tomography.* Scarborough, Ontario: Railfare Enterprises; 1981.)

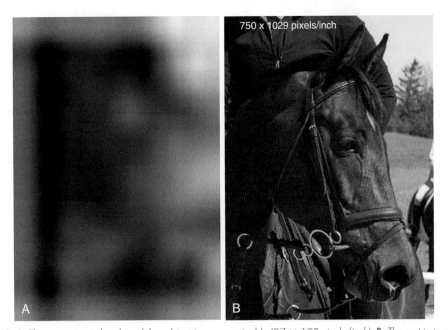

FIG. 12.6 **A,** The image is pixilated, and the subject is unrecognizable (37 × 123 pixels/inch). **B,** The matrix is enhanced, the pixels are smaller, and the resolution is superior (750 × 1029 pixels/inch).

structure)—a matrix of pixels or picture elements. (A *matrix* is a series of boxes or individual shades of information.) A computerized tomographic image is a three-dimensional image—a matrix of voxels—that includes the third dimension, depth. If a wide matrix is imaged, the result is said to be pixilated (Fig. 12.6A). If the boxes of information are very small, the image becomes clearer (Fig. 12.6B).

CT uses an x-ray machine that acquires images that look like slices in a loaf of bread. As with conventional tomography, the CT machine uses a moving x-ray tube to create the series of images, but it also requires the use of detectors moving synchronously with the x-ray tube and a computer receiving and interpreting the data.

Translation to the Computer

An x-ray tube emitting a fan-shaped beam of x-rays rotates 360 degrees around a gantry (or opening in the center of the machine) and the patient within it (Fig. 12.7A). Mounted directly across from the x-ray tube is a series of x-ray detectors that rotate at the same speed around the patient. The x-rays pass through the patient, and the attenuated beam is collected by detectors. The detectors convert the photons

FIG. 12.7 A, A CT scanner in a veterinary clinic. To the right of the scanner is a power injector, which is used for injecting contrast media as the scanner images the patient. **B,** The basic workings of a CT scanner. The x-ray tube rotates around the patient, and the data are sent to the computer. The resultant images look much like slices in a loaf of bread.

to an electrical signal that is fed into an analog-to-digital converter. The digital signal, or raw data (also known as *scan data*), is sent to a computer that reconstructs the images and presents them in the operator's chosen format. As the CT scanner is acquiring images, the table moves forward in increments set by the operator, enabling several images/slices to be taken at various levels for a complete examination. The computer reassembles the images and displays them on a monitor so that as the operator reviews the images, each "slice" is displayed in perfect focus independent of its neighbor (Fig. 12.7B).

◆ APPLICATION INFORMATION

As the x-ray beam passes through the patient, parts of it are absorbed by the tissues. Each tissue has its own density and thus absorbs the radiation differently. The measurement of the x-ray beam's absorption by each tissue is called the attenuation coefficient. In this text, the math is not important; the important part is that bone attenuates more x-rays than tissue, fat even less, and air attenuates very little of the beam. Thus, our image is made up of the various densities through which the x-ray beam has passed. Bone appears as white on an x-ray image because it absorbs more x-rays than the tissues or air around it.

The Hounsfield Genius

Normal x-ray practice is to take at least two views (90 degrees to each other) to display the anatomy free of superimposing structures. In CT, multiple views or projections are created by the rotation of the x-ray tube and detectors. The detectors are photodetectors that convert the x-ray photons into light and then into electric currents. Historically, the detectors were vacuum tubes containing xenon gas; however, modern-day CT scanners use solid-state detectors. The data or electric currents created by the detectors are fed into an analog-to-digital converter and then sent to the computer for reconstruction.

The primary method of reconstructing CT images is a process called *filtered back-projection*. Back-projection is a method of calculating an unknown value from multiples of known values. The multiple views performed by a CT scanner create a large number of calculations, so a computer is required to do it in a timely manner. Take a look at the simplified picture of the process in this example of a back-projection calculation:

by calculation $x = 1$

6	3	7	4
5	2	3	5
5	X	4	5
4	3	7	6

In this simple depiction, one can calculate the value of x by subtracting it from all the known values—both crosswise and diagonally. The calculated values appear in gray. The computer does a similar process in CT, but on the order of thousands of calculations. A mathematical filter or calculation is applied to the pixel calculations to cancel out any blurring artifact in the final image.

The numbers depicted in the example for back-projection can also be used to demonstrate another aspect of the CT image. When images are reconstructed for CT, they are constructed and displayed as a matrix. A matrix is made up of several pixels, or picture elements—the dots in a picture. (Look at Fig. 6B; the dots, or pixels, in that image are 750 across by 1029 in length.) The resolution of the image is tied to how many pixels are displayed in each field of view. In the previous example, the resulting image would have a matrix of 2. The size of a pixel depends on its relationship to the field of view that is displayed.

An image's resolution can be calculated in mm^2 as follows:

$$\text{Resolution (in millimeters)} = \text{Field of view (in millimeters)} \times \text{matrix}$$

In most modern-day CT scanners, the standard matrix used is 512 × 512.

Another factor in the setup of a CT scan image is the slice thickness (or, in the case of our seesaw, the fulcrum width).

The operator chooses the slice thickness according to the anatomy to be displayed. Each image in CT is a three-dimensional slice of the subject because the image has length, width, and height (or thickness). Because images in CT are created as slices, the pixels making up the image are actually voxels, or volume elements, and the density displayed is averaged into each pixel of each slice. When one looks at a single CT slice, the image has height and width, but one does not look at the picture from the top or bottom. Rather, the thickness of the image is whatever the collimation has been set at the time the slice is acquired. The concept of slice thickness is discussed in more detail later in this chapter.

Each voxel in a CT image is also calculated into a density measurement called a *Hounsfield unit (HU)* or *CT number*. The arbitrary scale is based on attenuation with pure water assigned a CT number of 0.

The value is calculated by this equation:

$$\text{Hounsfield unit} = K\frac{\mu p - \mu w}{\mu w}$$

where *K* is the constant (usually 1000), μp is the attenuation coefficient of the pixel, and μw is the attenuation coefficient of water. (An attenuation coefficient describes the ability of the pixel to absorb radiation. Bone absorbs more radiation, and fat and water absorb less radiation.) Based on this formula, the HU of pure water is zero, and any structure or tissue causing more x-ray attenuation than water will have a HU value above zero, whereas any structure or tissue causing less x-ray attenuation than water will have a HU value less than zero (negative).

This equation is significant to the CT scan for the following reasons:

1. It converts densities from tiny values of attenuation coefficients to usable units.
2. Every pixel can be interpreted as a unique density that can be used in diagnosis or postprocessing.

TABLE 12.1	Conversions for Attenuation Coefficients (AC) vs. Hounsfield Units (HU)	
SUBSTANCE	**AC**	**HU (AT 120 KV)**
Air	0.0004	−1000
Fat	0.185	−50 to −150
Water	0.206	0
Blood	0.208	+80
White matter	0.213	34
Gray matter	0.212	38

3. The Hounsfield unit sets up a direct relationship with creating and displaying the images.

Table 12.1 gives the conversions for various attenuation coefficients versus HUs. As shown in Table 12.1, the variances between the attenuation coefficients are very tiny (on the order of 10^{-3}), whereas the HU shows demonstrable and consistent differences for each of the tissue densities. This is also key for the visibility of various tissues in the body. On a normal x-ray, bone appears white because it is very dense, and soft tissues appear as shades of gray. It is difficult to see individual soft tissue organs on x-ray because their abilities to absorb x-rays are very similar; in addition, organs are superimposed on top of one another (Fig. 12.8A,B). However, as shown in Fig. 12.8C, a CT scan is able to show various soft tissue organs in cross-sections and in HUs.

Image Display

HUs also affect how images are displayed in terms of brightness and contrast. For CT images, the *window* of an image is the number of shades of gray making up the image (contrast). The *level* is the midpoint of the range of grays within a specific anatomical scanned area (density).

A brain, for example, may be windowed at 80 HU and leveled at 38 HU. This means that white and black make up the image, as well as 78 shades of gray in between. So how

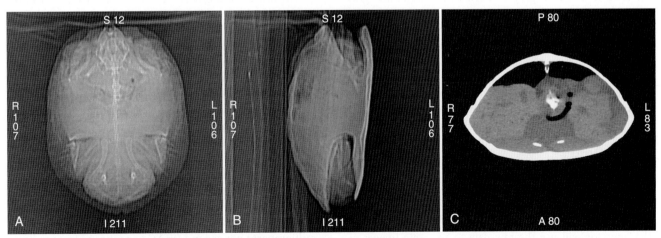

FIG. 12.8 A and B, Two x-ray images generated on a CT scanner showing how the turtle is not well demonstrated on simple x-rays. This is a classic issue for structures such as the brain and skull in other animals. C, The CT scanner allows the internal organs to be seen through the shell. Spleen, lungs, liver, and trachea are all visible on the CT scan.

FIG. 12.9 Same image of the turtle but with different window levels. **A,** The internal organs are best on abdominal windows (W350, L40). **B,** The bone is best on a bone window (W2500, L250). **C,** The lungs are shown on a lung window (W 2000, L−700).

does one come to this number? If 38 is the midpoint, it is half of the number for contrast. So, 80 is divided by 2 (or a half), which is 40. To calculate the number of shades of gray visible, you add and subtract 40 from the level of 38: $38 − 40 = −2$ and $38 + 40 = 78$. This means that all the shades of gray are visible from HUs −2 to 78. Bone, which is denser, simply appears as white because its HU is out of the visible range. Air and fat appear as black because, again, their HUs are less than what is visible as a gray level.

Let us try this calculation again. As stated before, bone is visible on a brain window only as white, so a different window/level (or contrast/brightness) is used to demonstrate bones. A typical window width is 2000, and a typical window level is 250. Half of 2000 is 1000. Now you add and subtract 1000 from 250 to get the visible range of grays. Because 250 is the midpoint, −750 to 1250 will be visible as shades of gray. Anything below −750 HU will be seen as black, and anything above 1250 will appear as white. This is a considerably wider window level. It is good for showing bone, but the brain is not as visible because there are very few HUs or shades of gray between white matter and gray matter (Fig. 12.9A–C).

HUs also can be measured with a cursor to help the veterinarian determine the nature of a lesion. For example, when a veterinarian sees a lesion in the lungs, if a cursor reading is −50 HU, then the lesion may be fat. If it is 160 HU, then it is calcium. Blood reads at about 80 HU. Some scanners even have a feature that allows the operator to apply a set cursor that will read all of the HUs for each voxel.

The CT Data

The operator uses two types of data on CT scanners. The scan data (raw data) collected from the detectors are used to create the images. These data sets tend to be very large, and so storage is usually temporarily on the CT scanner itself. The operator will use the raw data to re-create images as needed, even after the patient is no longer on the table. Once the raw data are removed from the scanner (most

scanners perform the removal automatically after a period), new images can no longer be produced. The image data are either photographed onto films or networked to a picture archival and communications system (PACS). Modern CT scanners are capable of producing hundreds, if not thousands, of images.

Just as in digital radiography, all images are stored, or archived, in a huge data bank. These banks may be local, or they may be anywhere on Earth.

For a CT scan operator, there are many ways that a scan or the images from it can be viewed. Some of the considerations that show the thinking behind the various methods are discussed in the following sections.

Field of View

In CT scanning, there are two types of field of view (the area seen in the image). The *scan field of view* (SFOV) is the number of detectors covered by the x-ray beam. This is important because if the patient's body part is outside the field of view (or chosen range of detectors), it cannot be reconstructed.

The *display field of view* (DFOV) is a key element in the resolution of CT images. DFOV will be either equal to or smaller than the SFOV. By decreasing the DFOV, one can increase the ability of the images to resolve structures. Although a maximum SFOV may be set by the manufacturer, the DFOV is a key factor that an operator chooses for his or her CT images (Fig. 12.10). Even after an animal has been removed from the CT scanner, a technologist can reconstruct the images using the scan or raw data to create images that have a desired DFOV.

Technical Factors Used in CT Scanning and Radiation Dose

As with x-ray units, CT scanners use kilovoltage (kV) and milliamperes per second (mAs) as scanning factors. Typically, the kV tends to be much higher than in standard radiography—from 80 to 140 kV. The mAs value also

FIG. 12.10 A Rabbit With a Tibial Fracture. **A,** This image was taken with a 22.0-cm display field of view. **B,** This image was acquired by magnifying the original scan. **C,** This image has the best resolution because the scan data were reconstructed into a 12.0 display field of view.

tends to be much higher, ranging from 10 to 400 mAs. The *scan time* depends on the method of scanning (spiral or conventional) and usually means the time it takes the x-ray tube to rotate 360 degrees around the patient for an exposure. By increasing the mAs, an operator can affect which structures are visualized.

Of course, increasing kV or mAs also increases the overall radiation dose emitted by the CT scanner. One unfortunate aspect of CT scanning is that the higher the technical factors, the prettier the images. CT has much more tolerance for high technical factors than does general radiography. In any imaging, the objective is to restrict dosage as much as possible and always adhere to the ALARA (as low as reasonably achievable) principle.

Slice Thickness

Slice thickness is a technical variable determined by the operator of the CT scanner and is a key factor in image resolution. Slice thickness is altered by prepatient and predetector collimators. The original CT scanners acquired images in slices 10 mm thick. If a lesion was less than 2 to 5 mm thick, it could be missed by the averaging of the 10-mm slice of anatomy. Modern-day CT scanners with multislice technology are able to acquire image slices thinner than 1 mm (Fig. 12.11A,B).

Algorithms/Kernels

An algorithm is a recurring mathematical calculation and is applied to each of the pixels creating the CT image to enhance certain structures. Some manufacturers give algorithms (or kernels) an actual number, whereas other manufacturers give these calculations a name. A soft or low-pass algorithm shifts the pixels to enhance structures that have very few increments of CT numbers (e.g., the brain). A high-pass or bone algorithm alters the images to enhance structures that have sharp edges. The use of an algorithm can be understood when comparing a soft tissue view to a bone view. Even with the proper window/level, a soft algorithm produces a blurry bone image,

FIG. 12.11 These Images Show How Slice Thicknesses are Determined on the CT Scanner. **A,** On a multislice scanner, ranges of detectors acquire multiple images in a collimation. **B,** The operator selects a slice thickness or detector range. The scanner's prepatient and predetector scanners maintain that slice thickness for the images.

and a bone algorithm on a brain image produces a very grainy, "noisy" image. In CT scanning, as long as there are raw data (or scan data), a user can postprocess the images multiple times to show various structures.

Table Movement and Pitch

A key working part in CT scanning is the movement of the table during the procedure. Three types of table motion can be chosen. When setting up the scans, a scout view (scanogram) may be taken. This looks much like a radiograph and allows the operator to choose the regions included in a scan. For the picture to be taken, the tube and the detectors remain in one location while the table passes through a chosen distance. For the actual CT scanning, the images are acquired in a conventional method or helical/spiral. The operator of the CT scanner has the ability to choose which type of scanning is best for a given image or pathology.

Conventional scanning refers to table motion as done by the original CT scanners. The scanner takes a slice (image) at one location. The table then moves a chosen distance, and another slice is taken (Fig. 12A). A whole stack of slices can be created in this manner. On older machines, the x-ray tube was connected by wires and cables to its generator and transformers in a separate box outside the gantry. The tube was therefore limited to moving in one rotation and then back. This motion also took time in CT scanners. Typically, the delay between slices on later-model conventional CT scanners was approximately 3.5 seconds.

In the late 1980s, a new phenomenon became available in CT scanning called *spiral* or *helical CT scanning*. The design of the scanner was changed to allow a slip ring and brushes (Fig. 12.12) to bring power to the CT gantry and x-ray tube. In turn, the same slip ring/brush assembly gave information back to the CT computers. This arrangement allowed the x-ray tube and detectors to rotate continuously, thus saving a delay between scans. In order for helical scanning to work, the CT scanners had to compensate for the motion of the scanner by using another calculation called an *interpolation algorithm*. Interpolation is the calculation of an unknown value based on two known values on either side. The scanner is thus able to calculate the slice in a straight plane rather than how it would appear (like a corkscrew). CT scanner manufacturers have used either a 180-degree or a 90-degree interpolation algorithm to correct helical images.

To lessen the CT dose, the helical scanner allows the technologist to choose a table motion greater than the slice thickness. Pitch is defined as the ratio between table movement (in millimeters) and CT slice thickness. How does this look in calculation?

$$\text{Pitch} = \frac{\text{Table movement (in mm)}}{\text{Slice thickness (in mm)}}$$

For example, if a table moves 5 mm for a 5-mm slice, then the pitch calculated is 1. If the CT operator chooses a pitch of 1.5 on a 5-mm slice, then the table will move 7.5 mm while scanning 5-mm-thick images.

FIG. 12.12 A, Photograph of slip ring and brushes. The brushes are mounted onto the slip ring. **B,** As the x-ray tube and gantry rotate around, the slip rings transfer electrical signals and receive data.

The plus in using pitch is that it drops the radiation dose for the patient while keeping the image resolution. On single-slice CT scanners, the pitch can be increased up to 1.8 with no visible effect on image resolution. Scanner design has changed further with the advent of multiple-slice CT scanners. Now, the table pitch must also take into account the numbers and width of the detectors chosen.

Prescribing a Scan and Protocols

The protocols or scan technical factors used in CT scanning are just as varied as the region or body area being scanned. All CT scanners allow operators to program protocols (labeled for body part or type of scan) and store them in the computer. Technologists can then enter the name (or select the name from a list created by the radiology information system) and then select the desired protocol, such as for a CT scan of the head. The technologist then completes a scanogram view or scout view (CT version of a radiograph) and from those images prescribes the actual CT scan.

The CT scanner always allows the technologist to make any desired change to a protocol setup as needed. On some protocols, an intravenous (IV) contrast agent may be required. IV contrast agents are iodine based and enhance veins, arteries, and some entire organs. Angiography can also be performed on CT; by rapidly injecting a contrast agent, an operator can show the arteries and veins in any given part of the body. Abdominal scans typically need a contrast agent so that the organs can be better seen. Contrast agents may also be used to demonstrate infection in extremities. In cases in which a spinal pathology is suspected, a veterinarian may inject a contrast agent into the spinal canal (via a lumbar puncture) to show any disturbances of the spinal cord. This procedure is called a *myelogram*. (Only special contrast agents are used in the spinal canal; see Chapter 23). Fluoroscopy, radiographs, and CT scans may all be part of the imaging of a spinal cord.

Multislice CT Scanners

Within the past 15 years, CT scanning has seen a further evolution in the design of the detectors. Most scanners available now have multiple detectors. Instead of a single detector array, the fan beam originating from the x-ray tube is now wider to radiate a larger array of detectors. Modern multislice scanners can have up to 256 detectors in the width of their array. Because of this new technology, larger sections can be obtained in one scan while the images are reconstructed into submillimeter thicknesses. This has allowed most CT scan data sets to be collected as volume scans that can be reconstructed into three-dimensional pictures afterwards.

Indications and Postprocessing for CT Scanning

CT scanning used to be the primary modality for imaging the head and spine, but magnetic resonance imaging has now supplanted it. However, CT scanning remains an excellent diagnostic tool for assessing trauma and for body imaging. It is also good at demonstrating the skeleton.

Because of the evolution of the technology, CT scans are performed so that the images can be reconstructed in multiple ways. A single conventional exposure through a multislice scanner can create 64 or more images of 0.5-mm to 0.625-mm thickness (depending on the design of the scanner). Whether the images are collected by a conventional scan or a spiral scan, they function as a volume if they have the same field of view, center, matrix, and algorithm. This means several slices can easily be stacked together and reconstructed into any two-dimensional plane or three-dimensional image.

In volume imaging, there are multiple ways to construct the objects. The simplest reconstruction is to angle the volume of images and reconstruct them into a two-dimensional view in a direction differing from the original scans. The operator can alter the slice thickness on the two-dimensional reconstruction and the window/level so that he or she can better demonstrate the affected anatomy. A spine is always reconstructed through the sagittal or longitudinal plane. Typically, several images are constructed along each plane (Fig. 12.13).

Three-dimensional images can simply be created by a process called *shaded-surface display*, whereby a three-dimensional object is created by limiting the number of HUs seen. For bone, 160 HU and higher is selected. For a skin surface, the range might include −200 HU and higher. These objects can be modified by well-designed software. Another type of three-dimensional imaging is called *volume rendering* (Fig. 12.14). This process takes the entire range of HUs and includes them in the picture. The operator can then select the range of voxels that are opaque and those that are transparent.

FIG. 12.13 A, Sagittal reconstruction of Waddle's spine from axial CT scans. **B,** A three-dimensional picture that is a shaded-surface display image demonstrating voxel values of 160 HUs and higher. Such three-dimensional images can be virtually angled and cut into to show various perspectives on anatomy.

FIG. 12.14 Tools such as three-dimensional imaging greatly assist in the understanding of pathology. Although the rabbit's fracture is visible in the two-dimensional coronal reconstruction or reformatted image (**A**), the severity is much more apparent on the volume-rendered three-dimensional reconstruction (**B**).

? POINTS TO PONDER

Basic Principles of CT
- The attenuation of each type of tissue forms the image. Bone attenuates more radiation than tissue. Various tissues attenuate differently. Air attenuates very little to not at all.
- The computer acquires the information and then interprets it as an algorithm depending on the request from the operator when the examination is set up.
- In general, radiography the image is static. The x-ray tube is static and the result is a two-dimensional image.
- With CT units, the x-ray tube and receptors move around the body in synchronicity so that a three-dimensional image can be interpreted by the computer.
- CT imaging systems move around the body part at a fixed location. The table is then moved forward and another "slice-image" is acquired.

- Attenuation information is obtained in multiple planes.
- This attenuation information is reconstructed into a simple grid.
- Within the computer, each body section is divided into three-dimensional boxes called voxels, which contain a two-dimensional grid of pixels.
- The attenuation is calculated in each direction.
- Add up all attenuations in each pixel and normalize them to a common scale.
- Each pixel represents a different density of structures within that section—the smaller the pixel, the higher the resolution.
- Repeat the attenuation information calculations for each slice.

Summary

Computed tomography is a modality that uses x-radiation to create images in cross-section. Slices of tissue are imaged and reconstructed. CT has the ability to demonstrate various densities of soft tissue and bone structures. Images can be reconstructed in many formats, including two-dimensional reformat, three-dimensional imaging, and volume rendering.

All these formats can aid the veterinarian in the assessment and diagnosis of patients.

Image Gallery

The CT scan images and reconstructions in Figs. 12.15 to 12.21 demonstrate various pathologies.

FIG. 12.15 Sagittal Reformat of Dog's CT Scan. Endotracheal tube has been placed in the trachea. A sagittal reformat of the dog's cranium and spine are seen in this reconstruction. (From Animage, LLC and the Animage FIDEX-FS advanced imaging system, with permission.)

FIG. 12.16 Axial Image of a Pelvic Mass That Is Pressing Against the Right Iliac Artery and Vein. (From Animage, LLC and the Animage FIDEX-FS advanced imaging system, with permission.)

FIG. 12.17 Contrast-Enhanced Reformat Demonstrating in the Coronal Plane a pelvic Mass Pressing Against the Right Iliac Artery and Vein. (From Animage, LLC and the Animage FIDEX-FS advanced imaging system, with permission.)

FIG. 12.18 Axial Reformat of an Arterial-Phase CT Scan. The aorta and renal arteries are well demonstrated. Because of multislice technology and spiral scanning, various phases of intravenous contrast enhancement can be taken. (From Animage, LLC and the Animage FIDEX-FS advanced imaging system, with permission.)

FIG. 12.19 Computerized Tomography Renal Angiogram. A nonenhancing tumor is seen within the patient's left kidney. Because of multislice technology and spiral scanning, various phases of intravenous contrast enhancement can be taken (arterial, capillary, and venous). Such imaging is helpful in characterizing tumors of the liver or kidney. (From Animage, LLC and the Animage FIDEX-FS advanced imaging system, with permission.)

FIG. 12.20 Dog Shot with Multiple Pellets. Coronal reformat reconstruction from volume of CT scan slices. Pellets are seen as high-density objects in the thorax and abdominal cavity below kidney and in pelvis. (From Animage, LLC and the Animage FIDEX-FS advanced imaging system, with permission.)

FIG. 12.21 Three-Dimensional Volume Rendering Demonstrating Multiple Pellets within the Body of a Dog. (From Animage, LLC and the Animage FIDEX-FS advanced imaging system, with permission.)

REVIEW QUESTIONS

1. A Hounsfield unit:
   a. Is a measurement of density on a CT scan
   b. Compares the density value of a pixel with that of water
   c. Is also called a CT number
   d. All of the above

2. If the scanning slice thickness is 5 mm and the table pitch is 2.0, the resulting table movement per rotation is:
   a. 5 mm
   b. 7.5 mm
   c. 10 mm
   d. 15 mm

3. Which method is the most common way to reconstruct CT scan images?
   a. Fourier transformation
   b. Filtered back-projection
   c. Back-projection
   d. Filtered optical transfer

4. What determines the slice thickness on the CT scanner?
   a. The prepatient collimators
   b. The predetector collimators
   c. The technician's choice
   d. All of the above

5. A technician has just finished scanning a patient. Which is the best way to magnify the images to show pathology?
   a. Magnify the picture using the scanner software.
   b. Use the raw data to magnify the picture.
   c. Decrease the field of view using the raw or scan data and reconstruct the images.
   d. Increase the field of view using the raw or scan data and reconstruct the images.

6. What does a slip ring assembly do in a CT scan?
   a. It allows the x-ray tube and detectors to rotate continuously.
   b. It allows for helical or spiral scanning.
   c. It makes the table move quickly.
   d. a and b
   e. b and c

7. Raw data or scan data:
   a. Are used to create more images
   b. Are archived regularly
   c. Are kept on the scanner for only a short duration
   d. Do not occupy much disk space on the scanner
   e. a and c

8. A CT scan of a patient's skull shows a fracture on the soft tissue images. The scan has been done on a multislice scanner. Which is the best way to show the skull fracture?
   a. Change the window/level to bone windows.
   b. Using the raw data, change the algorithm to bone or high-pass.
   c. Rescan the patient using thinner pictures.
   d. Reconstruct thinner pictures with a bone algorithm.

9. When may a veterinarian want contrast "on" for a CT scan?
   a. To show an infection
   b. To show a tumor
   c. To show the organs in the abdomen
   d. To show a fracture
   e. a, b, and c
   f. All of the above

10. What is the typical matrix used to show most CT scan images?
    a. 512
    b. 388
    c. 128
    d. 256

Chapter Review Question answers are located in the Instructor Resources on Evolve and can be provided to students at the discretion of the instructor.

Magnetic resonance imaging excels at demonstrating the brain, spinal cord, and soft tissue structures.

CHAPTER **13**

Magnetic Resonance Imaging

Stephanie Holowka, MRT(R), MRT(MR), MRSO(MRSC™)

The world is your mirror and your mind is a magnet. What you perceive in this world is largely a reflection of your own attitudes and beliefs.

— Michael LeBoeuf (1942), American author and management professor, University of New Orleans

OUTLINE

LEARNING OBJECTIVES

When you have finished this chapter, you will be able to:

1. Discuss the equipment necessary for magnetic resonance imaging.
2. Understand the principles of magnetic resonance imaging.
3. Know the MRI machine.
4. Describe how MRI is used in diagnosis.
5. List the safety issues in MRI.

APPLICATIONS

The application of the information in this chapter is relevant to the following area:

1. Imaging using magnetism and resonance to determine pathology.

KEY TERMS

Key terms are defined in the Glossary on the Evolve website.

Atom
Echo time
Faraday cage/Faraday shield

Magnet
Magnetic field
Radio frequency

Repetition time
Resonance

Signal intensity
Specific absorption rate

Introduction

Magnetic resonance imaging (MRI) came into existence in the early 1980s. Its creation was based on the principles of magnetic spectroscopy—the use of a magnetic field and radio frequencies to determine the chemical makeup of a substance. The chemical makeup of a substance can be determined by which radio frequencies are emitted by that substance and are received in response from the substance.

MRI has become increasingly common in human medicine and is now found in specialized veterinary centers as well (Fig. 13.1). Because it shows the concentration of free-floating hydrogen molecules in tissue, it has much better subject contrast than a computed tomography (CT) scan and conventional radiography. MRI is superior in demonstrating the brain, the spinal cord (Fig. 13.2), and soft tissue

structures such as the ligaments and cartilage in joints. MRI is also a desired modality in that it does not use any ionizing radiation in creating the images. This chapter gives an overview for understanding this fascinating and complex new technology.

Safety Notice

Magnets such as those used in MRI scanners are very dangerous, especially for untrained personnel (Fig. 13.3). Everyone entering an MRI room must be screened for unsafe implants and any loose metal. The highest danger to staff and patients is the projectile effect—the launching of a metallic object into the magnet by magnetic force. A person cannot predict how an object will project into a magnet. People have been severely injured and even killed by such accidents. Only magnetically safe or conditional devices and screened patients or staff should be allowed to enter an MRI room. Only safe stretchers, monitors, oxygen tanks, and similar equipment can be used in an MRI room. Every MRI site must have policies and procedures in place to ensure the safety of patients and staff. If there is any question of a device or patient's safety, it must be addressed through the most responsible MRI personnel—technologist or veterinary radiologist.

Principles

To understand the workings of MRI, one must start at the atomic level. All atoms have protons, neutrons, and electrons. The protons and neutrons are found in the center, or core (nucleus), of the atom, and the electrons spin around on the outside. Every atom also spins and wobbles in space as

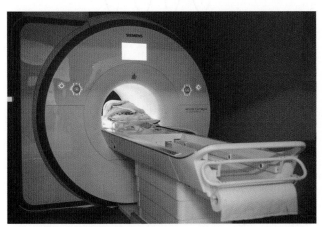

FIG. 13.1 An MRI Machine in a Veterinary Clinic. This is a high-field (3T) superconductor magnet. The higher field strength allows for higher resolution images of the brain and extremities. (Image courtesy Animal Health Partners in Toronto, Canada.)

FIG. 13.2 A Sagittal T2-Weighted Magnetic Resonance Image of a Dog's Spine. The scan shows that an intervertebral disc is bulging into the spinal canal and against the spinal cord. The compressed cord is brighter in that region, showing that it is swollen, or has edema. (Courtesy Thames Valley Imaging, London, Ontario, Canada.)

FIG. 13.3 An MRI Warning Sign. (Courtesy Magmedix, Inc., Ritchberg, Massachusetts.)

FIG. 13.4 Atoms in their normal random positions, spinning and wobbling. Arrows represent the positions of their magnetic polarities.

A

B

FIG. 13.6 **A,** What happens in magnetic resonance imaging. A radio antenna emits radio waves in a resonant frequency that causes certain atoms to go into a higher energy state. The hydrogen atoms respond to this frequency by aligning their magnetism *(black arrows)* to 90 degrees from their original orientation *(blue arrow)* within the magnet. They also wobble or precess together. **B,** When the radio waves are turned off, the atoms return to their original magnetization state and their energy state returns to equilibrium. The atoms give off radio waves, which are detected by the radio antenna.

well (Fig. 13.4). This wobble (much like how a top wobbles) is called *precession.*

Atoms join together to create molecules. All atoms and molecules (as in anything electrical) exhibit the ability to show magnetic polarity, or fields. When placed in a magnetic field, they will respond according to their own polarity (they align north and south).

How Does MRI Work?

In a most basic description, one puts a patient onto the table, which then enters the bore of the magnet. All the subject's molecules align on the basis of polarity and become magnetized (Fig. 13.5A,B). In performing a scan, a technologist applies a radio frequency tuned to the precessing frequency of hydrogen atoms (Fig. 13.6A). The hydrogen atoms in the subject respond by resonating (or responding) into a higher energy state. They also change the angle of their magnetization

and wobble together. The radio frequency is removed, and the molecules return to their normal energy state (Fig. 13.6B). In doing so, they give off a radio frequency that the MRI scanner calculates into an image. The actual method is quite a bit more complicated, but this is the basic concept of MRI.

Magnets and Magnetism

A magnet is any object that exhibits a magnetic field or force. Magnetic force can be created in an object in several ways. It can occur naturally in some substances, such as iron and malachite. It can be induced into an object; some metallic objects become magnetized if exposed to a strong magnetic field and, as a result, act as magnets. A magnet can be created by electricity. When an electrical current is applied through a series of copper windings, an electromagnet can be created. Magnetic force also exhibits polarity in that there are two poles, north and south, like positive and negative charges in electricity.

In magnetism, opposite poles attract each other and pull two magnets together. Like poles repel and push two magnets away from each other.

The imperial unit of measurement for magnetism is the gauss (G). For example, the earth has a magnetic field of 1 gauss. The most common measurement of magnetism is the metric equivalent, the tesla (T): 10,000 G = 1.0 T. The earth's magnetic field is 10^{-4} T. Tesla is the unit that people use in describing a medical magnet's field strength.

In medical MRI, three types of magnets can be in use. There are permanent magnets. These consist of two slabs of

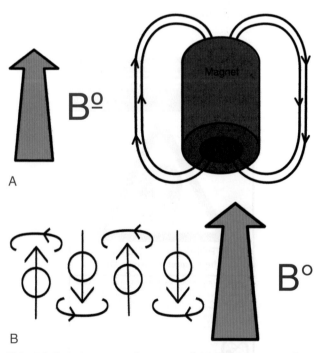

A

B

FIG. 13.5 **A,** A magnet and its magnetic field. The total magnetic force is represented by B⁰. **B,** What happens to atoms within a strong magnetic field. The atoms randomly align to their polarity, and B⁰ represents the total magnetization of the atoms.

FIG. 13.7 A Resistive Magnet MRI Unit Used to Image Horse Legs. The magnet covers only a specific field of view. A white spherical phantom (in between the two blue magnets) is covered by a surface coil.

Cross-section of an MRI

FIG. 13.8 A Basic Overview of the Components Needed to Make Up a Basic MRI Machine. A superconducting magnet would have a vacuum and helium chambers outside the actual magnet assembly but within the casing of the machine.

magnetic material facing each other (Fig. 13.7), and they tend to be lower field strengths—less than 0.3 T. There are electromagnets, or resistive magnets, created by an electrical charge applied through copper wire wrapped around a center. These also tend to be lower field magnets—less than 0.6 T. The most common medical magnets are called *superconducting magnets*. They are massive electromagnets made of windings that are superconductive in very low temperatures. Liquid helium (the coldest substance available on earth, with a temperature very close to absolute zero [−273° C/−459° F]) is used to keep the magnet active.

◆ APPLICATION INFORMATION

For the use of a superconducting magnet, great consideration is made in terms of the construction of the room surrounding the magnet. Special ventilation ducts must be created for quenching the magnet, a process whereby the liquid helium vents out rapidly and shuts off the magnet by increasing the resistance across the windings. Liquid helium has an expansion ratio of 1 to 700 L. There are at least 1000 L of liquid helium in a superconductor magnet, so the total expanded volume would rapidly exceed the size of any MRI room. It is these magnets (1.0 T or more field strength) that are never turned off. The very strong magnetic field is always on, even when the machine is not taking pictures.

? POINTS TO PONDER

For an MRI:
- The patient is placed in a strong magnetic field where signals are transmitted and received by surrounding coils.
- Gradients and radio waves stimulate protons in the patient to emit a signal and take advantage of the natural magnetic properties of hydrogen atoms to create an image used for reconstruction of the picture.

Aside from the magnet, many other parts work together to make an MRI unit function correctly (Fig. 13.8).

Magnetic Shims or Shim Coils

Shims are pieces or plates of metal used to correct the magnetic field within the magnet. For an MRI unit to work properly, the main magnetic field of the bore must be entirely homogenous. (All of the hydrogen atoms must synchronize exactly the same.) Any alterations of the main magnetic field could result in distorted images.

Gradients

Gradients are coils or assemblies within the magnetic bore that enable the machine to create images in any plane. An incremented current is applied across the gradient in an orientation chosen by the technologist, thus slightly varying the magnetic field in that direction. When the radio frequency is applied to the body, the variances in the frequency are calculated back to determine the "x-y-z" dimensions in space of each of the voxels of the image. The method used to reconstruct images from the gradients is called *two-dimensional Fourier transformation*. It is the design of the gradients that allows MRI to create images in any plane—axial (or transverse), coronal, or sagittal.

Radio Antenna

The radio antenna used in the MRI machine is quite strong, so strong that it could be used for a radio station. The antenna sends and receives radio waves to and from the patient. Radio waves are part of the electromagnetic spectrum, as are light, microwaves, and x-rays (see Chapter 1, Fig. 1.4). They are a form of energy but are not radioactive. Because the radio waves are important to the creation of images, MRI rooms must be shielded with a Faraday cage against any external radio signals. Outside radio waves can cause artifacts on the magnetic resonance images.

FIG. 13.9 Surface Coils are Used to Get Better Images of Smaller Structures in MRI. **A,** 3-inch coils. **B,** Cardiac coils. These coils demonstrate well any body part that can be contained within their dimensions.

Surface Coils

MRI machines are able to produce patient images from the main magnet (or body coil) itself; however, the radio signals received from smaller body parts have very poor resolution. Surface coils are devices that receive (and sometimes send) radio wave signals from a body part that is covered or contained by them (Fig. 13.9). There are specialized coils for many body parts, including the brain, spine, shoulders, head and neck, and hocks. These coils are made or adapted to each vendor's scanner and are not usually interchangeable because of the plug-in design for the coil, which is specific to each scanner. Typically, the smaller the coil, the better the image.

Use of surface coils depends on what needs to be seen. On a small dog brain scan, for example, one could use a chimney (human knee) coil because it may show a smaller field of view better than a human-sized head coil. Most superconductor magnets are designed for adult humans, and so other sites, including veterinary, may have to make their own adjustments as to which coils are used. They may also have to create their own specialized coils. Coils and MRI technology are constantly advancing. Now many coils have multiple channels and settings to decrease the time of the scan and to increase the signal obtained from the body part. One rule to keep in mind with MRI is that any coil within the active scanner must be plugged in. Coils that are on the table but unplugged during a scan can be damaged or could burn a patient.

Computers

MRI scanners require computers to perform the reconstructions of the radio signals into images. The computers also enable the technologist to photograph, network, and manipulate magnetic resonance images once formed. Unlike CT, no raw data can be kept or stored with MRI. The images are acquired in their chosen field of view (like CT), matrix, slice thickness, and other factors. One cannot go back after a 5-minute MRI scan and change the resolution of the images as one can in CT.

Physics and Technique

As stated earlier, an MRI scanner uses radio waves to manipulate hydrogen atoms in and out of an excited energy state. The actual application of this technique is quite a bit more complicated, and whole books are written on the physics and progress of this technology.

The frequency used by MRI to produce images is based on a calculation called the *Larmor equation*. All atoms have the ability to respond to radio waves in a magnetic field. This ability is called the *gyromagnetic ratio*. The frequency applied in MRI is calculated by the following equation:

$$W^0 = YB^0$$

where:

W^0 is the radio frequency

B^0 is the magnetic field (typically in field strength of Tesla)

Y is the gyrometric ratio

Medical MRI focuses on hydrogen, which also has the highest gyromagnetic ratio. The ratio for hydrogen is 42.56 MHz · T^{-1} or MHz/T. In a typical medical MRI, the field strength is 1.5 T. Using the previous equation yields the typical frequency for medical MRI, as follows:

$$42.56 \text{ MHz/T} \times 1.5\text{T} = 63.8 \text{ MHz}$$

When this frequency is applied by the radio antenna in a medical 1.5-T MRI scanner, the hydrogen atoms respond (or resonate) into a higher energy level and change the direction of their magnetization in the scanner. When the radio frequency is stopped, the atoms return to their equilibrium or prior state within the magnet. Because the atoms were excited into a higher energy state, they give off energy as they return in the form of radio waves that are detected by the radio antenna. The actual change of magnetic direction of the atoms on the return gives off two types of

FIG. 13.10. MR Images of a Dog's Brain. **A,** Sagittal T2 weighted image showing mass in hypothalamus and pituitary fossa. Cerebrospinal fluid surrounding brain and spinal cord appears bright on T2 weighting. **B,** A T2-weighted Fluid Attenuated Inversion Recovery (FLAIR) transverse image in the dorsal plane. The hypothalamic mass appears bright compared to the brain. **C,** Post contrast T1 weighted transverse image of hypothalamic tumor in dog brain. Slight enhancement of the lesion with gadolinium contrast. (Image courtesy Animal Health Partners, Toronto, Canada.)

signals. The first is called *T1 decay,* which is the direct magnetic movement of the center of the atom from its tipped position (90 degrees or whatever has been chosen) to its original state. The second is called *T2 decay,* the signal received from the spinning of the atom back into its original state. Tissues and molecules in the body have different responses with regard to T1 and T2 decay; this difference is what allows the MRI to show various tissues so well with all of the different settings.

The actual radio waves in these decayed signals are very small. During an MRI scan, the scanner applies the radio frequency in multiple pulses, which continue to "tip" the magnetic direction of the hydrogen molecules again and again. These repeated radio waves dramatically increase the radio signals received. One factor in an MRI technique is the time between the radio frequency pulses, which is referred to as *TR* or *repetition time.* A lower repetition time—699 milliseconds (ms) or less—shows the T1 decay response of the tissues. A higher repetition time—1500 ms or greater—shows the T2 decay response and changes the contrast of the images.

Another factor used in MRI is the echo time, or TE (in ms). This is the time between responses showing the maximum signal. As for TR, shorter TE times demonstrate the T1 response of tissues. Longer echo times show the T2 responses of tissues. MRI, like CT, shows images in slices. For an MRI, several slices are acquired in a single scan or sequence.

Signal Intensity and the Weighting of Images: T1 vs. T2

In MRI, the various shades of gray seen in an image are referred to as *signal intensities,* not densities. If a part of the image is shown as bright or closer to white, it is described as having a *high signal intensity.* The reverse is true for anatomy seen in darker shades of gray; they are called *low signal intensity.* When looking at images from an MRI, people also refer to the T1 or T2 appearance of the tissues as *weighting.* The most typical comparison are tissues that have opposite weightings—water and fat.

In a true T1-weighted image (TR < 699 ms, TE < 30 ms), cerebrospinal fluid (CSF) looks black (low signal intensity) (Fig. 13.10A). Fat (and skin) look bright or white (high signal intensity). A true T2-weighted image (TR > 2000 ms, TE > 80 ms) shows CSF as bright white and skin as black (Fig. 13.10B).

Signal-to-Noise Ratio

Many factors beyond TR and TE can be altered in MRI. Many can affect the quality, the resolution, and the amount of time it takes to obtain images. Technologists must take all these factors into account when entering a protocol for an MRI sequence. The goal in acquiring MRI images is to have a high signal-to-noise ratio. The higher the amount of signal, the better the pictures. Table 13.1 lists the effects of altering individual technical factors in MRI in a classic spin-echo image (see later discussion of sequences).

TABLE 13.1	Effects of Altering Technical Factors in MRI		
TECHNICAL FACTOR ALTERATION	**INCREASE OR DECREASE**	**EFFECT ON SIGNAL-TO-NOISE RATIO**	**EFFECT ON IMAGE RESOLUTION**
Field of view	Decrease	Decrease	Increase
Pixel size	Decrease	Decrease	Increase
Bandwidth	Increase	Increase	Decrease
Number of excitations or acquisitions	Increase	Increase	Increase
Slice thickness	Increase	Increase	Decrease
Image matrix size	Increase	Decrease	Increase

In radiography, a technologist balances radiation dose and resolution or image noise. In MRI, the trade-off is between time and image resolution. A technologist may, for example, want thinner slices, which will drop the signal, and therefore may have to increase the number of excitations, which doubles the time of a sequence.

Specialty Sequences

In MRI, specialty sequences can be used to image various parts of the body. It is possible to image blood vessels by MRI without the use of a contrast agent. A couple of sequences are able to capture the phases of moving blood, for example. These specialty sequences are called *magnetic resonance angiography* or *magnetic resonance venography*, and they can show the anatomy of blood vessels. These volumetric sequences enable the anatomy to be reconstructed in three-dimensional images, which are typically called *maximum intensity projections* (Fig. 13.11). Also, the naming of sequences varies from vendor to vendor. Charts are now available that translate these names from machine to machine. For example, "turbo spin-echo sequence" on one scanner is the same as "fast spin-echo" on another. A three-dimensional T1-weighted volume acquisition scan can be called "MPRAGE" by one vendor, "3D SPGR" by another, and an "FFE, or fast field-echo," by a third. MRI technologists must constantly learn and upgrade their knowledge about the physics and techniques of their scanning.

Another aspect of MRI is the ability to suppress the fat signal. This is desired in places where the fat may alter the ability to see pathology, such as the orbits and in soft tissue structures. The expression for this is *fat saturation,* for which various MRI methods can be used.

Contrast and MRI

MRI does require the use of a contrast agent to highlight infection, tumors, or vascular disease. The contrast agent used in MRI is called *gadolinium* (Fig. 13.12); various chemical formulas include this molecule. Gadolinium is a paramagnetic, meaning that it has partially magnetic qualities. It alters the T1 properties of tissues so that they enhance, or light up, in the picture. After contrast is injected into the patient, only T1-weighted sequences (with or without fat saturation) will show the enhancement of tissues.

Because gadolinium is removed by the kidneys, it is very important that a subject's kidney function is assessed before the MRI. In veterinary practice, because the patients are under general anesthesia when scanned, blood work assessing kidney

FIG. 13.11 A Noncontrast Magnetic Resonance Angiogram Performed on a Human Patient. The vessels are visible as a function of the blood flow within them. It is reconstructed as a maximum intensity project (MIP) and viewed from inferior to superior view.

FIG. 13.12 The Change in How a Tumor is Seen When Gadolinium Contrast is Administered. A, The T1-weighted image without contrast. B, The T1-weighted image with contrast. Usually, tissues enhance because the contrast decreases the T1 contrast of the pathology. (Image courtesy Animal Health Partners, Toronto, Canada.)

FIG. 13.13 Quick images in coronal (**A**), sagittal (**B**), and axial (**C**) planes showing the position of the horse's leg within the scanner.

function is always performed with the preanesthetic blood work. In humans, necrotizing systemic fasciitis, a very rare and irreversible complication, has occurred when gadolinium was given to patients with renal failure. In this condition, the skin and connective tissues permanently stiffen and retract, causing the patient to lose kidney function. For this reason, gadolinium is administered only to patients who have normal renal function.

Protocols

From this chapter, you have learned that there are many ways to scan a patient using MRI. Various surface coils and sequences can be used.

In a typical veterinary site, patients are accepted for MRI scans only when referred by specialists. The patient is prepared and evaluated before the MRI examination. These scans are not short in duration, with each sequence typically lasting around 5 minutes or so and an entire scan of body parts taking 20 minutes or longer. For this reason, patients are always anesthetized or sedated. The technologist or veterinarian chooses the most appropriately sized surface coils for the region to be covered. An MRI scan always starts with a low-quality, quick image called a *localizer*. The localizer allows the technologist to see the anatomy on subsequent images. Most MRI sites have specific protocols for each body part, using multiple sequences in at least two planes (Fig. 13.13).

MRI has a great advantage over other modalities. It has excellent subject contrast in that the soft tissues are better seen than even with CT. The images are also acquired in any plane or angle that the technologist may desire (see Figs. 13.13 to 13.16).

Decision Making: CT Scan vs. MRI

CT scan is much more easily available and less costly to manage in a veterinary office. This modality, although initially expensive, costs much less to maintain. Training on CT scan, because it involves x-ray, is simpler than the

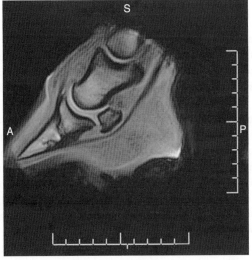

FIG. 13.14 A Sagittal T1-Weighted Image of the Horse's Left Forefoot. Several images in a plane were acquired in multiple settings.

FIG. 13.15 Coronal T1-Weighted Image Through a Horse's Forefoot.

FIG. 13.16 Axial T2-Weighted Image Taken Through the Horse's Forefoot. These images were acquired with the MRI unit shown in Fig. 13.7.

specialized training required for the practice of MRI. Both modalities also require the animal to be sedated or anaesthetized. Access to either machine within a clinic may be the biggest determinant as to how an animal may be initially imaged. In sites where both machines are available, the veterinarian may choose one modality over the other based on the symptoms and potential pathology in the animal. For trauma, CT scan is quickly able to show bleeding in the brain, broken bones and, with IV contrast, abdominal organ injuries. Images can also be taken of the brain and the sinuses. MRI, because of its greater ability to demonstrate soft tissues, is chosen when there is a brain or nervous system condition that needs to be diagnosed. MRI is also superior in the imaging of joints and ligaments.

Further Safety Considerations

As described previously, MRI uses a high-field-strength magnet to produce images, so the safety of patients and staff is of utmost importance. As mentioned, the most dangerous aspect of MRI is the projectile effect, whereby an object launches into a magnet. Injuries and deaths have occurred from such accidents. MRI applies radio frequencies to the entire body of the patient. Ferromagnetic (iron, containing) metal implanted into a patient may move out of position with exposure to the magnetic field. Another risk of implanted metal is heating, with possible burning of the patient. Everyone (patient, staff, or visitor) must be screened for MRI safety prior to entering the MRI room itself. This is accomplished with use of the written checklist that must be filled out by the animal handler (either owner or legal

designate) (Fig 13.17). Owners of veterinary patients must complete a questionnaire ascertaining that the animal has not had surgery involving metallic implants, clips, or other devices. They also must be asked if the animal has been shot with bullets or pellets or if the animal may have eaten objects that could be metallic. If there is any question about the potential for unknown metal, the animal will have to be radiographed to check for metal that could migrate in the MRI.

Another safety concern in MRI is the ability of the patient's body to dissipate heat from the interaction of the magnet and radio frequencies. Specific absorption rate (SAR) is a calculation made on the basis of the mass of the patient. Every written scan sequence in MRI lists the potential SAR value for the patient. This is much more significant in higher-field-strength magnets ($\geq$1.5T) than with the weaker ones. Because animals cannot dissipate or radiate the heat from the radio waves in the same way as humans do (perspiration), cooling packs should be applied to dogs who are larger with less surface area. MRI machines are also acoustically very noisy. Many MRI scans produce noise in excess of 60 to 90 decibels (dB). Ear shielding (ear plugs or specially rated headphones) is necessary for patients and anyone staying in the MRI room during a scan.

The static MRI field is not considered a risk for pregnant personnel. It is preferred to not have pregnant staff remain in the scan room during scanning, although prenatal MRIs are routinely performed on patients when necessary.

Further policies should be made within MRI departments in planning for emergencies. For situations such as fire, magnet quench, flood, and cardiac arrest, normal screening procedures cannot apply because it is impossible to rapidly screen everyone and every object entering the room to deal with an emergency.

Summary

Magnetic resonance imaging uses a very strong magnet and radio waves to create images. It has superior subject contrast because it demonstrates the molecular makeup of tissues. It is the best modality to image the brain, spinal cord, and other soft tissue structures such as the tendons and ligaments attached to joints. MRI should be performed only by trained individuals. For further reading, consult the bibliography at the end of this chapter.

Image Gallery

Figs. 13.18 to 13.29 demonstrate use of the invaluable tool of magnetic resonance imaging. **Please note:** These reports are given according to the entire scan, not just the images presented here. Some of the components would be viewed on adjacent scans within the procedure.

SickKids *MRI SCREENING OF PATIENTS*

THE HOSPITAL FOR SICK CHILDREN

> **WARNING:** The MR system has a very strong magnetic field that may be hazardous to patients entering the MR environment if they have certain metallic, electronic, magnetic, or mechanical implants, devices, or objects. Therefore, this form must be completed for all MRI requests. Be advised: **the MR system magnet is ALWAYS on and all metallic objects must be removed before the patient enters the MR environment.** If you have any questions or concerns regarding an implant, device, object, or MRI patient screening please call the MRI department at 416-813-5774 (press 7).

ADDRESSOGRAPH

Please complete all sections on the day of examination

1. Has patient ever worked with metal or operated welding or grinding equipment? Y ❏ N ❏

2. Has patient ever had a penetrating eye injury? **If yes** to #1 or #2, please arrange for orbit x-rays before MRI and include Radiology report with request. Y ❏ N ❏

3. Has patient ever been injured by a metallic object or foreign body (e.g. BB, bullet, shrapnel, etc.)? Y ❏ N ❏
If yes, please describe: _____

4. Could patient be pregnant? Y ❏ N ❏

5. Has patient ever had any kidney related problems? **If yes**, please indicate date and results of most recent blood work (creatinine): _____ Y ❏ N ❏

6. Has patient ever had a prior MRI examination? **If yes**, please describe if patient has experienced any problem related to previous MRI examination: _____ Y ❏ N ❏

7. Has patient had prior surgery / operation / invasive procedure (e.g. heart surgery, brain / eye surgery, orthopedic surgery, arthroscopy, endoscopy, etc.) of any kind? **If yes**, please indicate: Y ❏ N ❏

Date _____ Type of surgery _____ Implants used _____

Date _____ Type of surgery _____ Implants used _____

Date _____ Type of surgery _____ Implants used _____

Please indicate if patient has any of the following:

Surgical aneurysm clip(s)	Y ❏	N ❏	Artificial or prosthetic limb or joint	Y ❏	N ❏
Cardiac pacemaker / pacing wires	Y ❏	N ❏	Metal rods, plates, screws, nails, or wires	Y ❏	N ❏
Cochlear implant or implanted hearing device	Y ❏	N ❏	Wire mesh implant	Y ❏	N ❏
Implanted cardioverter defibrillator (ICD)	Y ❏	N ❏	Swan –Ganz or thermodilution catheterv	Y ❏	N ❏
Electronic implant or device	Y ❏	N ❏	Implanted insulin or infusion pump or device	Y ❏	N ❏
Magnetically-activated implant or device	Y ❏	N ❏	Transdermal medication patch	Y ❏	N ❏
Neuro or bio stimulator device	Y ❏	N ❏	Dental implants / dentures or braces	Y ❏	N ❏
Heart valve replacement	Y ❏	N ❏	G tube / C tube / J tube / gastric button	Y ❏	N ❏
Any type of intravascular coil, filter, or stent	Y ❏	N ❏	Intra-uterine device (IUD)	Y ❏	N ❏
Any vascular clip including PDA clips	Y ❏	N ❏	Tattoos or body piercing	Y ❏	N ❏
Myringotomy / ear tubes	Y ❏	N ❏	Programmable pump e.g. Baclofen **(confirm status pre and post MRI)**	Y ❏	N ❏
Orbital / eye prosthesis or implants	Y ❏	N ❏			
Coloured / tinted contact lenses	Y ❏	N ❏	Programmable shunt **(must be reprogrammed post MRI)**	Y ❏	N ❏
Hearing aid - **remove before entering MR system room**	Y ❏	N ❏			

ANY OTHER IMPLANT:

SCREENING

I attest that the above information is correct to the best of my knowledge. Form completed by (check): ❏ Patient ❏ Parent/Guardian

❏ Other _____ Date _____ Time _____

Name (print) _____ Signature _____

DI RN – if Sed/GA (sign) _____ DI Tech (sign) _____

Interpreter / Language Line Services used: Y ❏ N ❏   Interpreter signature / ID number (if applicable) _____

FIG. 13.17 The MRI Screening Checklist Used for Human Patients for an MRI at The Toronto Hospital for Sick Children. The checklist for patients is usually stricter than that for staff or visitors because the patient will be exposed to direct radio frequency.

FIG. 13.18 Incidental finding, right kidney cyst *(arrow)*. A 2.8-cm multilobulated cyst is present in the craniolateral aspect of the left kidney, without evidence of other renal anomaly. (Patient was being examined due to ataxic hind end.) (Courtesy Thames Valley Imaging, London, Ontario, Canada.)

FIG. 13.19 Skull and Cervical Spine. An aggressive soft tissue process that invades the left tympanic bulla and caudoventral portion of the left occipital bone, with regional fat alteration and severe ipsilateral retropharyngeal lymphadenopathy. (Courtesy Thames Valley Imaging, London, Ontario, Canada.)

FIG. 13.20 T2-Weighted Lumbar Spinal Tumor. Lobulated soft tissue mass infiltrating L6 and compressing the nerves of the cauda equina, with characteristics consistent with an aggressive neoplastic process. (Courtesy Thames Valley Imaging, London, Ontario, Canada.)

FIG. 13.21 A–C, Multiple views of a dog's paw. **A,** Sagittal T2 view of dog's paw. *Arrow* points to a foreign body on the inferior aspect between toes. **B,** T2 weighted dorsal view of paw showing the foreign body with a capsule forming around it. **C,** Transverse image of dog paw showing bright lesion where foreign body is present. (Courtesy Animal Health Partners, Scarborough, Ontario, Canada.)

FIG. 13.22 Lumbar Spine. Variable intervertebral disk degeneration throughout the spine in association with variable spondylosis deformans and endplate sclerosis. (Courtesy Thames Valley Imaging, London, Ontario, Canada.)

FIG. 13.23 Lumbar Spine Cyst at L3. Cyst-like lesion in the middorsal portion of the spinal cord at L3 that may communicate with the central canal and that is likely congenital in origin. (The dog is 4 months old.) (Courtesy Thames Valley Imaging, London, Ontario, Canada.)

FIG. 13.24 Coronal View, Spinal Tumor. Coronal view T1 fat saturation demonstrating a tumor at the caudal level of the lumbar spine *(arrow)*. (Courtesy Thames Valley Imaging, London, Ontario, Canada.)

FIG. 13.25 T2 spinal cord compression, sagittal view, T2 weighted demonstrating cord compression *(arrow)*. (Courtesy Thames Valley Imaging, London, Ontario, Canada.)

FIG. 13.26 Coronal Right Posterior Orbit, Porcupine Quill. Left retro-orbital soft tissue swelling with signs consistent with a migrating porcupine quill *(arrow)*, with mild to moderate local pyogranulomatous infection. (Courtesy Thames Valley Imaging, London, Ontario, Canada.)

FIG. 13.28 Sagittal Plane T2 Weighted Image of Dog's Brain. *Arrow* points to tumor pressing against the dog's brainstem. Hydrocephalus is seen in the ventricle. (Image courtesy Animal Health Partners, Toronto, Canada.)

FIG. 13.27 Second view, coronal right posterior orbit. Same patient as in Fig. 13.26, but different level. (Courtesy Thames Valley Imaging, London, Ontario, Canada.)

FIG. 13.29 Transverse Plane T1 Weighted Image of Dog's Brain. Tumor enhances with contrast *(arrow)*. Displacement of the brainstem and basilar artery by tumor can be seen. Enlarged ventricles are seen in black on the T1 weighted images. (Image courtesy Animal Health Partners, Toronto, Canada.)

REVIEW QUESTIONS

1. What part of the MRI machine is considered the most dangerous to anyone walking into the room?
   a. The radio antenna
   b. The magnet
   c. The shim coils
   d. The surface coils

2. What must be done for every person or patient entering into an MRI room?
   a. A screening form must be filled out to check for implants or operations.
   b. All loose metallic objects need to be removed.
   c. Pregnant workers cannot enter.
   d. a and b

3. What purpose are the magnetic shims in an MRI?
   a. They are used to create the images.
   b. They are used to make the field within the magnet homogenous.
   c. They are used to produce the images.
   d. They are used to create the radio waves.

4. What is a T1-weighted magnetic resonance image?
   a. An MR image on which fat appears black
   b. An image on which CSF appears white
   c. An image for which TR is 2000
   d. An image in which fat appears white

5. What method of reconstruction is used for magnetic resonance images?
   a. Filtered back-projection
   b. Back-projection
   c. Two-dimensional Fourier transformation
   d. Three-dimensional Fourier transformation

6. What happens to atoms when they are placed in a magnet?
   a. They start to spin or precess.
   b. They move randomly.
   c. They reposition themselves with regard to their magnetic polarity.
   d. They shift to the north pole of the magnet.

7. A superconductor magnet is filled with which substance?
   a. Hydrogen
   b. Helium
   c. Carbon
   d. Liquid helium

8. Which part of an MRI scanner obtains better images of smaller body parts?
   a. Gradient coils
   b. Shims
   c. Body coil
   d. Surface coils

9. Why is the word *resonance* used in the term MRI?
   a. It uses radio waves and they are musical.
   b. Atoms respond by resonating to their particular radio frequency as a function of the magnetic field strength.
   c. Resonance comes from the term used in spectroscopy.
   d. The atoms resonate to all of the radio waves.

10. For which atoms are MRI radio frequencies tuned to in order to create images?
    a. Hydrogen
    b. Carbon
    c. Oxygen
    d. Helium

11. What does "high signal intensity" mean in a magnetic resonance image?
    a. A high concentration of helium atoms is responding to the radio waves.
    b. More signal has been received from a tissue in an image with a given weighting.
    c. In a T2 image, the fat will show this.
    d. This refers to the dark part of an image.

Chapter Review Question answers are located in the Instructor Resources on Evolve and can be provided to students at the discretion of the instructor.

Bibliography

Hesselink JR. *Basic Principles of MR Imaging*. Available at: http://spinwarp.ucsd.edu/NeuroWeb/Text/br-100.htm.

MRI-Technology Information Portal. Available at: http://www.mr-tip.com/serv1.php.

Shellock FG. *MRI safety.com*. Available at: http://mrisafety.com.

Westbrook C, Roth CK, Talbot J. *MRI in Practice*. 4th ed. Hoboken: Wiley-Blackwell; 2011.

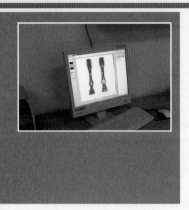

CHAPTER **14**

Nuclear Medicine and Introduction to Positron Emission Tomography

Lois C. Brown, RTR (Can/USA), ACR, MSc, P.Phys, Darryl Bonder, DVM, RSO, and Stephanie Holowka, MRT(R), MRT(MR), MRSO(MRSC)

*I can't change the direction of the wind, but I can adjust
my sails to always reach my destination*
—Jimmy Dean, American country music singer, 1928–2010

OUTLINE

LEARNING OBJECTIVES

When you have finished this chapter, you will be able to:

1. Understand the science of nuclear scintigraphy.
2. Know the etiology that indicates scintigraphy.
3. Define the term *isotope* and its use in nuclear scintigraphy.
4. Know the protocol for equine studies.
5. List the use of other isotopes for small animal studies.
6. Understand radiation protection in nuclear medicine.

APPLICATIONS

The application of the information in this chapter is relevant to the following area:

1. Diagnosis of skeletal trauma and pathology using an auxiliary diagnostic approach.

KEY TERMS

Key terms are defined in the Glossary on the Evolve website.

Annihilation
Attenuate
Attenuation profile
Cyclotron
Fludeoxyglucose

Half-life
Isotope
Millicuries
Nuclear scintigraphy
Osteoblastic activity

Photon
Positron
Positron emission
   tomography
Radioactive decay

Radioactive disintegration
Radioisotopes
Radionuclides
Scintigraphy

Introduction

When an equine partner demonstrates pain and is lame, the caregivers immediately strive to find a diagnosis being concerned with the where, what, and how of alleviating the pain.

When common diagnostics fail, other modalities such as nuclear medicine studies come into play.

Nuclear Medicine

In the first section of this book, the atom, the elements, and isotopes were briefly discussed. We will review isotopes, as the principle of nuclear medicine involves isotopes that congregate in an area of enhanced blood flow, allowing further diagnosis.

The Atom and Radioactivity

Each atom consists of three basic components: the electrons, which we manipulate in radiography; and protons and neutrons, which are contained in the nucleus. It is the neutrons that we will discuss now.

A stable atom such as helium, the second atom in the periodic table, has two protons, two neutrons, and two electrons. Most atoms are stable. The protons determine the characteristic of the element. If the number of neutrons differs in a substance, it is an isotope of the element. Barium, a contrast medium with which we are familiar, has seven naturally occurring isotopes.

> **? POINTS TO PONDER** Atoms that have the same atomic number but different atomic mass numbers are isotopes. Isotopes can occur naturally but also may be artificially produced in a laboratory.

Having excess neutrons may make isotopes radioactive. *Radioactivity* describes atoms that are in an abnormally excited state characterized by an unstable nucleus. To reach stability, these atoms spontaneously emit particles and energy to transform themselves into other atoms. This process is called *radioactive disintegration* or *radioactive decay*. The method of determining the activity of a radioisotope involves establishing how long it takes for the isotope to decay to half of its original radioactivity. This is called its *half-life*. The atoms involved in this process are called *radionuclides*. An atom with any rearrangement of the nucleus is called a *nuclide;* therefore, the atoms with nuclei that undergo radioactive decay are radionuclides.

In the 1940s and 1950s, a scientific branch of imaging was developed to examine radionuclides with respect to medical diagnosis. It was already known that infection produces heat, tumors attract cellular activity, and trauma causes an increase in blood supply around the wounded area. It was speculated that if a radioactive source was introduced within the patient either by swallowing or by injection, that source would gravitate to the area supplied by the most blood or with the highest cellular activity. The radiation emitted as the radionuclide decayed could then be imaged on a detection device that was connected to a camera. The substance ingested or injected had to be nontoxic, other than the amount of radiation introduced, and it had to be capable of being excreted through the urine or via the bowels.

One other criterion that was very important to this study was the half-life of the radionuclide. The half-life is described as the length of time necessary to reduce the intensity of the radiation emitted by half. In medicine it is important that a radionuclide administered to a person or animal must decay within a relatively short period so that the patient is not a radiation hazard to itself or to people working in the area.

The Isotopes
Small Animals

The most common radionuclides used in veterinary medicine today are iodine-131 and technetium-99m. Iodine-131 is mainly used to treat hyperthyroidism in felines and is not normally used for imaging, but nuclear scintigraphy might be utilized for before and after images of cat thyroid activity when treating hyperthyroidism.

Although it has been around for more than 50 years, nuclear scintigraphy is still relatively unused in small-animal veterinary medicine. The reason is because it uses radionuclides, which are both expensive and heavily regulated. In addition, the images derived from the studies are physiological in nature and therefore quite unfamiliar to most veterinarians. The heavy regulations and the high cost of the nuclides are also combined with the boarding and caring for animals while they are tested as the half-life of the nuclides disperse to a low enough level that they are not a risk to their owners and handlers. The other half of that equation then means that there are limited schools and courses for veterinarians to learn how to read the images produced by the cameras.

Another limiting factor is the half-life of the isotopes. The standing order of isotopes will quietly decay according to its half-life, assuming patients are available to fulfill this requirement.

Once it has decayed, it is no longer of use in the study.

Large Animals

Technetium-mdp is used for nuclear scintigraphy, particularly in equine studies. The quantity identifier for the radiation emitted by the isotopes is the curie (Ci), named after Marie and Pierre Curie, a husband-and-wife team who did very early research into radiation. The amount of radioisotope used for each examination is measured in millicuries (mCi).

The hospital or clinic that uses radioisotopes must be registered with the local atomic energy board. In Canada, it is the Canadian Nuclear Safety Commission (nuclearsafety.gc.ca). In the United States, it is the US Nuclear Regulatory Commission (www.nrc.gov). Internationally, it is the International Atomic Energy Agency (www.iaea.org) that provides information regarding the regulations for various countries.

The Science of Nuclear Medicine

Nuclear scintigraphy is the science of diagnosis by means of radioisotopes. The patient is injected with, or ingests, a radionuclide, and the nuclear medicine camera detects the emission of the radioactivity from the patient.

Nuclear medicine is a very effective way to localize pathology or the results of trauma because the radioisotope is carried to the area with the most active blood supply. Certain isotopes are more readily attracted to certain types of tissue. Technetium-99m is attracted to bone. Iodine-131 is attracted to the thyroid gland.

In nuclear medicine, the patient is the emitter and the detector is the camera. This imaging is just the opposite of radiography, in which the x-ray tube is the emitter and the detector is the image receptor. Nuclear medicine demonstrates function of a tissue or an organ, whereas radiography demonstrates the form of the anatomy.

Indications for Imaging With Nuclear Medicine

A subtle, severe, or multifocal lameness in horses may be very difficult to diagnose (Fig. 14.1). When regional anesthesia coupled with other imaging techniques does not demonstrate the abnormality, a very effective option is a nuclear scan. Bone scans can also be used to monitor the healing process of fractures. In addition, they are significant tools in a prepurchase examination of a horse.

In the equine patient, some of the areas of concern are quite large and difficult to image via the traditional methods of imaging—computerized tomography (CT), magnetic resonance imaging (MRI), and radiography. Nuclear medicine scanning can rule out abnormalities in these areas or identify pathology or the evidence of trauma. The animal does not have to be anesthetized to undergo the study.

Procedure

The average 450–500 kg horse is injected with 150 to 180 mCi technetium-99m, which has an affinity for localization in bone. After a period of 2 to 3 hours, the horse is brought to the camera, which is very large and has a room of its own (Fig. 14.2). The horse's body is brought within the field of range of the camera, which detects the emission of radiation known as *gamma photon bursts* from the horse and records the activity on a computer (Fig. 14.3A–C). The camera is moved around by a gantry system and electric hoist.

FIG. 14.1 The Nuclear Medicine Examination Room. The camera is ready to receive the emissions from the radionuclide. (Courtesy Darryl Bonder, Ontario Equine Hospital.)

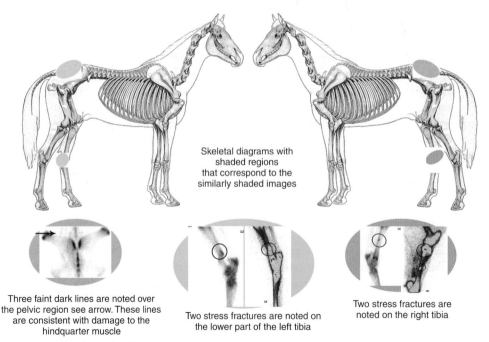

Skeletal diagrams with shaded regions that correspond to the similarly shaded images

Three faint dark lines are noted over the pelvic region see arrow. These lines are consistent with damage to the hindquarter muscle

Two stress fractures are noted on the lower part of the left tibia

Two stress fractures are noted on the right tibia

FIG. 14.2 A Case of Multifocal Lameness. This young horse had a history of being "off" in the hind end. Nuclear medicine studies revealed four stress fractures (two right and two left hind) and muscle damage over the hindquarters (arrow). (Courtesy Darryl Bonder, Ontario Equine Hospital.)

FIG. 14.3 A–C, A horse stands quietly while the gantry is moved into various positions. (Courtesy Darryl Bonder, Ontario Equine Hospital.)

An area of increased osteoblastic activity indicates accelerated metabolism within the bones, which will result in an indication of higher radiation emitted. It is termed a *hot spot.*

Phases of a Bone Scan

The vascular phase is not commonly used in horses unless a thrombosis is suspected. In this phase, the camera is positioned over the horse while the isotope is being injected. The course of the isotope can then be traced as it moves through the circulatory system.

The soft tissue phase (Fig. 14.4) occurs approximately 5 to 10 minutes after injection. It detects the pooling of the nuclide in tendons, ligaments and other soft tissue structures from the carpi (knees) and tarsi (hocks) distad (down). The larger, more proximal muscle masses are too large to image, resulting in "fogging" of the image (Fig. 14.5). The bone phase is the final phase as the nuclide is distributed throughout the bone (Fig. 14.4). This phase is usually performed 2 to 3 hours after the injection to ensure that the maximum amount of nuclide has gathered at the point of interest.

For the safety of the handlers regarding radiation exposure, the horse is then hospitalized for 48 hours post injection in order for the isotope to decay. The half-life of technetium-99m is about 6 hours, and it must go through several half-lives before the animal can be safely handled and sent home.

The Images

Because the images are demonstrating function and not anatomy, they are plotted out on the computer as a series of black dots. These dots indicate radioactive bursts emitted from the horse. The structure of the anatomy is visualized so that the area of interest is easily identified. Newer cameras count the radiation bursts and display the results in color. Various color combinations can be selected. In this image

FIG. 14.4 Exertional Rhabdomyolysis. An example of posttraumatic injury demonstrated in the soft tissue phase. (Courtesy Darryl Bonder, Ontario Equine Hospital.)

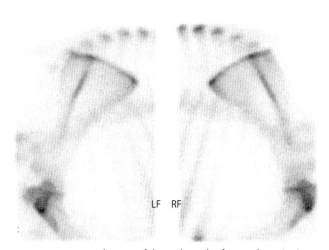

FIG. 14.5 Normal Scans of the Right and Left Scapulae. The bone phase of the scan reveals a normal set of scapulae in this case. (Courtesy Darryl Bonder, Ontario Equine Hospital.)

A   B

FIG. 14.6 A left humerus fracture **(A)** becomes more evident when color represents the location of the injury **(B)**. (Courtesy Darryl Bonder, Ontario Equine Hospital.)

(Fig. 14.6A,B), color red (hot) indicates high activity, and blue (cool) indicates low activity.

The following sections demonstrate normal and abnormal bone activity in horses and are identified as such.

Diagnosis

The veterinarian reading the scan compares the images from the left and right sides of the horse in order to make a diagnosis. Some areas of high activity are normal for certain breeds. Certain areas in young horses (the epiphyseal growth plates) should be highly active, and this is one reason why comparisons are essential. If one growth plate is not as active as the other, this finding could be a cause for concern (Fig. 14.7A,B). In Fig. 14.8A,B, the comparison view shows a complete fracture of the iliac crest with the left iliac wing completely displaced.

Nuclear medicine studies are often used to demonstrate subchondral joint disease. In Fig. 14.9A,B, the subchondral joint disease is verified on autopsy.

Radiation Protection

Nuclear medicine studies take place only at an approved site where radiation safety is ensured (Fig. 14.10). The patient is the radiation emitter, and the half-life of the radioisotope must be taken into consideration when patient care and length of stay are issues. The half-life of technetium-99m is 6 hours, which means that if you start with 160 mci at the time of injection, only 80 mci will be present 6 hours after the injection, and 40 mci will be present 12 hours after the injection. The typical equine protocol is to retain the horse at the hospital or clinic for a minimum of 24 hours or, more typically, for 48 hours in an isolation stall. Appropriate signage indicating radioactivity must be posted outside of the stall, including perimeter barriers.

When injecting the patient with a radioisotope, a lead syringe shield should be used to cover the syringe to reduce personnel exposure. Once the horse is injected with the isotope, its body and its waste products are radioactive. The waste products must be retained in a lead-lined container in a designated area for 48 hours. The staff handling the horses must wear laboratory coats, latex gloves, disposable boots, and dosimeters because of the risk of effluent contamination. Special procedures must be followed in the event of a spill. The scan room and the camera should be scanned with a survey meter before each examination to ensure that there is no contamination between examinations. The room is scanned at the start of the examination with a Geiger counter to establish a baseline. Fluorescent lights and concrete may emit a certain amount of radiation, which will be included in the count of a sensitive gamma camera (Fig. 14.11). The patient is scanned periodically during its stay in the hospital ward to ensure that it is no longer radioactive and is safe to go home (Fig. 14.12). Technicians working with an isotope are scanned out of the scintigraphy suite using a pancake probe, prior to disrobing.

If small animals are being imaged, similar procedures are followed. If patients are isolated in another area, patients should be transported by trolley or cat carrier covered with absorbent pads to avoid a urine spill. Both the trolley and carrier should remain in isolation for 72 hours and then wipe-tested to ensure there is no residual radio activity prior to return to general hospital use.

Summary of Nuclear Medicine

From the very early days of searching for a method to evaluate areas of heightened activity within the anatomy of their patients, scientists can now not only search the form of the pathology but also evaluate the function. This ability

FIG. 14.7 **A,** Right tibial stress fracture. The heightened activity (dark areas) in this scan demonstrates a fracture, whereas absence of activity could signify tissue necrosis. **B,** Comparison views of right and left knees, fetlocks, and tibiae. (Courtesy Darryl Bonder, Ontario Equine Hospital.)

is particularly valuable in equine studies, in which often the structures are so large that routine radiographs do not demonstrate the extent of trauma and pathology.

Further examples of the value in nuclear medicine diagnostics are illustrated in the PowerPoint presentation that accompanies this chapter online.

We can now move to small-animal imaging in a nuclear medicine field using the positrons emitted by a nuclide and combining them with either CT or MRI.

Positron Emission Tomography—Hybrid Imaging PET/CT, PET/MR

Introduction to PET

Imaging is a rapidly advancing field populated by the curious: If this works, what if I combine it with this? Such is the case with nuclear medicine. An imaging system that demonstrates function but not form needs to be paired with an imaging system (or systems) that demonstrate(s) form but not function. Now you have the best of both worlds. So nuclear medicine in the form of positron emission tomography (PET) is now paired with MRI, and in another facility it is paired with CT.

We have presented this science in this text as an introduction to the future of imaging. These units are available today to the veterinary market and are at times shared with the

medical market in the interests of costs and efficiency. It is beneficial for the veterinary community to understand superficially how these modalities function and how they can be of use to the patients. Fig. 14.13 is an illustration of a Siemens Electric Company PET/MR unit. This unit is used by human patients during the weekdays and by veterinary patients on evenings and weekends.

Principles of PET

PET (or PET scan) is an imaging modality that is a form of nuclear medicine technology. PET has been available since the 1970s and has become a hybrid technology that is normally combined with either CT or MRI.

PET uses the injection of a radioisotope that emits gamma rays (Fig. 14.14). The PET unit consists of a series of scintillating sensors (like nuclear medicine cameras) arranged in a ring, and this allows for the images to be acquired and then reconstructed like slices in a loaf of bread.

The most common isotope used is fludeoxyglucose (FDG), and it is used for the mapping of both brain function and malignant tumors. It is the glucose in FDG that is metabolized in active brain tissue and cancerous tumors, appearing as "hot spots" or places of increased activity on a PET scan. FDG and other PET isotopes must be produced with a device called a *cyclotron*. The FDG isotope

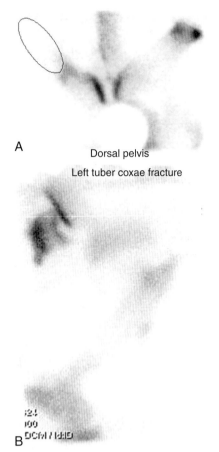

A

Dorsal pelvis

Left tuber coxae fracture

B

FIG. 14.8 A Particularly Serious Fracture of the Pelvis. This horse was discovered in the stall in the morning refusing to bear weight on the left hind leg. **A,** The oval area indicates the portion of the pelvis that is missing. **B,** The lateral view shows a tuber coxae fracture with displacement. (Courtesy Darryl Bonder, Ontario Equine Hospital.)

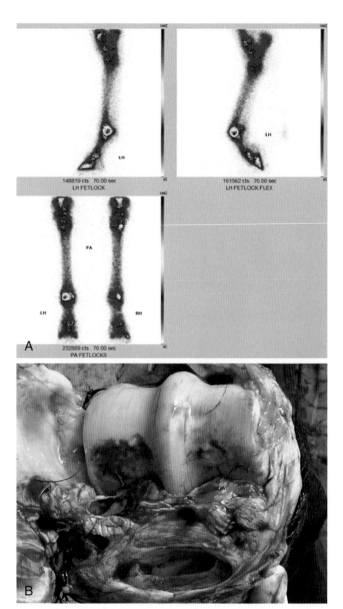

FIG. 14.9 A, Evidence of subchondral joint disease in the scan. **B,** Upon autopsy, subchondral joint disease. (Courtesy Darryl Bonder, Ontario Equine Hospital).

has a fairly short half-life of 110 minutes, which means that the place of its production must be located near the scanner. When an examination is scheduled, the isotope must be ordered and then delivered quickly.

Other isotopes can be used for PET studies, such as ammonia (for heart imaging). The reactions are the same as those in nuclear medicine; photons or beta decay with a predictable energy—511 keV. The positrons collide with electrons in the body, where they annihilate into two gamma photons that move away from one another at a 180-degree angle.

The PET scanners are designed to both detect photons and calculate their origin (in space and time) within the body. In PET imaging, the scintillation chambers (like gamma cameras) are arranged in multiple rows on a ring, and the table moves following the imaging of each slice. As with nuclear medicine, the photons are a form of radiation similar to x-rays with regard to body tissues. They can be attenuated or absorbed differently by various body tissues, especially bone.

In the original design of a PET machine, a special scan is performed using germanium to predict the absorption of the gamma ray photons. The data collected are then used to calculate an absorption correction (attenuation profile),

which would take into account various anatomical structures. A PET scan is then performed, and the computer of the scanner calculates the images using the attenuation profile it created on that specific patient. During both scans and in between, the patient must remain very still. The attenuation profile allows the images to more accurately show the slice-by-slice metabolism of the FDG isotope.

The slice data collected from PET scanners tend to be high in spatial resolution, 5 to 10 mm thick—much more accurate than a similar nuclear medicine scan.

How Did PET Become a Hybrid Technology?

One of the disadvantages of PET is that it produces images that look similar to those of nuclear medicine. Brain images show the uptake of the positron isotope (specifically glucose) but very little recognizable anatomy. Combining

FIG. 14.10 A Legal Door Sign Indicating the Presence of Radioactive Sources. In some countries the sign would read "Danger–RadioHazard Materials." (Courtesy Darryl Bonder, Ontario Equine Hospital.)

FIG. 14.12 A Radiation Dosimeter. The horse is kept at the facility until the dose count on this dosimeter is below 4 microsieverts/hour. Usually the count is less than 1 after 48 hours. (Image courtesy Harpell Associates, Oakville, Ontario, Canada.)

FIG. 14.11 A Geigver Counter Is Set to Measure in Kilocounts/Minutes (Kc/min). (Courtesy Darryl Bonder, Ontario Equine Hospital.)

FIG. 14.13 MR/PET Scanner Built by Siemens Electric Company. The two gantries are positioned one behind the other so that there is no interruption in the flow of the examination. (Courtesy Darryl Bonder, Ontario Equine Hospital.)

PET with CT accomplishes two aspects of the scans: 1) the x-ray radiation used in the CT scan has similar penetrating abilities to that of the produced photons, and therefore it can be used to create the attenuation profile; and 2) CT scans provide more anatomical information for the body part being imaged. The CT scans or PET/CT scans can also be fused together to correlate functional data with anatomical data (form and function in one image).

Several designs of CT/PET scanners have been created, but all machines feature a CT scanner, which can be used on its own, and a PET scanner, which is used in combination with the CT. For some vendors, the gantry is in one piece and appears like a CT scanner with a longer tunnel (Fig. 14.15); for others, the two units are separated and can be moved apart (Fig. 14.16). The gantries on CT/PET machines are not able to be angled, unlike a regular CT scanner. Still, the CT scanner does function much like a clinical multislice CT scanner, and so clinics and hospitals are able to use the machine for regular CT work in between PET studies.

PET/CT Studies

A PET/CT study starts with the injection of the isotope about 45 minutes before moving the patient onto the scanner. Because the FDG isotope may be taken up by active muscles, animals may be anesthetized so that they keep still. This

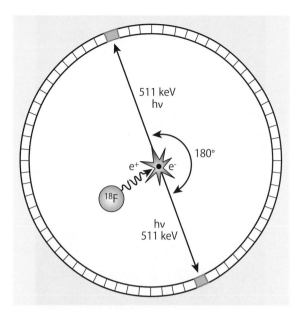

FIG. 14.14 The Production of Positrons From the Nucleus. When positrons join with electrons, they break apart in a fixed pattern. This is called *annihilation*. They break apart into two photons that move away from each other at a 180-degree angle. The PET unit is computed to detect where the particle originated and the timing of the annihilation. (From Hoppe R, Phillips T, Roach M. *Liebel and Phillips Textbook of Radiation Oncology*. 3rd ed. Philadelphia: Saunders; 2010.)

ensures that no false uptake occurs. The first part of the study is performed on the CT scan. The patient is positioned in a dorsoventral or ventrodorsal position. Intravenous contrast for the CT scan (for cancer detection) may be given. The anatomical images are now acquired. The computer is able to extract the density information from the CT detectors to create the attenuation profile for the PET study. The CT scan part takes less than a minute. Depending on the anatomy being imaged, the PET study can take from 20 to 40 minutes. The PET study can be seen both in its original state and then corrected by the attenuation profile. Ultimately, they can be fused against the CT scan images and show both comparable anatomical and functional data.

PET/MR Studies

MRI is the best modality to show soft tissues. Modern hybrid machines are able to provide both MRI and PET scans in the same examination (Fig. 14.17A,B).

The MRI/PET machine looks much like a regular MRI except that the tunnel or gantry is longer. The PET part is behind the MRI. The MRI will work much like a regular MRI scanner. Specialized surface coils have been created to work in MRI but not attenuate the gamma radiation used in PET. The patient is imaged with the MRI first. For the PET

FIG. 14.15 CT/PET Scanner by General Electric Company. (Courtesy Darryl Bonder, Ontario Equine Hospital.)

FIG. 14.16 CT/PET Scanner by Philips. Here the two units are clearly visible. (Courtesy Darryl Bonder, Ontario Equine Hospital.)

FIG. 14.17 A and B, Patient views from an MRI/PET scanner showing the degree of pathology in the left side of the skull. (Courtesy Darryl Bonder, Ontario Equine Hospital.)

portion of the scan, some machines have to be told which body part is imaged on the MRI, and the attenuation profile is calculated from that site's images. The PET scan is acquired in a set volume of slices from body section to body section and then merged with the MRI. The veterinarians can look at both the high-resolution MRI anatomy and the PET images—either fused together or separately—to see where the glucose is being metabolized. The main advantage of this type of hybrid imaging is that a lump of tissue may be seen as cancerous or as active disease.

Summary

The images here show that technology moves forward each year to more and more interesting imaging solutions. The veterinary community is moving rapidly with it. CT/PET and MR/PET are two new modalities that we can safely offer clients with a view to capturing an obscure diagnosis.

REVIEW QUESTIONS

1. The science of nuclear medicine uses:
   a. Isobars, which are emitted from technetium
   b. Isotopes, which are not radioactive
   c. Radiation to activate technetium
   d. Radioisotopes to image structures
2. The camera in nuclear medicine is used to:
   a. Help the technician obtain good pictures
   b. Detect any background radiation
   c. Detect the emissions of the isotope technetium-99m
   d. Promote the use of the isotope
3. The isotope that is most highly attracted to bone is:
   a. Iodine-131
   b. Technetium-99m
   c. Technetium-131
   d. Uranium-133
4. During the procedure, the equine patient:
   a. Is heavily sedated and usually does not react to the substance
   b. Is moved into several positions around the camera
   c. Stands and waits until a burst of radioactive activity is complete
   d. Stands quietly while its body emits radioactivity
5. The camera used in nuclear medicine:
   a. Is actually a gamma detector that collects bursts of activity
   b. Records the patient's internal movements as the isotope detects a signal
   c. Records the radioisotope as it collects in the area of interest
   d. Senses the radioactivity and reacts to it with light bursts

6. Once the horse has been injected with the isotope:
   a. It is then radioactive and needs special handling
   b. It is then radioactive but no protection is necessary
   c. The radioisotope emits just enough for the camera to detect
   d. The radioisotope is not very strong so it does not emit anything
7. The diagnosis from the images is made on the basis of:
   a. All the information from the chart and the monitor
   b. The camera images and the half-life of the isotope
   c. The collection of radioactive bursts by the camera
   d. The high-resolution images from the camera
8. After the examination, the patient must:
   a. Be isolated for at least 24 hours in order to allow the radioisotope to decay
   b. Be isolated for an hour and then sent home with special instructions
   c. Not be handled or fed until the radioisotope's half-life decays and it is safe to go home
   d. Not be ridden for at least 24 hours, until a diagnosis is made
9. Positron emission technology uses radioisotopes that must be created with a machine called a:
   a. Reactor
   b. Cyclotron
   c. Camera
   d. Scintillator
10. The process by which photons are created by positrons colliding with electrons is called:
    a. Decay
    b. Bremsstrahlung
    c. Annihilation
    d. Fusion
11. What calculation is used to compensate for the differences in absorption of gamma photons by various tissues?
    a. Attenuation profile
    b. Attenuation coefficient
    c. Absorption coefficient
    d. Interpolation

Chapter Review Question answers are located in the Instructor Resources on Evolve and can be provided to students at the discretion of the Instructor.

Radiographic Positioning and Related Anatomy

In the positioning chapters, the following will be stressed:

Describe the proper radiographic positioning techniques for all anatomic areas of small, large, and exotic animals so that for each position you are able to demonstrate:

- Normal views and protocol
- Ancillary views and protocol
- Where to measure
- Where to center the beam
- Correct collimation and peripheral boundaries
- A properly positioned patient
- Important concerns, idiosyncrasies, and anatomy

CHAPTER 15
Overview of Positioning

Marg Brown, RVT, BEd Ad Ed

Knowledge is of no value unless you put it into practice.
— Anton Chekhov, Russian playwright, 1860–1904

OUTLINE

LEARNING OBJECTIVES

When you have finished this chapter, you will be able to:

1. Understand the proper anatomical positioning terminology used in veterinary radiography.
2. Know the common rules for radiographic projections that are used when identifying and radiographing animals.
3. Focus on non-manual restraint.
4. Demonstrate radiation and patient safety procedures.
5. Describe required patient preparation before radiographic exposure.
6. Describe the advantages and disadvantages of the various positioning aids available.
7. Understand the required views.
8. List positioning guidelines to ensure production of high-quality diagnostic images.
9. Apply the three important tenets of radiation safety.
10. Understand the importance of collimation, particularly with the digital image.
11. Describe important issues for labeling and identifying an image.
12. Correctly display radiographs on a monitor or illuminator.
13. Determine whether a radiograph is diagnostic using a checklist.

KEY TERMS

Key terms are defined in the Glossary on the Evolve website.

Caudal (Cd)	Dorsopalmar (DPa)	Palmar (Pa)	Sagittal plane
Caudocranial (CdCr)	Dorsoplantar (DPl)	Palmarodorsal (PaD)	Skyline
Cranial (Cr)	Dose creep	Plantar (Pl)	Transverse plane
Craniocaudal (CrCd)	Lateral (L)	Plantarodorsal (PlD)	Ventral (V)
Distal (Di)	Lateromedial (LaM)	Proximal (Pr)	
Dorsal (D)	Medial (M)	Recumbent	
Dorsal plane	Oblique (O)	Rostral (R)	

TECHNICAL NOTE: To preserve space, the radiographs presented in this chapter do not show collimation. Always collimate so that the beam is limited to within the image receptor edges. In film radiography, you should see a clear border of collimation (frame) on every radiograph. In some jurisdictions, evidence of collimation is required by law. In digital imaging, the algorithm depends on proper collimation.

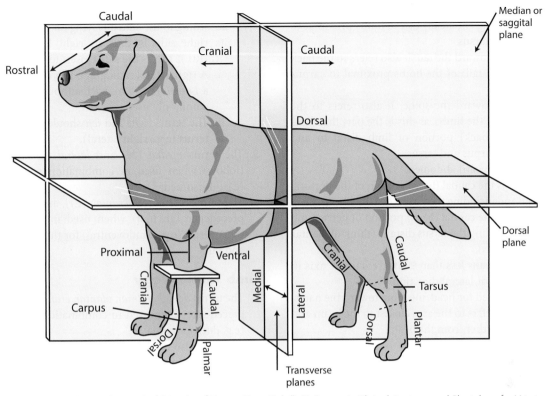

FIG. 15.1 Correct Anatomical Directional Terms. (From Colville T, Bassert J. *Clinical Anatomy and Physiology for Veterinary Technicians*. 3rd ed. St Louis: Elsevier; 2016.)

Part Two of this text educates the radiographer on how to properly position animals, with a focus on non-manual restraint. In no other diagnostic imaging jurisdiction is the patient held by the radiographer. The use of non-manual restraint using simple tools and common sense minimizes the radiographer to direct and secondary radiation, thereby limiting personnel to harmful radiation.

The patient is best immobilized by chemical restraint (sedation or general anesthesia) and/or positional devices. Please refer to a good anesthetic text for possible chemical agents. Knowledge of common behavior, restraint, and positioning principles are essential to minimize radiographer exposure even if chemical restraint is contraindicated. Always keep the welfare of both the patient and the radiographer in mind while producing accurate diagnostic images. A basic understanding of normal anatomy and proper terminology is also essential to produce diagnostic radiographic images that the veterinarian can accurately interpret and diagnose.

If manual restraint is necessary, the radiographer must take all available precautions to minimize exposure to ionizing radiation. All personnel in the radiographic suite must be shielded properly with the appropriate leaded apparel. See Chapter 3 for proper guidelines that minimize radiation exposure to the restrainer by stressing judicious adherence to distance from the beam, proper protection, and limited exposure time.

BOX 15.1	Positional Terminology
Dorsal (D)	Caudal (Cd)
Ventral (V)	Rostral (R)
Lateral (L)	Palmar (Pa, P)
Medial (M)	Plantar (Pl, P)
Left (L/Le)	Oblique (O)
Right (R/Rt)	Distal (Di)
Cranial (Cr)	Proximal (Pr)

Positional Terminology

It is important to understand the correct terminology. Most still use the *Nomina Anatomica Veterinaria* as the point of reference. The American College of Veterinary Radiology (ACVR) terms are also shown in Fig. 15.1. The basic terms used are listed in Box 15.1.

Rules of Positioning

There are a few rules to keep in mind based on ACVR (see Fig. 15.1):
1. Common terms and abbreviations used include:
   - Left (L, Le), right (R, Rt).
   - Medial (M), lateral (L) which is used in reference to limbs. The medial is the inside and the lateral is the outside of the limb.

- Cranial (Cr) is toward the head. It also refers to the front part (facing the head) of the limbs proximal to the carpus and tarsus.
- Caudal (Cd) is toward the tail. It also refers to the back part (facing the tail) of the limbs proximal to carpus and tarsus.
- Dorsal (D) is toward the spine. It also refers to the cranial (front of the limbs, as this is the part that faces the head and back) portion of limb distal to and including the carpus and tarsus.
- Ventral (V) is toward abdomen.
- Palmar (Pa) is the caudal (back) portion of the pectoral limb from and including the carpus distally (the "palm").
- Plantar (Pl) is the caudal (back) portion of pelvic limb from and including the tarsus distally (think of plantar warts in humans).
- Oblique (O) means less than 90 degrees to the axis in either a medial or lateral direction.
- Rostral (R) is used for head, meaning toward the nares.
- Proximal (Pr) refers to the area closest to the beam and distal (Di) is further from the beam.

2. Projections are named according to the direction in which the x-ray beam first enters the patient, then where the beam exits.
3. Combinations of basic directional terms accurately describe the point of entrance and point of exit. Consistency increases the standardization of the nomenclature.
4. Assuming an overhead vertical beam, if a patient is lying on its:
   a. Back (dorsal recumbency), the view is called *ventrodorsal (VD)*. The beam enters the ventral (V) portion—the abdomen or belly—and exits the dorsal (D) aspect, or the patient's spine (Fig. 15.2).
   b. Abdomen (ventral recumbency), the view is called *dorsoventral (DV)*. The beam enters the *dorsal (D)* portion—the spine—and exits at the *ventral (V)* aspect, or the abdomen.
   c. The abbreviated term indicates beam direction such that: the first letter is where the x-rays enter the body and the second letter is where x-rays leave the body (part that lies against the image receptor)

> **✎ TECHNICIAN NOTES**   According to etymological rules, when two terms are combined, the combining vowel (generally "o") is used to connect them.

FIG. 15.2 Patient Lying in Ventrodorsal Recumbency. The beam enters the abdomen and exits out the back or spine.

   d. Side or lateral recumbency, the patient is labeled according to the side it is lying on. An animal lying on its right side is thus in right lateral recumbency (RL/RtL). This is the side closest to the image detector.
      i. A right lateral radiograph is properly referred to as a *Le-RtL (entry to exit)*, although this term is not commonly used.
      ii. The terms *right* and *left* should precede any other terms (e.g., right lateral).
5. The terms *medial (M)* and *lateral (L)* are subservient (follow) when used in combination with other terms (e.g., dorsomedial).
6. The terms *rostral (R), cranial, (Cr),* and *caudal (Cd)* take precedence (go first) when used in combination with other terms (e.g., caudoventral) for the head, neck, trunk, and tail.

Limb Terminology

1. The terms *dorsal, palmar, plantar, cranial,* and *caudal* take precedence when used in combination with other terms (e.g. dorsoproximal).
2. Lateral is also used for limbs.
   a. Small animals usually lie on their side with the affected limb against the image receptor. Technically, this is a medial-lateral (ML) view as the beam enters the inside of the limb and exits the outside of the limb, but the view is generally referred to as a lateral (L).
   b. Large animals are weight bearing. The beam enters from the outside of the limb (lateral aspect) and exits on the inside of the limb (medial) where the image detector is placed. Technically, this is a lateral-medial (LM) view but is also generally referred to as a lateral. This is opposite of small animals in lateral recumbency.
3. *Oblique (O)* projection is taken with the central ray at an angle of less than 90 degrees to any of the body planes in a medial or lateral direction. The term *oblique* is commonly used in equine limbs.
   a. The major directional axes of mediolateral (ML), dorsopalmar/dorsoplantar (DP), or craniocaudal (CrCd) are combined to describe the position.
      i. For example: dorsolateral-palmaromedial oblique (DLPMO) of the metacarpus: the central ray faces the dorsal (front) part of the limb 45 degrees laterally from the midline and parallel to the ground. The point of entry is the dorsolateral aspect of the limb. The point of exit is the palmaromedial (medial) aspect of the limb and is perpendicular to the image receptor, which is placed here (Fig. 15.3). Insert a hyphen to separate the point of entry and point of exit.
      ii. Note that when the abbreviation DLPMO is used, the first two letters show beam entry (DL) while the next two letters show beam exit (PM) and placement of image detector. The first letter of each pair will be cranial/dorsal or caudal/palmar/plantar and the second letter of each pair will be either medial or lateral.

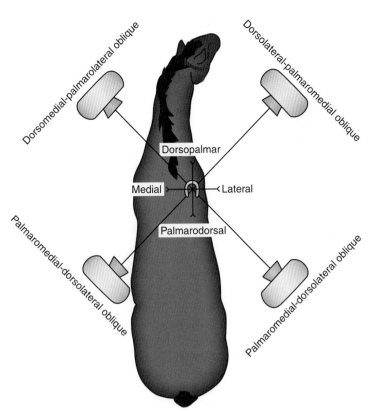

FIG. 15.3 Correct Anatomical Directional Terms for Oblique Views.

iii. DLPMO is often referred to as a *medial oblique* because the medial aspect is against the film.

iv. The most accurate description of the example above is Dorsoproximal 45-degree lateral-palmarodistomedial oblique (DPr45°L-PaDiMO). This will be expanded upon in Chapter 24.

4. Tangential or skyline: Refers to the central ray entering and exiting the same side of the limb so that the bone is in profile.

a. For example, palmaroproximal-palmarodistal (PaPr-PaDi) in reference to an equine forelimb navicular region, means that the beam is aimed at the palmar-(back) aspect of the foot starting at the top (proximo-), remains on the palmar side, and exits at the sole of the hoof (disto-). The horse's foot is centered on the image receptor, which is on the ground. Further terminology will be discussed in Chapter 24.

Patient Positioning

The Patient

The comfort and welfare of the patient should be considered at all times. Patience is vital, especially with patients who cannot be sedated, are critically ill, are compromised in any way, or are in pain. Make sure that any required supplies or monitoring equipment are close at hand. Constantly assess and monitor all patients.

Patients will tolerate abnormal positions if they feel secure. To minimize anxiety, handle them in a slow, quiet manner in a darkened room. They often respond to a calm, soft voice and gentle stroking. Quick, loud movements and severe restraint usually result in a frightened, tense, and even aggressive patient. Permit the patient time to settle, either with or without sedation. Do not underestimate the value of a muzzle. Muzzles often distract the patient, as well as being a "technician saver." Cats especially do not respond to over-restraint. The combination of patience with mild sedation and strategically placed positioning aids produces well-positioned images.

The rotor noise (spinning of the rotating anode) of the x-ray tube often startles animals. When working with patients who exhibit signs of anxiety, consider starting and releasing the rotor switch just before taking the radiograph so the patient becomes accustomed to the noise. Be careful not to cause rotor damage by depressing the switch incorrectly.

Prevent retakes by making sure proper exposure factors are used and the patient is correctly positioned. A border of collimation (frame) on each image should be noted; only include the full anatomy of the area of interest plus the peripheral borders (e.g., the thorax should include the shoulder joint and diaphragm). Peripheral borders will be stressed for each position in the relevant chapters. Proper collimation further protects the patient and positioner from secondary radiation as well as increasing detail and radiographic contrast of the image (Fig. 15.4).

FIG. 15.4 Limit the image receptor to include the area that is being radiographed and its peripheral borders to prevent unnecessary radiation and excess secondary radiation.

FIG. 15.5 It is important to remove any object that could interfere with the image. The halter was not removed from this horse's head before exposure.

Keep the safety rules of time, distance, and shielding in mind at all times. Always wear protective equipment if you must hold the patient or be in the room when an exposure is made. Keep as far from the central beam as possible. For film/screen systems, use a fast combination to lessen the milliamperage (mA) and exposure time needed.

There are further safety concerns in digital radiography, such as the temptation to obtain more, rather than fewer, images because digital images are easy to delete. An increased number of images means increased exposure to the patient and personnel. Limit the number taken by being correct the first time. Minimize dose creep, which is the tendency to increase your kilovolts (kV) and mAs.

Carefully plan and prepare for the exposure as much as possible before positioning the patient on the table to minimize the restraint time. Preparation includes measuring the patient, setting the exposure technique on the machine console, positioning the cassette/image receptor, making the label (if needed), collimating the beam, gathering positional aids, and donning any protective gear.

Proper preparation may allow you to temporarily step away from the beam and secondary radiation even without chemical restraint.

> ✎ **TECHNICIAN NOTES**   Always measure the animal in the position it is to be radiographed. Aim for excellent diagnostic images the first time.

Patient Preparation

The patient should be clean and free of any debris. If the hair coat of the patient is wet or full of debris, confusing artifacts can appear on the image. Collars, harnesses, and leashes of any sort, especially those made of metal, should be removed (Fig. 15.5). Remove bandages, splints, and casts before imaging unless there is a definite medical reason for leaving them

in place. Pedal radiography of the horse may require removing the shoe and cleaning the frog of the foot to minimize any artifacts that may obscure an area of interest.

For radiography of the small animal abdomen, the gastrointestinal tract must be free of ingesta and fecal material. A cathartic such as an enema or a laxative may be indicated to remove the obstructive material. A more detailed discussion of patient preparation for abdominal studies is provided in Chapter 23.

> ✎ **TECHNICIAN NOTES**   Always remember the tenets of safety—time, distance, and shielding—when working with x-rays. What you don't see can cause future damage, impairing your health. Protect yourself.

Positioning Aids for Human Safety

Devices such as sandbags, foam blocks, wedges, radiolucent troughs, tape, gauze, rope, bungee cords, Velcro, or compression bands can be used (Fig. 15.6) to assist in the positioning of the patient. Any reusable aids should be waterproof, washable, stain resistant, and easy to store.

Prepared sandbags are generally pre-filled with clean silica sand, permanently sealed, and often made of vinyl or nylon with plastic linings. Other material, such as bean bags, which are filled with polyester beads, can also be used; however, they do not offer the same weight as sand. Sand-and-bean bags are radiopaque and should not be in the field of interest. Empty sealable bags filled with sand can be used. If you are making your own sandbags, consider canvas (legs of jeans work well) or thick vinyl, making sure to use very

FIG. 15.6 A, Positioning devices available for nonmanual restraint. They should be covered for easy cleaning and sanitation. B, Set of small and large foam V-troughs that can be used in conjunction with Velcro strapping. (Courtesy Julia Bitan, http://handsfreexrays.com, Toronto, ON.)

FIG. 15.7 Use of tape to secure the head out of the field of view.

FIG. 15.8 Soft Velcro strapping can be attached to the table for easy patient positioning of any body part. (Courtesy Ashley Jenner/Julia Bitan, http://handsfreexrays.com, Toronto, ON.)

narrow stitching so the sand will not leak out. Fabric sand bags are not easily disinfected, so before each use, wrap them in disposable plastic.

U- and V-shaped troughs are essential to maintain a patient in dorsal recumbency. Generally, they are clear plastic or vinyl-covered commercial foam (Fig. 15.6B). The plastic/acrylic troughs are radiolucent, lightweight, and easy to clean. U-shaped troughs offer good head support. Those with acrylic rods can be used to maintain the shape of the skull. When using troughs for abdominal or thoracic images, keep in mind that if the partial or entire field of view is on the trough, the radiograph may display distortion artifacts or asymmetry.

Further commercial foam positioning devices are available in various shapes, including triangular and rectangular, as well as in various sizes. Foam positioning devices can also be made by cutting foam purchased from fabric stores into desired shapes with a scalpel blade or electric knife. Properly covered wedges are essential for disinfection between patients and for keeping the devices dry to minimize radiographic artifacts. Foam can produce an air density shadow on the processed radiograph and if not properly covered, absorbs and retains liquids that may be radiopaque when dry.

Tape (Fig.15.7), gauze, hook-and-loop tape (Velcro) (Fig.15.8), and compression bands are extremely effective but must be functional to be satisfactory. They can be used to extend and hold limbs, rotate limbs, secure the patellae and femurs for a hip dysplasia view, widen the space between the

toes, temporarily secure a head out of the field of view, and so on. Velcro on the underside of the table that allows straps to stick, is effective for many views and should be considered as a standard method of non-manual restraint for radiography. Sedation can be very minimal because the straps are quickly released. Rope and gauze, using a half-hitch knot (a simple overhand knot, bringing the working end over and under the standing part) or variation, can be tied to the table if the patient is sedated. If necessary, a restrainer can hold the ends standing at a distance from both the primary beam and secondary radiation. A wooden spoon can even be used to keep a cat's head out of the field of view so the radiographer is farther away from the primary beam.

Clothes pegs/clothes pins for cats, commercially available cat scruffers, or nylon towel clamps applied to the dorsal neck region (a feline behavior principle that the queen uses with her kittens) can be effective if the positioning is quick and the patient is not in pain. Place the sandbag over the device to keep in position. However, the American Animal Hospital Association (AAHA) and American Association of Feline Practitioners (AAFP) have made statements that

FIG. 15.9 Positioning of an untranquilized feline using towel, sandbag, and Velcro straps. (Courtesy Ashley Jenner/Julia Bitan, http://handsfreexrays.com, Toronto, ON.)

scruffing cats does not allow a sense of control, often increasing fear and fear aggression.

Wrapping a cat in a towel ("cat burrito") can be effective if you need to pull out the limbs or for imaging the abdomen and thorax. Sandbagging the towel keeps cats in position. Wrapping does allow many angry cats to become compliant (Fig. 15.9).

These devices, along with sedation if necessary, effectively minimize manual restraint. Non-manual restraint must always focus on the safety and comfort of the patient. Devices must be quickly applied and released and should never compromise the patient. Correct use of positioning aids gives the patient the illusion it is being held. Strategically placed sandbags or compression devices over the neck and limbs, judicious use of tape or a compression band and Velcro, a dimly lit room, calm and deliberate movements, or a gloved hand placed over the head and pelvis held until the rotor is depressed, may keep patients, especially dogs in lateral recumbency, calm long enough for the restrainer to step back (leaving the glove) at least 6 feet as the image is taken. Keep talking to the patient as you quietly step back. Move forward as soon as the image has been taken. Another person should be depressing the exposure buttons on the console; if you are using the foot pedal, step back as far as possible. Increasing your distance from the beam drastically reduces your exposure.

If there is no alternative but to restrain a patient, it is imperative to look away from the field of view and lean back as far as possible while taking the image. At no point should any part of your body be in the field of view, as protective equipment protects you from secondary radiation, not from the primary beam.

Acrylic tubes, stockinette material, pillowcases, paper bags, and plastic containers can also be strategically used for the positioning of exotic animals and pocket pets. Please see Chapter 25 for more detail on this subject.

Equine radiographers are less likely to practice non-manual restraint because of perceived physical safety for both the handler and the horse. However, every effort should be made to always practice the three essential components of radiation safety (time, distance, and shielding). See Chapter 24 for further information on equine positioning.

✏ **TECHNICIAN NOTES**   Have everything ready before taking the exposure. This includes measuring the animal, turning on the machine, setting the main voltage calibration if required, having proper source image distance, use of a grid if needed, collimating, and setting the exposures. Have the cassettes or plates ready. Positioning devices should be close at hand, but remove any objects or distractions. The patient should be clean and have no artifacts in the area of interest.

Required Views and Positioning Guidelines

The following guidelines assist in producing high-quality images:

- Minimum recommended exposures are two views of each anatomical area taken at right angles to each other. You are trying to visualize a three-dimensional body on a two-dimensional image; details will be missed if two perpendicular views are not taken (Fig. 15.10). There may be exceptions to positioning the patient in two views perpendicular to each other if the patient is debilitated or in trauma, or if the position will cause undue stress to the animal. If a vertical beam for a VD is not possible, consider both a horizontal and vertical beam in lateral recumbency so that you still have two perpendicular views (Fig. 15.11).
- Position the area of interest closest to the image receptor to reduce distortion and magnification (Fig. 15.12).
- In general, the central ray should be centered directly over the area of interest to minimize distortion and misdiagnosis. If there is a known lesion, however, it is important to center the beam directly over this area, especially if there are healing fractures or spinal lesions.
- Measure using an inexpensive caliper that measures part thickness in centimeter increments over the thickest part for any anatomical region so that the full area of interest will be penetrated with sufficient exposure factors.
  - The patient must be measured in the same position used for the radiographic image; if the animal is measured while standing, the tissue thickness measurement will be greater than when the animal is recumbent, especially for soft tissue studies (Fig. 15.13A,B).
  - If there is a large difference in tissue thickness between the cranial and caudal borders, two separate exposures

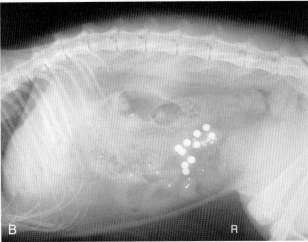

FIG. 15.10 A and **B**, It would be difficult to determine exactly where the barium-impregnated polyurethane spheres (BIPS) are positioned without the two perpendicular views. Note the proper placement for viewing of ventrodorsal (VD) and lateral radiographs.

FIG. 15.11 Horizontal Beam of a Dog in a Standing Lateral View.

FIG. 15.12 Note the difference in magnification between the left limb, which is closer to the plate, and the opposite right limb, which is raised from the image receptor. Also note that the bone edges are not as defined on the right limb.

may need to be taken. This is not uncommon in the abdomen and thorax of a deep-chested dog. If there is only a small difference in tissue density, it is best to compromise the difference.

- The thickest part of the area of interest should be toward the cathode side so that the most penetrating x-rays can assist in proper exposure (Fig. 15.14; see Chapter 2).
- Use an image receptor that is large enough to cover the body area being imaged. All required anatomy must be included for each anatomical area such as abdomen, thorax, skull, and vertebrae.
  - All images of long bones (humerus and femur) should include the shaft of the bone, as well as the joints both distal (Di) and proximal (Pr) to the bone.
  - For joint radiography, the central ray must be centered over the joint space, and the beam should include a portion of the long bones distal and proximal to the joint.
  - Proper centering and inclusion for limbs is further expanded in Chapters 18 and 19.
- Image the opposite corresponding limb in immature or older patients to allow the pathological structure of one limb to be compared with the normal anatomy of the other.

FIG. 15.13 A, Measuring with a caliper in this position may lead to extra tissue thickness. **B,** Calipers are properly used when the patient is measured lying in the radiographic view to be projected. This patient measures 17 cm.

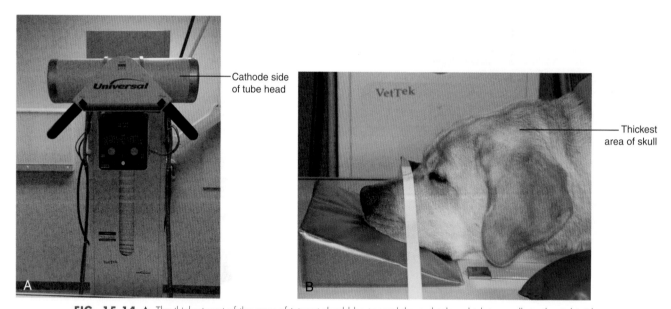

Cathode side of tube head

Thickest area of skull

FIG. 15.14 A, The thickest part of the area of interest should be toward the cathode, which is usually to the right side of the tube head. **B,** Positioning with the thickest part to the cathode.

- An image receptor can be divided to include two separate images on one radiographic film during tabletop technique (Fig. 15.15).
  - Place a lead sheet over the half not being imaged (called a cassette mask) to prevent exposure while the other side is being radiographed.
  - Lead sheets can be purchased from most x-ray supply companies and are usually supplied in preselected sizes; larger sheets can be purchased and cut to the desired size.

- The lead should be at least 2 mm thick. If a lead sheet is unavailable, a lead glove can be placed over the area to be shielded.
- Collimate to the image to prevent secondary radiation from causing unnecessary fogging.
- Both views should be facing the same direction so that toes or nose are facing the same side of the cassette on each view.
- A nonslip pad, such as a rubber shelf liner placed under the cassette, keeps it from slipping (Fig. 15.16) when using the tabletop technique.

FIG. 15.15 Divided Image Receptor View of a Dog Extremity in Film Radiography. Through the use of a lead shield, both views can be exposed on one plate. The receptor is not divided when a grid is used.

FIG. 15.16 Placing a grip pad under the image receptor helps keep the cassette from sliding when using tabletop technique. Note also how the beam is collimated inside the cassette.

Image Identification

Identification (ID) of the radiographic images is important, both for legal purposes and identifying that the images belong to the patient you are radiographing. Please see Chapter 7 for further details. Each radiographic image should contain the following information: owner and patient ID, date of examination, name and location of the facility, veterinarian, and other state or provincial requirements. The radiography log includes this information along with additional information including age, breed, and sex of the patient that could be helpful for future retrieval and identification.

Positioning markers (right, left, front, hind) should be used to assist in correct interpretation of the images, especially for equine images of areas distal to the carpus and tarsus or symmetrical anatomical areas such as a skull. Conventionally, markers are placed laterally (as opposed to medially) for DP, CrCd, or CdCr and oblique limb radiographs.

FIG. 15.17 The patient is in right lateral recumbency, lying on its right side. Note that the marker is placed cranially and ventrally.

Place the markers cranially for lateral radiographs. In DV or VD views, place the appropriate L or R marker on the correct side of the patient. In a lateral body projection, the marker indicates the side that is directly on the table or image receptor. Thus, an R indicates a patient lying in right lateral recumbency or on its right side. The marker or label would generally be placed cranially and ventrally (Fig. 15.17).

Use markers for special procedures such as a gastrointestinal contrast study that is part of a series to indicate time elapsed or order of images taken. In film radiography, this designation can be made on the lead tape label. Specialized time clocks can be used to easily adjust the time lapse (Fig. 15.18). Gravity markers that indicate a standing patient are also available, although not frequently used.

> **TECHNICIAN NOTES** Quickly go through a mental checklist such as this one before pushing the exposure button:
> - Are the settings correct?
> - Is the plate/cassette/machine/grid in position?
> - Is the thickest part toward the cathode, if applicable?
> - Are the markers and ID (if using) in the proper location and not obstructing relevant anatomy?
> - Do you have the correct body part and view?
> - Is the patient properly centered? Are the peripheral borders correct?
> - Is the x-ray beam correctly collimated?
> - Is the patient properly prepared, positioned, and restrained so that the body part is parallel to the image receptor and the central ray is perpendicular to both?
> - Is the patient in the correct phase of respiration if applicable?

Viewing Radiographs

To assist in understanding normal radiographic anatomy, you should always view radiographs on the illuminator or monitor in the following manner (see Fig. 15.10):

Lateral radiographs: The cranial part of the patient is to your left.
Dorsoventral/ventrodorsal radiographs: The cranial part of the animal points up, and the animal's left side is on your right (as if you are going to shake its paw).

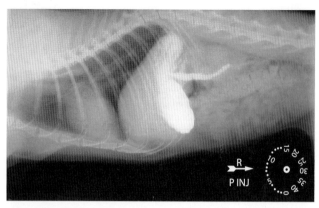

FIG. 15.18 The time clock indicates that the radiograph was taken 7 minutes after administration of barium. The feline patient is lying on its right side.

FIG. 15.19 Mystery Radiographs. What do you think the different objects are in this image? (Courtesy Julia Bitan, http://handsfreexrays.com, Toronto, ON.)

Lateromedial/mediolateral or oblique radiographs of the limbs: The proximal part of the limb points up, and the cranial or dorsal aspect of the limb is to your left.

DP/PD/CrCd/CdCr radiographs of the limbs: The proximal end of the extremity is at the top of the illuminator or monitor or pointing up.

Consistency is important. When labeling film radiographs, consider how the labels and markers are positioned so that they can easily be read when the radiographs are viewed in the proper positions. For proper illumination specifications and concerns see Chapter 7.

Fig. 15.19 is a mystery radiograph. Review it and answer the question presented with it.

Radiographic Checklist

Before submitting the images to the veterinarian, ask yourself the following questions to ensure that you have optimal diagnostic and legal radiographic images:

- Do you have good exposure with appropriate contrast and density?

- Is your image properly centered?
- Is the body part properly positioned, with no rotation?
- Are the appropriate borders included, and is there evidence of collimation?
- Is the image label present and legible, and are positional lead markers present?
- Is there no evidence of a human exposure, such as a glove?
- Is the film properly processed (if applicable)?
- Have artifacts been kept to a minimum to prevent interference with the image?

If the answer is no to any of these questions, consider:

- Is the image diagnostic?
- Does the image need to be repeated?

> ✎ **TECHNICIAN NOTES** Your image must have the correct exposure, include the entire anatomy, have no rotation, and be displayed correctly.

> ✷ **KEY POINTS**
>
> 1. Describe the radiographic projection from where the beam first enters and then where it exits the area of interest.
> 2. Label the side that the animal is lying on for lateral radiographic images.
> 3. The terms *dorsopalmar (DPa)/palmarodorsal (PaD)* is used for pectoral limbs to designate the area distal to and including the carpus. For pelvic limbs, dorsoplantar (DPl)/plantarodorsal (PlD) is used to designate the area distal to and including the tarsus. Craniocaudal (CrCd)/caudocranial (CdCr) is used for areas proximal to the carpus and tarsus.
> 4. The area of interest should be closest to the image receptor.
> 5. Keep human safety in mind at all times, utilizing the three important safety principles of time, distance, and shielding.
> 6. Minimize retakes by preparing and planning carefully.
> 7. Use non-manual and chemical restraint if possible.
> 8. Be creative and know proper positioning techniques to effectively use positioning aids and non-manual restraint.
> 9. Utilize slow and deliberate movements in a dimly lit room to keep a patient calm.
> 10. Place the markers laterally for DP, CrCd, or CdCr views and cranially for lateral views of limbs.
> 11. Position a VD/DV image/radiograph on the monitor/viewer so that you are "shaking its paw" and looking at the ventral aspect. For a lateral view, the animal's head will be to your left.

REVIEW QUESTIONS

1. A cat is lying on its abdomen with its limbs extended. The view of the tarsus in this position would be called:
   a. Palmarodorsal (PaD)
   b. Plantarodorsal (PlD)
   c. Craniocaudal (CrCd)
   d. Caudocranial (CdCr)

2. Sandbags are considered:
   a. Radiolucent and can be in the field of view
   b. Radiolucent and should not be in the field of view
   c. Radiopaque and can be in the field of view
   d. Radiopaque and should not be in the field of view

3. It is important to collimate the beam as much as possible so that there is less:
   a. Contrast and density on the image
   b. Secondary exposure to the patient and restrainer
   c. Chance of magnification or distortion
   d. Likelihood that the patient will move

4. An image of the radius/ulna of a Dachshund has been collimated to include the humerus and metacarpus. This is:
   a. Correct, as the joints above and below the area of interest have been included
   b. Incorrect, as not enough of the limb has been included
   c. Incorrect, as it should be collimated to include from the elbow to the carpus
   d. Incorrect, as only the radius and ulna should be included

5. The lateral and DV feline skull will be imaged on one film. You should:
   a. Have the nose in each view pointing in the same direction
   b. Do so when utilizing a grid
   c. Use a lead sheet to cover the side being radiographed
   d. Place the marker at the caudal aspect of the skull in each case

6. You are radiographing a right craniocaudal humerus of a Standard Poodle. The "R" marker is best placed:
   a. Under the humerus
   b. At the toes on the right side
   c. Along the medial side of the humerus
   d. Along the lateral side of the humerus

7. You can be farther from the beam during exposure if you:
   a. Wear appropriate apparel and hold your patient
   b. Use the shortest exposure time possible
   c. Utilize positioning aids whenever possible
   d. Measure at the thickest part

8. You are to radiograph the full abdomen of a sedated Doberman. The thickest part measures 20 cm. You are best to image the:
   a. Cranial aspect and then remeasure and radiograph the caudal aspect
   b. Full abdomen on one large image receptor using the cranial measurement
   c. Average of both the cranial and caudal measurements of the abdomen
   d. Thickest part only and not include the caudal abdomen

9. When placing an image of a DP extremity on the illuminator for the veterinarian to read, you should position it so that the digits are pointing:
   a. Upward
   b. Downward
   c. To the left
   d. To the right

10. The veterinarian required a follow-up radiograph of the abdomen of a patient. The technique chart was correctly followed, but your image was darker than the one taken by your colleague a month ago. This could be because:
    a. Your patient has gained weight
    b. You measured at the thickest part while the patient was on the table
    c. You collimated more than your colleague did
    d. You measured while the patient was standing

11. The veterinarian requests a right lateral of the thorax of a Pomeranian. The patient will be:
    a. Lying on its right side
    b. Lying on its left side
    c. Standing so that its right side is against the plate
    d. Positioned so that the beam enters from the right side

12. The collimation for this Pomeranian patient in Question 11 will extend to the:
    a. Thorax and abdomen, because both will fit on the image
    b. Heart and lungs, as this is the area that the veterinarian is interested in
    c. Third rib cranially and the 12th rib caudally, as this is the area of interest
    d. Diaphragm and shoulder joint, as the full thorax should be included

13. You are to radiograph a lateral abdomen of a well-behaved Golden Retriever. To keep your patient in position so you can move away from the beam, you should place:
    a. Sandbags over the chest and abdomen
    b. Sandbags over the head/neck, pelvis, and limbs
    c. Foam pads over the head/neck, pelvis, and limbs
    d. A scruffer over the neck region behind the ears

14. A dorsoproximal 60-degree lateral-palmarodistomedial oblique (DPr60°L-PaDiMO) of an equine right carpus means that the beam is entering the right limb at 60 degrees from the:
    a. Front and lateral side of the limb
    b. Front and medial side of the limb
    c. Back and lateral side of the limb
    d. Back and medial side of the limb

15. The (DPr60°L-PaDiMO) of an equine right carpus in Question 14 means that the image receptor is against the:
    a. Dorsal and medial side of the limb
    b. Dorsal and lateral side of the limb
    c. Palmar and medial side of the limb
    d. Palmar and lateral side of the limb

Chapter Review Question answers are located in the Instructor Resources on Evolve and can be provided to students at the discretion of the instructor.

Bibliography

Aspinall V, Cappello M. *Introduction to Veterinary Anatomy.* London: Butterman-Heineman; 2009.

Colville T, Bassert J. *Clinical Anatomy and Physiology for Veterinary Technicians.* 3rd ed. St. Louis: Elsevier; 2016.

Dyce KM, Sack WO, Wensing CJG. *Textbook of Veterinary Anatomy.* 5th ed. St. Louis: Saunders; 2018.

Evans H, de Launta A. *Guide to the Dissection of the Dog.* 8th ed. St. Louis: Saunders; 2017.

Fauber TL. *Radiographic Imaging and Exposure.* St. Louis: Elsevier; 2017.

Han C, Hurd C. *Practical Diagnostic Imaging for the Veterinary Technician.* 3rd ed. St. Louis: Mosby; 2005.

Jenner A. Non-manual radiography: radiation and patient safety. *RVT Journal, Ontario Association of Veterinary Technicians.* 2016;39(2).

Romich J. *An Illustrated Guide to Veterinary Medical Terminology.* 4th ed. Stamford, CT: Cengage Learning; 2015.

Sirois M. *Principles and Practice of Veterinary Technology.* 4th ed. St. Louis: Elsevier; 2017.

Smallwood JE, Shively MJ, Rendano VT, Habel RE. A standardized nomenclature for radiographic projections used in veterinary medicine. *Vet Radiol.* 1985;26:2-9.

Thrall DE. *Textbook of Veterinary Diagnostic Radiology.* 7th ed. St. Louis: Elsevier; 2017.

Tighe M, Brown M. *Mosby's Comprehensive Review for Veterinary Technicians.* 5th ed. St. Louis: Mosby; 2019.

CHAPTER **16**
Small Animal Abdomen

Marg Brown, RVT, BEd Ad Ed

Never regard study as a duty but as an enviable opportunity to learn to know the liberating influence of beauty in the realm of the spirit for your own personal joy and to the profit of the community to which your later works belong.
— Albert Einstein, German-born theoretical physicist, 1879–1955

OUTLINE

LEARNING OBJECTIVES

When you have finished this chapter, you will be able to:

1. Properly and safely position a dog or cat for the common abdominal views, with an emphasis on non-manual restraint.
2. Correctly measure and center the patient to include the peripheral borders.
3. Keep the abdomen parallel to the image receptor and perpendicular to the central ray.

4. Be familiar with alternative positions for abdominal radiography as required.
5. Identify normal radiographic abdominal anatomy and variations in different positions.

KEY TERMS

Key terms are defined in the Glossary on the Evolve website.

Brachycephalic
Cachexic
Chondrodystrophic
Coxofemoral joint

Decubitus
Field of view (FOV)
Focal radiograph
Horizontal beam

Intervertebral foramina
Positioning terminology
Sagittal
Spinous process

Transverse process
Vertebral bodies
Xiphoid

TECHNICAL NOTE: To preserve space, the images presented in this chapter do not show collimation. For safety, always collimate so that the beam is limited to within the image receptor edges. In film radiography, you should see a clear border of collimation (frame) on every radiograph. In some jurisdictions, evidence of collimation is required by law. In digital imaging the algorithm depends on proper collimation.

Positioning for the abdomen is relatively straightforward, but image visualization can be difficult due to the similarity in densities of multiple organs. The subtle differences in tissue densities of the abdomen offer significantly less natural contrast than in the thorax. Visualization of contrast depends on the gas and ingesta within the gastrointestinal (GI) tract and the fat in the peritoneal and retroperitoneal areas. Contrast media are often required to visualize differences.

Radiographic Concerns

- In film-screen radiography, use low kilovoltage (kV) and high milliampere-seconds (mAs) to differentiate the various shades of gray between organs and structures. Because of the minimal difference in opacity between abdominal fat and soft tissues in the abdominal parenchyma, a short scale of contrast with more blacks and whites and fewer grays is more diagnostic.
  - Use the highest mA and lowest kV that will produce the highest-quality film. Higher mA means shorter exposure with less chance of motion artifacts.
- The "enhanced contrast resolution of digital imaging" makes digital exposure factors less critical, but a technique chart needs to be adhered to.[1]
- Deep-chested dogs exhibit a marked difference in density between the cranial and caudal halves of the abdomen, which is especially evident in the ventrodorsal (VD) view. Use a 14- × 17-inch (35.5 × 43 cm) image receptor for large dogs. A very large dog will likely require two radiographs measured at the cranial and caudal abdomen, respectively. If there is only a minimal difference in anatomical thickness, a compromise can be made. The thickest area is generally the liver. If interested in another area, measure and center on that location.
- Using the same technique with digital radiography may be possible for the entire abdomen of such dogs.
- Take advantage of the anode heel effect (the thickest part toward the cathode) in deep-chested dogs to help reduce density differences, especially in the VD or dorsoventral (DV) views.
- A grid should be used if the measurement exceeds 10 cm to prevent scatter that causes fogging, which further decreases the contrast in film radiography.
- In digital radiography, many companies do not supply a grid. Proper collimation is essential.

Other Concerns

- The two positions commonly viewed are the right and/or left lateral and ventrodorsal (Box 16.1). The right lateral (RL) is the most common, but consistency is important so that abnormalities can quickly be visualized. Contrast studies and other situations may also require a left lateral. Utilizing both laterals takes advantage of bowel gas

| BOX 16.1 | Protocol for Abdominal Radiography |

Routine Views
- Right or left lateral
- Ventrodorsal

Ancillary Views
- Dorsoventral
- Lateral decubitus
- Modified lateral/lateral oblique

redistribution that provides inherent contrast medium and valuable additional information that can assist diagnosis. If duodenal gas as a contrast medium is desired, first place the patient in left lateral recumbency for the radiographic series as the incidence of duodenal gas will be greater.[1] See Table 16.1 for further differences between left and right lateral, as well as between VD and DV.

- In a right lateral view, the patient is lying on its right side. Technically, the correct terminology is *left-right lateral (Le-RtL)*, if one considers the "point of entrance of the beam to point of exit"; however, this term is not generally used in small animals.
- It is important to expose the image at the end of expiration, when a brief pause often occurs before inspiration. During expiration, there is a maximum amount of space for the abdominal contents as the lungs contract and the diaphragm relaxes cranially.
- Routine abdominal studies generally do not require fasting or an enema. Chapter 23 outlines preparation for contrast studies or specific concerns.
- Non-manual restraint should be utilized whenever possible to minimize radiation exposure to personnel. Use of a sedative or tranquilizer may be needed. Non-manual restraint is illustrated in the following positions.
- Try to give the patient the illusion that it is being held by appropriate use of sandbags, tape, behavioral strategies, and other methods. For further suggestions, please see Chapter 15.

> **TECHNICIAN NOTES** Measure the animal in the position in which it is to be imaged to calculate the settings from the technique chart.

> **TECHNICIAN NOTES** Before positioning the patient: turn on the machine, set the main voltage calibration if required, have proper source image distance, measure the abdomen in the correct position, and set the exposures. Have the image receptors ready. Positioning devices should be close at hand.
> Lastly, position your patient. To minimize scattered radiation, remove any objects or distractions not utilized.
> The patient should have no artifacts in the area of interest and should be chemically restrained if possible.

Routine Positions

Lateral—Routine

Positioning

Place in: Lateral recumbency.

Head: Keep in a natural position.

Place a sandbag over the neck appropriately, being careful not to restrict breathing.

Forelimbs: Pull cranially, tying limbs with Velcro straps secured to the table. Alternatively, a sandbag can be used to restrain the limbs.

Hindlimbs: Pull together slightly caudally to prevent superimposition of the femoral muscles over the abdomen.

Tie limbs with Velcro straps secured to the table.

Alternatively, use a sandbag to restrain the limbs.

Place a foam pad of suitable thickness between the femurs to help eliminate rotation of the caudal abdomen and pelvis.

Sternum: Elevate with wedged sponges so the sternum is at the same plane as the thoracic vertebrae. See Figs. 16.1, 16.2, and 16.3.

Comments and Tips

- Place any ID or markers at the cranial ventral aspect of the abdomen.
- Ensure that the sternum and spine are on the same plane and are parallel to the image receptor; the central ray is perpendicular to the tabletop.
- The cranial border for routine abdominal views can also be determined by palpating the xiphoid process of the sternum. Place the cranial portion of the collimator light two finger widths cranial to the xiphoid process.
- The horizontal line of the collimator light should bisect the abdominal cavity into equal dorsal and ventral portions.
- Minimize skin folds to prevent overshadowing folds of tissue.
- If the hindlimbs are kept more 90 degrees to the spine, organ crowding in the caudoventral abdomen is reduced.[1]
- Focal radiographs or compression radiographs are produced by using gentle pressure with a compression paddle such as a wooden spoon or plastic paddle. This may effectively isolate organs such as the kidneys or move an obscured organ to improve the visualization of a suspected pathology in a VD position.[1] This decreased thickness also means less scatter with a lower kVp and thus more contrast. Measure the reduced thickness to obtain the proper settings.
- A right lateral offers better longitudinal separation of the kidneys,[1] less duodenal gas, and a more consistently identifiable spleen. Left lateral is preferable in vomiting patients, as the fluid will be in the fundus and gas rises to better define the pyloric antrum. This contrast between the gas and the structure may potentially highlight a foreign body that may not be as obvious on the right lateral. A left lateral view may also be required in contrast studies after the administration of contrast media.

FIG. 16.1 A, Proper positioning for the lateral abdomen view of a canine with the use of sandbags. Velcro straps can also be used. **B,** Feline positioning for lateral abdomen. (Image courtesy and permission of Julia Bitan, RVT, http://handsfreexrays.com, Toronto, ON.)

Example

MEASURE: Caudal aspect of 13th rib at the thickest area (unless interested in a specific region).

CENTRAL RAY:

Canine: Over caudal aspect of 13th rib at level of L2 to L3.

Feline: Two to three finger widths caudal to 13th rib.

BORDERS:

Cranially: About 1 inch cranial to the xiphoid of the sternum to include the full diaphragm and heart apex.

Caudally: To the greater trochanter to include the coxofemoral joints.

Include the entire abdomen.

> ✎ **TECHNICIAN NOTES** Remember to go through your mental checklist before pushing the exposure button (see Chapter 15). Always be conscious of radiation safety.

Continued

Lateral—Routine—cont'd

> **TECHNICIAN NOTES**   Expose immediately at the end phase of expiration so the diaphragm is positioned cranially and the abdominal contents are not compressed. To get maximum expiration:
> - For a panting patient: cup or blow on the nose to momentarily stop breathing, being careful as this may trigger some animals to bite.
> - Apply light pressure on the abdomen to facilitate expiration.
>
> Breathe with the patient for a few breaths. If a two-step rotor is available, breathe with the patient, depress the exposure switch (initial button of the two-step process) at inspiration if possible. The moment breathing is paused, make the exposure.

> **TECHNICIAN NOTES**   To determine whether an anatomically normal patient is properly positioned[1–3]:
> ### Lateral View
> - Rib heads are superimposed.
> - Intervertebral foramina are the same size.
> - Transverse processes are superimposed at the origin from the vertebral bodies, appearing as Nike swooshes.[4]
> - Coxofemoral joints and wings of the ilia are superimposed.
>
> ### Ventrodorsal View
> - Relevant spinous processes are aligned in the center of the vertebral bodies appearing tear-dropped in shape.
> - Rib and abdominal symmetry.
> - Wings of the ilium are symmetrical.
> - Obturator foramina are symmetrical.

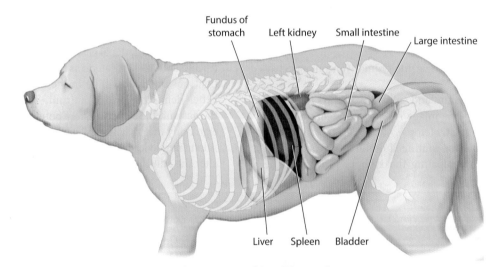

FIG. 16.2 Right Lateral (Le-RtL) View of the Abdomen Showing Major Organs.

FIG. 16.3 **A,** Right lateral radiograph of the abdomen of a dog. **B,** Right lateral radiograph of the abdomen of a 17-year-old domestic shorthair. (**A** Courtesy Vetel Diagnostics, San Luis Obispo, California, and Seth Wallack, DVM, DACVR, AAVR, director and CEO of Veterinary Imaging Center of San Diego; **B** Courtesy Rosedale Animal Hospital.)

Ventrodorsal—Routine

Positioning

Place in: Dorsal recumbency in a foam V-trough.

Head: Keep the muzzle straight, forward, and parallel to the table.

Carefully position a sandbag over the head and neck, taking care not to restrict breathing.

Forelimbs: Pull cranially to the comfort of the patient, individually tying limbs with Velcro straps secured to the table.

Alternatively, place a sandbag, just proximal to the elbows or at the carpus.

Hindlimbs: Keep in a natural frog-leg position, individually tying limbs with Velcro straps secured to the table.

Alternatively, place a sandbag over each limb. (See Figs. 16.4 and 16.5)

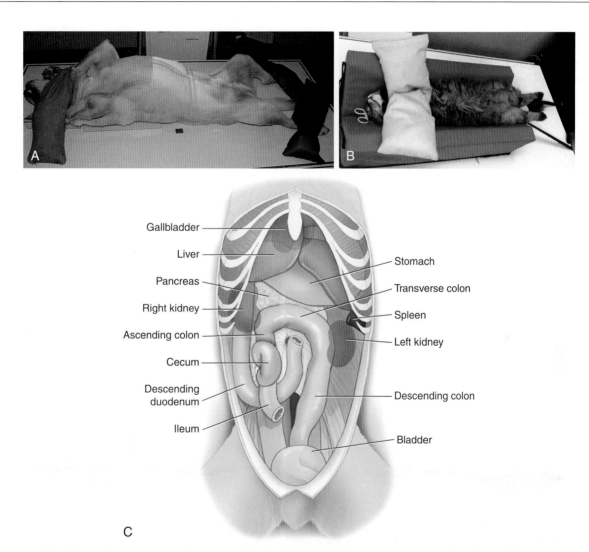

C

FIG. 16.4 **A,** Proper positioning for the ventrodorsal abdomen view of a canine with the use of sandbags. **B,** Positioning of a feline in VD position with the use of trough and Velcro straps. **C,** Ventral anatomy of the canine abdomen. (Image courtesy and permission of Ashley Jenner, RVT, and Julia Bitan, RVT, http://handsfreexrays.com, Toronto, ON.)

Continued

Ventrodorsal—Routine—cont'd

Comments and Tips

- Place any ID or markers adjacent to the corresponding side of the abdomen.
- The body should be evenly positioned so that the two sides of the rib cage appear equidistant; the sternum and spine are superimposed. The foam V-trough may be better placed under the thorax to minimize distortion and artifacts.
- Imagine a straight line connecting the point of the nose with the caudal midline. It may be difficult in brachycephalic or chondrodystrophic breeds to position the muzzle almost parallel with the table. Keep the head and neck of these breeds straight in front of the body with no rotation.
- If the pelvic limbs are pulled too caudally, crowding will be increased and skin folds noticed in the lateral thigh and/or caudal abdomen region. These may interfere with assessment of the caudal aspect of the abdomen.[1]

MEASURE: Caudal aspect of the 13th rib at level of umbilicus (about L2–L3).

CENTRAL RAY:

Canine: Center on midline over caudal aspect of 13th rib at level of umbilicus (L3).

Feline: Two to three finger widths caudal to 13th rib.

BORDERS: *Cranially*: T9 vertebrae (about 1 inch cranial to the xiphoid of the sternum—full diaphragm).

Caudally: Greater trochanter to include the coxofemoral joints (pubic symphysis).

Include the full abdomen.

> **✎ TECHNICIAN NOTES**   The positioning is the same for the lateral views of the thorax and abdomen; only the central ray and borders change. Thus, if both lateral abdomen and thorax are required, separately image both lateral views prior to the VD views.

FIG. 16.5 A, Ventrodorsal radiograph of the abdomen of a canine. B, Ventrodorsal radiograph of the abdomen of a 17-year-old feline.

Ancillary Positions

Other views can be added for injury, gastric contrast studies, or to assess fluid or free air.

Dorsoventral—Ancillary

Though DV views are rarely made, they can be used if the animal is compromised in the VD position or if an additional view is required for regular studies due to gravitational dependence of gas or when required in contrast studies (Fig. 16.6).

Positioning

Place in: Ventral recumbency.

Head: Keep straight and forward, carefully placing a sandbag over the neck and head, taking care not to restrict breathing.

Forelimbs: Extend slightly forward in a natural position.
Individually tie limbs with Velcro straps secured to the table or place sandbags over each elbow.

Hindlimbs: Keep in a natural position.
Place a sandbag over each limb near the stifle or tie with Velcro straps secured to the table.

Comments and Tips

- Place any identification or markers adjacent to the correct side of the abdomen.
- Evenly position the body so the two sides of the rib cage appear equidistant.
- Ideally, a straight line should be imagined connecting the point of the nose with the caudal midline.
- Superimpose the sternum and spine. The image receptor and central ray are perpendicular to both.

MEASURE, CENTRAL RAY, BORDERS: Same as for the VD view.

> ✎ **TECHNICIAN NOTES** Collimate; include labels/markers and have a clear frame in every film image.

FIG. 16.6 A, Dorsoventral positioning. **B,** Dorsoventral radiograph of the abdomen of a canine. (**A** Courtesy Seneca College, Toronto, ON; **B** Courtesy Joshua Schlote, BS, LVT, Northeast Community College, Norfolk, NE.)

Lateral Decubitus (Ventrodorsal View with Horizontal Beam)—Ancillary

The lateral decubitus should be considered if fluid or free gas, gas-capped fluid levels in an abscess or in a bowel loop, is suspected, or if the animal will be harmed when placed in a VD or DV position. Small amounts of fluid may not be identified radiographically (Fig. 16.7).

Place in: Right lateral recumbency on a thick foam pad or equivalent (to allow the dependent portion of the abdomen to be in the field of view).
- The position is described according to the side on which the patient is lying (i.e., right decubitus if the patient is in right lateral recumbency).

Head, Forelimbs, Hindlimbs: Positioned as described for a lateral.
- Ensure that the sternum and spine are on the same plane and parallel to the image receptor; the central ray is perpendicular.

Image receptor: Placed vertically behind the patient.

Horizontal beam: Directed ventrodorsally, entering the sternum and exiting the vertebrae.
- If free gas is suspected, wait at least 5 minutes once the patient is in position before imaging to allow dorsal collection of the gas.[5]

MEASURE, CENTRAL RAY, BORDERS: As for the ventrodorsal view.

TECHNICIAN NOTES   Collimate only to the required borders for safety and to minimize scatter.

FIG. 16.7 Positioning of a Dog for Lateral Decubitus—Ventrodorsal View with a Horizontal Beam. (Courtesy Seneca College, Toronto, ON.)

Modified Lateral—Ancillary

This position is used in male dogs to provide an unobstructed view of urethral calculi in the ischial arch and os penis without superimposition of the pelvic limbs (Fig. 16.8).[1,3,5]

Positioning

Place in: Right lateral recumbency.

Head: Keep in a natural position and restrain appropriately with a sandbag over the neck.
Be careful not to restrict breathing.

Forelimbs: Extend cranially, tying limbs with Velcro straps secured to the table. Alternatively, a sandbag can be used to restrain the limbs.

FIG. 16.8 Positioning for a Modified Lateral View of a Male Dog for Contrast Studies. The hindlimbs are pulled cranially as far as possible for evaluation of the membranous and penile urethra.

Modified Lateral—Ancillary—cont'd

Hindlimbs: Extend both limbs as cranially as possible to the comfort of the patient without causing rotation of the body off the table.

Tie limbs with Velcro straps secured to the table.

Alternatively, use a sandbag to restrain the limbs.

An appropriately sized foam pad placed between the femurs may help eliminate rotation of the pelvis.

Sternum: Elevate the ventral abdomen with wedged sponges so the sternum is at the same plane as the vertebrae.

Comments and Tips

- The pelvic limbs should not be superimposed over the caudal aspect of the os penis or the urethra.
- Decrease radiographic technique for soft tissue. Low kVp will create high-contrast radiographic film.

Lateral Oblique—Ancillary

This view may be needed for specialized studies in male dogs to prevent superimposition of the os penis over the bladder in the VD view (Fig. 16.9).

Positioning

Place in: Right lateral recumbency.

Head: Keep in a natural position and support appropriately with a sandbag over the neck.

Forelimbs: Extend cranially and secure.

Hindlimbs: Pull the dependent limb caudally.

Tie limbs with Velcro straps secured to the table.

Alternatively, use a sandbag to restrain the limb.

Raise the contralateral limb and secure dorsally out of the field of view by placing Velcro straps or a bungee cord around the tarsus/metatarsus and securing to the table or tube stand.

Comments and Tips

- Do not superimpose pelvic limbs over the os penis.
- For male dogs, this view may be needed for specialized studies to prevent the penis from being superimposed over the bladder in the VD view.
- Oblique view positioning can also be achieved by placing the patient in the VD or DV positions and rotating the body 15 to 30 degrees. This moves the esophagus, stomach, colon, and urinary bladder away from the vertebrae to allow better visualization of these organs.
- The criteria for proper symmetry will not apply to the oblique views.

FIG. 16.9 A, Positioning for lateral oblique view of the canine abdomen. The pelvic limbs should not be superimposed over the caudal aspect of the os penis. **B,** Lateral oblique radiograph of the abdomen of a feline patient during an excretory urography using iodine.

Modified Lateral and Lateral Oblique Positions

MEASURE: Over the acetabulum/ischium.

CENTRAL RAY: Over the cranial wing of the ilium unless the rectum is of interest; in that case, have the central beam over the pelvis.

BORDERS: For a caudal contrast study:

Cranial: L4

Caudal: Caudal aspect of the rectum to image a bladder or prostate.

Anatomical Abdominal Radiographic Concerns

Figs. 16.10 to 16.12 and Table 16.1 demonstrate that radiographic anatomy changes as the patient's position changes. Figs. 16.2, 16.4C, 16.13, and 16.14 show further anatomical features of the abdomen.

✎ **TECHNICIAN NOTES**   Strategically used positioning aids give the patient the illusion it is being held. A sandbag over the neck and limbs and/or the use of Velcro straps or alternatives is essential if the patient is not appropriately sedated. Avoid holding the patient and step away from the primary beam. Reducing your x-ray exposure depends on your diligence.

FIG. 16.10 Normal Canine and Feline Stomach Variations Due to Position Changes. The major areas of the stomach are *F*, fundus; *B*, body; *A*, pyloric antrum; *P*, pyloric canal; *C*, cardia. **A**, Canine stomach in lateral recumbency. **B**, Feline stomach in lateral recumbency. The gastric axis is parallel with the ribs. **C**, Canine stomach in dorsal or ventral recumbency. The gastric axis is perpendicular to the spine, and the stomach is slightly U-shaped. **D**, Feline stomach in dorsal or ventral recumbency. The pylorus is located at the midline, and the stomach has more of an acute angle, appearing J-shaped.

FIG. 16.11 Effects of Positional Changes as Shown in the Canine Stomach. Remember air rises. **A**, Right lateral (RtL); gas is in the fundus (F) and dorsal body of the stomach (B). **B**, Left lateral (LeL); gas is in the main to distal body, pyloric antrum (A) and canal (P), and duodenum. **C**, Ventrodorsal (VD); gas is in the pyloric antrum, body near the midline, and descending duodenum. **D**, Dorsoventral (DV); gas is in the fundus and cardia (C).

- A brief overview of normal radiographic anatomy is presented in Appendix A on the Evolve website in order for the imager to understand the implications of failure to properly position the patient.
  - Radiographic changes may be seen that are not attributable to disease processes or other findings.
  - The term *"normal"* may not be straightforward because every organ or structure has particular normal findings based on the shape, size, location, position, margins, number, and opacity, as well as being affected by superimposition of other tissues. Factors such as age and body condition also affect the interpretation of the peritoneum and retroperitoneal space.
- Fat in the abdomen serves as a contrasting translucency to help identify the structures. Thus, you see various body images much better in a fat cat than in an emaciated one because of the various types of fat present.
  - Fat types include subcutaneous fat, retroperitoneal fat, and fat within the falciform ligament ventral to the liver. If there is no body fat, such as in immature or cachexic patients, it will be hard to distinguish the peritoneal or retroperitoneal organs.

FIG 16.12 Normal Variations in Fluid (Barium) and Gas Distribution in the Stomach with Different Patient Positions. **A,** Dorsoventral view, in ventral recumbency. Gas rises to the fundus and fluid settles dependently to fill pyloric portions and part of the body. The diaphragm has a slightly "bumpier" appearance than in the ventrodorsal view because the trilobed crura are lateral to the central cupula. **B,** Ventrodorsal view, in dorsal recumbency. Gas is located in the body and pyloric antrum. Fluid settles dependently to fill the fundus and body. In this dog, there is a small amount of barium trapped in the pyloric antrum. **C,** Left lateral view. Gas rises to the pyloric portion, and fluid settles dependently to fill the fundus and body. **D,** Right lateral view. Gas rises to the fundus and body, when there is some barium adherent to the mucosa. Fluid settles dependently to fill the pyloric portion. (From Thrall DE. *Textbook of Veterinary Diagnostic Radiology.* 7th ed. St Louis: Elsevier; 2017.)

- Retroperitoneal and peritoneal fluid and gas also change the extent to which kidneys and other organs are obscured. Keep in mind that not all normal structures present anatomically are visible radiographically. However, abnormalities such as enlargements and increased opacities may cause these organs to become visible and may cause variations in positions of other organs.

See Appendix A on the Evolve website for specific organ overview (see also Figs. 16.13 and 16.14).

Fig. 16.15 is a mystery radiograph. Review it and answer the question presented with it.

Note

See Chapter 23 for further contrast studies and Chapters 10 to 14 for alternative modes of imaging.

TABLE 16.1	Radiographic Anatomy with Position Changes Using a Vertical Beam*
RADIOGRAPHIC ANATOMY	**POSITIONAL CHANGE(S)[1-5]**

Right Lateral View (See Figs. 16.2, 16.3, 16.11A, 16.12D, 16.15)

Fundus and body of the stomach	Fundus caudal to the left crus of the diaphragm Gas filled and in the dorsal and cranial aspects of the abdomen
Pyloric antrum	Just caudal to the liver—soft tissue opacity ventrally Contains fluid and ingesta
Axis of stomach	Appears vertical
Liver	Appears larger than in left lateral; appears smaller in expiration
Spleen	Distal extremity more noticeable in dogs (caudal and slightly ventral to pylorus or liver) but may not be seen as separate structure due to overlap of the liver
Left kidney (upper)	Caudal to right kidney Appears more bean shaped, is slightly magnified
Crura of diaphragm	Appear parallel

Left Lateral View (See Figs. 16.11B, 16.12C)

Fundus	Fluid filled and difficult to identify unless filled with contrast medium
Duodenum, pyloric antrum, and canal (± body)	Gas filled
Axis of stomach	Appears vertical
Liver	Appears smaller than in right lateral
Entire shadow of spleen	May be hidden under small intestines
Right kidney (upper)	Cranial to left kidney Appears larger, is more bean-shaped
Crura of diaphragm	Sometimes appear to cross

Ventrodorsal View (See Figs. 16.4B, 16.5, 16.11C, 16.12B, 16.14)

Body near midline, pyloric antrum/descending duodenum (±)	Gas filled
Cardia, fundus	Partially fluid filled and may be difficult to see
Axis of stomach	Appears horizontal
Ascending colon and cecum	On patient's right
Descending colon	On patient's left
Colon	Question mark shape
Spleen	Left craniodorsal abdomen, under liver The proximal extremity appears as a small triangle caudolateral to fundus of stomach, medial to the body wall, and craniolateral to left kidney
Right kidney	Cranial to left kidney

Dorsoventral View (See Figs. 16.11D, 16.12A, 16.14)

Fundus and cardia	Gas filled and caudal to the left diaphragmatic crus
Ventral part of the body and the pyloric antrum	Difficult to see; filled with fluid
Axis of stomach	Appears horizontal
Ascending colon and cecum	On patient's right
Descending colon	On patient's left
Colon	Question mark shape
Spleen	On left, under liver; appears as small triangle caudal to fundus of stomach
Right kidney	Cranial to left kidney

*Due to a variety of other factors, the appearance may not always be as described in the table.

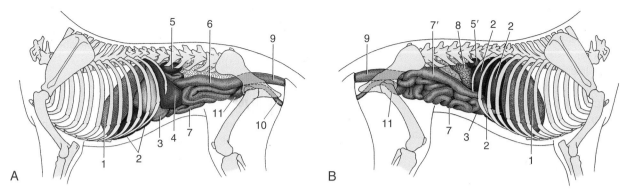

FIG. 16.13 Visceral projections on the left **(A)** and right **(B)** canine abdominal walls. *1*, Diaphragm; *2*, liver; *3*, stomach; *4*, spleen; *5* and *5'*, left and right kidneys, respectively; *6*, descending colon; *7*, small intestine; *7'*, descending duodenum; *8*, pancreas; *9*, rectum; *10*, female urogenital tract; *11*, bladder. (From Singh B. *Dyce, Sack and Wensing's Textbook of Veterinary Anatomy.* 5th ed. St Louis: Elsevier; 2018.)

FIG. 16.14 A, Transverse section of the patient abdomen at the level of the first lumbar vertebra to show location. **B,** Corresponding computerized tomography (CT) scan slightly more caudal than the section shown in A; the patient was lying on its back during the CT procedure. *1*, First lumbar vertebra; *2*, last rib; *3*, descending colon; *4*, transverse colon; *5*, lymph nodes and blood vessels in mesentery, with the jejunum ventral to them; *6*, caudal vena cava; *7*, aorta, between crura of diaphragm; *8*, right kidney; *8'*, cranial pole of left kidney; *9*, descending duodenum and pancreas; *10*, greater omentum; *11*, linea alba; *12*, liver; *13*, spleen. (From Singh B. *Dyce, Sack and Wensing's Textbook of Veterinary Anatomy.* 5th ed. St Louis: Elsevier; 2018.)

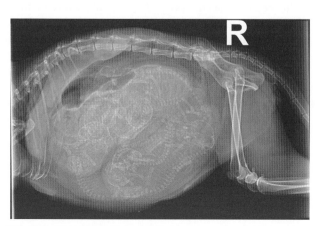

FIG. 16.15 Mystery Radiograph. How many fetuses do you see in this image of a pregnant cat?

> ✳ **KEY POINTS**
>
> 1. The lack of natural contrast inherent in the abdomen necessitates particular attention to appropriate exposure factors for proper diagnosis.
> 2. Routine positions for the abdomen are the right lateral (generally) and VD.
> 3. Correct positioning and technique are required for proper interpretation. This includes measuring and centering, inclusion, and proper symmetry.
> 4. Proper positioning is essential to minimize misdiagnosis. Knowledge of normal radiography assists in ensuring that perfect images are presented.
> 5. Not all abdominal organs are visible radiographically. Ultrasound, magnetic resonance imaging, and computerized tomography may be required for proper diagnosis.

REVIEW QUESTIONS

1. The normal radiographic views of the abdomen are generally the:
   a. Left lateral and ventrodorsal
   b. Left lateral and dorsoventral
   c. Right lateral and dorsoventral
   d. Right lateral and ventrodorsal

2. Normal preparation of routine abdominal radiographs generally include:
   a. Fasting but not an enema
   b. No fasting or an enema
   c. An enema but no fasting
   d. Use of contrast media

3. A VD abdomen radiograph is required for a Doberman pinscher. The head is best placed toward the:
   a. Cathode
   b. Anode

4. How should the hindlimbs be positioned for a regular right lateral abdomen view?
   a. The right limb should be slightly forward and the left limb as far back as possible.
   b. The left limb should be slightly forward and the right limb as far back as possible.
   c. Both limbs should be pulled cranially and superimposed.
   d. Both limbs should be pulled slightly caudally and superimposed.

5. To ensure symmetry in your final ventrodorsal radiograph of the abdomen:
   a. The rib heads, transverse processes, and coxofemoral joints should be superimposed
   b. The intervertebral foramina should be the same size
   c. The wings of the ilium are symmetrical
   d. The transverse processes are superimposed and appear as Nike swooshes

6. When measuring and centering for a ventrodorsal abdomen of a Cocker Spaniel, you should:
   a. Measure and center over the caudal aspect of the 13th rib
   b. Measure and center at the level of T13
   c. Measure at T13 but center over the caudal aspect of the 13th rib
   d. Center at T13 but measure over the caudal aspect of the 13th rib

7. You have collimated for this VD radiograph 1 inch cranial to the xiphoid of the sternum and have included the coxofemoral joints. This is:
   a. Correct because the VD should include these peripheral borders
   b. Incorrect because the cranial border does not need to include the diaphragm
   c. Incorrect because the image does not need to extend caudally to the hip joint
   d. Incorrect because the image only needs to be from the edge of the liver to the bladder

8. You are ready to take the image and are breathing with your patient so that you will properly depress the final exposure button during this VD canine abdomen at:
   a. Mid-expiration
   b. Peak inspiration
   c. The beginning of inspiration
   d. The end of expiration

9. The veterinarian had asked you to apply gentle pressure in this VD abdomen with a wooden paddle to isolate what she suspects might be a tumor. You do so and find the radiograph is darker with less contrast than your original one without any applied pressure. This is because you used:
   a. A grid for this image and not the first one
   b. Less kVp than your first image
   c. The same setting for both images
   d. A thicker measurement than the first image

10. The veterinarian asks you to image a beagle in which he suspects peritonitis. You do have an adjustable tube head unit. In order to properly evaluate whether there is fluid in the abdomen, you should place your patient in:
    a. VD position and utilize a vertical beam
    b. Dorsal recumbency and utilize a horizontal beam
    c. Ventral recumbency and utilize a horizontal beam
    d. Right lateral recumbency and utilize a horizontal beam

11. The veterinarian wants you to take a modified lateral of a male golden retriever. The hindlimbs should be:
    a. Pulled as cranially as possible to cause rotation of the body off the table
    b. Positioned perpendicular to the spine to prevent crowding in the caudoventral abdomen
    c. Pulled as cranially as possible without causing rotation of the body off the table
    d. Caudally with the upper limb raised and out of the field of view

12. The settings for your 12-cm abdomen of a bulldog that will not be sedated are 60 kV and 10 mAs. You are best to use:
    a. 400 mA and 1/40 of a second
    b. 300 mA and 1/30 of a second
    c. 200 mA and 1/20 of a second
    d. 100 mA and 1/10 of a second

13. In a right lateral view as opposed to a left lateral abdomen:
    a. There is greater longitudinal separation of the kidneys
    b. The fundus and body of the stomach are closer to the film
    c. The liver appears slightly smaller
    d. The axis of the stomach is more vertical

14. The veterinarian asks you to complete a ventrodorsal view with a horizontal beam. If the patient is lying on its right side, this view is properly termed:
    a. Right lateral
    b. Right decubitus
    c. Left decubitus
    d. Ventrodorsal

15. The veterinarian asks you to complete a series of abdominal radiographs. You inadvertently forgot the markers. The image in front of you shows the duodenum, pyloric antrum, and distal body of the stomach filled with gas and the axis of the stomach appearing vertical. This view is likely a:
    a. Ventrodorsal
    b. Left lateral
    c. Right lateral
    d. Dorsoventral

Chapter Review Question answers are located in the Instructor Resources on Evolve and can be provided to students at the discretion of the instructor.

References

1. Thrall DE. *Textbook of Veterinary Diagnostic Radiology.* 7th ed. St. Louis: Elsevier; 2017 [chapters 36-46].
2. Muhlbauer MC, Kneller SK. *Radiography of the Dog and Cat*: Guide to Making and Interpreting Radiographs. Oxford: Wiley-Blackwell; 2013 [chapter 6].
3. Holloway A. *BSAVA Manual of Canine and Feline Radiography and Radiology*: A Foundation Manual. Suffolk: BSAVA; 2013 [chapter 6].
4. Morgan JP, Doval J, Samii V. *Radiographic Techniques*: The Dog. Hannover: Schlutersche GmbH & Co.; 1998.
5. Owens JM, Biery DN. *Radiographic Interpretation for the Small Animal Clinician.* St. Louis: Ralston Purina; 1999.

Bibliography

Aspinall V, Cappello M. *Introduction to Veterinary Anatomy.* 3rd ed. London: Butterman-Heineman; 2015.

Ayers S. *Small Animal Radiographic Techniques and Positioning.* Oxford: Wiley-Blackwell; 2013.

Colville T, Bassert J. *Clinical Anatomy and Physiology for Veterinary Technicians.* 3rd ed. St. Louis: Mosby; 2016.

Done SH, Goody PC, Evans SA, Stickland NC. *Color Atlas of Veterinary Anatomy, the Dog and Cat.* London: Mosby; 2009.

Singh B. *Dyce, Sack and Wensing's Textbook of Veterinary Anatomy.* 5th ed. St. Louis: Elsevier; 2018.

Evans H, de Launta A. *Guide to the Dissection of the Dog.* 8th ed. St. Louis: Saunders; 2017.

Han C, Hurd C. *Practical Diagnostic Imaging for the Veterinary Technician.* 3rd ed. St. Louis: Mosby; 2005.

Owens JM, Biery DN. *Radiographic Interpretation for the Small Animal Clinician.* St. Louis: Ralston Purina; 1999.

Romich J. *An Illustrated Guide to Veterinary Medical Terminology.* 4th ed. Stamford, CT: Cengage Learning; 2015.

Sirois M. *Principles and Practice of Veterinary Technology.* 4th ed. St. Louis: Mosby; 2017.

Tighe M, Brown M. *Mosby's Comprehensive Review for Veterinary Technicians.* 5th ed. St. Louis: Mosby; 2019.

(Courtesy Jennifer White, Mississauga Oakville Veterinary Emergency and Specialty Hospital, ON)

CHAPTER 17
Small Animal Thorax

Marg Brown, RVT, BEd Ad Ed

A good head and a good heart are always a formidable combination.
— Nelson Mandela, South African antiapartheid activist and president, 1918–2013

OUTLINE

LEARNING OBJECTIVES

When you have finished this chapter, you will be able to:

1. Properly and safely position a dog or cat for the common thoracic views, with an emphasis on non-manual restraint.
2. Produce diagnostic images of the thorax using correct measurements, exposure, centering, borders, positioning, and symmetry.
3. Be familiar with alternative views and why they are required.
4. Identify normal thoracic radiographic anatomy.

KEY TERMS

Key terms are defined in the Glossary on the Evolve website.

Atelectasis
Dependent
Diaphragmatic crura
Heel effect

Hemithorax
Hilar region
Horizontal beam
Mediastinum

Object-film distance (OFD)
Opaque/radiopaque
Orthogonal

Parenchyma
Positional terminology

TECHNICAL NOTE: To preserve space, the images presented in this chapter do not show collimation. For safety, always collimate so that the beam is limited to within the image receptor edges. In film radiography, you should see a clear border of collimation (frame) on every radiograph. In some jurisdictions, evidence of collimation is the law. In digital imaging, the algorithm depends on proper collimation.

Thoracic radiography is a common diagnostic procedure in small-animal practice. Specific indications include suspicion of heart disease, pneumonia, neoplasia (primary or metastatic), treatment, or disease follow-up. Computed tomography (CT) or echocardiography may be needed for further diagnosis.

Radiographic and Positioning Concerns

- In film/screen systems, the thorax is best radiographed using a long contrast scale with many shades of gray. Obtain this with higher kilovoltage (kV) and lower milliampere-seconds (mAs). The large volume of air within the lung already creates an inherently high contrast.
  - Correct exposures are critical. Underexposure may lead to an incorrect diagnosis of interstitial opacification. Overexposure or images taken with oversaturated digital systems can hide subtle lung lesions or lead to a false diagnosis.
  - Exposures may need to be changed, such as with the presences of a mediastinal mass or pleural fluid. Increase the kVp exposure by 15% to 20% in these cases.
- Contrast and density in the digital system can be manipulated after the image is obtained, making exact digital exposures not as critical; however, the closer to the correct technique, the better the image. As with film radiography, it is essential to measure the patient in the position it is to be imaged.
- Once the mAs have been determined, use the highest mA and shortest time possible to minimize respiratory motion artifacts that can induce blurring.
- Consider grids in film radiography for measurements over 10 cm to minimize the scattered radiation on film that further decreases contrast.
- Exposure should be taken at peak inspiration. This increases aeration of the lung field, allowing maximum contrast between the gas-filled lungs and soft tissue pulmonary structures. At peak inspiration, there is greater separation of the cardiac silhouette and diaphragm, especially in the lateral views.
- Along with exposure factors and peak inspiration, high-quality thoracic images require emphasis on accurate positioning and centering. A symmetrical image is essential because any displacement of the x-ray beam or rotation of the patient will produce marked changes in the imaging of the thoracic anatomy, causing possible misdiagnosis.
- There should be a minimum of two orthogonal views: minimally, one lateral view and a ventrodorsal/dorsoventral (VD/DV) view. However, further views are often required for proper diagnosis. Diagnosis can be missed if enough views are not taken.
- Because of the increased opacity of the dependent lateral lung due to recumbency-associated atelectasis, the lateral view appears more opaque than the VD/DV views. If there is suspected lung disease noted on the laterals, orthogonal views are required to first rule out atelectasis.[1] Consider taking the DV/VD view first to minimize the

length of time that the patient has been lying in lateral recumbency.
- Both right and left laterals are recommended if pneumonia or metastasis is suspected.[1-3] In addition, image a VD view for pneumonia, DV for cardiac disease, and a VD or DV view for metastasis.
- On rare occasions, the DV/VD oblique view, made at 20 to 30 degrees from center, may be required. The area of interest is moved away from the spine or cardiac shadow, which may help identify rib lesions or pulmonary lesions in the hilar region. Decubital views may also be required as needed to rule out disease process.
- The protocol and patient preparation are the same for both dogs and cats. Make sure the patient has a clean, dry hair coat, and remove collars or leashes (Fig. 17.1). A thick hair coat, such as the matted hair of cats, can cause prominent artifacts.
  - Sedation may assist in avoiding manual restraint and obtaining more diagnostic images.
- Patients in respiratory distress or geriatric patients may require more sternal time, flow-by oxygen, and breaks. Critically ill patients can decompensate at any time, so it is essential to have any supplies and emergency drugs specific to their needs easily accessible. Vigilant assessment and monitoring is critical for these patients.
- Sedated and overweight animals often do not ventilate as fully as nonsedated animals, leading to possible misinterpretation of alveolar or interstitial patterns. If the patient is connected to the anesthetic machine, positive ventilation can be applied to synchronize inspiration with the exposure time to create more contrast in the lungs.
- The full lung field needs to be included, from the cranial thoracic inlet to the most caudodorsal lung field. Keep in

FIG. 17.1 Make sure the patient has a clean, dry hair coat, and remove collars or leashes. Artifacts on this radiograph include incorrect marker placement, sandbags, and leash clip.

mind that the thorax is inside the rib cage so include the full rib cage. Generally, a 14- × 17-inch (35.5- × 43-cm) plate will accommodate most large dogs, but if a dog is too large to allow full inclusion of the lung field on one image, each view may have to be divided into cranial and caudal sections. If more than one plate is required, make sure that the full cardiac silhouette is included in at least one image.

- Because the massive shoulder muscles cause underexposure of the cranial thoracic vertebrae, use the anode heel effect to advantage by having the thickest part toward the cathode, especially in medium and larger dogs.
- Any image is only an instantaneous picture of the thorax in a particular point in time.

> ✎ **TECHNICIAN NOTES**   Always measure the patient in the position in which it is to be imaged to avoid incorrect settings.

> ✎ **TECHNICIAN NOTES**   Strategically used positioning aids give the patient the illusion that it is being held. A sandbag over the neck and limbs and/or the use of straps is essential if the patient is not properly sedated. Have the room darker; use slow, methodical movements, especially for cats; keep speaking in a low, calm voice; and take advantage of the behavioral characteristics of the patient.

TABLE 17.1	Protocol for Thoracic Radiography
VIEW	**PROTOCOL**
Routine	Right and/or left lateral Ventrodorsal (VD) (generally for lungs) Dorsoventral (DV) (generally for heart)

Ancillary	Lateral decubitus view
	Alternate lateral views with a horizontal beam:
	   DV or VD decubitus view
	   Standing lateral
	Dorsoventral or ventrodorsal 20–30 degrees
	   oblique
	Expiratory radiographic images

Table 17.1 lists the protocol for thoracic radiography.

> ✎ **TECHNICIAN NOTES**   The thorax is inside the rib cage, so include the full rib cage on each thoracic image.

> ✎ **TECHNICIAN NOTES**   Diagnostic-quality thoracic images are obtained by using short exposure times, obtaining peak inspiration, and using strict symmetry and positioning.

Routine Positions

Lateral Thorax—Routine

- Technically, the correct terminology for the right lateral is *left-right lateral* if one considers "point of entrance to point of exit"; however, this term is not generally used in small animals. Label the patient for the side it is lying on—it would be lying on its right side for a right lateral.
- If only one lateral is required, personal preference dictates the view. Most right-handed imagers prefer the patient lying on its right side, producing a right lateral view. However, it is highly recommended that both laterals be obtained due to atelectasis, especially if a lesion is small and not visible in the VD or DV view, such as commonly occurs with a lung nodule or small mass.[1]
- When a patient is in lateral recumbency, the dependent lung is more opaque and less inflated than the nondependent (upper) lung. This may obscure lesions in the dependent lung, due to atelectasis that occurs in any patient at any state of consciousness in lateral recumbency, and is related to the body mass of the patient.
- Atelectasis of the downward lung occurs in less than 5 minutes and is due to not only the effects of gravity,[3] but also to the heart compressing the lung, compression causing less movement of the dependent rib cage, and less cranial movement of the dependent portion of the diaphragm.[1] Thus, if a lesion is suspected in the right lung, image the left lateral. The aeration of the upper lobes also enhances contrast.
- In addition, the advantage of increased object-film distance (OFD) magnifies the lesion, which may further assist diagnosis.

- The right cranial lobe pulmonary artery and vein are commonly used to assess pulmonary circulation. The left lateral view better distinguishes these vessels, more accurately determining the relative vessel size[3] because there is no superimposition of other structures (see Table 17.2 for variations between right and left lateral).
- Images should be taken at maximum inspiration. If required, images taken during expiration may aid in detection of small amounts of pleural fluid, pneumothorax, or diagnosis of tracheal or bronchial collapse[1]

(Figs. 17.2 through 17.8).

Positioning

Place In: Right or left lateral recumbency.

Head: Keep in a natural position.
  Maintain appropriately with a sandbag over the neck so as not to restrict breathing.

Forelimbs: Pull as far cranially as possible without rotating the thorax, tying limbs with Velcro straps secured to the table. Alternatively, a sandbag can be used to restrain the limbs.

Hindlimbs: Pull together slightly caudally.
  Tie limbs with Velcro straps secured to the table or alternatively use a sandbag to restrain the limbs.
  Place a foam pad of suitable thickness between the femurs if needed to eliminate rotation.

Sternum: Elevate with wedged sponges so the sternum is at the same plane as the thoracic vertebrae to eliminate rotation.

MEASURE: Caudal border of the scapula over the thickest part of the thorax.

CENTRAL RAY: At the caudal border of the scapula, between the fifth and sixth ribs (where you feel the strongest heartbeat), approximately midway between the spine and sternum.

BORDERS: The thorax is inside the ribcage, so include the full ribcage.

CRANIAL: Palpate from the cranial point of the scapulohumeral articulation (include thoracic inlet).

Caudal: A few centimeters caudal to the last rib.

Dorsal: Include thoracic vertebrae.

Ventral: Include sternum.

Lateral Thorax—Routine—cont'd

FIG. 17.2 A, Positioning for the lateral thorax view. Place positioning devices appropriately to eliminate rotation of the thorax. The marker should be placed cranially and ventrally. It can be placed under the foam pad. **B,** Positioning for a feline lateral with non-manual restraint with the use of straps, sandbags, and towel. Collimation, centering, and borders are the same as for the canine. (**A,** Courtesy Seneca College of Applied Arts and Technology, King City, ON. **B,** Courtesy Ashley Jenner and Julia Bitan, http://handsfreexrays.com, Toronto, ON.)

🖉 **TECHNICIAN NOTES** Inspiration is required to inflate the lungs and provide better contrast between the soft tissues of the thorax and air in the lungs.

To obtain maximum inspiration from the patient:
- Breathe with the patient and depress the rotor of a two-step system at the point of either expiration or partial inspiration (depending on the patient's respiratory rate). Press the second stage at maximum inspiration.
- If the patient has an endotracheal tube (ET), squeeze the anesthetic bag or use an Ambu bag (bag valve mask).

Comments and Tips
- Place any identification (ID) or markers on the ventral aspect of the abdomen near the axilla.
- Ensure that the sternum is parallel to the table and at the same level as the vertebrae; the beam is perpendicular to both. Rotation of the sternum may separate the mainstream bronchi, mimicking left atrial enlargement or a heart mass.[3]
- Extend the forelimbs as much as the patient will comfortably allow to prevent any superimposition of the brachium muscles over the cranial lung field. Do not cause any rotation.
- Expose immediately at full inspiration.
- In addition to positioning devices, folds of skin, nipples, and fatty masses ventral to the sternum can cause artifacts (see Fig. 17.5).

🖉 **TECHNICIAN NOTES** Quickly go through your mental checklist before depressing the exposure button. The checklist includes, but is not limited to the following:
- Settings correct
- Image receptor/grid in position
- Proper location of markers and ID (if using at this stage)
- Correct body part and view
- Thickest part to the cathode
- Properly measured and centered (Fig. 17.8)
- Borders correct and collimated
- Patient properly prepared, positioned, and supported with the thorax perpendicular to the central ray and parallel to the image receptor
- Maximum inspiration

Lateral Thorax—Routine—cont'd

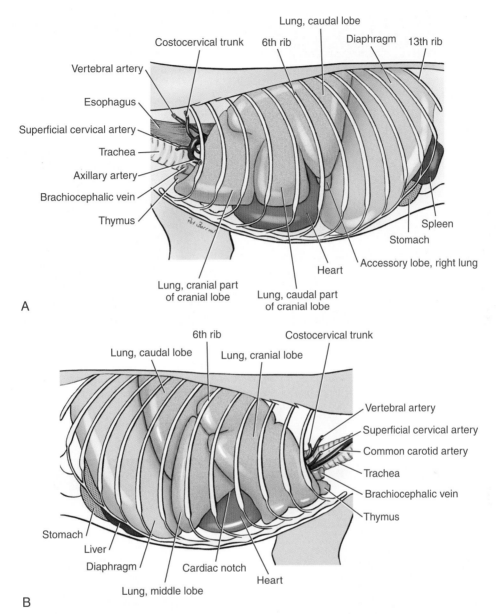

A, Diagram of the left thoracic viscera within the rib cage of this left-to-right lateral projection (RtL).

FIG. 17.3 A, Diagram of the left thoracic viscera within the rib cage of this left-to-right lateral projection (RtL). **B,** Diagram of the right thoracic viscera within the rib cage of this right-to-left lateral projection (LeL).

Lateral Thorax—Routine—cont'd

FIG. 17.4 A, Radiograph of the right lateral thorax in inspiration. The thorax is inside the rib cage. In a normal average dog, the heart measured at the base is about 2½ to 3½ times the width of an intercostal space, depending on the breed. In comparison with the left lateral view, the heart base appears more conical or oval on the right lateral view. **B,** Radiograph of the left lateral thorax in inspiration. Note that on the left lateral view, the apex of the cardiac silhouette is displaced from the sternum, making the overall cardiac shape appear more rounded than on the right lateral view. In both cases there is a triangular region of lung between the caudal vena cava, heart, and diaphragm.

FIG. 17.5 The parallel horizontal lines over the ventral portion are folds of skin. Nipples, papillomas, or fatty masses can also cause artifacts.

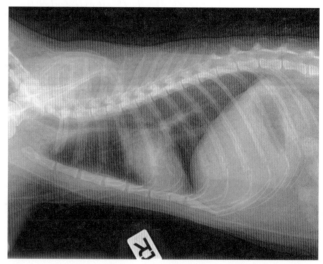

FIG. 17.6 Right Lateral Image of the Feline Thorax. The apex is usually more pointed in a cat than in a dog. Normal heart width is two intercostal spaces. (Courtesy Jennifer White, Mississauga Oakville Veterinary Emergency and Specialty Hospital, ON.)

Lateral Thorax—Routine—cont'd

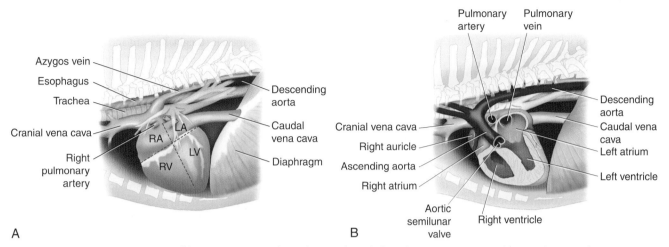

Azygos vein
Esophagus
Trachea
Cranial vena cava
Right pulmonary artery

RA
LA
RV
LV

Descending aorta
Caudal vena cava
Diaphragm

Pulmonary artery
Pulmonary vein
Cranial vena cava
Right auricle
Ascending aorta
Right atrium
Aortic semilunar valve
Right ventricle

Descending aorta
Caudal vena cava
Left atrium
Left ventricle

A

B

FIG. 17.7 Anatomy of the Canine Heart and Vessels. **A,** Left-to-right lateral (RtL) projection. Note the vertical waist at the junction of the cranial vena cava and the right atrium, and the horizontal waist at the atrioventricular groove at the junction of the left atrium and left ventricle, dividing the heart into the four chambers. *A,* atrium; *L,* left; *R,* right; *V,* ventricle. **B,** Right-to-left lateral projection (LeL).

FIG. 17.8 Measure at the caudal border of the scapula over the thickest part with the patient in the proper position. In a thick, muscled dog, the thickest part should be toward the cathode to take advantage of the heel effect.

Ventrodorsal Thorax—Routine

- The VD thorax view is suggested for images of the lung, ventral pulmonary fields, cranial and caudal mediastinum, accessory lung lobes, and caudal vena cava as well as in cases of pleural effusion.
- In the VD, changes in the descending aorta and great vessels are more noticeable than in the DV. The accessory lung lobe is better aerated to allow for more accurate assessment of the caudal mediastinal or accessory lobe pathology. (See Table 17.2 for further variations between VD and DV.)
- In severely ill animals, a VD view may cause compression of remaining functional lung fields. If your patient is critically ill or compromised, make sure to have any emergency supplies or equipment close at hand and constantly assess and monitor the patient.
- The VD is often easier to position more symmetrically than the DV, especially in cats.
- The amount of dependent atelectasis that occurs in VD or DV views is much less than in the lateral views.

Positioning

Place in: Dorsal recumbency in a foam V-trough.

Head: Keep the muzzle straight, forward and parallel to the table.

Carefully position a sandbag over the head and neck, taking care not to restrict breathing.

A straight line should be imagined, connecting the point of the nose with the caudal midline.

Forelimbs: Pull cranially to the comfort of the patient, keeping the nose between the limbs. Individually tie limbs with Velcro straps secured to the table.

Alternatively, place a sandbag just proximal to the elbows or at the carpus, which can also support the head.

Hindlimbs: Keep in a natural frog-leg position, individually tying limbs with Velcro straps secured to the table, or alternatively, place a sandbag over each limb.

Sternum and spine: Superimposed—they should not be seen as separate structures.

Body: Evenly positioned so that the two sides of the rib cage appear equidistant.

Symmetry is essential (Figs. 17.9 through 17.13).

MEASURE: Over the caudal border of the scapula at the highest point of the sternum.

CENTRAL RAY: Midline over the superimposed spine and sternum at the caudal margin of the scapula or between the fifth and sixth ribs.

BORDERS: *The thorax is inside the ribcage, so include the full ribcage.*

Cranial: Cranial point of the scapulohumeral articulation (include thoracic inlet).

Caudal: a few centimeters caudal to the last rib.

Dorsal: Include thoracic vertebrae.

Ventral: Include sternum

FIG. 17.9 A, Positioning of the ventrodorsal (VD) thorax is generally suggested for views of the lung. The forelimbs are pulled cranially. Make sure there is no rotation of the thorax. **B,** Positioning for a feline VD thorax. (**A,** Courtesy Seneca College of Applied Arts and Technology, King City, ON; **B,** Courtesy Julia Bitan, http://handsfreexrays.com, Toronto, ON.)

Ventrodorsal Thorax—Routine—cont'd

Comments and Tips

- Place any ID or markers adjacent to the appropriate side of the thorax near the axilla.
- Positioning devices in the area of interest may affect the image.
- Expose immediately at full inspiration.
- A nonroutine (humanoid) VD thoracic view can also be taken with the thoracic limbs pulled caudally. This view rotates the scapula and associated muscles away from the cranial thorax to aid in evaluation of the mediastinum, lungs, and pleura.[3]

- In large-breed dogs, separate cranial and caudal images may be required. Make sure that the full cardiac silhouette is included on at least one image.

> **✎ TECHNICIAN NOTES** With exceptions, consider the DV view to image the heart and the VD view to image the lungs.

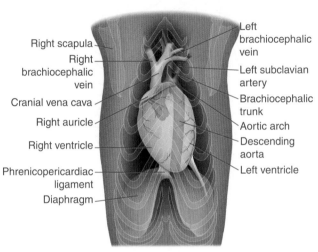

FIG. 17.10 Diagram of the Ventral View of the Canine Thorax Showing the Heart (VD).

Labels: Right scapula, Right brachiocephalic vein, Cranial vena cava, Right auricle, Right ventricle, Phrenicopericardiac ligament, Diaphragm, Left brachiocephalic vein, Left subclavian artery, Brachiocephalic trunk, Aortic arch, Descending aorta, Left ventricle

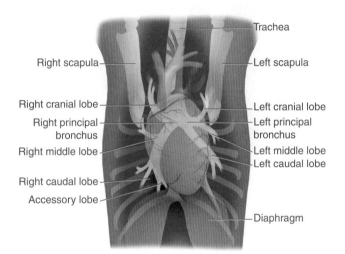

FIG. 17.11 Diagram of the Ventral View of the Canine Bronchial Tree in the Ventrodorsal Position.

Labels: Right scapula, Right cranial lobe, Right principal bronchus, Right middle lobe, Right caudal lobe, Accessory lobe, Trachea, Left scapula, Left cranial lobe, Left principal bronchus, Left middle lobe, Left caudal lobe, Diaphragm

Ventrodorsal Thorax—Routine—cont'd

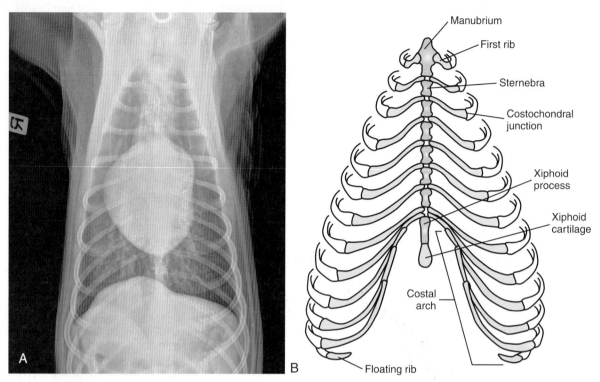

Manubrium

First rib

Sternebra

Costochondral junction

Xiphoid process

Xiphoid cartilage

Costal arch

Floating rib

FIG. 17.12 A, Ventrodorsal (VD) radiograph of the thorax in inspiration. The cardiac silhouette appears more elongated in the VD than the dorsoventral (DV) because of increased object-film distance (OFD), and the cardiac apex shifts to the left laterally and dorsally. The diaphragm appears as three humps—right and left crura and the cupula project into the thorax. **B,** Canine costal cartilages and sternum. Include the full rib cage in thoracic images.

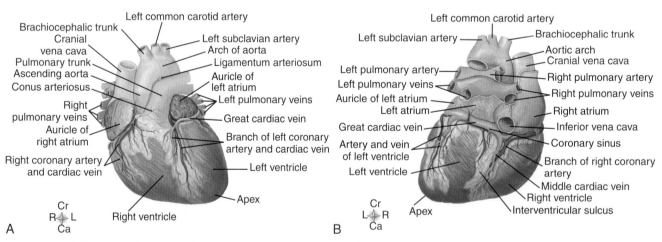

Brachiocephalic trunk
Cranial vena cava
Pulmonary trunk
Ascending aorta
Conus arteriosus
Right pulmonary veins
Auricle of right atrium
Right coronary artery and cardiac vein
Left common carotid artery
Left subclavian artery
Arch of aorta
Ligamentum arteriosum
Auricle of left atrium
Left pulmonary veins
Great cardiac vein
Branch of left coronary artery and cardiac vein
Left ventricle
Apex
Right ventricle
Cr
R L
Ca

Left common carotid artery
Left subclavian artery
Left pulmonary artery
Left pulmonary veins
Auricle of left atrium
Left atrium
Great cardiac vein
Artery and vein of left ventricle
Left ventricle
Apex
Brachiocephalic trunk
Aortic arch
Cranial vena cava
Right pulmonary artery
Right pulmonary veins
Right atrium
Inferior vena cava
Coronary sinus
Branch of right coronary artery
Middle cardiac vein
Right ventricle
Interventricular sulcus
Cr
L R
Ca

FIG. 17.13 Diagrams of the Heart and Great Vessels. **A,** Ventral view. **B,** Dorsal view. (From Patton KT, Thibodeau GA. *Anatomy and Physiology*. 9th ed. St Louis: Saunders; 2016.)

Dorsoventral Thorax—Routine

The DV thorax view is generally considered the best position for the heart as it lies in a more natural position. This offers a consistent cardiac silhouette, evaluation of the pulmonary lobar vessels, and better evaluation of the structures in the dorsal thorax, such as hilar lymph nodes, the caudal dorsal lungs, trachea, mainstem bronchi, and left atrium.[3] However, some sources suggest that the DV may not always be indicated to evaluate heart disease provided that the difference in positioning is accounted for.[1] The DV view is also helpful for evaluating pneumothorax and should be used for patients in respiratory distress (Figs. 17.14 and 17.15).

Positioning

Place In: Ventral recumbency in a radiolucent V-trough if needed.

Head: Gently position forward, and carefully place a sandbag over the neck and head, taking care not to restrict breathing. Keep the sandbag out of the field of view.

The chin can be supported on a pad to keep the cervical vertebrae at the same plane.

Keep the head straight. A straight line should be imagined, connecting the point of the nose with the caudal midline.

Forelimbs: Extend cranially.

Slightly supinate the paws so that the elbows are together and the scapulae lie lateral to the lung field.

Either tie Velcro straps to each limb and secure to the table, or place sandbags over the limbs to maintain position.

Hindlimbs: Keep in a natural position, and secure with Velcro straps or sandbag.

Sternum and spine: Superimposed—they should not be seen as separate structures.

Body: Evenly positioned so that the two sides of the rib cage appear equidistant. Symmetry is essential.

MEASURE: Over the caudal border of the scapula or at the highest point.

CENTRAL RAY: Midline at the caudal margin of the scapula or between the fifth and sixth ribs.

BORDERS: *The thorax is inside the ribcage, so include the full ribcage.*

Cranial: Cranial point of the scapulohumeral articulation (thoracic inlet).

Caudal: A few centimeters caudal to the last rib.

Dorsal: Include thoracic vertebrae.

Ventral: Include sternum.

FIG. 17.14 Dorsoventral Radiograph of the Thorax in Inspiration. The right side of the heart appears more rounded due to upright position than in a ventrodorsal (VD) position. It has the appearance of a lopsided egg, with the cardiac silhouette often displaced to the left by the cranially displaced diaphragm, making the left side look almost straight and the cranial and right borders rounded. The diaphragm is displaced cranially and generally only has one convex shape (the cupula) projecting into the thorax. (Courtesy Jennifer White, Mississauga Oakville Veterinary Emergency and Specialty Hospital, ON.)

FIG. 17.15 Positioning for the Dorsoventral Thorax View. Because the heart lies in a more natural position, this view is generally preferred over the ventrodorsal (VD) for the heart. Make sure there is no rotation.

Dorsoventral Thorax—Routine—cont'd

Comments and Tips

- Place any ID or markers near the axilla in the collimated area on the correct side.
- Expose immediately at full inspiration.
- If the limbs cannot be supinated, the forelimbs can be positioned with the elbows lateral to the thoracic inlet. Positioning is easier, but the scapulae will be superimposed over the lung field.
- A slippery table may make a patient anxious, so consider using a radiolucent foam mat, towel, or sandbags surrounding the paws to help the patient feel more secure.
- If the patient is critically ill or compromised, make sure to have any emergency supplies or equipment close at hand; constantly assess and monitor the patient.

> **TECHNICIAN NOTES** A common mistake is to center too far caudally. Center directly over the heart (palpate) and make sure to include cranially from the shoulder joint caudal to the last rib. The thorax is inside the rib cage, so include the full rib cage.

> **TECHNICIAN NOTES** Good-quality thoracic images[1,3] have the following characteristics:
> - Primary x-ray beam centered on the heart
> - All the ribs are included
> - No rotation
> - No motion artifacts
> - Exposed at peak inspiration
> - Proper contrast and density to evaluate the heart and lungs adequately
>
> **The lateral view is properly positioned when[1-3]:**
> - Rib heads are superimposed and ribs do not extend dorsal to the spine
> - Dorsal spinal processes are faintly visible through scapulae
> - Intervertebral foramina are the same size
> - Transverse processes are superimposed at the origin from the vertebral bodies, appearing as Nike swooshes[1]
> - Ribs over the heart are superimposed and faintly visible over the cardiac silhouette
> - Costochondral junctions are at the same level
>
> **The DV/VD view is properly positioned when[1-3]:**
> - Sternum and spine are superimposed
> - Ribs and thorax are symmetrical so that the distance from the central spine is equidistant to both sides of the thoracic wall
> - The intervertebral spaces are underexposed over the heart but visible cranial to the heart
> - Vertebral bodies are visible over the cardiac silhouette
> - Dorsal spinous processes do not extend beyond the lateral edges of the vertebral bodies

> **TECHNICIAN NOTES** In peak inspiration, the diaphragmatic crura are farther apart. There is greater separation of heart and diaphragm as evidenced by the larger triangular region of lung between the caudal vena cava, heart, and diaphragm (see Table 17.2 for further criteria).

Ancillary Positions

Horizontal Beam Radiography—Ancillary

The patient may be in lateral, ventral, or dorsal recumbency, or may be standing. The x-ray tube is positioned so that the x-ray beam is horizontal across the table. The horizontal beam is used to verify fluid or free air, or for a patient that would be compromised if placed in the VD or DV position. The horizontal beam can be helpful if fluid is to be removed from an area or to identify a mass. Sharp fluid lines will be noticed in horizontal beam radiographs only if there is a free fluid–free gas interchange.[1] If free air is suspected, keep the patient in position at least 5 minutes before exposure to allow dorsal collection of the air.[3] If the x-ray tube head does not rotate horizontally, these views cannot be completed. These views are not possible in digital units unless the plate is removable.

General Comments and Tips for the Horizontal Views

- The side or position that the patient is lying on is referred to as *decubitus*. The beam is parallel to the horizon.
- Place the image receptor vertically behind and close to the patient, using a positioner if needed. In some cases, it is easier to drop the cassette slightly below the level of the table top.
- Place the marker cranial to the axilla, indicating the side closest to the image receptor within the collimated area.
- Expose at full inspiration.
- The correct source image distance must be used.

> **TECHNICIAN NOTES** The term *decubitus* means lying down, so in radiology a right lateral decubitus view means the patient is lying on its right side and the x-ray beam is parallel to the horizon. Thus, you are imaging for a VD (beam enters at the sternum) or DV view (beam enters at the vertebrae).
>
> A ventral decubitus means the patient is in the DV position, lying on its sternum. The x-ray beam will be parallel to the table with the cassette vertically placed on the opposite side of the patient, so you are imaging for a lateral.

Lateral Decubitus View—Ancillary

Also referred to as Lateral Recumbent Horizontal-Beam VD or Ventrodorsal View with Horizontal Beam.

Positioning, Comments, and Tips

- This position is an alternative for the ventrodorsal view.
- Position as for lateral recumbency (Fig. 17.16), except that the patient should be on a thick foam pad or equivalent to allow the dependent portion of the thorax to be in the field of view.
- The position is described according to which side of the patient is closer to the table (i.e., right decubitus if it is lying on its right side).
- The horizontal beam will be directed in a VD direction, entering the sternum and exiting the vertebrae.
- Ensure that the sternum and spine are on the same plane.
- The opacity in this position is significantly less as compared to that seen with the atelectasis effect of the lateral imaged with a vertical beam.

> **TECHNICIAN NOTES** Collimate, ensuring that labels/markers are included and borders are visible for every image.

FIG. 17.16 Positioning for the Lateral Decubitus View (Ventrodorsal [VD] View with Horizontal Beam). The beam enters as for a VD. The patient is best raised with a foam pad, or the cassette can be positioned lower than the table.

Dorsoventral or Ventrodorsal Decubitus View—Ancillary

Also referred to as Ventral/Dorsal Recumbent Horizontal—Beam Lateral.

Positioning, Comments and Tips

Dorsoventral Decubitus View: Position as for a DV view with the patient in ventral recumbency on a thick foam pad or equivalent. Use a radiolucent V-trough if needed.

Ventrodorsal Decubitus View: Position as for a VD view with the patient in dorsal recumbency on a thick foam pad or equivalent. Use a radiolucent V-trough if needed.

- Use gravitational markers such as a Mitchell marker.
- This is an alternate lateral view.

- The beam will be directed horizontally through the patient in a lateral direction with the cassette vertically placed on the opposite side.
- Ensure that the body is evenly positioned so that the sternum and vertebrae are superimposed; the image receptor and central ray are perpendicular to both.
- A straight line should be imagined, connecting the point of the nose with the caudal midline.

Standing Lateral View (With a Horizontal Beam)—Ancillary

Positioning, Comments, and Tips

- Have the patient in a natural standing position (Fig. 17.17).
- There will be superimposition of the shoulder musculature over the cranial lung field.
- The beam will be directed horizontally through the patient in a lateral direction.

- The position is described as a standing right or left lateral. The marker indicating the side against the image receptor is placed cranial to the axilla within the collimated area.
- Use gravitational markers such as a Mitchell marker.

For All Decubitus Views:

MEASURE: Caudal border of the scapula over the thickest part of the thorax.

CENTRAL RAY: At the caudal border of the scapula, between the fifth and sixth ribs.

BORDERS: *The thorax is inside the ribcage, so include the full ribcage.*

Cranial: Palpate from the cranial point of the scapulohumeral articulation (thoracic inlet).
Caudal: A few centimeters caudal to the last rib.
Dorsal: Include thoracic vertebrae.
Ventral: Include sternum.

FIG. 17.17 Positioning for a standing Lateral (LeL) View with a Horizontal Beam and the use of a Portable Cassette Holder.

Ventrodorsal Oblique View—Ancillary

This position views lesions of the thoracic wall and pleura that may be obscured because of overlying tissue or due to the tangential or perpendicular angle of the beam.[3]

Positioning, Comments, and Tips

- Measure and position as for VD.
- Then rotate the sternum away from the side of interest about 20 to 30 degrees. The x-ray beam is centered on the lesion.
- Utilize peripheral borders as needed.

Further Information

Patient Positioning Changes and Anatomy Concerns

Variation in patient position, as well as the phase of respiration, does alter the radiographic appearance (Figs. 17.18 through 17.21). These changes are more prominent in medium and larger dogs and less so in cats and small dogs. Being familiar with these changes will assist you in providing diagnostic images.

Effect of Positional Changes and Phase of Respiration on Thoracic Radiographic Images

See Table 17.2.

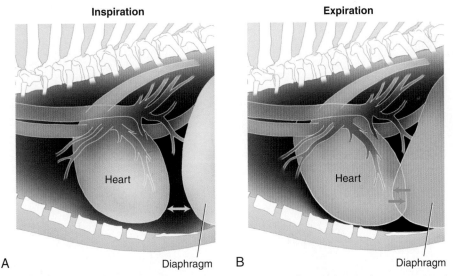

Inspiration

Expiration

Heart

Heart

A Diaphragm   B Diaphragm

FIG. 17.18 A, During inspiration in a lateral view, the heart appears smaller and the vessels appear more elongated. There is increased distance from the apex of the heart to the diaphragm and less sternal contact. The intrathoracic portion of the trachea widens, and the lungs appear more inflated and less radiopaque. B, During expiration, the heart appears larger and the lung lobes smaller and more radiopaque. There is increased sternal contact of the right side of the heart and superimposition of the apex over the diaphragm with dorsal elevation of the trachea and a smaller triangular region of lung between the caudal vena cava, heart, and diaphragm.

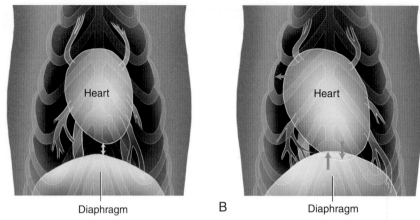

FIG. 17.19 A, During inspiration in either the ventrodorsal (VD) or dorsoventral (DV) view, the heart appears smaller and the vessels appear more elongated. There is increased distance from the apex to the diaphragm. **B,** During expiration in either the VD or DV view, the heart appears larger. There is increased sternal contact on the right side. The diaphragm is superimposed on the caudal cardiac border. The lungs appear more radiopaque.

FIG. 17.20 Right lateral in inspiration **(A)**, right lateral in expiration **(B)**, left lateral in inspiration **(C)**, and left lateral in expiration **(D)**. In inspiration, among other factors, there is increased distance from the apex of the heart to the diaphragm, less sternal contact, the vessels are more elongated, the lungs appear larger and more inflated and the heart appears smaller, and the caudal vena cava is more parallel to the spine. (Courtesy Jennifer White, Mississauga Oakville Veterinary Emergency and Specialty Hospital, ON.)

FIG. 17.21 Ventrodorsal in inspiration **(A)**, ventrodorsal in expiration **(B)**, dorsoventral in inspiration **(C)**, and dorsoventral in expiration **(D)** of different patients. In inspiration, the heart generally appears smaller, the vessels more elongated, and increased distance from the apex to the diaphragm as compared to expiration. In deep inspiration, the apex of the heart is nearer the midline. (Courtesy Jennifer White, Mississauga Oakville Veterinary Emergency and Specialty Hospital, ON.)

TABLE 17.2	Effect of Positional Changes and Phase of Respiration on Thoracic Radiographic Images[1-3]
RIGHT LATERAL THORAX	**LEFT LATERAL THORAX**

(See Figs. 17.3A, 17.4A, 17.5, 17.6, 17.7, 17.20A,B, 17.22A, 17.27A) • Heart is more "conical" or oval—the cardiophrenic ligament prevents the heart from moving to dependent portion of pleural cavity. • Diaphragmatic crura are parallel to each other—the dependent right crus will be more cranial. • The caudal vena cava will merge with cranial right crus, so it is only visible between the cardiac silhouette and diaphragm. • Right lateral recumbency causes more superimposition of the right and left pairs of cranial lobe vessels. • Overlap between the right and left cranial lobe pulmonary vessels so more difficult to assess the size of pulmonary arteries and veins. • Air in the fundus of the stomach behind the left diaphragmatic crus.	(See Figs. 17.3B, 17.4B, 17.20C,D) • Overall cardiac shape appears more rounded—the apex of the cardiac silhouette is displaced from the sternum. • The right and left crura diverge from each other ventrally to dorsally (appear to cross). • The dependent left crus of the diaphragm is more cranial. • Caudal vena cava silhouettes with right crus, usually caudal to the left crus. • The right cranial lobar artery and vein are best seen because the contralateral right lung is better inflated. • Easier to determine vessel size and to distinguish between right and left cranial lobe pulmonary vessels. • The fundic portion of the stomach is fluid filled and caudal to the left crus.

TABLE 17.2	Effect of Positional Changes and Phase of Respiration on Thoracic Radiographic Images[1–3]—cont'd
RIGHT LATERAL THORAX	**LEFT LATERAL THORAX**

Inspiration for Both Laterals (See Figs. 17.4, 17.6, 17.18A, 17.20A,C)

- Heart appears smaller because the lungs are more inflated so they appear larger.
- Vessels appear more elongated.
- There is increased distance from the apex of the heart to the diaphragm (more noticed in cats, and medium and large-breed dogs).
- The size of the triangular region of lung between the caudal vena cava, heart, and diaphragm is larger.
- Diaphragmatic crura at about T12–T13 (depending on breed, cats to L1)
- Cupula at T8–T10, depending on breed.
- Less sternal cardiac contact because the lungs extend to the sternum.
- Intrathoracic portion of trachea widens, and the cervical portion of the trachea narrows.
- The dependent diaphragm is displaced more cranially.
- In extreme inspiration, the diaphragm is more vertical—its shape moves from convex to straight.
- Caudal vena cava is horizontal or parallel with the spine.

Expiration for Both Laterals (See Figs. 17.18B, 17.20B,D, 17.22A)

- Heart appears larger while lung lobes are less inflated, so are smaller and more radiopaque.
- Increased sternal contact of the right side of the heart.
- Superimposition of apex over the diaphragm.
- Dorsal elevation of trachea.
- Intrathoracic portion of the trachea narrows, and cervical portion widens.

DORSOVENTRAL (DV) THORAX	**VENTRODORSAL (VD) THORAX**

(See Figs. 17.14, 17.19B, 17.21C,D)

- Cardiac shape more rounded due to upright position.
- Appearance of lopsided egg as the cardiac silhouette is often displaced to the left by the cranially displaced diaphragm, making the left side look almost straight. The cranial and right borders are rounded.
- The cranially displaced diaphragm pushes the heart cranially and into the left hemothorax, which is more evident in medium and large dogs than in cats or small dogs.
- The diaphragm appears as a single convex shape with a clear left and right crura and medially located cupula. If the x-ray beam is centered caudally, it may appear as three humps, which is especially noted in deep-chested patients.
- Accessory lung lobe region is less aerated due to cranial diaphragm placement.
- There is improved pulmonary inflation in the DV view and better visualization of the caudal lobar pulmonary vessels and bronchi—more magnified and perpendicular to the beam than in the VD view.
- Caudal lobar vessels are significantly magnified due to increased object to film distance.
- Superimposition of cardiac silhouettes, great vessels, trachea, and esophagus.[1]
- Vertebrae appear more magnified.

(See Figs. 17.10, 17.11, 17.12, 17.19A, 17.21A,B, 17.22B)

- The cardiac silhouette is more elongated (increased OFD), and the cardiac apex shifts to the left laterally and dorsally. In dogs with deep and narrow chests, the heart may appear more rounded than oval because of upright orientation.
- Minor changes in size and shape of the cardiac silhouette are not as accurate in VD because of magnification, especially in large-breed dogs.
- Changes of descending aorta and great vessels are more noticeable.
- The diaphragm appears as three humps—right and left crura and the cupula project into the thorax. If the x-ray beam is centered caudally, the diaphragm will appear as a single convex shape.[3]
- Accessory lung lobe region is better aerated and is elongated between the cardiac silhouette and diaphragm; less air is noted in the dorsocaudal lungs.
- Pulmonary arteries sometimes superimposed over the heart.
- Thymus in puppies appears as a triangular-shaped soft tissue opacity in cranial mediastinum.

Inspiration for VD and DV (See Figs. 17.12, 17.19A, 17.21A,C)

- Heart appears smaller and lungs less opaque.
- Vessels appear more elongated.
- There is increased distance from the apex to the diaphragm.
- DV images produced during deep inspiration show the apex of the heart nearer to the midline.
- The diaphragmatic cupola is centered at T8–T10, depending on breed.
- The costrophrenic angle is located at 10th–12 rib, depending on breed.

Expiration for VD/DV (See Figs. 17.19B, 17.21B,D, 17.22B)

- Heart appears larger and lungs appear more radiopaque.
- Increased sternal contact on the right side.
- The diaphragm superimposes the caudal cardiac border.

Normal Thoracic Radiographic Anatomy

The four basic anatomical regions of the thorax are generally considered to be the extrathoracic region, the pleural space, the pulmonary parenchyma, and the mediastinum (Figs. 17.23 and 17.24). The mediastinum divides the thorax into right and left sides and is formed by the parietal pleura of the right and left hemithoraces. The mediastinum contains important structures, including the trachea, esophagus, heart, aorta and its major branches, thoracic duct, lymph nodes, and nerves. Please see Table 17.2 for the effect of positional changes and phase of respiration on thoracic radiographic images. Knowledge of basic anatomy is important to provide the veterinarian with diagnostic images because radiographic changes may be

seen that are not attributable to disease processes or other findings. Figs. 17.10, 17.11, 17.13, and 17.18 through 17.26 show further anatomy of the related areas. Fig. 17.25 indicates anatomy identification in the VD/DV position using the face clock analogy. Fig. 17.27 shows how the heart is visualized on a radiographic image compared with two types of ultrasound images. See Chapter 10 for information on ultrasound.

Appendix B on the Evolve website outlines an overview of normal thoracic radiography and further radiographic concerns in order for the imager to understand the implications of failure to properly position the patient.

Fig. 17.28 is a mystery radiograph. Review it and answer the question presented with it.

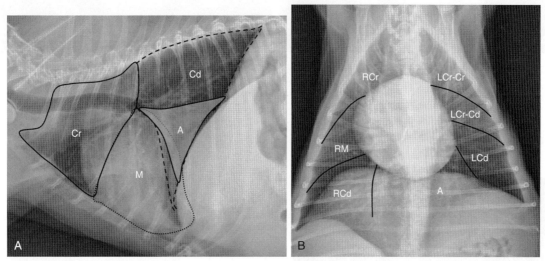

FIG. 17.22 A, Lateral canine thoracic radiograph where the approximate location of lung lobes is indicated. *A,* Accessory lobe; *Cd,* right and left caudal lobes; *Cr,* right cranial lobe and cranial segment of left cranial lobe; *M,* right middle lobe and caudal segment of left cranial lobe. **B,** Ventrodorsal (VD) canine thoracic radiograph where the approximate location of lung lobes is indicated. *A,* Accessory lobe; *LCd,* left caudal lobe; *LCr-Cd,* caudal segment of left cranial lobe; *LCr-Cr,* cranial segment of left cranial lobe; *RCd,* right caudal lobe; *RCr,* right cranial lobe; *RM,* right middle lobe. (Thrall DE. *Textbook of Veterinary Diagnostic Radiology.* 7th ed. St. Louis: Elsevier; 2017)

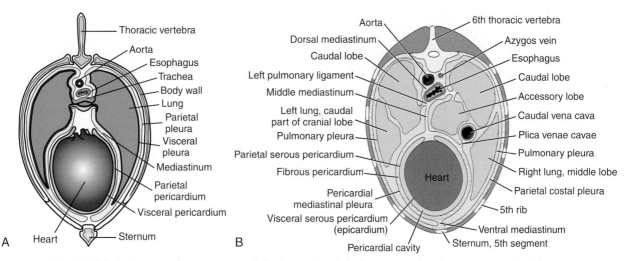

FIG. 17.23 A, Diagram of a cross-section of the thorax through the heart to visualize thoracic contents. **B,** Schematic transverse section of thorax through the heart, caudal view. (**A** From Colville T, Bassert J. *Clinical Anatomy and Physiology for Veterinary Technicians.* 3rd ed. St Louis: Elsevier; 2016.)

FIG. 17.24 A, Computerized tomography (CT) scan at midthorax. *1,* Esophagus; *2,* right principal bronchus; *3,* carina of trachea; *4,* ventral mediastinum–phrenicopericardial ligament; *5,* heart; *6,* left pulmonary artery; *7,* aorta. **B,** CT scan at caudal thorax. *1,* Right caudal lobe; *2,* caudal vena cava; *3,* accessory lobe; *4,* plica venae cavae; *5,* heart; *6,* caudal mediastinum; *7,* left caudal lobe; *8,* esophagus; *9,* aorta.

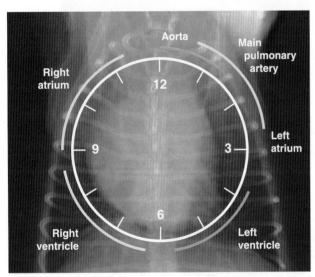

FIG. 17.25 The cardiac silhouette can be evaluated with a clock face analogy. In either the dorsoventral or ventrodorsal position of the cat, the left atrium forms the left heart border from 2 to 3 o'clock and the left ventricle from about 3 to 6 o'clock. In the dog, the left atrium is not visible in this area and does not make up the heart border. The left ventricle forms the left heart border from 2 to 6 o'clock in the dog. The right atrium is at 9 to 11 o'clock. When evident, the main pulmonary artery is noted at 1 to 2 o'clock. The left pulmonary artery extends beyond the heart at about 4 o'clock, and the right pulmonary artery is found at about 8 o'clock.[1] The lateral radiograph would show the aorta at about 10 to 11 o'clock, the main pulmonary artery and right atrium at 9 to 10 o'clock, the right ventricle at 5 to 9 o'clock, and the left ventricle at 2 to 5 o'clock.

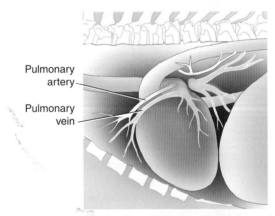

FIG. 17.26 In the lateral radiographic projection of the normal canine thorax, it is difficult to differentiate pulmonary arteries from the veins. The artery is always dorsal to the vein in the cranial lung lobes. In general, the size of the pulmonary arteries should have the same size and shape as that of the corresponding pulmonary veins at the same level.[1] (Thrall DE. Textbook of Veterinary Diagnostic Radiology. 7th ed. St. Louis: Elsevier; 2017.)

FIG. 17.27 Three Different Images of the Heart. **A,** Right lateral radiograph. **B,** An ultrasound scan shows the right-sided short axis of heart chambers and vessels. *AO,* aorta; *LA,* left atrium; *PA,* pulmonary artery; *PV,* pulmonary vein; *RA,* right atrium; *RV,* right ventricle. **C,** Pulsed wave Doppler ultrasonograph (see Chapter 10) evaluating blood flow across the aortic valve. There is normal velocity across the valve (approximately 1 m/s) and a normal high-resistance flow pattern. The flow of blood can be tracked: blue indicates blood flowing away from the transducer, and red shows blood flowing toward the transducer (remember BART: blue away/red toward). Further color shows greater variances that detect abnormal blood flows.

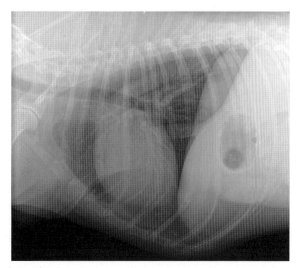

FIG. 17.28 Mystery Radiograph. There is no marker on this image. How can you tell which view it is and whether it is in inspiration or expiration?

✳ KEY POINTS

1. Proper positioning and technique are essential for proper interpretation of thoracic images. This includes where to measure and center, what to include, and correct positioning and symmetry.
2. A change in patient position, central ray, inaccurate positioning, or phase of respiration affects the radiographic appearance, so it is essential that the technician is aware of the changes that could occur if the view is not accurately imaged.
3. A long scale of contrast, obtained by higher kVp and lower mAs, is suggested for film-screen imaging; underexposure or overexposure may lead to misdiagnosis.
4. Lateral and DV thorax views are generally completed for evaluation of the heart, whereas lateral and VD views are suggested for visualization of lung parenchyma.
5. Additional and alternative views may be needed, depending on the suspected conditions.
6. In the lateral view, lung lesions are best identified in the nondependent position (lesions in the left lung will be more noticeable in right lateral recumbency).
7. Measurement is made over the caudal border of the scapula; the central ray is over the heart, and the full rib cage is included.
8. The exposure is generally taken at maximum inspiration but there are exceptions, such as diagnosing tracheal or bronchial collapse.
9. The four basic anatomical regions of the thorax are generally considered to be the extrathoracic region, the pleural space, the pulmonary parenchyma, and the mediastinum, including the heart and great vessels. Knowing the normal anatomy of these areas helps the technician take proper radiographic images and, ultimately, enables the veterinarian to make the correct diagnosis.
10. Other modalities such as ultrasound, echocardiography, or computerized tomography (CT) are more diagnostic and may be required to properly view the thoracic anatomy or augment diagnosis of radiographically visible structures.

REVIEW QUESTIONS

1. The veterinarian requests that you image a beagle for routine thoracic images before surgery. For proper diagnosis your image should have a:
   a. Long scale of contrast produced by higher kVp and lower mAs
   b. Long scale of contrast produced by lower kVp and higher mAs
   c. Short scale of contrast produced by higher kVp and lower mAs
   d. Short scale of contrast produced by lower kVp and higher mAs

2. The veterinarian requires thoracic images of a beagle, which should be measured at the thickest part, or the:
   a. Thoracic inlet
   b. Point of the heart
   c. Cranial border of the scapula
   d. Caudal border of the scapula

3. The peripheral borders for the beagle thoracic image are the:
   a. Caudal border of the scapula to the first lumbar vertebral body
   b. Point of the heart to the first lumbar vertebral body
   c. Shoulder joint to just past the 13th rib
   d. First thoracic vertebra to the 13th thoracic vertebral body

4. You will expose the thoracic images for the beagle:
   a. At maximum expiration
   b. At maximum inspiration
   c. Halfway between maximum inspiration and expiration
   d. At any point in the respiratory cycle

5. You check that you have taken proper inspiration images for this beagle. On the image, the heart in either lateral or DV taken during inspiration will appear:
   a. Smaller. The vessels are more elongated, and there is increased distance from the apex of the heart to the diaphragm.
   b. More conical or oval. The diaphragm is more caudal, and there is dorsal elevation of the trachea.
   c. Smaller. The vessels are more shortened, and there is decreased distance from the apex of the heart to the sternum.
   d. Larger. The vessels are larger, and there is greater sternal contact and a clear left and right crus with a medially located cupula.

6. To minimize rotation when positioning for the lateral for this beagle, you should:
   a. Not place any foam pads between the limbs or under the sternum
   b. Place thick foam pads between the limbs and under the sternum to rotate vertebrae
   c. Place foam pads only under the sternum because none are required between the limbs
   d. Place foam pads to elevate the sternum and between the hindlimbs if needed

7. When positioning for the lateral view, you want to ensure that the front limbs are pulled as far:
   a. Cranially as possible without rotating the thorax
   b. Cranially as possible with slight rotation of the thorax
   c. Caudally as possible with a wedge between if needed
   d. Caudally as possible, causing the sternum and vertebrae to be on the same plane

8. You forgot to include a marker, but you know that you did provide the right lateral image of this beagle because on the image you note that:
   a. The diaphragm is not touching the heart
   b. The heart is more conical
   c. The heart is rounder
   d. Air is noted in the pyloric antrum

9. You are confident that you are presenting the veterinarian with well-positioned DV images of this beagle because on the image you see:
   a. Superimposition of the sternum and vertebrae
   b. Intervertebral foramina are the same size
   c. Ribs over the heart are superimposed
   d. The "Nike swoosh" of the transverse processes

10. A routine VD is required on a feline patient. It is generally best to pull the front limbs:
    a. Caudally and have the nose pointing up equidistant between the front legs
    b. Caudally and have the nose parallel to the table equidistant between the front legs
    c. Cranially and have the nose pointing up equidistant between the front legs
    d. Cranially and have the nose parallel to the table equidistant between the front legs

11. The veterinarian suspects a lesion in the right lung of a poodle. She would like you to complete both laterals, but the most important one in this case is the:
    a. Right lateral
    b. Left lateral

12. The veterinarian would like you to complete a DV decubitus view on a springer spaniel, as fluid is suspected. This means that the patient should be in:
    a. DV position using a vertical beam
    b. Lateral recumbency using a horizontal beam
    c. Dorsal recumbency using a horizontal beam
    d. Ventral recumbency using a horizontal beam

13. In the DV decubitus view of the springer spaniel with fluid, exposure factors without fluid are 72 kV and 10 mAs. You are best to:
    a. Keep the same exposure factors
    b. Increase the kV to 80 and keep the mAs at 10
    c. Increase the kV to 80 and decrease the mAs to 5
    d. Increase the source image distance and keep the same factors

14. Pneumonia is suspected in a retriever. The recommended views are:
    a. Both laterals and a ventrodorsal
    b. Both laterals and a dorsoventral
    c. The right lateral and a ventrodorsal
    d. The right lateral and a dorsoventral

15. The mediastinum contains the:
    a. Heart solely
    b. Heart, trachea, esophagus, aorta and major branches, thoracic duct, lymph nodes, and nerves
    c. Trachea, esophagus, aorta and major branches, thoracic duct, lymph nodes, and nerves
    d. Stomach, liver, kidneys, diaphragm, gallbladder, intestines and bladder

Chapter Review Question answers are located in the Instructor Resources on Evolve and can be provided to students at the discretion of the instructor.

References

1. Thrall DE. *Textbook of Veterinary Diagnostic Radiology*. 7th ed. St. Louis: Elsevier; 2017.
2. Ayers S. *Small Animal Radiographic Techniques and Positioning*. Oxford: Wiley-Blackwell; 2013.
3. Muhlbauer MC, Kneller SK. *Radiography of the Dog and Cat: Guide to Making and Interpreting Radiographs*. Ames, IA: Wiley Blackwell; 2013.

Bibliography

Colville T, Bassert J. Clinical *Anatomy and Physiology for Veterinary Technicians*. 3rd ed. St. Louis: Mosby; 2016.

Done SH, Goody PC, Evans SA, Stickland NC. *Color Atlas of Veterinary Anatomy: the Dog and Cat*. 2nd ed. London: Mosby; 2009.

Evans H, de Launta A. *Guide to the Dissection of the Dog*. 8th ed. St. Louis: Saunders; 2017.

Han C, Hurd C. *Practical Diagnostic Imaging for the Veterinary Technician*. 3rd ed. St. Louis: Mosby; 2005.

Jenner A. Non-manual radiography: radiation and patient safety. *RVT J Ont Assoc Vet Tech*. 2016;39(2).

Owens JM, Biery DN. *Radiographic Interpretation for the Small Animal Clinician*. St. Louis: Ralston Purina; 1999.

Romich J. An *Illustrated Guide to Veterinary Medical Terminology*. Clifton, NY: Delmar Cengage Learning; 2015.

Singh B. *Dyce, Sack and Wensing's Textbook of Veterinary Anatomy*. 5th ed. St Louis: Elsevier; 2018.

Sirois M, Schlote J. *Diagnostic Imaging for Veterinary Technicians*. Minneapolis MN: Bluedoor, LLC, 2017.

Sirois M. *Principles and Practice of Veterinary Technology*. 4th ed. St. Louis: Mosby; 2017.

Tighe M, Brown M. Mosby's *Comprehensive Review for Veterinary Technicians*. 5th ed. St. Louis: Mosby; 2019.

CHAPTER 18

Small Animal Forelimb

Marg Brown, RVT, BEd Ad Ed

Four legs good, two legs bad.
—George Orwell, English novelist, 1903–1950

OUTLINE

LEARNING OBJECTIVES

When you have finished this chapter, you will be able to:

1. Properly and safely position a dog or cat for common forelimb positions with an emphasis on non-manual restraint.
2. Correctly measure and center the patient to include the peripheral borders.
3. Keep the bone or joint parallel to the image receptor and the central ray perpendicular to the field of view (FOV) and receptor.
4. Identify views that may need to be completed as an alternative.
5. Identify the normal anatomy found on a radiographic image.

KEY TERMS

Key terms are defined in the Glossary on the Evolve website.

Articular margin	Hyperextended	Occult	Skyline
Caudocranial/craniocaudal	Hyperflexed	Osteochondritis dissecans	Stress Radiographs
Craniodistal-cranioproximal	Mediolateral	Positional terminology	
Flexed	Oblique		

TECHNICAL NOTE: To preserve space, the images presented in this chapter do not show collimation. For safety, always collimate to limit the beam within the image receptor. In film radiography, you should see a clear border of collimation (frame) on every radiograph. In some jurisdictions, evidence of collimation is required by law. In digital imaging, the algorithm depends on proper collimation.

Diseases of the musculoskeletal system most often affect the patient's mobility. Skeletal and joint disorders are the most common, but other problems in the musculoskeletal system do occur. The emphasis in this and the next chapter will be the imaging of the appendicular skeleton (Fig. 18.1A) to detect potential pathology. Bone disorders can be developmental, infectious, nutritional, due to trauma or neoplasia, or be of unknown etiology. Bone diseases are generally present at birth or are the result of nutritional deficiencies or injuries. Movable joints are vulnerable to joint diseases or disorders affecting their membranes, as well as related ligaments, cartilage, and bone.

There can be a large number of incidental findings and anatomical variants. Often it is not possible to determine the significance of lesions based on radiological appearance alone. High-quality images are essential to minimize misdiagnosis. Joint studies are generally completed non–weight bearing, making it difficult to overtly evaluate joint space on the images. Radiographic changes are often subtle because bone is a matrix of different tissues that continuously remodel through life as animals mature and respond to disease and trauma. Immature bones have an open physis between the epiphysis and the metaphysis, seen as a translucent line that should not be confused with a fracture.

> ✏ **TECHNICIAN NOTES** Mentally place the patient in sternal recumbency for the distal portion of the limb and in dorsal recumbency for the proximal portion, and the positional terms will make sense.

Radiographic and Patient Concerns

- There are many factors to consider in the production of high-quality images.
- Except for the shoulder and scapula in some dogs, most projections are completed tabletop. A grid is not generally used because the tissue thickness of the forelimb is less than 10 cm.
- It is important to collimate the field as tightly as possible to reduce scatter radiation. This also achieves higher contrast, both in analog and digital imaging (see Chapter 8).
- Use a small focal spot to maximize spatial resolution.
- Use low kV and high mAs technique to maximize radiographic contrast and not overexpose the image. One should clearly see the soft tissues and trabecular pattern of the bones.
- When a joint is to be imaged, always center on the joint; otherwise, there will be geometrical distortion due to the divergence of the x-ray beam.
- The field of view:
  - Long bones: include the proximal and distal joints.
  - Joints: include one-third each of the long bones, proximal and distal to the joint.
- Along with ensuring that the required anatomy is included, it is also essential to achieve symmetry for proper diagnosis. There should be no rotation.
- The marker is placed at the dorsal or cranial aspect of the limb for lateral views and on the lateral aspect of the limb for the opposite views.
- Most digital systems have a software scaler for orthopedic measurements. If the unit does not, consider a scaler for

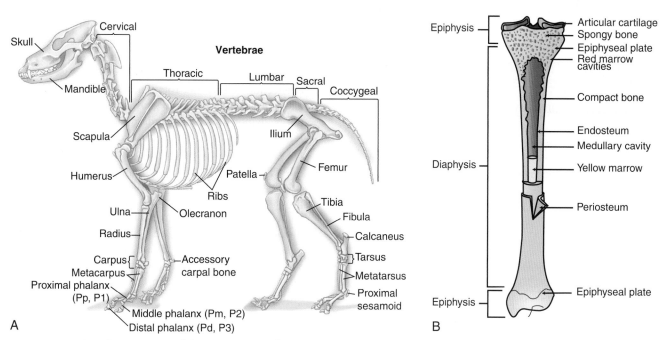

FIG. 18.1 A, Canine skeleton. B, Structure of a long bone (tibia). (B, From Colville T, Bassert JM. *Clinical Anatomy and Physiology for Veterinary Technicians.* 3rd ed. St Louis: Elsevier; 2016.)

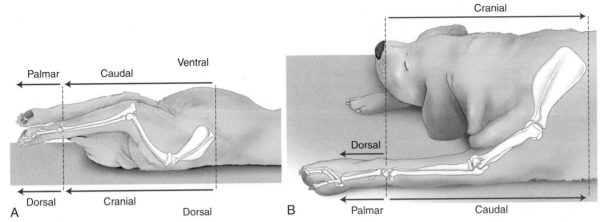

FIG. 18.2 A, Patient in dorsal recumbency for the contralateral image of the proximal limb: scapula, shoulder, and humerus. The humerus is referred to as the caudocranial (CdCr) view in this position. The thorax is termed ventrodorsal in this view. **B,** For positioning of the distal forelimbs (elbow, radius/ulna, carpus, metacarpus, and digits), the patient is generally in sternal recumbency. Note that the terminology changes at and including the carpus. Thus in this position, the view of the elbow is craniocaudal (CrCd) and the carpus is dorsopalmar (DP or DPa).

digital images, such as a coin or object of known size, for orthopedic templating.[1]

- Obtain orthogonal views in all cases to properly diagnose three-dimensional objects. Therefore, in addition to a lateral (L) view, the patient is generally placed in dorsal recumbency to acquire a view of the proximal portion of the limb (shoulder, scapula, and humerus) or in sternal recumbency for the distal portion (elbow, radius and ulna, carpus, metacarpus, and digits) (Fig. 18.2). Thus, for the pectoral limb, along with the lateral view of each part, the common views are termed (Table 18.1):
  - Caudocranial (CdCr) for the shoulder, scapula, and humerus—patient lying on its back
  - Craniocaudal (CrCd) for the elbow, radius and ulna—patient lying on its abdomen

TABLE 18.1	Protocol for Pectoral Limb Radiography	
ANATOMICAL LOCATION	**ROUTINE VIEWS**	**ANCILLARY VIEW(S)**
Scapula	Lateral, Caudocranial	Lateromedial
Shoulder	Lateral, Caudocranial	Extended or flexed lateral Skyline for the bicipital groove Craniocaudal
Humerus	Lateral, Caudocranial	Craniocaudal
Elbow	Lateral, Craniocaudal	Caudocranial (horizontal beam), hyperflexed lateral, obliques
Radius/ulna	Lateral, Craniocaudal	
Foot: carpus, metacarpus, and digits	Lateral, Dorsopalmar	Extended or flexed lateral, obliques

- Dorsopalmar (DP/DPa) for the carpus, metacarpus and digits—patient lying on its abdomen (Sometimes this is referred to as *anterior/posterior [AP]*; however, this is a human term and not correct for animals.)
- The lateral views are relatively straightforward to image.
- The CrCd/CdCr views can be especially challenging in dogs because it can be difficult to keep the bones parallel to the table to minimize geometrical distortion. In cats, it is generally easier to obtain symmetry with CrCd/CdCr views. Chemical restraint is highly suggestive for diagnostic CrCd/CdCr views to keep the area of interest parallel to the table.
- Further ancillary views such as oblique positioning are not common in small animals but they may be useful for the humerus, elbow, carpus, metacarpus, or digits. Obliques project different edges of a joint or region that may be overlooked. The tangential projection allows peripheral visibility.[2] Flexed views of the elbow and carpus may also be taken. Stress radiography of joints involves application of traction, rotation, or a wedge to the joint and is useful for sprains to show subluxation that might not be demonstrated on standard radiographic views.[2]
- If it is too painful for the patient to complete the orthogonal view, consider a horizontal beam, if the unit allows.
- Radiographs of the opposite limb are a valuable reference if there are any anatomical variant concerns, such as in physically immature patients. Many joint conditions are bilateral (e.g., osteochondritis dissecans, cranial cruciate disease, elbow dysplasia), so occult pathology might be missed if contralateral limbs are not imaged. A comparison with the opposite limb is often suggested in lameness of younger or older dogs. In this case, a survey of both limbs from the shoulder joint to the elbow is recommended.
- Cats generally do not have developmental dysplasia of the bones and joints that leads to lameness; trauma is the most likely reason for imaging feline limbs.

- In tabletop views for analog radiographs, both positions can be placed on the cassette if the size of the animal and body part allow. It is essential to center on one limb at a time. In a split cassette, point the toes of each view in the same direction. Collimate tightly and use a lead shield to cover the side not being imaged to prevent scatter radiation from fogging the contralateral side of the cassette. Splitting the detector is not possible in digital, but tight collimation is essential.
- Unless otherwise indicated, a vertical beam is used.
- Musculoskeletal images are often performed on patients in pain. Sedation and analgesics are often required due to painful manipulation. If trauma is suspected, address any concurrent issues such as thoracic pathology before radiography.
- In non-manual restraint, it is essential to give the patient the illusion that it is being held with judicious use of sandbags, V-troughs, soft Velcro straps, compression bands, tape, etc.
- Positioning devices in the field of view may affect exposure or cause image artifacts. Hair coat should be clean, dry, and free from dirt because debris may mimic foreign bodies.
- Compensate with increased exposure factors for splints and casts.
- Review the suggestions in Chapter 15 on techniques that can be used to assist in non-manual restraint.
- See Box 18.1 for terms relating to radiographic anatomy associated with bones.
- Other imaging modalities that are commonly available are ultrasonography, computerized tomography (CT), and magnetic resonance imaging (MRI). MRI is particularly useful when evaluating tendons and ligaments around joints. Nuclear medicine or scintigraphy is used in equines and is expanded on in Chapter 14.

TECHNICIAN NOTES To produce high-quality orthopedic images:
- Use low kV and high mAs technique with a small focal spot
- Utilize tabletop technique except for proximal limbs of large dogs.
- Measure the patient at the thickest part and in the position it is to be radiographed.
- Minimize object-film distance (OFD).
- Center on the area of interest.
- Collimate and include only what is required.
- Keep the bone parallel to the image receptor and the central ray perpendicular to both.
- Have no rotation.
- Minimize superimposed structures.
- Label correctly.
- Obtain orthogonal views.
- Radiograph the contralateral limb for comparison when required.

BOX 18.1 | Terms Related to Radiographic Anatomy Associated with Bones[3]

- Condyle—rounded projection on the bone for articulation with another bone.
- Diaphysis—the shaft or body of the long bone.
- Epicondyle—a projection of bone on the lateral edge above its condyle.
- Epiphysis—the end of the long bone, with each long bone having a distal and proximal epiphysis.
- Epiphyseal plate or growth plate—plate of cartilage at the junction of the proximal and distal epiphysis with the diaphysis that ossifies as the animal matures.
- Foramen—opening or passage into or through a bone.
- Fossa—hollow or depressed area on a bone, usually filled with muscles or tendons.
- Metaphysis—the wide portion of a long bone between the epiphysis and the narrow diaphysis that contains the growth plate.
- Trochlea—usually, grooves in bone that allow tendons to act as pulleys.
- Tuberosity/trochanter/tubercle—protuberances on the bones, usually for muscle attachment.
- A long bone is described as having a head, shaft (body), and neck.

From Aspinall V, Cappello M. *Introduction to Veterinary Anatomy.* London: Butterworth-Heineman; 2009.

TECHNICIAN NOTES The label or marker is placed on the lateral aspect of the limb for orthogonal views and when possible for lateral views.

TECHNICIAN NOTES For efficiency and ease of positioning, position and secure the body parts that are not in the beam. Then position the area of interest.

TECHNICIAN NOTES Collimate and include labels/markers and visible borders for every film image taken.

TECHNICIAN NOTES Always collimate as closely as possible.

Scapula

Lateral (Mediolateral) View of the Scapula—Routine

Positioning to View Body of Scapula

Place in: Lateral recumbency with the affected side down.

Head and Neck: Arch the head and neck dorsally so they are at 135 degrees to the thoracic spine, placing sandbags over the neck to keep it in position and taking care not to restrict breathing.

Think of the head and limbs as being in a T-shaped position—the head and contralateral limb form the top of the T, and the affected limb its main stem (Fig. 18.3A).

Hindlimbs: Leave in a natural position and support with Velcro/sandbags if needed.

Forelimbs: To visualize the body of the scapula, pressure is forcibly applied to the affected limb to position the full scapula dorsal to the vertebral column.

Pull the contralateral limb ventrally and caudally so the thorax will rotate slightly and further isolate the scapular body (Fig. 18.3).

Tie in place or use a sandbag. Grasp the affected limb below the elbow joint, keeping the joint extended so it cannot flex. Push the limb perpendicular to and dorsally toward the line of the neck and upper limb until the spinous processes can be seen bulging dorsal to the thoracic vertebral spinous processes. Use a heavy sandbag over the elbow to keep the limb in position. Manual restraint may be required.

Comments and Tips

- The goal is an unobstructed view, positioning the scapula dorsal to the vertebral column.
- Pulling the opposite limb slightly rotates the thorax, which further isolates the scapula dorsal to the body.
- If the upper limb is overextended dorsally, the upper shoulder musculature will be over the area of interest.

MEASURE: Dorsally at the cranial border of the scapula approximately at about the site of T1 to T2 spinous process or thickest area where scapula is noted.

CENTRAL RAY: Center of the scapula.

BORDERS: *Cranial:* Proximal to shoulder joint.

Caudal: Past Caudal border of the scapula.

Dorsally and ventrally: Include the entire scapula.

FIG. 18.3 A, Line drawing to show the correct alignment or T-position for mediolateral images of the shoulder and scapula. B, Positioning for the mediolateral scapula dorsal to the vertebral column. The affected limb is pushed up dorsally to image the full scapula above the thoracic spine.

Lateral (Mediolateral) View of the Scapula—Routine—cont'd

FIG. 18.3, cont'd C, Mediolateral image of the scapula, dorsal to the vertebral column. **D,** Medial view of the right shoulder joint and scapula. (**A,** Redrawn from Muhlbauer MC, Kneller SK. *Radiography of the Dog and Cat: Guide to Making and Interpreting Radiographs.* Oxford: Wiley-Blackwell; 2013; **B,** Courtesy Seneca College of Applied Arts and Technology, King City, ON.)

Lateral (Lateromedial) View of the Scapula—Ancillary

Positioning[4]

Place in: Lateral recumbency with the affected side up.

Head and Neck: Position the skull and neck parallel to the short edge of the table, using a sandbag to keep the nose pointing forward. The shoulder should be below the level of the thoracic spinous processes.

Hindlimbs: Leave in a natural position and support with sandbags or Velcro straps if needed.

Forelimbs: Pull the lower contralateral limb distally away from the thorax slightly cranially and secure with Velcro straps or a sandbag.

Secure the upper affected limb with ties or Velcro around the mid to lower radius and pull dorsally so the carpus is above the skull (Fig. 18.4).

Comments and Tips

- The goal is an unobstructed view, positioning the scapula dorsal to the vertebral column to more easily visualize the spine of the scapula and the proximal border.

- The elbow will be slightly flexed and the scapula dorsal to the thoracic spinous processes.
- The pulling of the lower limb and pushing of the affected upper limb rotates the patient's torso to position the affected scapula dorsal to the cervical and thoracic spinous processes. The entire scapular spine can be palpated when the affected limb is away from the table.
- Geometric distortion will result with rotation of the torso and magnification will be noted of the affected scapula due to increased object film distance (OFD).
- To avoid confusion in labeling, it may be advantageous to use both markers, keeping the affected scapula marker at the cranial dorsal aspect of the image receptor and the recumbent limb marker at the cranial distal portion.

Lateral (Lateromedial) View of the Scapula—Ancillary—cont'd

MEASURE: Dorsally at the cranial border of the scapula approximately at about the site of T1 to T2 spinous process or thickest area where scapula is noted.

CENTRAL RAY: Center of the scapula.

BORDERS: *Cranial:* Proximal to shoulder joint.
Caudal: Past Caudal border of the scapula.

  Dorsally and ventrally: Include the entire scapula.

FIG 18.4 A, Positioning of the lateromedial view of the scapula with the affected limb up. Secure and pull the affected limb dorsally so the carpus is above the skull **B,** Image of the lateromedial scapula. (**A,** Courtesy Jocelyn Affleck, Golf Glen Veterinary Clinic, Aurora, ON; **B,** Courtesy Jennifer White, Mississauga Oakville Veterinary Emergency and Specialty Hospital, ON.)

Lateral (Mediolateral) View of the Scapula—Ancillary

- To better visualize the distal scapula and scapular neck ventral to the trachea over the radiolucent lung fields, if the patient is in pain or manipulation is not possible, position the patient in lateral recumbency with the affected limb pulled caudally and dorsally while the upper unaffected limb is extended cranially. Force is not applied to push the limb dorsally.
- Note that as compared to the previous position, this is a mediolateral so the affected limb is against the table and pulled caudally and dorsally.

- The sternum can be slightly rotated up to allow the scapula to be better visualized.
- This view also causes less pain to the patient.
- Measuring, central ray, and borders as above.

✎ TECHNICIAN NOTES   Remember to go through your mental checklist before pushing the exposure button (see Chapter 15).

Caudocranial View of the Scapula[4]—Routine

Positioning

Place In: Dorsal recumbency in a trough or with the use of tape if needed.

Head and Neck: Push the head slightly laterally from the affected limb to avoid superimposition of the cervical spine over the joint.

Place a sandbag over the neck if required, taking care not to restrict breathing.

Hindlimbs: Leave in a natural position and support with Velcro/sandbags if needed.

Forelimbs: Secure each limb separately and extend cranially, especially the affected limb (Fig. 18.5).

Use sandbags or Velcro to attach the affected limb to the table so that the humerus is almost parallel to the table.

Comments and Tips

- Rotate the patient's sternum from the scapula about 10 to 12 degrees to avoid superimposition of the scapula and ribs. Keep the spine of the scapula perpendicular to the table.
- Tape or Velcro placed over the distal portion of the humerus that is pulled medially helps the olecranon point straight up so the scapula and humerus are straight.
- Place the marker lateral to the limb imaged.

MEASURE: At the level of the scapulohumeral articulation (shoulder joint) so that the calipers are extended over the first thoracic vertebral body.

CENTRAL RAY: Center of the scapula.

BORDERS: *Cranial*: 1 inch cranial to acromion process of scapular spine.

Caudal: Caudal border of scapula (about level of eighth rib).

Laterally: On either side of the palpated scapular spine.

Greater tubercle of humerus
Acromion of scapula
Spine of scapula
Lesser tubercle of humerus
Humeral (scapulohumeral) joint

R

FIG. 18.5 A, Positioning of the caudocranial scapula. B, Caudal view of the right shoulder joint and scapula. C, Caudocranial image of the scapula, humerus, and shoulder joint. (A, Courtesy Seneca College of Applied Arts and Technology, King City, ON.)

Shoulder Joint

Lateral (Mediolateral) View of the Shoulder—Routine

Positioning

Place in: Lateral recumbency with the affected limb down.

Head and Neck: Arch the head and neck dorsally so they are 135 degrees to the thoracic spine to avoid superimposition of the cervical spine over the shoulder joint.

Place sandbags over the skull and out of the field of view.

Hindlimbs: Leave in a natural position and support with Velcro/sandbags if needed.

Forelimbs: Flex and pull the contralateral limb caudodorsally in line with the thorax wall and neck to prevent superimposition (Fig. 18.6).

Secure with a sandbag or Velcro.

The affected limb is extended cranially and distally away from and perpendicular to the line of the neck allowing the shoulder joint to be ventral to the sternum.

Support with a sandbag or secure with Velcro strap.

Comments and Tips

• Think of the head and limbs as being in a T-shaped position—the head and contralateral limb form the top of the T, and the affected limb its main stem (Fig. 18.3A).

• Place the marker of the lower affected limb cranial to the shoulder joint.

• Extension of the head and neck places the shoulder joint ventral to the sternum and air-filled trachea, and puts the trachea dorsal to the scapulohumeral articulation, separating the joint surfaces.

• Palpate the shoulder joint by feeling along the humerus. The shoulder joint should be cranial to the manubrium and ventral to the trachea on the final image.

• The sternum will be slightly rotated from the thorax. Avoid overrotation of the thorax, which would place the shoulder joint in an oblique position and make evaluation of the articular surfaces of the shoulder joint difficult.[2]

• To visualize the articular margin of the humeral head, which aids in better determining osteochondrosis lesions, the affected limb can be slightly pronated and then slightly supinated[5] to cause slight obliquity.

• Shoulder instability can be assessed by comparing two laterals: one with and one without pulling on the limb (applied traction).

MEASURE: At the level of the shoulder joint.

Extend the caliper to the point of the unaffected shoulder, being careful not to include that limb.

CENTRAL RAY: At the scapulohumeral articulation[6] (shoulder joint) by palpating the proximal head of the humerus and the glenoid fossa of the scapula.

BORDERS: *Distally*: Distal third of the scapula.

Proximally: Proximal third of the humerus.

FIG. 18.6 A, Positioning of the lateral projection of the shoulder joint. The limb is fully extended to avoid superimposition, and the unaffected limb is pulled caudally in line with the neck. **B,** Mediolateral image of the shoulder joint. (Courtesy Jennifer White, Mississauga Oakville Veterinary Emergency and Specialty Hospital, ON.)

Caudocranial View of the Shoulder—Routine

Positioning

Place in: Dorsal recumbency in a trough or with the use of tape/Velcro if needed. Foam pads can also be placed under the midthoracic and midabdominal regions.

Head and Neck: Push the head slightly laterally from the affected limb to avoid superimposition of the cervical spine over the joint. Support as needed.

Hindlimbs: Leave in a natural position and support with Velcro/sandbags if needed.

Forelimbs: Extend both forelimbs cranially.

Use sandbags or tie/tape the affected limb to the table, keeping the humerus almost parallel to the table (Fig. 18.7 A,B).

Comments and Tips

- The patient should be maintained in a true ventrodorsal position.
- The dog's or cat's body and ribs should fall slightly away from the scapula to avoid superimposition and keep the spine of the scapula perpendicular to the table.
- Overrotation of the humerus produces an oblique shoulder joint.
- If the joints need to be compared, both can be included and the beam centered between the joints. However, separate views may be required for broad-chested patients.
- Craniocaudal images (ancillary view), with the patient in dorsal recumbency and the limbs pulled caudally along the side of the thorax, can be taken to eliminate superimposition of the scapula over the cranial thorax.

MEASURE: At the level of the scapulohumeral articulation (shoulder joint).

Extend the calipers over the caudal cervical vertebral bodies, but do not include the opposite limb.

CENTRAL RAY: Palpate the proximal head of the humerus and the acromion of the scapula at the center of the scapulohumeral articulation (shoulder joint).

BORDERS: *Distally*: Distal third of the scapula. *Proximally*: proximal third of the humerus.

> **TECHNICIAN NOTES**   Using a modified abdomen technique chart for the scapula, shoulder, and humerus in film radiography may produce a more diagnostic image if the bone chart images are too dark and the thorax settings images are not dense enough.

FIG. 18.7 A, Positioning of the caudocranial shoulder joint. B, Caudocranial image of the shoulder joint.

Skyline (Cranioproximal-Craniodistal) View of the Shoulder for the Bicipital Groove—Ancillary

Positioning

To find calcified bodies in the bicep brachii or supraspinatus tendon,[2,5] the skyline view of the shoulder may be required with the patient in sternal recumbency.

Place In: Sternal recumbency

Head and Neck: Move the head and neck slightly away from the affected shoulder without any thorax rotation.

Place the head and neck on foam pads and place sandbags over the neck to maintain the position, taking care not to restrict breathing.

Hindlimbs: Leave in a natural position and support with sandbags if needed.

Forelimbs: Keep the unaffected limb in a fairly natural position with a sandbag.

Flex the elbow joint of the affected limb to project the flexed shoulder joint over the proximal third of the radius and ulna.

Place sandbags lateral to the limb to prevent adduction.

The film/screen cassette rests on the cranial surface of the antebrachium and is placed in the crook of the elbow joint. Use foam wedges to support cassette (Fig. 18.7C, D).

Comments and Tips

- The decreased source image distance (SID) will affect exposure factors.
- Most digital receptor (DR) panels are locked in place beneath the table, so this procedure is not feasible with digital units.

MEASURE AND CENTER: At the head of the humerus, palpating for the bicipital groove.

BORDERS: Proximal humerus with tight collimation.

C

D

FIG. 18.7, cont'd C, Skyline positioning for the bicipital groove with film cassette. D, Radiograph of the skyline view (cranioproximal-craniodistal) of the shoulder/proximal humerus to project the bicipital groove *(white arrows)*. *H,* Humeral head; *T,* greater tubercle). (**B,** Courtesy Jennifer White, Mississauga Oakville Veterinary Emergency and Specialty Hospital, ON; **D,** from Thrall DE. *Textbook of Veterinary Diagnostic Radiology.* 6th ed. St Louis: Elsevier; 2013.)

Humerus

Lateral (Mediolateral) View of the Humerus—Routine

Positioning
Place In: Lateral recumbency with the affected limb down.

Head and Neck: Position and support the head and neck upward with sandbags, taking care not to restrict breathing.

Hindlimbs: Leave in a natural position and support with Velcro/sandbags if needed.

Forelimbs: Extend and secure the contralateral limb caudally to avoid superimposition.

The affected limb should be extended downward and cranially.

Secure with a sandbag or tie (Fig. 18.8).

Comments and Tips
- Larger dogs may require two views if there is a significant difference in tissue density between the elbow and the shoulder. Measure each area separately.

MEASURE: Toward the proximal humerus at the level of the scapulohumeral articulation (shoulder joint).

CENTRAL RAY: Midshaft of the humerus.

BORDERS: *Proximal:* To shoulder. *Distal:* To elbow.

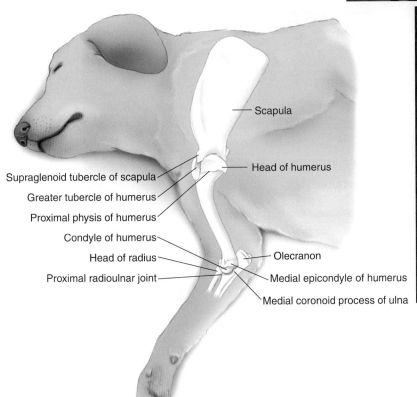

Scapula

Head of humerus

Supraglenoid tubercle of scapula

Greater tubercle of humerus

Proximal physis of humerus

Condyle of humerus

Head of radius

Proximal radioulnar joint

Olecranon

Medial epicondyle of humerus

Medial coronoid process of ulna

B

Anconeal process of ulna

Lateral coronoid process of ulna

FIG. 18.8 **A,** Positioning for the mediolateral (lateral) view of the humerus. **B,** Medial view of the right humerus. **C,** Mediolateral (lateral) image of the humerus. (**A,** Courtesy Seneca College of Applied Arts and Technology, King City, ON.)

Caudocranial View of the Humerus—Routine

Positioning

Place In: Dorsal recumbency in a trough or Velcro in position if needed.

Head and Neck: Keep the head and neck fairly parallel to the humerus.

Secure with a sandbag if needed, taking care not to restrict breathing.

Hindlimbs: Leave in a natural position so that the spine is perpendicular to the table. Support with sandbags or Velcro if needed.

Forelimbs: Tape/Velcro, extend and sandbag or tie both forelimbs cranially, especially the affected limb.

Keep the humerus almost parallel to the table (Fig. 18.9).

Comments and Tips

- Increased OFD will cause some distortion. To minimize, pull the limb as cranially and as close to the image receptor as possible.
- This positioning may not be tolerated by patients with fractures or severe degenerative joint disease. Consider using a horizontal beam if required in these situations.

MEASURE: Midshaft toward the proximal aspect; across at the level of T1.
CENTRAL RAY: Midshaft of the humerus.
BORDERS: *Proximal*: Include shoulder joint. *Distal*: Include elbow joint.

Scapula
Greater tubercle of humerus
Lesser tubercle of humerus
Deltoid tuberosity
Medial epicondyle of humerus
Supratrochlear foramen of humerus
Trochlea of humeral condyle
Lateral epicondyle of humerus
Medial coronoid process of ulna
Capitulum of humeral condyle
Ulna
Olecranon
Radius

B   C

FIG. 18.9 A, Positioning for the caudocranial view of the humerus. B, Caudal view of right canine humerus. C, Caudocranial image of the humerus. (B and C, From Thrall DE. *Textbook of Veterinary Diagnostic Radiology.* 7th ed. St. Louis: Elsevier; 2017.)

Caudocranial View of the Humerus—Routine—cont'd

Horizontal Beam of the Humerus—Ancillary

- The lateral decubitus view (caudocranial view with horizontal beam) may be useful for a compromised patient due to extensive trauma or other concerns.
- Center, measure, and include as for the caudocranial view.
- The affected limb will be placed uppermost on a large sponge and extended.

- The film-screen cassette is positioned against the cranial aspect of the affected forelimb.
- The tube head is directed horizontally from the caudal aspect of the limb and perpendicular to the humerus and image receptor.
- In cats, it may be difficult to place the cassette proximally enough to view the humeral head and the shoulder with a horizontal beam.

Craniocaudal View of the Humerus—Ancillary

Positioning

Place In: Dorsal recumbency in a trough or secured if needed.

Head and Neck: Keep the head and neck straight.

Secure with a sandbag if needed, taking care not to restrict breathing.

Hindlimbs: Leave in a natural position and support with sandbags if required.

Forelimbs: Extend both limbs caudally, being sure that the affected limb is flexed at the shoulder and pulled far enough caudally to keep the humerus parallel to the table. Tie to the table or carefully place a sandbag over the limbs (Fig. 18.10A).

Comments and Tips

- Use the craniocaudal view when adequate extension of postoperative patients cannot be achieved for the caudocranial view.
- The humerus in this position is more parallel to the table as compared to caudocranial view, but there is increased OFD.
- If the veterinarian suspects incomplete ossification of the humeral condyle, a CrCd is the best view, with a slight 15-degree craniomedial to caudolateral oblique.[2]
- Alternatively, the patient can be placed in sternal recumbency with the limbs pulled forward. Extend the affected limb (Fig. 18.10B).

MEASURE: Midshaft of the humerus toward the proximal aspect.

CENTRAL RAY: Midshaft of the humerus.

BORDERS: *Proximal:* Include shoulder joint. *Distal:* Include elbow joint.

> ✎ **TECHNICIAN NOTES** The lateral and caudocranial views of the scapula, shoulder, and humerus positioning procedures are all similar, with slight variations.

FIG. 18.10 A, Positioning for the craniocaudal view of the humerus in dorsal recumbency. B, Alternative positioning for the craniocaudal humerus view. (A/B, Courtesy Seneca College of Applied Arts and Technology, King City, ON.)

Elbow

Lateral (Mediolateral) View of the Elbow—Routine

The lateral view of the elbow joint can show a fragmented process.[7]

Positioning

Place In: Lateral recumbency with the affected limb down.

Head and Neck: Position dorsally, placing sandbags over the neck to keep in position, taking care not to restrict breathing.

Hindlimbs: Leave in a natural position and support with Velcro/sandbags if needed.

Forelimbs: Extend the contralateral limb caudally and secure with ties or sandbag.

Place the affected limb cranially and ventrally so that the degree of flexion is between 45 and 90 degrees, depending on veterinarian preference (Fig. 18.11).

Depending on the patient type, a small foam wedge can be placed under the metacarpus and/or the shoulder region.

Comments and Tips

- A small foam pad under the shoulder and distal region of the affected limb helps maintain lateral symmetry of the structures.
- Avoid rotation and superimposition of adjacent structures.
- A properly positioned elbow shows superimposition of the distal humeral condyles and a clear view of the olecranon.

MEASURE: Thickest part of the elbow at the distal humerus.

CENTRAL RAY: Palpate and center on the distal humeral condyles (elbow).

BORDERS: *Distal:* Distal third of the humerus.

Proximal: Proximal third of the radius/ulna.

FIG. 18.11 **A,** Positioning for the mediolateral (lateral) view of the elbow joint. **B,** Medial view of the elbow joint. **C,** Mediolateral (lateral) image of the elbow joint. (B and C, Courtesy Jennifer White, Mississauga Oakville Veterinary Emergency and Specialty Hospital, ON.)

Craniocaudal View of the Elbow—Routine

Positioning

Place In: Sternal recumbency.

Hindlimbs: Leave in a natural position to keep the spine straight and support with Velcro/sandbags if needed.

A V-trough may be used for stability of the caudal portion of the body.

Forelimbs: Extend both front legs forward.

Pull the unaffected limb, placing a small foam pad under the elbow to prevent rolling and rotation.

Extend the affected forelimb and secure it with Velcro/tape or a sandbag distally.

Head and Neck: Push away from the affected limb and the beam so they are not in the field of view.

Support the head at a natural height with foam pads.

Tape/Velcro can be placed around the head to keep it out of the field of view. (Fig. 18.12).

Comments and Tips

- Symmetry is essential.
- Move the patient's body slightly until palpation reveals the olecranon of the ulna to be in the center of the joint midway between the lateral and medial humeral epicondyles on the finished image.
- The slight raising of the opposite limb also helps place the olecranon between the humeral epicondyles. This keeps the radius and ulna parallel and the humerus at a slight angle to the tabletop.
- The paw of the affected limb will not be flat on the table in a true craniocaudal elbow view.
- A craniocaudal view can also be completed with the patient in dorsal recumbency and the affected limb pulled caudally.
- Keep the humerus parallel to the table.
- To prevent superimposition of the ribs, abduct the affected limb slightly away from the thorax.

MEASURE: Thickest part of the elbow at the distal humerus.

CENTRAL RAY: Palpate and center on the humeral condyles at the level of articulation. Angle the beam distoproximally 10 to 20 degrees to visualize the joint surfaces if full extension is not possible.

BORDERS: *Distal:* Distal third of the humerus.
Proximal: Proximal third of the radius/ulna.

> ✐ **TECHNICIAN NOTES** Remember when positioning for the contralateral view of the distal portion of the limb, the patient is usually lying in sternal recumbency.

Supratrochlear foramen of humerus

Lateral epicondyle of humerus

Head of radius

Medial epicondyle of humerus

FIG. 18.12 A, Positioning for the craniocaudal projection of the elbow joint. Putting a sponge under the opposite elbow and head helps keep the olecranon in true CrCd position. **B** and **C,** Cranial views of the right elbow. **D,** Craniocaudal image of the elbow joint.

Craniocaudal View of the Elbow—Routine—cont'd

C

D

FIG. 18.12, cont'd

Hyperflexed (Mediolateral) View of the Elbow—Ancillary

- Hyperflexion allows evaluation of the ulnar anconeal process. This view is indicated when an ununited anconeal process (failure of the anconeal process to unite with the ulna, resulting in a fracture through the growth plate), a fragmented coronoid, or osteochondrosis is suspected.
- Elbow dysplasia is seen primarily in young dogs of large breeds, causing varying degrees of weight-bearing lameness and arthritis.
- Extreme flexion of the medial to lateral view is required if images are being sent to the Orthopedic Foundation of Animals for elbow dysplasia evaluation.[8]

Positioning

Place In: Lateral recumbency with the affected limb down.
Head and Neck: Move dorsally, placing sandbags over the neck to keep in position.
Hindlimbs: Leave in a natural position and support with Velcro/sandbags if needed. (Fig. 18.13).

Forelimbs: Secure the unaffected limb caudodorsally.
Keep the carpus of the affected limb in a true lateral position as you move it toward the neck.
Flex the affected elbow as much as possible by bending the limb dorsally.
Secure the paw under the head with tape/Velcro placed on the lateral aspect of metacarpal region.
Affix to the table under the cranial cervical region.

Comments and Tips

- A sponge under the shoulder assists in preventing the flexed elbow from moving medially.
- The limb should be flat on the table in a true lateral position with no rotation.
- If the tape was secured on the medial aspect, upward rotation would occur, causing the site of interest to be oblique.
- The elbow is positioned directly over the center of the digital plate. Tight collimation is essential.

MEASURE: At the distal humerus with the elbow in the flexed position.
CENTRAL RAY: Palpate and center on the humeral condyles.
BORDERS: *Distal:* Distal third of the humerus.
Proximal: Proximal third of the radius/ulna.

TECHNICIAN NOTES   Flexion assists in full examination of the joint.

Hyperflexed (Mediolateral) View of the Elbow—Ancillary—cont'd

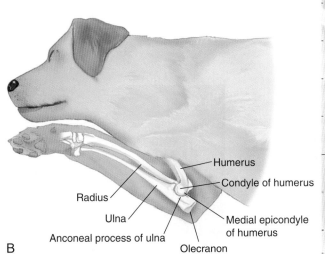

Humerus
Condyle of humerus
Radius
Ulna
Medial epicondyle
of humerus
Anconeal process of ulna
Olecranon
B

C

FIG. 18.13 A, Positioning for the mediolateral (lateral) flexed view of the elbow joint. B, Medial projection of the right flexed elbow. C, Mediolateral (lateral) image of the flexed elbow. (B and C, Courtesy Jennifer White, Mississauga Oakville Veterinary Emergency and Specialty Hospital, ON.)

Craniocaudal View with a Horizontal Beam of the Elbow—Ancillary

The CrCd elbow view could also be taken with a horizontal beam (lateral decubitus or CdCd view with horizontal beam) if required and if available:

- Measure, center, and include as for the craniocaudal view of the elbow joint.

- Place the patient in opposite lateral recumbency with the extended affected side uppermost, resting on a large sponge and the image receptor against the caudal aspect.
- The tube head is directed horizontally from the cranial aspect of the limb and perpendicular to the elbow and the image receptor. (Fig. 18.17 is an example of using the CrCd view with a horizontal beam for the radius/ulna.)
- Place the label on the lateral aspect.

Oblique View of the Elbow—Ancillary

An oblique view may be needed to properly visualize the supratrochlear foramen of the humerus and the anconeal and coronoid process of the ulna (Fig. 18.14).

Head, Neck, Hindlimbs: Support the patient and limb with foam pads and sandbags.

Front limbs: Pull and support the affected limb as cranial as possible and rotate the elbow joint:

- Laterally about 30 degrees for the medial oblique and to see the medial coronoid process (craniolateral-caudomedial oblique) view.

- Medially (toward the patient) about 30 degrees for the lateral oblique (craniomedial-caudolateral oblique) view.
- Include only the structures making up the articulation.

Comments and Tips

- To visualize increased joint space and to see the medial coronoid process, extend the limb and angle the x-ray beam 20 degrees craniodistal to caudoproximal.[5]

MEASURE, CENTRAL RAY, BORDERS:

- Measure, center, and include as for the craniocaudal view.

✎ TECHNICIAN NOTES For a true craniocaudal view, palpate the olecranon, making sure that it rests midway between the humeral epicondyles and is perpendicular to the central ray.

A

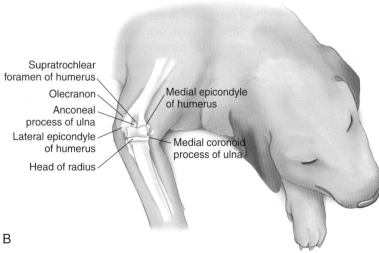

B

Supratrochlear foramen of humerus
Olecranon
Anconeal process of ulna
Lateral epicondyle of humerus
Head of radius
Medial epicondyle of humerus
Medial coronoid process of ulna

R

Olecranon

Sesamoid bone of supinator muscle (inconstant)

C

FIG. 18.14 A, Positioning for an oblique projection of the elbow joint. This is the craniolateral-caudomedial (medial) oblique position. Ideally, the limb should be pulled more cranially. B, Medial oblique view of the right elbow joint. C, Craniolateral-caudomedial (medial) oblique image of the right elbow. (B and C, Courtesy Jenn White, Mississauga Oakville Veterinary Emergency and Specialty Hospital, ON.)

Radius/Ulna

Lateral (Mediolateral) View of the Radius/Ulna—Routine

Positioning

Positioning is the same as for the lateral extended elbow view (Fig. 18.15):

Place In: Lateral recumbency with the affected limb down.

Head and Neck: Move the head and neck dorsally, placing sandbags over the neck to keep in position, taking care not to restrict breathing.

Hindlimbs: Leave in a natural position and support with sandbags if needed.

Forelimbs: Extend the contralateral limb caudodorsally securing with a sandbag or tying.

Place the affected limb parallel to the edges of the image receptor and support.

Slightly flex the carpus to avoid supination of the limb.

A small foam wedge placed under the metacarpal region or the shoulder region keeps a true lateral view of the elbow depending on the patient anatomy.

Comments and Tips

- Foam placed under the humerus and cranial thorax helps keep proper alignment.
- The image receptor must be large enough to include both the proximal row of carpal bones and the proximal olecranon.
- If the distal portion of the radius and ulna is the area of interest, measure at the midshaft of the bone to minimize overexposure.

A

MEASURE: Site of the distal humerus.
CENTRAL RAY: Midshaft of the radius and ulna.
BORDERS: *Proximal*: Include elbow joint.
Distal: Include carpal joint.

> ✏ **TECHNICIAN NOTES** Note the similarity in positioning for the elbow, radius and ulna, and foot.

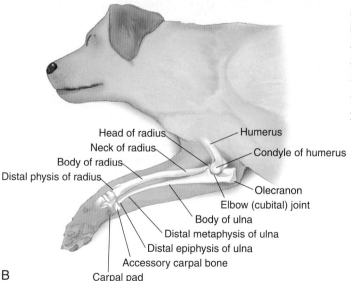

B

Head of radius
Neck of radius
Body of radius
Distal physis of radius
Humerus
Condyle of humerus
Olecranon
Elbow (cubital) joint
Body of ulna
Distal metaphysis of ulna
Distal epiphysis of ulna
Accessory carpal bone
Carpal pad

C

FIG. 18.15 A, Positioning for the mediolateral (lateral) projection of the radius and ulna. **B,** Medial view of the right radius and ulna. **C,** Mediolateral (lateral) image of the radius and ulna. (B and C, Courtesy Jennifer White, Mississauga Oakville Veterinary Emergency and Specialty Hospital, ON.).

Craniocaudal View of the Radius/Ulna—Routine

Positioning

Same as for the CrCd elbow view.

Place In: Sternal recumbency.

Head and Neck: Move away from the affected limb and beam. Support the head in a comfortable position with foam pads. Sandbags or Velcro/tape can keep the head out of the field of view.

Hindlimbs: Leave in a natural position to keep the spine straight and support with Velcro/sandbags if needed.

A V-trough may be used for stability of the caudal half of the body.

Forelimbs: Place a small foam pad under the elbow of the unaffected limb to prevent rolling or rotation.

Extend the affected forelimb and secure with a sandbag or tie to the table or to a sandbag (Fig 18.16).

Comments and Tips

- Palpate to confirm that the olecranon is positioned midway between the humeral epicondyles for a true CrCd view of the radius/ulna.
- A thin foam pad placed between the point of the elbow and the image receptor may stabilize the elbow.
- The image receptor must be long enough to incorporate the carpus, elbow, and radius/ulna.
- If the distal portion of the radius and ulna is the area of interest, measure at the midshaft of the bone to minimize overexposure.
- A CrCD view with horizontal beam (lateral decubitus) can also be taken for the radius and ulna (Fig. 18.17).

MEASURE: Site of the distal humerus.

CENTRAL RAY: Midshaft of the radius and ulna.

BORDERS: *Proximal:* Include elbow joint. *Distal:* Include carpal joint.

FIG. 18.16 A, Positioning for the craniocaudal view of the feline radius and ulna. Tape can be used to keep the head out of the field of view. B, Positioning for the craniocaudal view of the canine radius and ulna.

Craniocaudal View of the Radius/Ulna—Routine—cont'd

Lateral epicondyle of humerus
Elbow (cubital) joint
Head of radius
Medial epicondyle of humerus
Body of ulna
Body of radius
Distal metaphysis of radius
Distal epiphysis (styloid process) of ulna
Ulnar carpal bone
Intermedioradial carpal bone

C

Olecranon
Medial coronoid process of ulna
Sesamoid bone

D

FIG. 18.16, cont'd C, Cranial view of the right canine radius and ulna. D, Craniocaudal image of the right canine radius and ulna.

FIG. 18.17 Positioning for a Craniocaudal View of the Radius/Ulna Using a Horizontal Beam.

The Foot: Carpus, Metacarpus, and Digits

The carpus, metacarpus, and digits are typically radiographed in one view. If there is a particular area of interest, center and measure on this site. See Fig. 24.29C for anatomy of the carpal joints of various species.

> ✎ **TECHNICIAN NOTES** Use positioning aids strategically to give the patient the illusion that it is being held. A sandbag over the neck and limbs and/or the use of tape/Velcro is essential if the patient is not properly sedated. Speak to your patient in a calm, low voice and back away as the exposure is taken.

Lateral (Mediolateral) View of the Foot—Routine

Positioning

Place In: Lateral recumbency with the affected limb down.

Hindlimbs: Leave in a natural position and support with Velcro/sandbags if needed.

Head and Neck: Move the head and neck dorsally, placing sandbags over the neck to keep the position, taking care not to restrict breathing.

Forelimbs: Extend the contralateral limb caudally, and secure with Velcro sandbag.

Extend the affected limb cranially, placing sandbags on the proximal portion of the limb.

Tie or support the distal metacarpus to the table or a sandbag.

Radiographing the Digits: Separate the digits to prevent superimposition. This is best completed by:

- Separately taping/applying Velcro around the toenail of the lateral (fifth) phalanx and the medial (second) phalanx.

- Then pull the lateral phalanx slightly cranially and laterally, and the medial phalanx slightly caudally and laterally.

Tape/Velcro can also be put around the digit itself, and cotton or foam (manicuring pads) can be placed between the toes. The phalanges are not separated as effectively. (Fig. 18.18).

Comments and Tips

- A wooden or plastic paddle supported with a sandbag can assist in keeping the carpus straight (Fig. 18.18A).
- The foot can be flexed by applying slight dorsal pressure to the digits.

MEASURE, CENTER, BORDERS OF THE FOOT: **SEE BOX 18.2**

> ✎ **TECHNICIAN NOTE** The film cassette can be split to include both views on the image if the grid is not used. Point the toes in the same direction and collimate tightly. Place a lead shield on the side not being imaged to prevent scatter radiation from affecting the contrast. Splitting the detector is not possible in digital but tight collimation is essential

BOX 18.2	Measure, Center, Borders of the Foot

MEASURE: At the site of interest:
  Carpus: At the carpal joint.
  Metacarpus or Phalanges: At the site of the phalangeal-metacarpal articulation.
CENTRAL RAY: Centered on the area of interest:
  Carpus: Middle row of carpal bones.
  Metacarpus or Phalanges: Center of the phalangeal-metacarpal articulation.
BORDERS:
  Carpus: Distal third of the radius and ulna to proximal third of the metacarpus.
  Metacarpus or Phalanges: Carpus proximally to the distal phalanges.
LABEL
  Lateral: Cranial to the joint or bone.
  Orthogonal views: Lateral to the limb.

Lateral (Mediolateral) View of the Foot—Routine—cont'd

Distal epiphysis of radius

Antebrachial joint

Distal epiphysis (styloid process) of ulna

Accessory carpal bone

Ulnar carpal bone

Carpal pad

Proximal sesamoid of bone digit I

Pd of digit I

Dorsal sesamoid bone

FIG. 18.18 **A,** Positioning for the mediolateral (lateral) projection of the canine carpus, metacarpus, and digits. Tape can also be used to secure the limb. **B,** Medial view of canine carpus, metacarpus, and digits. **C,** Mediolateral (lateral) image of the canine, metacarpus, and digits. **D,** Flexed lateral image of the carpus when pressure is applied to the dorsal surface of the digits. (**B,** Courtesy Jennifer White, Mississauga Oakville Veterinary Emergency and Specialty Hospital, ON; **D,** Courtesy Rosedale Animal Hospital, Toronto, ON.)

Lateral (Mediolateral) Hyperextended View of the Foot—Ancillary

Hyperextended Lateral View of the Foot (Stressed View)[6]

- Position, measure, center and borders as for the mediolateral view.
- Keep the carpus in a true lateral projection.
- Hyperextend the carpus by bending the toes upward.

- Apply tape/Velcro at the radius and ulna, and secure to the table laterally (Fig. 18.19).
- Apply tape/Velcro at the distal metacarpus/digits; extend the limb and secure the tape/Velcro in the opposite direction of the tape on the radius/ulna.
- This view diagnoses joint involvement or lesions that might not be visible if the joint is not stressed.

FIG. 18.19 Positioning for the hyperextended lateral view of the carpus.

Lateral (Mediolateral) Hyperflexed View of the Carpus—Ancillary

Positioning

Place In: Lateral recumbency with the affected limb down.

Head and Neck: Move dorsally, placing sandbags over the neck to keep in position, taking care not to restrict breathing.

Hindlimbs: Leave in a natural position and support with Velcro/sandbags if needed.

Forelimbs: Extend the contralateral limb caudally, and secure with a sandbag or tie.

Extend the affected limb and hyperflex the carpus by either:
- Taping or using Velcro in a figure-eight pattern around the metacarpus and radius and ulna (best).

- Keeping the carpus flexed by (1) bending the toes caudally toward the radius and ulna, (2) applying pressure with a wooden or plastic paddle at the phalanges, and (3) securing with a sandbag. (Fig. 18.20).

Comments and Tips

- Do not extend the carpus beyond the patient's available range of motion.
- This position helps evaluate the carpal articulation when joint laxity is noted.

MEASURE: At the carpus joint while in the flexed position.

CENTRAL RAY: On the middle row of carpal bones.

BORDERS: Distal third of the radius/ulna to proximal third of the metacarpus, including the digits if needed.

FIG. 18.20 Positioning for the flexed mediolateral projection of the canine carpus, metacarpus, and digits.

Dorsopalmar View of the Foot—Routine

Positioning

Place In: Sternal recumbency.

Head and Neck: Extend and support the head laterally with foam pads, sandbags, or Velcro/tape away from the affected limb and the beam.

Hindlimbs: Extend in a natural position to keep the spine straight and support with Velcro/sandbags if needed.

A V-trough may be used for stability of the caudal half of the body.

Forelimbs: Extend both forward keeping the unaffected limb extended.

Sandbag/Velcro the affected forelimb proximally.

Tie the metacarpus/digits at the distal portion securing to the table or sandbag. (Fig. 18.21).

MEASURE, CENTER, BORDERS OF THE FOOT: **SEE BOX 18.2**

FIG. 18.21 A, Positioning for the dorsopalmar projection of the canine carpus, metacarpus, and digits. B, Dorsal view of the canine carpus, metacarpus, and digits. C, Dorsopalmar image of the canine carpus, metacarpus, and digits. (C, Courtesy Jennifer White, Mississauga Oakville Veterinary Emergency and Specialty Hospital, ON.)

Dorsopalmar View of the Foot—Routine—cont'd

Comments and Tips

- Abduct the affected elbow slightly to straighten the carpus.

Stress View:

- If joint laxity of the carpus is present and evaluation of the joint space is required:

- Apply stress to the carpus by securing tape/Velcro to the midradius/ulna and the distal metacarpus.
- Pull in opposite directions, as for the hyperextended lateral view of the carpus (Fig. 18.22).[7]

FIG. 18.22 Stress images of the carpus may be completed if joint laxity is to be determined. The position and pulling of the tape change where pressure is applied on the carpus: **A**, Medial stress; **B**, lateral stress.

Oblique Views of the Foot—Ancillary

The two oblique views of the foot are the dorsolateral palmaromedial oblique (DLPMO), the medial oblique view, and the dorsomedial palmarolateral oblique (DMPLO), the lateral oblique view.

Positioning

Place In: Sternal recumbency.
Head and Neck: Displace and support the head laterally, with foam pads, sandbags, or tape, away from the affected limb and beam.
Hindlimbs: Extend caudally in a natural position to keep the spine straight supporting with sandbags or Velcro if needed. A V-trough may be used for stability of the caudal half of the body.

Forelimbs: Extend both forward. Secure the affected distal metacarpus/digits and pull cranially.
- For the medial oblique view: rotate the elbow joint 45 degrees laterally and support it with tape and sandbag.
- For the lateral oblique view: rotate the elbow joint 45 degrees medially and support it with tape and sandbag.

Comments and Tips

- Rotate the elbow to allow the beam to enter the limb 45 degrees from the midsagittal plane either laterally or medially.

MEASURE, CENTER, BORDERS OF THE FOOT: **SEE BOX 18.2**
LATERAL OBLIQUE (PMDLO) VIEW: Center the beam 45 degrees medially from the midsagittal plane (Fig. 18.23).
MEDIAL OBLIQUE (PLDMO) VIEW: Center the beam 45 degrees laterally from the midsagittal plane (Fig 18.24).

Oblique Views of the Foot—Ancillary—cont'd

Radius

Ulna

Accessory carpal bone

Carpal pad

MCI

MCII

Pp of digit I

MCV

Pd of digit I

MCIV

MCIII

Pp of digit V

Pp of digit II

Pd of digit V

Pp of digit III

Pm of digit V

Pm of digit II

Pd of digit II

Pp of digit IV

Pm of digit III

Pm of digit IV

Pd of digit III

Pd of digit IV

FIG. 18.23 **A,** Positioning for the dorsomedial-palmarolateral oblique (DMPLO or lateral) projection of the canine metacarpus and digits with the digits separated. **B,** Dorsomedial-palmarolateral (lateral) oblique view of the canine carpus, metacarpus, and digits. **C,** Radiograph of the DMPLO projection of the canine metacarpus and digits.

Oblique Views of the Foot—Ancillary—cont'd

Ulna
Distal radioulnar joint
Accessory carpal bone
Ulnar carpal bone
CIV

Radius
Antebrachiocarpal joint
Radial carpal bone
Middle carpal joint
CI
CIII

B

FIG. 18.24 A, Positioning for dorsolateral-palmaromedial (DLPMO or medial) oblique image. **B,** Medial oblique radiographic anatomy of the canine carpus. **C,** Medial oblique image of the metacarpus and digits. (**A** and **B,** Courtesy Joshua Schlote, BS, LVT, Northeast Community College; **C** Courtesy Jennifer White, Mississauga Oakville Veterinary Emergency and Specialty Hospital, ON.)

Examples (Figs. 18.23 and 18.24)

> ✎ **TECHNICIAN NOTES** The beam is described
> as "point of entrance to point of exit." For the DLPMO,
> the beam enters dorsally on the lateral side and exits at
> the palmar aspect on the medial side. The "point of exit"
> is where the image receptor is placed, which in this case
> is on the palmar medial side. Because the beam does
> not exit perpendicular to the midline, the view is called
> *oblique*. In this case, it is a medial oblique because the
> beam exits medially. (This concept is further described in
> Chapter 24).

KEY POINTS

1. The patient will generally be in dorsal recumbency for the proximal limb (scapula, shoulder, and humerus) and in sternal recumbency for the distal limb (elbow, radius/ulna, and foot) when views perpendicular to the midsagittal plane are required.
2. Correct positioning and techniques are required for proper interpretation. This includes measuring, centering, inclusion, and proper symmetry.
3. The label is placed cranially for the lateral projections and laterally for the orthogonal projection.
4. Peripheral borders for joints are one-third of the bones proximal and distal to the joint. Borders for long bones include the proximal and distal joints.
5. Consider the patient when positioning and use good-quality radiographic techniques.
6. There is similarity in positioning, with slight variations, between the proximal views (scapula, shoulder, and humerus) and among the distal views (elbow, radius/ulna, and foot).

Fig. 18.25 is a mystery radiograph. Review it and answer the question presented with it.

REVIEW QUESTIONS

1. A lateral radius/ulna radiograph of a Doberman is required. The marker should be placed at the:
   a. Cranial radius/ulna
   b. Lateral radius/ulna
   c. Caudal radius/ulna
   d. Medial radius/ulna
2. You are to image the lateral shoulder joint of a feline patient. The field of view should include the:
   a. Shoulder joint only
   b. Distal third of the humerus and proximal third of the scapula
   c. Distal third of the scapula through the proximal third of the humerus
   d. Distal third of the humerus and proximal third of the scapula

FIG. 18.25 Mystery Radiograph. Identify the artifacts.

3. The veterinarian requests complete images of the shoulder joint of a 6-month-old Great Dane limping on its right side that worsens after exercise. He suspects osteochondrosis and wishes a lateral image to confirm. It is best to complete the position so that:
   a. The shoulder joint is not superimposed over the trachea
   b. There is no pronation or supination of the affected limb
   c. Only a right lateral is taken as the left lateral is not needed
   d. The left lateral is taken to see the magnified lesion on the right limb
4. The caudocranial scapula image of an Akita is best taken with the patient lying in:
   a. Dorsal recumbency
   b. Ventral recumbency
   c. A right lateral oblique position
   d. A left lateral oblique position
5. What is the primary disadvantage of the CrCd view of the humerus versus the CdCr view?
   a. The limb is positioned parallel to the image receptor.
   b. Superimposition over the ribs is likely.
   c. The limb must be abducted slightly from the thorax.
   d. Increased object-film distance can cause magnification.
6. The best views of routine elbow radiography of a Bichon Frise are the lateral and the:
   a. Caudocranial
   b. Craniocaudal
   c. Palmarodorsal
   d. Dorsopalmar

7. Proper symmetry for the elbow view of the Bichon Frise in the previous question requires:
   a. Slightly raising the opposite limb
   b. Keeping the opposite limb flat on the table
   c. Keeping the patient on its back
   d. Positioning and raising the head toward the affected limb

8. The best view for evaluation of the ulnar anconeal process of a Bernese Mountain Dog is a(an):
   a. Extended mediolateral view of the elbow
   b. Natural mediolateral view of the elbow
   c. Hyperflexed mediolateral view of the elbow
   d. Craniocaudal view of the radius/ulna

9. The peripheral borders of the ulnar anconeal process of the Bernese Mountain Dog elbow would be:
   a. Two-thirds of the bones distal and proximal
   b. The carpus and the shoulder joint
   c. Proximal third of the humerus and distal third of the radius/ulna
   d. Proximal third of the radius/ulna and distal third of the humerus

10. When radiographing either a lateral shoulder or humerus of a Boxer:
    a. Keep the head and limbs in as natural a position as possible
    b. Keep the patient in dorsal recumbency
    c. Raise the head and keep the affected and contralateral limbs in a natural position
    d. Raise the head and neck dorsally, and pull the affected limb cranially

11. Measure a craniocaudal view of the radius and ulna of a Retriever at the:
    a. Proximal radius
    b. Distal humerus
    c. Distal radius
    d. Elbow joint

12. The veterinarian requires an orthogonal view of a Retriever with a severe fracture of the right humerus showing thoracic pathology. If your unit allows, you are best to consider a:
    a. Caudocranial view with a vertical beam
    b. Right lateral decubitus view with a horizontal beam
    c. A horizontal beam with the patient lying on its left side
    d. A horizontal beam with the patient lying on its right side

13. The patient in the previous question requiring the orthogonal view of the humerus should be positioned:
    a. With the right limb uppermost on a large sponge
    b. With the right limb on the table on a small sponge
    c. In ventral recumbency
    d. In dorsal recumbency

14. Fractured toes are suspected in a German Shepherd. In a medial oblique view, center on the:
    a. Dorsomedial aspect and place the lateral side of toes against the image receptor
    b. Palmarolateral aspect and place the medial side of toes against the image receptor
    c. Palmaromedial aspect and place the lateral side of toes against the image receptor
    d. Dorsolateral aspect and place the medial side of toes against the image receptor

15. For the medial oblique view in the previous question, include:
    a. Radius ulna to the distal digits
    b. Metacarpus to the distal digits
    c. From the carpus to the distal digits
    d. First to fifth digits

16. To prevent superimposition of the scapula and ribs in the caudocranial scapula of a Borzoi:
    a. Rotate the patient's sternum from the scapula about 40 degrees
    b. Rotate the patient's sternum from the scapula about 10 to 12 degrees
    c. Have the scapula perpendicular to the table and parallel to the sternum
    d. Have the forelimbs pulled caudally and separate the affected limb from the body

Chapter Review Question answers are located in the Instructor Resources on Evolve and can be provided to students at the discretion of the instructor.

References

1. Holloway A, McConnell F. *BSAVA Manual of Canine and Feline Radiography and Radiology: A Foundation Manual.* Suffolk: BSAVA; 2013: [Chapter 7].
2. Thrall DE. *Textbook of Veterinary Diagnostic Radiology.* 7th ed. St. Louis: Elsevier; 2017.
3. Aspinall V, Cappello M. *Introduction to Veterinary Anatomy.* London: Butterman-Heineman; 2009.
4. Mauragis D, Berry C, Clifford R. Small animal radiography of the scapula, shoulder and humerus. *Today's Veterinary Practice.* May/June 2012, p 46-51.
5. Muhlbauer MC, Kneller SK. *Radiography of the Dog and Cat: Guide to Making and Interpreting Radiographs.* Oxford: Wiley-Blackwell; 2013: [Chapter 2].
6. Sirois M, Anthony E, Mauragis D. *Handbook of Radiographic Positioning for Veterinary Technicians.* Clifton Park, NY: Delmar Cengage Learning; 2010.
7. Han C, Hurd C. *Practical Diagnostic Imaging for the Veterinary Technician.* 3rd ed. St. Louis: Mosby; 2005.
8. Orthopedic Foundation for Animals. Application for Hip/Elbow Dysplasia Database; 2016. http://www.offa.org/pdf/hdedapp_bw.pdf.

Bibliography

Ayers S. *Small Animal Radiographic Techniques and Positioning.* Oxford: Wiley-Blackwell; 2013.
Colville T, Bassert J. *Clinical Anatomy and Physiology for Veterinary Technicians.* 3rd ed. St. Louis: Mosby; 2016.
Done SH, Goody PC, Evans SA, Stickland NC. *Color Atlas of Veterinary Anatomy, the Dog and Cat.* London: Mosby; 2009.
Evans H, de Launta A. *Guide to the Dissection of the Dog.* 8th ed. St. Louis: Saunders; 2017.
Holloway A. *BSAVA Manual of Canine and Feline Radiography and Radiology: A Foundation Manual.* Suffolk: BSAVA; 2014.
Singh B. *Dyce, Sack and Wensing's Textbook of Veterinary Anatomy.* 5th ed. St Louis: Elsevier; 2018.
Sirois M, Schlote J. *Diagnostic Imaging for Veterinary Technicians.* Minneapolis MN: Bluedoor, LLC; 2017.
Tighe M, Brown M. *Mosby's Comprehensive Review for Veterinary Technicians.* 5th ed. St. Louis: Mosby; 2019.

CHAPTER 19

Small Animal Pelvis and Pelvic Limb

Marg Brown, RVT, BEd Ad Ed

Animals when in company walk in a proper and sensible manner, in single file, instead of sprawling all across the road and being of no use or support to each other in case of sudden trouble or danger.

—Kenneth Grahame, author of *The Wind in the Willows*, 1859–1932

OUTLINE

LEARNING OBJECTIVES

When you have finished this chapter, you will be able to:

1. Properly and safely position a dog or cat for the various common positions of the pelvic limb with an emphasis on non-manual restraint.
2. Correctly measure and center the patient to include the peripheral borders.
3. Ensure that the body part is parallel to the image receptor and the central ray is perpendicular to the field of view (FOV) and receptor.
4. Identify views that may need to be completed as an alternative.
5. Identify normal anatomy of the pelvis and hindlimb found on an image.

KEY TERMS

Abduction
Axial rotation
Cavitation
Congruence
Degenerative joint disease
Distraction index
Dysplasia
Frog-leg VD
Hip dysplasia
Laxity
Legg-Calve-Perthes (LCP) disease
Luxation
PennHIP
Positional terminology
Stance phase
Subluxation
Ventrodorsal extended leg view, OFA

TECHNICAL NOTE: To preserve space, the images presented in this chapter do not show collimation. For safety, always collimate so that the beam is limited to within the image receptor edges. In film radiography, there should be a clear border of collimation (frame) on every radiograph. In some jurisdictions, evidence of collimation is required by law. In digital imaging, the algorithm depends on proper collimation.

Overview

Please review Chapter 18 for radiographic and patient concerns common to the pectoral and pelvic limbs because the same principles of proper imaging apply. See Fig. 18.1 and Box 18.1 for terms relating to radiographic anatomy associated with bones.

Imaging of the pelvis is generally performed to evaluate dysplastic or degenerative changes of the coxofemoral joints (Box 19.1). Fractures, joint-associated neoplasia, and arthritis are further reasons for radiographing not only the pelvis but also the femur, stifle, tarsus, metatarsus, and phalanges, which make up the remaining portion of the hindlimb of the appendicular skeleton.

A perpendicular view of the pelvis and pelvic limbs is required in addition to the lateral (L) view (Table 19.1). The general rule for both pectoral and pelvic limbs is to have the patient in:

- Dorsal recumbency for the proximal portion of the pelvis and limb (pelvis and femur) (Fig. 19.1)

BOX 19.1 | Normal Coxofemoral Anatomy

Breed variations must be kept in mind, but generally:
- The cranial third of each coxofemoral joint space is equal in width.
- At least half of the femoral head should be positioned within the acetabulum.
- The angle of the femoral neck should be about 130 degrees.
- Femoral heads should be rounded and smooth; the fovea capitis is a normal flattened area on the femoral head.
- The femoral neck should be smooth, with no proliferative remodeling changes.

- Sternal recumbency for the distal portion (stifle, tibia/fibula, tarsus, metatarsus, and digits) (Fig. 19.2)
- Keeping this positioning in mind, it is easy to remember the proper names for routine orthogonal views:
- The patient is in dorsal recumbency for views of the pelvis and femur:
  - This is the ventrodorsal (VD) view for the pelvis.
  - The femur in dorsal recumbency is termed craniocaudal (CrCd).
- The patient is in sternal recumbency for views of the limb distal to and including the stifle:
  - The stifle, tibia, and fibula are referred to as caudocranial (CdCr).
  - Views distal to and including the tarsus are plantarodorsal (PlD/PD).
- The Orthopedic Foundation of Animals (OFA) requires that for submissions, "image contrast should be such that the microtrabecular pattern of the femoral head and neck are readily seen. The dorsal-lateral margin of the acetabulum must also be visible."[1]
- Most canine pelvis film radiographs require a grid because of the greater thickness. Similar to the pectoral limb, a grid is not generally used because the tissue thickness is usually less than 10 cm. Grids may or may not be incorporated into digital units and their technique charts.
- Review the suggestions in Chapter 15 on techniques that can be used to assist in obtaining high-quality radiographs with the use of non-manual restraint, including sandbags, tape, soft Velcro strapping, rope, etc. Try to give your patient the illusion it is being held without actually holding. Analgesia and chemical restraint are highly recommended.

TABLE 19.1 | Protocol for the Pelvis and Pelvic Limb Radiography

ANATOMICAL LOCATION	ROUTINE VIEWS	PATIENT RECUMBENCY	ANCILLARY VIEWS	PATIENT RECUMBENCY
Pelvis	Lateral, Ventrodorsal extended -Leg	Lateral, Dorsal	Ventrodorsal: frog-leg	Dorsal
			PennHIP*: compression, distraction	Dorsal
Femur	Lateral, Craniocaudal	Lateral, Dorsal	Caudocranial	Lateral–horizontal beam
Stifle	Lateral, Caudocranial	Lateral, Sternal	Craniocaudal	Dorsal
			Proximodistal (skyline)	-Sternal -Lateral–horizontal beam
Tibia/fibula	Lateral, Caudocranial	Lateral, Sternal		
Foot: tarsus, metatarsus, and digits	Lateral, Plantarodorsal	Lateral, Sternal	Flexed and extended lateral	Lateral
			Dorsoplantar Flexed Dorsoplantar	Dorsal
			Obliques	Sternal/Dorsal

*Requires certification and training.

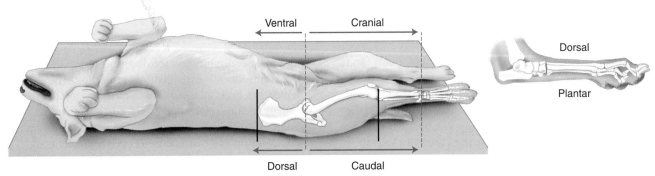

FIG. 19.1 Patient in dorsal recumbency (VD) for the proximal portion of the orthogonal image of the pelvis, acetabulum, and femur (within the black lines). In this position, the projection for the pelvis is ventrodorsal (VD) and craniocaudal (CrCd) for the femur. The VD position is less used for views of and distal to the stifle due to increased magnification. Terminology for anatomy distal to and including the tarsus is dorsoplantar (DPl/DP).

FIG. 19.2 The patient is generally in sternal recumbency (DV) for positioning of the distal rear limbs—stifle, tibia, fibula, tarsus, metatarsus, and digits (within black lines). Terminology changes to plantarodorsal (PlD/PD) at and distal to the tarsus. In this position, the femur, stifle and tibia/fibula are termed caudocranial (CdCr). This DV position is not used for the pelvis and femurs.

TECHNICIAN NOTES For high-quality orthopedic radiographs:
- Low kV and high mAs technique
- Tabletop technique except for the pelvis and proximal limb of large dogs
- Small focal spot
- Measure at the thickest part of the area to be radiographed
- Measure the patient in the position in which it is to be imaged
- Minimize object-film distance (OFD)
- Center at the area of interest: either the center of the bone or at the joint
- Collimate and include only what is required—full bone to the joints or one-third of bones proximal and distal for the joints
- Keep the bone parallel to the image receptor
- Keep the central ray perpendicular to the bone and image receptor
- Ensure there is no lateral rotation of the pelvis
- Minimize superimposed structures
- Label correctly
- Place the label at the dorsal/cranial limb for the lateral views and laterally for orthogonal views
- Obtain required views
- Radiograph the contralateral limb for comparison when required

TECHNICIAN NOTES Proper terminology will be easier to remember if you mentally place the patient in dorsal recumbency for the proximal portion and in sternal recumbency for the distal portion of the limb.

For long bones, the field of view includes the joints proximal and distal.

For joints, the field of view includes one-third each of the bones proximal and distal.

Pelvis

- The pelvis consists of paired ilia, acetabula, pubis, and ischia.
- The ventrodorsal extended-leg (hip-extended) and lateral views are the standard positions used to evaluate the small-animal pelvis. The frog-leg VD position can be used when it is too painful for the patient to tolerate a ventrodorsal extended-leg radiograph or for assessing the coxofemoral joint if there is suspicion of capital physeal or femoral neck fracture.[2]

- The most common view for diagnosis of hip dysplasia is the ventrodorsal extended-leg projection (Box 19.2), which has been adopted for coxofemoral joint certification by the OFA (Orthopedic Foundation of Animals). In addition to this view, PennHIP evaluation also requires compression and distraction VD pelvis projections.

> ✎ **TECHNICIAN NOTES** Have the thickest part of the pelvis toward the cathode to take advantage of the heel effect.

Lateral View of the Pelvis—Routine

Positioning

Place In: Lateral recumbency with the affected area down (Fig. 19.3).

Head: Keep in a natural position and, if needed, support appropriately with a sandbag over the neck, being careful not to restrict breathing.

Forelimbs: Pull the forelimbs cranially, and secure with a sandbag, or Velcro to the table.

Hindlimbs: Slightly scissor the limbs so that the limb closest to the receptor is in a neutral position, pulled slightly cranially.

Flex the stifle naturally as if the patient was standing.

Pull the upper limb caudally enough to differentiate between the femurs.

Place a foam pad under the uppermost stifle to keep the femur parallel to the table and the tuber ischii superimposed (Fig. 19.3B) and parallel.

Place sandbags or secure over the distal portion of the limbs to keep them in place.

Comments and Tips

- Keep the chest and abdomen in a true lateral position using positioning wedges as needed.
- For true pelvic symmetry on the image: the femoral heads, the iliac wings, and the transverse processes of the caudal lumbar vertebrae are respectively superimposed.
- The uppermost limb will be more magnified because of increased OFD (Fig. 19.3D).
- Separation of the limbs is particularly important if hip luxation is suspected.
- A lateral oblique view may be required to visualize the hip joints without superimposition. If the machine allows, the patient is positioned the same way and the x-ray tube head is angled cranially about 20 degrees to separate the hip joints on the image.[3] Alternatively, the patient can be slightly rotated if the tube head remains stationary at 90 degrees.

MEASURE: At the level of the trochanter or the thickest part.

CENTRAL RAY: Greater trochanter of the femur.

BORDERS: *Cranially*: Wing of the ilium to include at least one lumbar vertebra.
Caudally: Caudal ischium.
Dorsally: To dorsum.
Ventrally: One-third of the femur.

> ✎ **TECHNICIAN NOTES** Remember to go through your mental checklist before pushing the exposure button: settings correct; image receptor/machine/grid in position; proper location of markers and ID (if using at this stage); correct body part and view; properly centered; borders correct and collimated; patient properly prepared, positioned, and restrained so that the pelvis or limb being imaged is perpendicular to the beam and parallel to the image receptor.

BOX 19.2	Radiographic Signs of Hip Dysplasia as Evidenced on a Standard Ventrodorsal Extended-Leg View

- Subluxation or luxation occurs.
- There is increased width of the joint space (only cranial portion is evaluated).
- A shallow acetabulum is noted.
- Secondary degenerative joint disease is noted:
- There is subchondral bone sclerosis and/or exostosis on the rim of the acetabulum (specifically, the dorsal cranial margin).

- Proliferative remodeling degenerative changes can be seen on the femoral neck at the site of the joint capsule attachment.
- The angle of the femoral neck is less than 130 degrees (coxa vara) or more than 130 degrees (coxa valga).

Lateral View of the Pelvis—Routine—cont'd

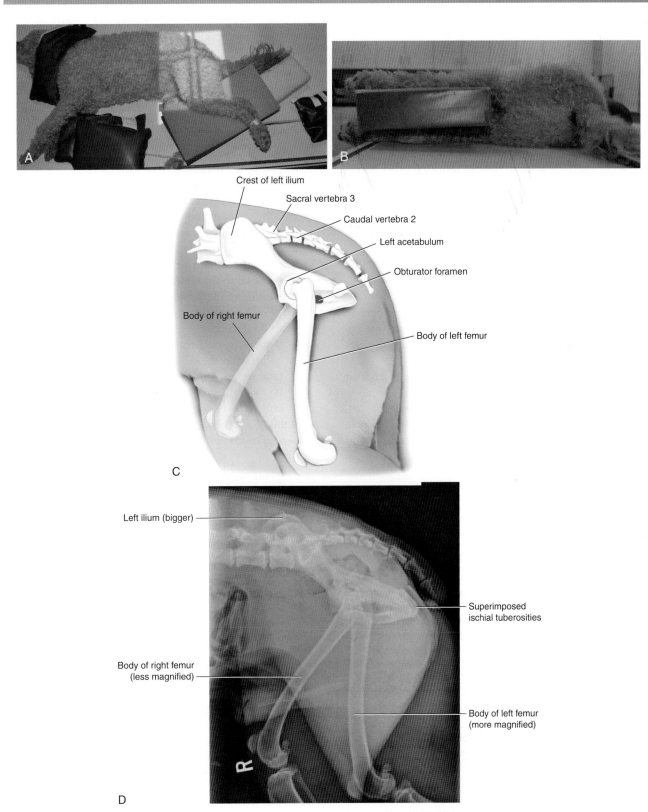

FIG. 19.3 **A,** Positioning for the canine lateral pelvis projection with the femurs slightly scissored. **B,** Make sure to place a foam wedge between the limbs to correct any rotation of the pelvis, to keep the wings of the ilia and the tuber ischii superimposed, and the femurs parallel to the table. **C,** Lateral terminology of the pelvis. **D,** Radiograph of the right canine lateral pelvis. (**A** and **B,** Courtesy Seneca College, King City, ON; **D,** Courtesy Jennifer White, Mississauga Oakville Veterinary Emergency and Specialty Hospital, ON.)

Ventrodorsal Extended-Leg View of the Pelvis—Routine

Positioning

Place In: Dorsal recumbency.

A V-trough can be used for the cranial portion of the body.

Head: Point forward and secure with a sandbag over the neck if needed, being careful not to restrict breathing.

Forelimbs: Pull the forelimbs cranially and secure with a sandbag, or Velcro/tie to the table.

Hindlimbs: The hindlimbs should be positioned as follows:

- Stand behind the patient and grasp each hindlimb at the level of the metatarsus so thumbs face each other on the medial aspect of the patient's limb.
- Rotate the femurs inward so that the patellae are centered over the trochlear groove of the stifle—the femurs are parallel to each other and the long axis of the spine and are level with the table.
- A second person places a piece of tape under both stifles long enough to overlap on the lateral aspect of the opposite femurs as the femurs are rotated.
- Take each end of the tape and forcibly pull to the opposite limb at the level of the proximal stifle to ensure that the femurs are maintained in a medial rotation when they are released.
- Additional tape can be placed around the pelvis just cranial to the acetabulae if needed.
  - Slowly lower the limbs until a point of resistance is felt. Place a pad underneath the tarsus to maintain this level.
  - Each limb can be individually taped at the metatarsus and secured to the table so that the digits of each limb are even.

- Place a sandbag over the distal portion of the limbs to further keep them parallel with the table (Fig. 19.4).

Comments and Tips

- Sedation or anesthesia that permits muscle relaxation is required for proper positioning.
- Label appropriately. A positional marker should be included and placed at the cranial aspect of the pelvis.
- If the pelvis is included in the V-trough, there will be magnification because of increased OFD.
- To minimize any rotation of the body, make sure the nose is equidistant between the forelimbs and in line with the tail. The sternum and vertebrae are superimposed.
- Keep the tail aligned with the spine—there should be one line from nose to tail.
- Palpate the greater trochanter of each femur, making sure each is level to the table.
- Any tilting of the pelvis will alter the perceived size and shape of the obturator foramina, iliac wings, and sacroiliac joints on the image.
  - If there is axial rotation, the side of the pelvis that is closest to the table will show the smaller obturator foramen and the larger iliac wing.
  - If one of the limbs appears shorter than the other, this limb is raised slightly and is not parallel to the table.
- If this view is needed for an injury or suspected fractures, be very cautious with internal rotation and caudal traction.

MEASURE: Thickest part of the pelvis.

CENTRAL RAY: Midline between the ischial tuberosities.

BORDERS: The tip of iliac wings (last two lumbar vertebrae) to the distal patella.

🖉 **TECHNICIAN NOTES** It is important to snugly secure the tape around the proximal stifles for the ventrodorsal extended-leg view so that the femurs are parallel to each other and the patellae appear superimposed over the centers of the femoral condyles. It is better to err on the side of having the tape too snug. Heavy sedation or general anesthesia is required.

🖉 **TECHNICIAN NOTES** Axial rotation causes the side of the pelvis closest to the table to show a smaller obturator foramen and a larger iliac wing. If the image shows that the obturator foramina are of unequal size, for the subsequent image, slightly lower the side of the pelvis that has the larger circular obturator foramen (big is up) for the next image. This repositioning will result in the truer oval shape of each obturator foramen

If one of the limbs appears shorter than the other, slightly lower this limb and make sure it is parallel to the table for the next image.

🖉 **TECHNICIAN NOTES** To properly evaluate the VD extended-leg pelvis image, make sure that:

- The radiograph is legally labeled, and positioning markers are included.
- The entire pelvis, femurs, and stifles are included.
- The femurs are extended, parallel to each other and to the ilia.
- The patellae are superimposed on the midline of each femur and positioned over the centers of the femoral condyles.
- There is no rotation—the wings of the ilia, the sacroiliac joints, and the obturator foramina are all equal in size and mirror images of each other.

Ventrodorsal Extended-Leg View of the Pelvis—Routine—cont'd

Right sacroiliac joint

Sacral vertebra 2

Caudal vertebra 1

Fovea capitis of right femur

Acetabulum

Right obturator foramen

Right ischial tuberosity

Right femur

Crest of left ilium

Wing of left ilium

Body of left ilium

Head of left femur

Greater trochanter of femur

Body of left pubis

Left ischium

B

FIG. 19.4 A, Positioning for the canine ventrodorsal extended-leg projection. Secure tape over the distal femurs. In addition, tape/Velcro can be placed around the metatarsus and pulled caudally to keep the limbs as parallel to the table as possible. With enough support in the sandbag, tape may not be necessary. **B,** Ventral view of the canine pelvis. **C,** Radiograph of a standard ventrodorsal extended-leg projection. Note that the femurs are parallel to each other; the patellae are positioned over the center of the femoral condyles; there is no rotation; and the entire pelvis, femurs, and stifles are included. (**C,** Courtesy GK Smith, DVM, and Mandy Wallace, DVM, Veterinary School of the University of Pennsylvania.)

Ventrodorsal Frog-Leg View of the Pelvis—Ancillary

Positioning

Place In: Dorsal recumbency. A V-trough can be used for the cranial portion of the body but avoid including the pelvis to prevent increased OFD.

Keep sternum and spine superimposed.

Head: Keep in a natural position with the nose pointing forward.

If needed, support appropriately with a sandbag over the neck, being careful not to restrict breathing.

Forelimbs: Pull the forelimbs cranially and secure with a sandbag or tie to the table.

Hindlimbs: Leave the hindlimbs in a naturally flexed position.

For most patients, the femur is positioned at 45 degrees to the spine. In some larger dogs, the femur may be 90 degrees to the spine.

Place a sandbag over the tarsal joints (Fig. 19.5).

Comments and Tips

- Keep the limbs positioned identically to maintain symmetry.
- Locate the ischium by palpating for the right and left ischial tuberosity.
- This view is used in case of injury or for assessing acetabular depth and coxofemoral fit.[4]
- If the acetabular rim and femoral head are of interest, tilt the pelvis slightly toward the affected side, keeping the unaffected limb out of the field of view.[4,5]

MEASURE: Thickest part of the pelvis or over acetabulum.

CENTRAL RAY: Midline at the caudal portion of the pubis.

BORDERS: The wings of the ilia to the caudal border of the ischium. Include at least one-third of each femur.

FIG. 19.5 A, Positioning for the canine ventrodorsal frog-leg pelvis projection. B, Ventral view of the canine pelvis in a frog-leg position. C, Radiograph of the canine ventrodorsal frog-leg pelvis. (C, Courtesy Jennifer White, Mississauga Oakville Veterinary Emergency and Specialty Hospital, ON.)

OFA Evaluation of Hip Dysplasia

Hip dysplasia is the abnormal development of the femoral joint that results from a lack of conformity between the acetabulum and the femoral head. Hip dysplasia is a heritable disease manifested as hip joint laxity that leads to the development of osteoarthritis (OA). This polygenic and multifactorial disease is the most commonly inherited orthopedic disease in dogs. All breeds are affected, and in some cases more than 50% of the breed has canine hip dysplasia (CHD).

If exact duplicates are required for film radiography, two films can be placed in the cassette and the mAs increased. However, for optimum film quality, it is still best to take two separate exposures.

In order for film radiographs to be eligible for OFA registration, there must be permanent patient identification on the film emulsion, which could include use of lead letters, radiopaque tape/label holder, or darkroom imprinter. The information required is the hospital or veterinarian's name, the date the radiograph was taken, and the registered name or number of the patient. Digital radiographs already include all the identifying information through Digital Imaging and Communications in Medicine (DICOM) standards.

Only dogs that are 24 months of age to the day or older at the time of radiography can qualify for an OFA hip number. A consultation report can be issued for younger dogs, but the hips are not certifiable.

OFA recommends that the patient be in good physical condition with radiographs taken at least 1 month after weaning puppies or before or after a heat cycle, due to hormonal variations that may cause increased joint laxity.[1]

Three board-certified radiologists independently evaluate the phenotype of the hips on a standard ventrodorsal extended-leg view. The radiograph is reviewed, and a report verifies the abnormal radiographic findings if radiographs reveal borderline, mild, moderate, or severe hip dysplasia grades.

The seven possible categories are normal (excellent, good, fair), borderline, and dysplastic (mild, moderate, severe).[1] Excellent, good, and fair hip grades are within normal limits and are given OFA numbers. This information is in the public domain and is accepted by the American Kennel Club and the Canadian Kennel Club for dogs with permanent identification (tattoo, microchip). Dysplastic hip grades are not in the public domain, unless the owner has chosen the open database.

Alternative authorized identification, further information, and forms can be found on the OFA's website (https://www.ofa.org/diseases/hip-dysplasia).

Other hip registries are maintained by the Fédération Cynologique Internationale (FCI; European) in which the Norbert angle is used; British Veterinary Association/Kennel Club (BVA/KC; Britain, Ireland, Australia, and New Zealand), and the Verein für Deutsche Schäferhunde (SV; Germany); each has its own grading system.[1,4]

Toy and small breeds 12 months of age or older can register with the Legg-Calve-Perthes database. Legg-Calve-Perthes (LCP) disease is a disorder of hip joint conformation most often seen in the miniature and toy breeds between the ages of 4 months and 1 year. Because there is a genetic component, it is recommended that dogs affected with LCP not be used in breeding programs.[1]

> ✎ **TECHNICIAN NOTES** Patients must be a minimum of 24 months of age to receive OFA hip registration and 16 weeks for PennHIP certification.

PennHIP Radiographs of the Pelvis—Ancillary

The ventrodorsal extended-leg view has been shown to tighten the joint capsule and the surrounding soft tissue, an effect that may mask evidence of joint laxity in mild-to-moderate hip dysplasia.[6] This finding has led to greater attention to dynamic pelvic radiographic studies such as was developed by the University of Pennsylvania School of Veterinary Medicine's Hip Improvement Program (PennHIP) to document the degree of laxity in coxofemoral joints.[2,7,8]

PennHIP is a radiographic screening method that quantitatively measures canine hip joint laxity through the use of stress radiographs to determine how likely a dog is to develop CHD and hip arthritis later in life.[9,10] The PennHIP method of evaluation is more accurate than the current standard in its ability to predict the onset of OA.[7,8,10] OA, also known as degenerative joint disease (DJD), is the hallmark of hip dysplasia.

For quality assurance of the submissions to the database, veterinarians are required to be trained and certified. Qualified technical personnel are allowed to accompany the veterinarian to the training seminars or to take online seminars and, like the veterinarian, may become certified to perform the procedure. Alternatively, a PennHIP-certified veterinarian may train technical staff in his or her practice, who may then complete quality assurance radiographs for the certification process (Fig. 19.6).[10] At the time of writing, on-line certification is free for qualified individuals. Conventional and digital PennHIP images are submitted for evaluation and for storage in an ever-expanding database that collects information on the etiology, prediction, and genetic basis of CHD.

Dogs can be screened using PennHIP as early as 16 weeks of age, which can assist breeders, service or working dog organizations, and veterinarians to recommend appropriate strategies such as diet, medication, or activities to delay or minimize the disease.

The degree of laxity in an individual dog is ranked relative to others of the same breed, which allows the animals that have tighter hips within each breed to be identified and to be considered suitable for breeding.

A distraction index (DI) ranging from 0 to 1 compares the amount of laxity in each hip between the compression and distraction radiographs. The closer the DI is to 0, the less joint laxity is present and the less likelihood for predisposition to DJD or OA. Hips scoring close to 1 are considered to be very loose and thus highly likely to develop hip dysplasia. Average DI does vary by breed. Dogs with hip laxity less than the respective breed average are considered appropriate for

FIG. 19.6 A, Radiograph of a ventrodorsal extended-leg projection with an Orthopedic Foundation of Animals (OFA) rating of "good." **B,** Radiograph of a PennHIP distraction projection of the same dog with an index of 0.92 shows marked laxity that is not evident on the ventrodorsal extended-leg view. The dark lines are normal and caused by the air between the foam and acrylic rods. **C,** Radiograph of a PennHIP compression view of the same patient. (Courtesy GK Smith, DVM, and Mandy Wallace, DVM, Veterinary School of the University of Pennsylvania.)

breeding. Generally, dogs with DI values less than 0.3 have very low "risk" for development of OA later in life.[9,10] Conversely, there is a direct relation when the DI is greater than 0.3 in breeds such as German Shepherds or greater than 0.4 for Labrador Retrievers and Rottweilers.[2]

Because the dog is anesthetized or deeply sedated and is not weight bearing, the laxity as determined by the DI is actually passive hip laxity as opposed to functional hip laxity, which to date is not measurable.[9]

PennHIP recommends waiting 8 weeks post lactation or 16 weeks post whelping before a PennHIP evaluation, due to relaxin and prolactin hormones possibly increasing hip laxity. The rise in hormone levels during the female heat cycle does not affect hip laxity as measured by PennHIP.[9,10]

Information regarding radiographic requirements for PennHIP can be found at https://antechimagingservices .com/antechweb/pennhip.

Other radiographic stress techniques described in the literature do not require certification, such as the ventrodorsal view with limbs extended using fulcrum positioning and the ventrodorsal view with limbs flexed for the distraction positioning.[2,4] These are not discussed in this chapter.

Radiographs

Three radiographs are part of the PennHIP evaluation.

Ventrodorsal Extended-Leg View of the Pelvis

The first required image is the standard ventrodorsal extended-leg view, which has been described. The ventrodorsal extended-leg view is made so that secondary signs of hip dysplasia such as DJD and existence of OA of the hip joint can be evaluated.

Distraction View of the Pelvis

The second required submission is the distraction view, which requires specialized acrylic distractor rods to be placed between the hindlimbs at the femoral heads (Figs. 19.6B and 19.7). The rods act as a fulcrum at the proximal femurs to lateralize the femoral heads when a small adduction force is applied, creating maximum lateral displacement of femoral heads.

Position the patient in dorsal recumbency. Keep the limbs in a neutral stance such that the femurs are positioned between 10 degrees of flexion and 30 degrees of extension, 10 to 30 degrees of abduction, and 0 to 10 degrees of external rotation.[4] This neutral position avoids the main disadvantage

FIG. 19.7 Positioning for the PennHIP Distraction View, Utilizing Distractor Rods with the Limbs in a Natural Stance.

of the extended hip projection, which is the spiral tensioning of the joint capsule that forces the femoral head into the acetabulum, reducing subluxation.[2]

This position is optimal for the measurement of hip joint laxity, which is the primary risk factor that predicts the development of DJD.

Cavitation occurs infrequently when the distractor device imposes a lateral distractive force on the hips, creating negative pressure that causes a void to form in the synovial fluid, shown as an air bubble. Cavitation is not painful and does not cause short- or long-term damage to the joint. It resolves within 24 hours, and then the distraction image can be repeated. If cavitation occurs, that particular hip joint (if unilateral cavitation) or both (bilateral) cannot be evaluated.

Compression View of the Pelvis

The patient is also in dorsal recumbency and in a neutral or standing orientation referred to as the *"stance phase"* of weight bearing. Medial pressure is applied lateral to the greater trochanters to compress the coxofemoral joints and obtain an image at their most congruent position. The femoral heads are fully seated in the acetabular fossae (see Fig. 19.6C). Congruency is measured.

> **TECHNICIAN NOTES**   All dogs have some degree of joint laxity—even Greyhounds and Borzois—so if you do not see any laxity, check the technique and the level of sedation.

Pelvic Limb Positions

Femur

Lateral (Mediolateral) View of the Femur—Routine

Positioning

Place In: Lateral recumbency with the affected limb down.

Head: Keep the head in a natural position, and support the neck with a sandbag, being careful not to restrict breathing.

Forelimbs: Pull the forelimbs cranially and support with a sandbag/Velcro.

Hindlimbs: Flex the unaffected limb, abduct and pull laterally with a bungee cord or Velcro, and secure.

Extend the lower affected limb and secure with a sandbag over the distal limb. Place a thin foam pad under the proximal tibia to prevent rotation of the femur (Fig. 19.8).

Comments and Tips

- Abducting the affected limb eliminates superimposition of the proximal femur over the tuber ischium. The beam may have to be angled distoproximally if the upper limb is not out of the field of view.
- Be sure to palpate and include the femoral joint to radiograph the full affected femur.
- In thickly muscled dogs, two views may be required (measure accordingly at each end).
- A fluid bag positioned over the distal end to emulate soft tissue may prevent overexposure to the distal aspect. Measure at the proximal femur.
- Position the patient so that the femoral head is pointing toward the cathode of the x-ray tube.
- Place the label cranially.

MEASURE: Midshaft of the femur (to compensate for the difference in tissue thickness at either end of the femur).

CENTRAL RAY: Midshaft of the femur.

BORDERS: The coxofemoral joint to the stifle.

> ✎ **TECHNICIAN NOTES** You will be more efficient if you first position and secure the body parts that are not radiographed, then position the area of interest.

FIG. 19.8 A, Positioning for the mediolateral (lateral) view of the canine femur. **B,** Medial view of the femur. **C,** Radiograph of the right canine mediolateral (lateral) femur. (**C,** Courtesy Jennifer White, Mississauga Oakville Veterinary Emergency and Specialty Hospital, ON.)

Acetabulum
Head of femur
Neck of femur
Lesser trochanter of femur
Body of femur
Patella
Tibial tuberosity
Sesamoid bones
Medial condyle of femur

Lateral condyle of femur
Tibia

Craniocaudal View of the Femur—Routine

Positioning

Place In: Dorsal recumbency in a V-trough or secure with the use of tape/Velcro or a sandbag if needed.

To ensure symmetry, it is usually best if the patient can be positioned as for a ventrodorsal extended-leg view. Center on the affected limb.

Head: Keep in a natural position and, if needed, support appropriately with a sandbag over the neck, being careful not to restrict breathing.

Forelimbs: Pull the forelimbs cranially and secure with a sandbag or tie/Velcro to the table.

Hindlimbs: Rotate both femurs inward so that the patellae lie over the patellar grooves.

Tape around both femurs just proximal to the stifle, keeping the femur parallel to the table and the patella between the femoral condyles.

Place a small sponge under the tarsus to prevent rotation of the stifle and a sandbag over the distal portion of the limbs (Fig. 19.9).

Comments and Tips

- Securing both limbs helps minimize rotation.
- Complete extension and fastening of the affected limb is essential.

MEASURE: Midshaft of the affected femur.
CENTRAL RAY: Midshaft of the affected femur.
BORDERS: The coxofemoral joint to the stifle.

FIG. 19.9 A, Positioning for the craniocaudal view of canine femur. Securing limbs together as in a VD extended view assists in symmetry. Placing a sandbag over the tarsus will help straighten the limbs.

Craniocaudal View of the Femur—Routine—cont'd

Acetabulum

Head of femur

Greater trochanter of femur

Neck of femur

Lesser trochanter of femur

Body of femur

Medial sesamoid

Lateral sesamoid

Medial epicondyle of femur

Patella

Medial condyle of femur

Lateral epicondyle of femur

Lateral condyle of femur

Medial condyle of tibia

Tuber ischium

B

C

FIG. 19.9, cont'd B, Cranial view of the canine femur. C, Radiograph of the canine craniocaudal femur. (C, Courtesy Jennifer White, Mississauga Oakville Veterinary Emergency and Specialty Hospital, ON.)

Caudocranial View (Horizontal Beam) of the Femur—Ancillary

Positioning

Place In: Lateral recumbency with the affected limb uppermost and supported on a sponge.

Head: Keep in a natural position and, if needed, support appropriately with a sandbag over the neck. Be careful not to restrict breathing.

Forelimbs: Pull the forelimbs cranially and secure with a sandbag or Velcro/tie to the table.

Hindlimbs: Position a cassette vertically against the cranial aspect of the affected limb. Extend the limb as much as possible, fastening it well with a sandbag or tie to a secure object (Fig. 19.10).

Comments and Tips

- The horizontal beam is directed caudocranially.
- It is difficult to include the proximal portion of the femur and acetabulum with this position. Positioning is identical for the caudocranial stifle using a horizontal beam.

🖉 **TECHNICIAN NOTES** Remember to place the label and markers on the cranial aspect of the limb for the lateral views and on the lateral aspect for the orthogonal views.

MEASURE: Midshaft of the femur.

CENTRAL RAY: Midshaft of the femur.

BORDERS: The coxofemoral joint to the stifle.

FIG. 19.10 Positioning for the Caudocranial (Horizontal) View of the Canine Femur.

Stifle

Lateral (Mediolateral) View of the Stifle—Routine

Positioning

Place In: Lateral recumbency with the affected leg down.

Head: Keep in a natural position and support appropriately with a sandbag over the neck, being careful not to restrict breathing.

Forelimbs: Pull the forelimbs cranially and secure with a sandbag or Velcro/tie to the table.

Hindlimbs: Flex the unaffected limb, abduct, and pull laterally with a bungee cord or rope to a secure object

Alternatively, tape/Velcro around the stifle and tarsus and secure to the table.

Extend the affected limb, keeping the stifle in a relatively natural position so the patella is flat on the table.

Place a sandbag over the distal limb or secure with tape/Velcro (Fig. 19.11).

Comments and Tips

- The unaffected limb needs to be extended only dorsally enough to be out of the field of view. Avoid overrotation.

- Place a sponge pad under the affected tarsus so the tibia is parallel to the image receptor, which slightly rotates the stifle but keeps the femoral condyles aligned cranially to caudally.

- In a true lateral view, there will be superimposition of the femoral condyles.

- As an alternative, the unaffected leg may be pulled forward and secured to the table, being careful to avoid superimposition over the area of interest. This is particularly applicable to severe degenerative joint disease of the coxofemoral joints.

- A flexed lateral radiograph (ancillary view) with tibial compression is used if interested in cranial drawer movement (to note cranial displacement of the proximal tibia in relation to the distal femur).

- Flex the stifle 90 degrees and flex the tarsus as much as possible so the metatarsus is parallel to the humerus.

MEASURE: At the distal end of the femur.

CENTRAL RAY: Palpate and center on the indentation of the stifle joint (intercondylar fossa of the femur).

BORDERS: Proximal third of the tibia and distal third of the femur.

Medial and lateral condyles of femur

Cartilage between tibial tuberosity and body of tibia

Patella Femur

Medial condyle of femur

Tibial tuberosity Sesamoids

Tibia Body of fibula

FIG. 19.11 A, Positioning for the mediolateral view of the canine stifle. **B,** Medial view of the canine stifle joint. **C,** Radiograph of the canine mediolateral (lateral) stifle. (**C,** Courtesy Jennifer White, Mississauga Oakville Veterinary Emergency and Specialty Hospital, ON.)

Caudocranial View of the Stifle—Routine

The stifle is closer to the image receptor, so there is less magnification and geometric distortion. (Fig. 19.12).

Positioning

Place In: Sternal recumbency in a V-trough, or secure with sandbags if needed. (A feline patient will not likely need further support.)

Head: Keep in a natural position and support appropriately with a sandbag over the neck, being careful not to restrict breathing.

Forelimbs: Pull the forelimbs cranially and secure with a sandbag or Velcro/tie to the table.

Hindlimbs: Allow the unaffected limb to lie flexed and raised with a foam pad.

Extend the affected limb and support with tape/Velcro or a sandbag.

Place a small sponge under the tarsus to prevent rotation of the stifle.

Comments and Tips

- It is essential that the affected limb rests on the patella. Palpate the femoral condyles to ensure proper placement in the patellar groove.

- Raising the unaffected limb will image the affected patella in the patellar groove. The patient will be slightly rotated.
- If able, the x-ray tube head may need to be angled in a cranial direction about 5 to 10 degrees to avoid superimposition of the femur and tibia over the stifle joint.
- Ensure that the affected limb is pulled caudally and there is no rotation of the limb. This positioning may not be possible in dogs with severe hip dysplasia, trauma, or degenerative changes of the lumbar or lumbosacral spine without heavy sedation or general anesthesia.
- If a true caudocranial view of the stifle is not possible, an ancillary CdCr view with a horizontal beam can be substituted. This view may be more desirable in medium to large breed dogs.
  - Follow the positioning for the CdCr (horizontal beam) femur (Fig. 19.10).
  - Measure, center, and utilize borders as for the routine CrCd stifle.

MEASURE: At the distal end of the femur.

CENTRAL RAY: On the stifle joint. Angle the beam 5 to 10 degrees cranially.

BORDERS: Distal third of the femur and proximal thirds of the tibia/fibula.

> ✎ **TECHNICIAN NOTES** Collimate. Include labels and markers. Have visible borders for every image.

> ✎ **TECHNICIAN NOTES** Strategically used positioning aids give the patient the illusion it is being held. A sandbag over the neck and limbs and/or the use of tape/Velcro is essential, especially if the patient is not properly sedated. Keep talking to your patient in a calm, low voice and slip away just as the image is taken.

Caudocranial View of the Stifle—Routine—cont'd

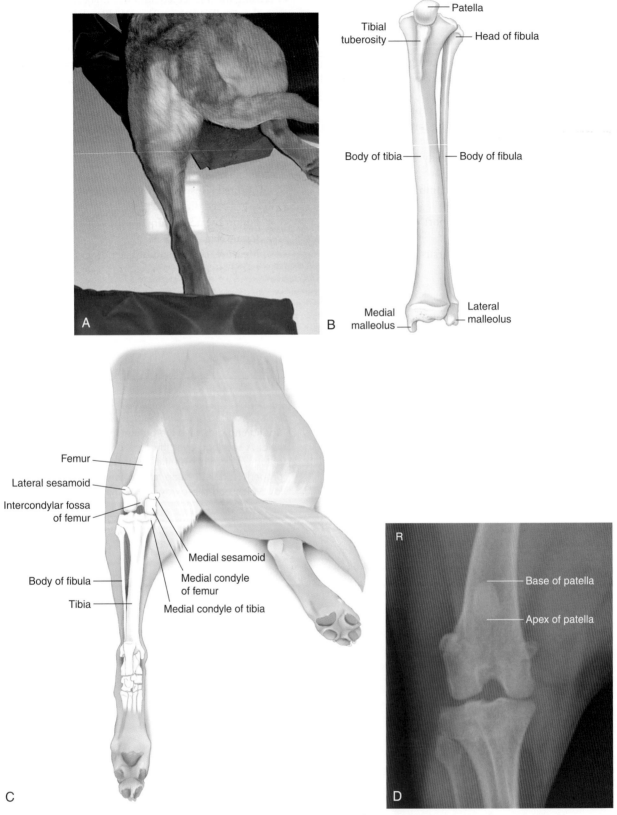

FIG. 19.12 **A,** Positioning for the caudocranial view of the canine stifle. **B and C,** Caudal view of canine stifle joint, tibia and fibula. **D,** Radiograph of the canine caudocranial stifle. (**D,** Courtesy Jennifer White, Mississauga Oakville Veterinary Emergency and Specialty Hospital, ON.)

Craniocaudal Stifle Joint—Ancillary

This view results in greater magnification than the caudocranial view and may be difficult if the patient has restricted extension of the pelvis. (Fig. 19.13).

Positioning

Place In: Dorsal recumbency in a V-trough, or secure with sandbags if needed. (A feline patient will not likely need further support.)

Head: Keep in a natural position and support appropriately with a sandbag over the neck, being careful not to restrict breathing.

Forelimbs: Pull the forelimbs cranially and secure with a sandbag or Velcro/tie to the table.

Hindlimbs: Allow the unaffected limb to lie flexed, raised with a foam pad next to the body.

Extend the affected limb, making sure to keep the limb straight (palpate the femoral condyles so they are in the mid patellar groove) and closer to the table.

Slightly tilt the thorax away from that limb and rotate the femurs inward.

Support with tape/Velcro or a sandbag over the tarsus and femur if needed.

MEASURE: At the distal end of the femur.

CENTRAL RAY: On the stifle joint.

BORDERS: Distal third of the femur and proximal third of the tibia/fibula.

FIG. 19.13 Positioning for the craniocaudal view of the stifle. There may be some magnification depending on the patient size.

Skyline View of the Stifle—Ancillary

Proximodistal (Cranioproximal-Craniodistal) with a Vertical Beam
Positioning

Place In: Sternal recumbency in a V-trough or secure with sandbags if needed. (The feline patient will not likely need further support.)

Head: Keep in a natural position with the nose pointing forward and, if needed, support appropriately with a sandbag over the neck, being careful not to restrict breathing.

Forelimbs: Pull the forelimbs cranially and secure with a sandbag or tie to the table.

Hindlimbs: Allow the contralateral limb to flex partially and position itself laterally.

Place a sandbag or sponge under the nonaffected limb to keep it slightly elevated, which will straighten the affected stifle.

Flex the affected pelvic limb lateral to the caudal abdomen, with the foot flexed to slightly elevate the patella (Fig. 19.14A) and keep the tibia under the femur to push the stifle joint away from the body.

Rotate the pelvis toward the affected limb, keeping the femur perpendicular to the image receptor.

Comments and Tips

- Measure, center, and use borders as per routine stifle but angle the beam 5 to 10 degrees in a cranial direction.
- It is essential that the affected limb rest on the tibia. Palpate so the patella is centered over the trochlear groove.
- A small foam pad may be placed beneath the patella for more comfort, although there will be some OFD.
- The skyline is used to visualize trochlear groove and patellar alignment.
- Skyline views can assist in further diagnosis of osteochondrosis, fractures, neoplasia, or ligamentous instability.[2]

FIG. 19.14 A, Positioning for the proximodistal (cranioproximal-craniodistal) view of the canine patella with a vertical beam.

Skyline View of the Stifle—Ancillary—cont'd

Distoproximal (Craniodistal-Cranioproximal) with a Horizontal Beam

Place In: Lateral recumbency with the affected limb uppermost and supported on a sponge.

Head: Keep in a natural position and, if needed, support appropriately with a sandbag over the neck, being careful not to restrict breathing.

Forelimbs: Pull the forelimbs cranially and secure with a sandbag or tie to the table.

Hindlimbs: Completely flex the affected limb as much as possible. Secure with Velcro or a cord around the metatarsus and fasten to the tube stand (Fig. 19.14B).

Alternatively, tape a figure-of-eight–type bandage around the midtibia and femur to hold the stifle in place.

Comments and Tips

- Measure, center and borders as per routine stifle.
- Place the cassette against the cranial surface of the upper limb and direct the beam in a CdCr direction.
- KV should be reduced to account for the decreased tissue thickness as compared to a regular CdCr or proximodistal stifle view.

FIG. 19.14, cont'd B, Alternative positioning for the skyline view of the canine stifle joint (patella) using a horizontal beam. Referred to as distoproximal (craniodistal-cranioproximal). C, Radiograph of the canine proximodistal patella view or skyline view.

Tibia and Fibula

Lateral (Mediolateral) View of the Tibia/Fibula—Routine

Positioning
Place In: Lateral recumbency with the affected limb down.

Head: Keep in a natural position and, if needed, support appropriately with a sandbag over the neck, being careful not to restrict breathing.

Forelimbs: Pull the forelimbs cranially and secure with a sandbag or Velcro/tie to the table.

Hindlimbs: Flex the unaffected limb, abduct, and pull dorsally, Extend the affected limb in a natural position, and either fasten the metatarsus with a sandbag or tie/tape/Velcro the metatarsus to the table or to a sandbag (Fig. 19.15).

Comments and Tips
- If needed, place a sponge under the tarsus to elevate it and to prevent obliquity of the limb.
- If a cranial cruciate ligament tear is suspected and tibial plateau leveling osteotomy (TPLO) to be completed, both the stifle and tarsal joints are to be flexed 90 degrees.[5]

MEASURE: Midshaft of the tibia and fibula (to compensate for the difference in tissue thickness at either end).

CENTRAL RAY: Midshaft of the fibula and tibia.

BORDERS: The tarsus and the stifle.

A

Body of femur

Patella

Medial condyle of femur

Body of tibia

Sesamoid bones

Trochlea of talus

Tarsocrural joint

Tuber calcanei

Proximal intertarsal joint

B

— Body of fibula

C

FIG. 19.15 A, Positioning for the mediolateral (lateral) view of the canine tibia and fibula. B, Medial view of canine tibia and fibula. C, Radiograph of the canine mediolateral (lateral) tibia and fibula. (C, Courtesy Jennifer White, Mississauga Oakville Veterinary Emergency and Specialty Hospital, ON.)

Caudocranial View of the Tibia/Fibula—Routine

Positioning

Place In: Sternal recumbency in a V-trough and secure with a sandbag or use tape/Velcro if needed. (The feline patient will not likely need further support.)

Head: Keep in a natural position and, if needed, support appropriately with a sandbag over the neck, being careful not to restrict breathing.

Forelimbs: Pull the forelimbs cranially and secure with a sandbag or Velcro/tie to the table.

Hindlimbs: Allow the unaffected limb to lie flexed next to the body and slightly raised with a foam pad.

Secure the affected limb over the metatarsus with a sandbag, or tie/Velcro and secure.

Place a small sponge under the tarsus to prevent rotation of the stifle if needed (Fig. 19.16).

Comments and Tips

- It is essential that the affected limb rest on the patella.
  - If you place a foam pad under the unaffected stifle, the raised limb helps to keep the affected patella in the patellar groove.
  - The body will be slightly rotated.
- A lateral decubitus view (as shown in Fig. 19.10 for the femur) can be substituted if a true caudocranial view of the tibia/fibula is not possible.
  - The horizontal beam is directed caudocranially. Completely extend and secure the affected limb.
  - Position as per the description for the caudocranial view (horizontal beam) of the femur but focus on the tibia/fibula.

MEASURE: Midshaft of the tibia and fibula (to compensate for the difference in tissue thickness at either end).

CENTRAL RAY: Midshaft of the tibia and fibula.

BORDERS: The tarsus and the stifle.

FIG. 19.16 A, Positioning for the caudocranial view of the canine tibia/fibula.

Caudocranial View of the Tibia/Fibula—Routine—cont'd

Femur

Lateral condyle of tibia

Head of fibula

Body of fibula

Body of tibia

Tuber calcanei — Medial malleolus of tibia

B

L

C

FIG. 19.16, cont'd B, Caudal view of the canine tibia and fibula. C, Radiograph of the canine caudocranial tibia/fibula. (C, Courtesy Jennifer White, Mississauga Oakville Veterinary Emergency and Specialty Hospital, ON.)

The Foot: Tarsus, Metatarsus, and Digits

The tarsus, metatarsus, and digits are typically radiographed in one view. If there is a particular area of interest, center and measure on this site.

Lateral (Mediolateral) Views of the Foot—Routine/Ancillary

Positioning

Place In: Lateral recumbency with the affected limb down.

Head: Keep in a natural position and, if needed, support appropriately with a sandbag over the neck, being careful not to restrict breathing.

Forelimbs: Pull the forelimbs cranially and secure with a sandbag or tie to the table.

Hindlimbs: Abduct the unaffected limb, pull dorsally.

Secure with tape/Velcro around the stifle and tarsus or support with a bungee cord to the x-ray tube stand.

Place a small foam pad or gauze under the calcaneus to keep the tibia parallel to the table.

Minimize any rotation of the affected limb and secure in place, flexing as required below.

Positioning for a Natural Lateral View of the Tarsus/Metatarsus—Routine

- Place the affected limb in a natural position and secure (Fig. 19.17).

Positioning for an Extended Lateral View of the Tarsus—Routine

- Extend the affected limb fully by pulling away from the body and secure (Fig. 19.18).

FIG. 19.17 A, Positioning for the mediolateral (lateral) view of the canine tarsus. **B,** Radiograph of the mediolateral (lateral) natural projection of the canine tarsus, metatarsus, and digits. A Robert Jones bandage has been applied. (**B,** Courtesy Jennifer White, Mississauga Oakville Veterinary Emergency and Specialty Hospital, ON.)

FIG. 19.18 Positioning for the Mediolateral (Lateral) Extended View of the Canine Tarsus, Metatarsus, and Digits.

Lateral (Mediolateral) Views of the Foot—Routine/Ancillary—cont'd

Positioning for a Flexed Lateral View of the Tarsus—Ancillary

- Flex the affected foot at 90 degrees, and support with a paddle or sandbag at the plantar aspect of the digits (Fig. 19.19).
- Alternatively, place a figure-of-eight–tape around the distal tibia and proximal metatarsus to achieve full flexion of the tarsus.

Positioning for a Lateral View of the Digits—Routine

- Separate the digits to prevent superimposition (Fig. 19.20).

- This is best completed by separately taping around the toenail of the lateral (fifth) phalanx and the medial (second) phalanx.
- Pull the lateral phalanx slightly cranially and laterally, and the medial phalanx slightly caudally and laterally.
- Tape can also be put around the digit itself.
- Cotton or manicure pads can be placed between the toes, although this alone does not separate the phalanges as effectively.

FIG. 19.19 **A,** Positioning for the mediolateral (lateral) flexed view of the canine tarsus. **B,** Medial flexed view of the canine foot. **C,** Radiograph of the mediolateral (lateral) flexed canine tarsus view. (**C,** Courtesy Jennifer White, Mississauga Oakville Veterinary Emergency and Specialty Hospital, ON.)

Lateral (Mediolateral) Views of the Foot—Routine/Ancillary—cont'd

FIG 19.20 A, When positioning for the digits, the toes should be separated if they are of interest. **B,** Radiograph with the toes separated. (Courtesy Jocelyn Affleck, Golf Glen Clinic, Aurora, ON.)

Plantarodorsal View of the Foot—Routine

Positioning

Place In: The patient is placed in sternal recumbency in a V-trough or secured with the use of a sandbag if needed. (The feline patient will not likely need further support.)

Head and Forelimbs: Secure the head and forelimbs with a sandbag or tie the limbs to the table.

Hindlimbs: Allow the unaffected limb to lie flexed next to the body.

Extend the affected foot and support with a sandbag, or tie at the metatarsus/digits and secure.

Keep the femur, stifle, and tibia in true alignment and the calcaneus vertical for true plantardorsal tarsus (Fig. 19.21).

Comments and Tips

- If you place a foam pad under the unaffected stifle, the raised limb will assist in keeping the calcaneus image more centered. The body is slightly rotated.
- Palpate for the tibial tuberosity to obtain a true plantarodorsal view.

MEASURE, CENTER, BORDERS, LABEL OF THE FOOT: **SEE BOX 19.3**

Plantarodorsal View of the Foot—Routine—cont'd

Tarsocrural joint

Calcaneus

Talus

Proximal intertarsal joint

Tarsometatarsal joint

Mt2

Mt3

Mt4

Mt5

Metatarsophalangeal joint of digit 2

Proximal phalanx of digit 2

Middle phalanx of digit 2

Distal phalanx of digit 2

Metatarsal pad

FIG. 19.21 A, Positioning for the plantarodorsal view of the canine tarsus, metatarsus, and digits. B, Plantar view of tarsus, metatarsus, and digits. C, Radiograph of the plantarodorsal view of the canine tarsus, metatarsus, and digits. (C, Courtesy Jennifer White, Mississauga Oakville Veterinary Emergency and Specialty Hospital, ON.)

BOX 19.3	For All Pelvic Foot Views

MEASURE: At the site of interest:
  Tarsus: At the tarsus joint.
  Metatarsus or Phalanges: On the joint.
CENTRAL RAY: Center on the area of interest:
  Tarsus: At the tarsus joint.
  Metatarsus or Phalanges: On the central bone.
BORDERS:
  Tarsus: Proximal third of metatarsus to distal third of the tibia and fibula.

Metatarsus or Phalanges: Tarsus proximally to the distal phalanges.
LABEL
  Lateral: Cranial to the joint or bone
  Orthogonal views: Lateral to the limb

Dorsoplantar View of the Foot—Ancillary

A dorsoplantar view is not routinely completed. If this view is required, there are 3 options:

- Place in dorsal recumbency for a dorsoplantar projection view of the foot.
  - Support body, head/neck, and front limbs as described for the craniocaudal view of the stifle, and extend and secure the affected foot.
  - There may be greater magnification and possible geometric distortion depending on the size of the patient.
- Secondly, the patient is placed in sternal recumbency with the plantar aspect of the foot against the image receptor and the tarsus flexed (Fig. 19.22A). The beam is centered vertically over the area of interest. There will be no magnification or distortion.

- This flexed dorsoplantar position can also be used to position for the skyline of the tarsus to detect osteochondrosis lesions by better visualizing the tibiotarsal joint without superimposition of the calcaneus. The beam is centered vertically over the stifle.
- Alternatively, the patient can be placed in dorsal recumbency with the tarsus of interest on the image detector and raised so it is positioned on a wooden or cardboard box.
  - Flex the tarsus so the foot is perpendicular to the cassette and parallel with the x-ray beam to prevent superimposition of the tuber calcus.
  - Exposure factors may need to be modified due to the variation in source image distance (Fig. 19.22B).

MEASURE, CENTER, BORDERS OF THE FOOT: **SEE BOX 19.3**

FIG 19.22 A, Positioning for the dorsoplantar view of the canine metatarsus and digits. A dorsoplantar view taken in this position has less object-film distance than that with the patient in dorsal recumbency. This position can also be used to view the calcaneus skyline. B, An alternative for a flexed dorsoplantar position of the tarsus with the limbs raised.

Oblique Views of the Foot—Ancillary

Many tarsal fractures and some OCD lesions require oblique views. With the patient in sternal recumbency, the oblique views of the hind foot are labeled plantarolateral-dorsomedial (PLDMO) (medial oblique) view and the plantaromedial-dorsolateral (PMDLO) or a (lateral oblique) view.

Positioning

Place In: Sternal recumbency.

Rotate the thorax and abdomen towards the affected limb for a lateral oblique but away from the affected limb for a medial oblique.[3]

Head: Keep in a natural position and, if needed, support appropriately with a sandbag over the neck, being careful not to restrict breathing.

Forelimbs: Pull the forelimbs cranially and secure if needed.

Hindlimbs: Keep the unaffected limb in a natural position. Extend and secure the affected metatarsus/digits as far caudally as possible.

Medial oblique (PLDMO) view: Keep the unaffected limb extended caudally, allowing slight rotation of the body away the unaffected limb. This will permit the affected foot to lie obliquely with the lateral aspect toward the beam and the medial portion on the image receptor.

The tarsus/foot should be rotated 35 to 45 degrees. Support as needed.

Lateral oblique (PMDLO) view: Rotate and elevate slightly laterally the unaffected pelvic limb with a large sponge so that the medial aspect of the foot is directed to the beam and the lateral aspect is against the image receptor. The thorax and abdomen are rotated towards the affected limb. The tarsus/foot should be rotated 35 to 45 degrees. Support as needed (Fig. 19.23).

Alternative Positioning

- Alternatively place the limb in a true plantarodorsal position and angle the beam if the tube head is movable.
- **Lateral oblique** (plantaromedial-dorsolateral (PMDLO)) view: Angle the tube head 10 to 15 degrees toward the medial side of the tarsus so the lateral aspect is on the image detector.
- **Medial oblique** (plantarolateral-dorsomedial (PLDMO)) view: Angle the beam 10 to 15 degrees toward the lateral side of the tarsus so the lateral aspect is on the image detector.

Comments and Tips

- The medial oblique view provides an unobstructed view of the lateral trochlea of the talus if osteochondrosis is suspected as the calcaneus is not superimposed.[2]
- The patient may also be positioned in dorsal recumbency to obtain oblique views but there will be greater magnification and possible geometric distortion.
  - The beam will be angled 15 to 20 degrees[11] in either direction.

MEASURE, CENTER, BORDERS OF THE FOOT: **SEE BOX 19.3**

FIG. 19.23 A, Positioning for the plantaromedial-dorsolateral (lateral) oblique view of the canine tarsus, metatarsus, and digits. B, Radiograph of the oblique metatarsus and digits. (B, Courtesy Jennifer White, Mississauga Oakville Veterinary Emergency and Specialty Hospital, ON.)

✏ **TECHNICIAN NOTES** The beam is always described as "point of entrance to point of exit." For the PMDLO, the beam enters at the plantar aspect on the medial side and exits dorsally on the lateral side. The "point of exit" is where the image receptor is placed, which in this case is next to the dorsal surface on the lateral aspect. Because the beam does not exit perpendicular to the midline, the view is called an *oblique*. This example is a lateral oblique because the beam exits laterally. (This concept is further described in Chapter 24.)

Fig. 19.24 is a mystery radiograph. Review it and answer the question presented with it.

FIG. 19.24 Mystery radiograph. How can you tell which side of the pelvis is slightly raised in this image? What has caused the different density at the right acetabulum?

✳ **KEY POINTS**

1. For views perpendicular to the midsagittal plane, the dog or cat generally lies in dorsal recumbency for the pelvis and the proximal limb (femur), and in sternal recumbency for routine views of the distal limb (stifle, tibia and fibula, and foot).
2. Correct positioning and technique are required for proper interpretation. This includes accurate measuring and centering of the beam, correct inclusion, and proper positioning and symmetry.
3. The label is placed lateral to the limb for the orthogonal projections and at the cranial aspect for the lateral projections without obscuring anatomy.
4. For joints, borders include one-third each of the limbs proximal and distal. For long bones, the joints proximal and distal are included.
5. Always consider the patient in the process of utilizing high-quality radiographic techniques.

REVIEW QUESTIONS

1. You are positioning for a right lateral pelvis of a Belgian Sheepdog. The femur that will be more magnified on the image is:
   a. The right, because of decreased object-film distance
   b. The left, because of increased source-image distance
   c. The left, because of increased object-film distance
   d. The right, because of increased source-image distance
2. When positioning for this right lateral pelvis of the Belgian Sheepdog, you should position the hindlimbs so that:
   a. The right limb is pulled slightly cranially and the left slightly caudally
   b. The left limb is pulled slightly cranially and the right slightly caudally
   c. Both limbs are superimposed and pulled cranially
   d. Both limbs are superimposed and pulled caudally

3. A Poodle is exhibiting severe pain with trauma in the pelvis. Using a vertical beam, you should position so that your patient is in:
   a. Lateral recumbency with the limbs superimposed
   b. Dorsal recumbency with the hindlimbs in a frog-leg position
   c. Dorsal recumbency in a VD extended-leg view
   d. Sternal recumbency with the hindlimbs in a frog-leg position
4. Center the VD frog-leg view of the Poodle:
   a. Midline at the caudal pubis
   b. Between the obturator foraminae
   c. Midline at the caudal portion of the ischium
   d. On the greater trochanters

5. The hindlimbs of this VD frog-leg view of the Poodle should be:
   a. Pulled so that the femur is 90 degrees from the spine
   b. Left in a naturally flexed position
   c. Extended as much as possible
   d. Raised and placed in a neutral stance

6. When positioning for a VD extended-leg pelvic radiograph in a German Shepherd, it is best to place the stifles:
   a. At an angle to the table
   b. Toward either the cathode or the anode
   c. Toward the cathode
   d. Toward the anode

7. The right marker for this VD extended-leg pelvis will be placed beside the:
   a. Left patella
   b. Right patella
   c. Wing of the left ilium
   d. Wing of the right ilium

8. The OFA label requirements for evaluation of hip dysplasia must include:
   a. Only the owner's name
   b. The name of the person taking the radiograph
   c. Only the positional marker
   d. All required identification to be permanent

9. The field of view for this VD extended-leg pelvis will be from the:
   a. Tip of the ilia to the ischia
   b. Body of the ilia to the ischial tuberosities
   c. Tip of the ilia to the distal patella
   d. Body of the ilia to the distal patella

10. The obturator foramina on this image are not of equal size. This means that to obtain a symmetrical image, you should raise the side of the pelvis with the:
    a. Larger circular obturator foramen
    b. Narrower obturator foramen

11. You also notice on this VD extended-leg radiograph of the German Shepherd that the right femur appears shorter than the left. This is because the:
    a. Left limb is slightly raised and not parallel to the table
    b. Right limb is slightly raised and not parallel to the table
    c. Patient is shifted to the right
    d. Patient has shifted to the left

12. The main principle of PennHIP is to:
    a. Subjectively measure canine hip joint laxity
    b. Subjectively measure canine hip joint irregularities
    c. Quantitatively measure canine hip joint irregularities
    d. Quantitatively measure canine hip joint laxity

13. A horizontal beam is being used for the proximodistal patella of a Retriever. The patient should be placed in:
    a. Lateral recumbency with the affected limb closer to the table
    b. Lateral recumbency with the affected limb uppermost
    c. Sternal recumbency with the image receptor underneath the patella
    d. Dorsal recumbency with the image receptor laterally to the patella

14. The field of view for the stifle joint of a feline is the:
    a. Stifle joint
    b. Proximal third of the femur to the distal third of the tibia
    c. Proximal third of the tibia to the distal third of the femur
    d. Femur, tibia, and digits

15. Measurement for the tibia and fibula of a cat should be taken at the:
    a. Center of the tibia/fibula
    b. Stifle joint
    c. Tarsal joint
    d. Distal femur

16. In a plantarodorsal view of the right tarsus of an Irish Terrier, the patient is routinely placed in:
    a. Dorsal recumbency
    b. Ventral recumbency
    c. Right lateral recumbency
    d. Left lateral recumbency

Chapter Review Question answers are located in the Instructor Resources on Evolve and can be provided to students at the discretion of the instructor.

References

1. Orthopedic Foundation of America; 2012. Available at: https://www.ofa.org/diseases/hip-dysplasia, 2020.
2. Thrall DE. *Textbook of Veterinary Diagnostic Radiology*. 7th ed. St. Louis: Elsevier; 2017.
3. Holloway A. *BSAVA Manual of Canine and Feline Radiography and Radiology: A Foundation Manual*. Suffolk: BSAVA; 2013 [chapter 7].
4. Muhlbauer MC, Kneller SK. *Radiography of the Dog and Cat: Guide to Making and Interpreting Radiographs*. Oxford: Wiley-Blackwell; 2013 [chapter 4].
5. Ayers S. *Small Animal Radiographic Techniques and Positioning*. Oxford: Wiley-Blackwell; 2013 [chapter 10].
6. Smith GK, Karbe GT, Agnello KA, McDonald-Lynch MB. Pathogenesis, diagnosis, and control of canine hip dysplasia. In: Tobias KM, Johnston SA, eds. *Veterinary Surgery: Small Animal*. St. Louis: Elsevier; 2011:824-848.
7. Powers MY, Karbe GT, Gregor TP, et al. Evaluation of the relationship between Orthopedic Foundation for Animals'

hip joint scores and PennHIP distraction index values in dogs. *J Am Vet Med Assoc*. 2010;237:532-541.

8. Verhoeven GEC, Fortrie RR, Duchateau L, et al. The effect of a technical quality assessment of hip-extended radiographs on interobserver agreement in the diagnosis of canine hip dysplasia. *Vet Radiol Ultrasound*. 2010;51:498-503.

9. *PennHIP—Antech Imaging Services*: home page. Available at: http://info.antechimagingservices.com/pennhip/index.html. Retrieved March 25, 2021.

10. PennHIP information courtesy of Drs. GK Smith and M Wallace, University of Pennsylvania. 2015

11. Morgan JP. *Techniques of Veterinary Radiography*. Ames, Iowa: Iowa State University Press; 1993.

Bibliography

American College of Veterinary Radiology (ACVR). *Radiology 2—equine*. ACVR; 2016.

Aspinall V, Cappello M. *Introduction to Veterinary Anatomy*. 3rd ed. London: Butterworth-Heinemann; 2013.

Colville T, Bassert J. *Clinical Anatomy and Physiology for Veterinary Technicians*. 3rd ed. St. Louis: Mosby; 2016.

Evans H, de Launta A. *Guide to the Dissection of the Dog*. 8th ed. St. Louis: Saunders; 2017.

Fauber TL. *Radiographic Imaging and Exposure*. St. Louis: Elsevier; 2017.

Han C, Hurd C. *Practical Diagnostic Imaging for the Veterinary Technician*. 3rd ed. St. Louis: Mosby; 2005.

Orthopedic Foundation for Animals. *Hip Dysplasia,* 2020. Available at: https://www.ofa.org/diseases/hip-dysplasia.

Orthopedic Foundation for Animals. *Elbow Dysplasia,* 2020. Available at: https://www.ofa.org/diseases/elbow-dysplasia.

Owens JM, Biery DN. *Radiographic Interpretation for the Small Animal Clinician*. 2nd ed. Baltimore: Williams & Wilkins; 1999.

Romich J. *An Illustrated Guide to Veterinary Medical Terminology*. 4th ed. Stamford, CT: Cengage Learning; 2015.

Singh B. *Dyce, Sack and Wensing's Textbook of Veterinary Anatomy*. 5th ed. St. Louis: Elsevier; 2018.

Sirois M. *Principles and Practice of Veterinary Technology*. 4th ed. St. Louis: Elsevier; 2017.

Sirois,M, Schlote J. Diagnostic Imaging for Veterinary Technicians. Minneapolis MN, Bluedoor, LLC; 2017.

Smallwood JE, Shively MJ, Rendano VT, Habel RE. A standardized nomenclature for radiographic projections used in veterinary medicine. *Vet Radiol*. 1985;26:2-9.

Tighe M, Brown M. *Mosby's Comprehensive Review for Veterinary Technicians*. 5th ed. St. Louis: Mosby; 2019.

CHAPTER 20
Small Animal Vertebral Column

Marg Brown, RVT, BEd Ad Ed

If something goes wrong, don't whine about it.
Have a spine about it. Adjust, adapt, and move forward.
—Ralph Marston, author of *The Daily Motivator*, b. 1955

OUTLINE

LEARNING OBJECTIVES

When you have completed this chapter, you will be able to:

1. Describe the common positions and protocols used to radiograph the small-animal vertebral column.
2. Properly and safely position a dog or cat for routine positions of the vertebral column with an emphasis on non-manual restraint.
3. Correctly measure and center the patient to include the peripheral borders.
4. Keep the body part parallel to the image receptor and perpendicular to the central ray.
5. Identify ancillary views that may be required.
6. Identify normal spinal anatomy found on a radiographic image.

KEY TERMS

Key terms are defined in the Glossary on the Evolve website.

Coned-down view
Diverge
Dynamic
Flexed lateral
Hyperextension
Hyperflexion
Kyphosis
Orthogonal
Positioning terminology
Survey
Vertebral formula

TECHNICAL NOTE: To preserve space, the images presented in this chapter do not show collimation. For safety, always collimate so that the beam is limited within the image receptor edges. In film radiography, you should see a clear border of collimation (frame) on every radiograph. In some jurisdictions, evidence of collimation is required by law. In digital imaging, the algorithm depends on proper collimation.

Survey axial skeletal imaging has limited diagnostic value in neurological disease and may be insufficient in conditions of the vertebral column, such as trauma. Definitive evidence may need to be obtained by myelography, computerized tomography (CT), or magnetic resonance imaging (MRI).[1,2] When these modalities are available, they have largely replaced radiography for spinal disease/trauma diagnosis in referral practices.

However, despite the limitations, proper survey vertebral radiographs are a valuable tool for patients who have suffered spinal injuries and present with paresis or paralysis, either partial or complete. In addition, survey radiographs can demonstrate many of the signs consistent with intervertebral disk protrusion. Common intervertebral disk protrusion sites are T12 to T13, T13 to L1, C2 to C3, and C3 to C4.[1]

High-quality images are needed to see subtle changes in bone opacity, shape, and angulation of the vertebrae or vertebral column[1,2] (Table 20.1). It is essential that the patient be symmetrically positioned. Because of the anatomical complexity, sedation or general anesthesia should be used to achieve accurate positioning with muscle relaxation. As an example, false narrowing of the intervertebral disk spaces due to muscle spasm may occur and impede diagnosis.[1,2] Because most feline patients requiring vertebral radiography likely present with spinal injury, sedation or general anesthesia and gentle handling are needed. If trauma is suspected, ensure that any concurrent issues such as thoracic pathology are addressed before radiography.

See Appendix C on the Evolve website for information on the vertebral number and characteristics of the vertebrae of some common species.

Radiographic and Positioning Concerns

- The common views of this portion of the axial skeleton are the lateral (L) and ventrodorsal (VD) views of the cervical, thoracic, thoracolumbar, lumbar, lumbosacral, sacral, and caudal vertebrae. Depending on the size of the patient, a full survey study is either four or five images of each orthogonal view. Survey radiographs of small to medium-sized dogs generally center at C3 to C4, T6 to T7, L4, and lumbosacral. A large dog survey generally includes centering at the thoracolumbar region, whereas cat studies of the vertebrae are often part of the whole-body view.
- Correct positioning and attention to detail are essential to produce images of diagnostic value. Center the primary beam on the specific area of interest and tightly collimate immediately adjacent to the spine to increase the detail and contrast.
- The x-ray beam diverges from the central ray, so it is important to limit the number of vertebrae examined so that the intervertebral disk spaces are more perpendicular to the central beam. The farther away the area of interest is from the central ray, the greater the geometrical variation and the more inaccurate the interpretation of that area. Intervertebral spaces at the periphery of radiographs often appear falsely narrowed.[3] Coned-down views give further high-quality images especially for areas of interest.
- As terminology is based on entrance of central ray to its exit, technically the correct term for a right lateral, for example, is a left to right lateral, though right lateral is commonly used.
- The directional and identification labels should be in the field of view, but not overlapping important anatomy, especially in VD views.
  - For lateral views, place the label along the dorsum.
  - In the VD views, the label may have to be taped to the patient in lieu of being placed on the image receptor.
- For all laterals, it is essential that the sternum and spine are on the same plane parallel to the tabletop with no sagging of the area of interest.
- This usually means that the sternum will be elevated slightly to position the sternum and spine on the same plane and that foam may be needed under areas such as cervical vertebrae. To obtain symmetry in some patients such as those with a round thorax, the sternum may need to be displaced slightly ventrally. Always inspect visually and palpate for precise symmetry.[1]
- Tape placed along the spine may assist in proper alignment[4] (Fig. 20.1).

TABLE 20.1	Protocol for Spinal Radiography	
ANATOMICAL LOCATION	**ROUTINE VIEWS**	**ANCILLARY VIEWS**
Cervical vertebrae	Lateral, Ventrodorsal Center at C3–C4	Hyperextended or hyperflexed lateral, lateral oblique, Coned down
Thoracic vertebrae	Lateral, Ventrodorsal Center at T6–T7	Oblique, dorsoventral Coned down (T6–T7)
Thoracolumbar vertebrae	Lateral, Ventrodorsal Center at thoracolumbar junction	Oblique
Lumbar vertebrae	Lateral, Ventrodorsal Center at L3–L4	Oblique
Lumbosacral vertebrae	Lateral, Ventrodorsal Center at lumbosacral junction	Hyperextended or flexed lateral

FIG. 20.1 Placing tape along the vertebrae helps maintain correct alignment and position. A line drawn between the greater trochanters should be perpendicular to the table. A small foam pad under the nose may be required.

- Use sponges or cotton padding between the limbs, under the sternum and vertebrae, to keep the spine parallel to the tabletop, avoid any sagging, and prevent axial rotation.
- Sandbags can also be used for positioning on areas that will not be in the field of view.
- Extending the front and hindlimbs in opposite directions in patients without spinal cord injuries keeps the thoracolumbar vertebral column extended to a near-parallel position, as well as opening the intervertebral spaces,[1-3] being careful to avoid injury.
- Generally, it is more comfortable for right-handed radiographers to place the dog or cat in right lateral recumbency, but either side can be dependent.
- For ventrodorsal views, the sternum and vertebrae must be superimposed with a straight line from nose to tail.
- If the patient is compromised and the machine allows, VD views can also be made using the horizontal cross-table beam with the patient in lateral recumbency. This is especially useful if vertebral body fractures are suspected. Dorsoventral (DV) views (ancillary view) are not as accurate because of the increase in object-film distance (OFD) as well as difficulty in obtaining a parallel technique.
- Hyperflexion and hyperextension views (ancillary views) can further evaluate the caudal aspect of the lateral cervical and the lumbosacral vertebrae if the patient is chemically restrained and will not be traumatized by such handling. Be extremely gentle with handling. Veterinarians should perform these procedures.
- The hair coat should be clean and dry. Remove the collar for any cranial and cervical views. The bladder and colon should be emptied, especially for VD views, as material within the colon or a distended bladder can create multiple superimposed shadows that might interfere with diagnosis.

- Choose a high-detail cassette/film combination if film is used. Low kilovoltage (kV) and high milliampere-seconds (mAs) provide better radiographic contrast, and the use of a grid further increases the contrast. Ensure there is enough kV for penetration and mAs for film density or signal (digital film).
- If using digital imaging, use appropriate algorithms to process raw data to prevent a sudden transition between bone and soft tissue that can create an artificial dark halo around the vertebrae.[2]

TECHNICIAN NOTES   Try this: Evenly place a row of pennies on a 5-cm sponge about half an inch (1.5 mm) apart along the center length of the image receptor. Take an x-ray (suggested technique of 50 kV and 2 mAs) and look at the image. Notice how the spacing between the pennies narrows toward the outer edges of the film.

TECHNICIAN NOTES   A vertebra is generally made up of a body (the denser ventral portion, which is separated from the bodies of adjacent vertebra by intervertebral disks), vertebral arch (located dorsal to the body), and various processes (the cranial and caudal articular processes, the dorsal spinous process, and the lateral transverse process) (see Figs. 20.3, 20.9, 20.15, 20.16, and 20.17).

TECHNICIAN NOTES   The vertebral column is divided into five regions: cervical (neck), thoracic (chest), lumbar (abdomen), sacral (pelvis), and caudal (tail). To refer to a specific vertebra, use abbreviations for the region followed by the number within the region, beginning at the cranial end. For example, T12 is the twelfth thoracic vertebra. The abbreviation for caudal vertebrae is Cd (although sometimes the tail vertebrae are referred to as coccygeal and the abbreviation is Cy).

The vertebral formula is made up of the first letter of each region, followed by the number of vertebrae in that group. The vertebral formula for a dog and cat is $C_7T_{13}L_7S_3Cd_{6-20}$.

TECHNICIAN NOTES   Note that the positioning itself is fairly similar for most of the lateral and ventrodorsal views of the vertebrae. Keep basic principles in mind and maintain symmetry.

TECHNICIAN NOTES   Remember to collimate tightly to the vertebrae. Place the label/marker on the dorsal aspect for the lateral views. For VD views, tape the marker on the body or place it on the table in an area that will not obscure important anatomy.

Cervical Vertebrae

Lateral View of the Cervical Vertebrae—Routine

Positioning

Place In: Lateral recumbency.

Hindlimbs: Superimpose and place the pelvic limbs caudally; secure with Velcro/sandbag.

Forelimbs: Position and superimpose the forelimbs caudally; secure with Velcro/sandbag.

A small foam pad can be placed between the limbs.

Head/Neck/Sternum: Extend the head and elevate the nose using a sponge.

Keep the head in a true lateral position—draw an imaginary line between the medial canthi and make sure this line is perpendicular to the table.

Place a flat positioning device under the midcervical area if it is sagging. Support the cranial area of the head with a sandbag, or secure it with tape/Velcro strapping.

Place sponges under the sternum to achieve true alignment with the vertebrae.

Vertebrae: Use foam pads or cotton beneath the cervical vertebrae to keep them parallel to the table (Figs. 20.2 and 20.3).

Comments and Tips

- The head must be in a true lateral position as any obliquity of the head can change the position of the cranial cervical vertebrae.

- Try to keep true lateral positioning of the entire body, even if radiographing only the cervical area. Keep the spine parallel to the table—the sternum and vertebrae should be on the same plane. The transverse processes of each vertebra should be superimposed on the image.

- Too much or too little padding can cause false narrowing of the intervertebral disks.

- Overextending the limbs might cause rotation of the spine.

- Do not flex or extend the head.

- To help align the cervical vertebrae with the long axis of the image receptor, position the pelvis region dorsally in a line with the head.

- A separate image of the cervicothoracic junction may be required to better evaluate this region.[1]

- Larger canine patients may have to be radiographed in two sections for the lateral and ventrodorsal cervical vertebrae:
  - *Radiograph 1:* Central ray at C2 to C3; include from the base of the skull to C4; measure at C2 to C3.
  - *Radiograph 2:* Central ray at C5 to C6; include from C4 to the center of the spine of the scapula; measure at the level of C6 to C7.

MEASURE: Across the shoulder at the level of C6 to ensure adequate penetration of the caudal cervical vertebrae, though a slight overexposure may occur with the cranial cervical vertebrae.

CATS AND SMALLER DOGS: C3 to C4.

CENTRAL RAY: C3 to C4.

BORDERS: *Cranial:* Base of the skull.

Caudal: Spine of the scapula (just past the shoulder joint, ~T2).

Dorsally and Ventrally: Collimate tightly to the edge of the wings of the atlas and the center of the spine of the scapula.

TECHNICIAN NOTES Strategically used positioning aids give the patient the illusion that it is being held.

TECHNICIAN NOTES Pulling the front limbs caudally prevents shoulder soft tissue from overlapping the spine.

TECHNICIAN NOTES Be extra careful when manipulating small-breed dogs that present with apparent neck pain.

TECHNICIAN NOTES Quickly go through your mental checklist *before* pushing the exposure button:
- Settings correct
- Image receptor/machine/grid in position
- Proper location of markers and ID (if using at this stage)
- Correct body part and view
- Properly centered
- Borders correct and collimated
- Patient properly prepared, positioned, and restrained so the vertebrae are in the same horizontal plane as the sternum for the lateral and superimposed for the VD, and parallel to the image receptor
- The central ray is perpendicular to the field of view and the receptor

Lateral View of the Cervical Vertebrae—Routine—cont'd

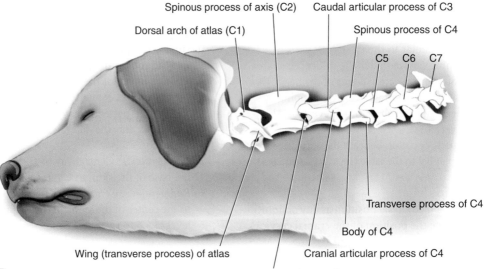

Spinous process of axis (C2)   Caudal articular process of C3

Dorsal arch of atlas (C1)   Spinous process of C4

C5   C6   C7

Transverse process of C4

Body of C4

Wing (transverse process) of atlas   Cranial articular process of C4

B

Intervertebral space (disk) between C2 and C3

1. Lateral vertebral foramina (left and right) of atlas; emergence of CN I
2. Dorsal arch of atlas (C1)
3. Spinous process of axis (C2)
4. Synovial joints between articular processes of C2 and C3
5. Spinous process of C3
6. Caudal articular processes of C3
7. Spinous process of C4
8. Vertebral canal of C4
9. Spinous process of C5
10. Spinous process of C6
11. Spinous process of C7

18. Transverse processes of C4
19. Cranial articular processes of C4
20. Intervertebral foramina between C2 and C3
21. Intervertebral disk space between C2 and C3
22. Endotracheal tube
23. Wings (transverse processes) of atlas
24. Ventral tubercle of atlas

12. Trachea
13. Expanded ventral laminae of transverse processes of C6
14. Cranial extremity (head) of C6
15. Caudal physis of C5
16. Caudal extremity (fossa) of C4
17. Body of C4

C

FIG. 20.2 A, Positioning for the lateral view of the cervical vertebrae. B, Left-to-right lateral anatomy of the cervical vertebrae. C, Lateral radiograph of cervical vertebrae. (A, from Evans H, de Lahunta A. *Guide to the Dissection of the Dog*. 7th ed. St Louis: Saunders; 2010; C, from Thrall DE. *Textbook of Veterinary Diagnostic Radiology*. 7th ed. St. Louis: Elsevier; 2017.)

Ventrodorsal View of the Cervical Vertebrae

Positioning

Place In: Dorsal recumbency in a V-trough or supported by tape/Velcro strapping or sandbag if needed.

Hindlimbs: Place the pelvic limbs in a neutral position and secure with Velcro/sandbags.

Forelimbs: Evenly position the forelimbs caudally and secure with Velcro/sandbag.

Head/Neck/Sternum: Keep the head in a natural position with the nose slightly up to minimize the curvature of the cervical spine. Secure with padding lateral to the head and neck. Keep the sternum superimposed over the vertebrae.

Vertebrae: Use padding beneath the rostral neck to keep the cervical vertebrae parallel to the table (Figs. 20.3 and 20.4).

Comments and Tips

- If the unit allows, angle the beam in a slight caudocranial direction (20 degrees) between the intervertebral spaces to improve visualization of the disk spaces because they slope caudally in the VD position.
- Minimize rotation by making sure the sternum and vertebrae are superimposed and perpendicular to the image receptor.
- The nose should be in line with the base of the tail and the limbs evenly positioned.
- To image the occipital bone, point the nose upward and secure with sandbags lateral to the head and neck so that there is no bone superimposition of C1 to C2 with the occipital bone.
- If there is an endotracheal tube in place, it should be removed if possible before the image is taken to avoid artifacts that might interfere with diagnosis.
- An open-mouth view of the odontoid process can be made as described in Chapter 21.

MEASURE: Level of C6 near the manubrium.

CENTRAL RAY: C3 to C4.

BORDERS: *Cranial*: Base of the skull.

Caudal: Just past the shoulder joint (~T2)

Laterally: Tightly collimate.

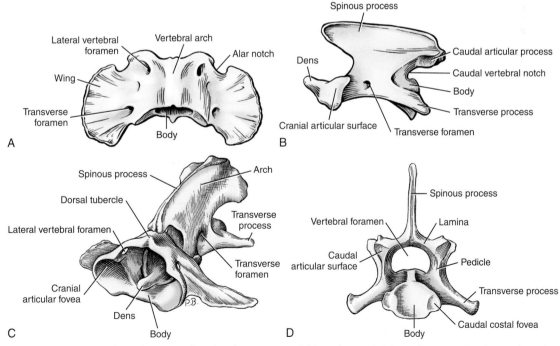

FIG. 20.3 Cervical Vertebrae. **A,** Atlas, dorsal view. **B,** Axis, left lateral view. **C,** Atlas and axis articulated, craniolateral aspect. **D,** Seventh cervical vertebrae, caudal aspect.

Ventrodorsal View of the Cervical Vertebrae—cont'd

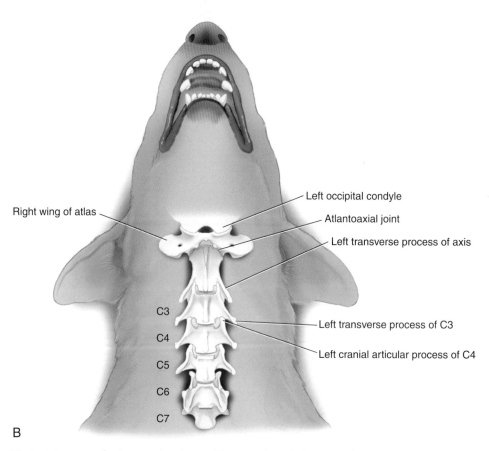

Right wing of atlas

Left occipital condyle

Atlantoaxial joint

Left transverse process of axis

C3

C4

C5

C6

C7

Left transverse process of C3

Left cranial articular process of C4

FIG. 20.4 A, Positioning for the ventrodorsal view of the cervical vertebrae. B, Ventrodorsal radiographic anatomy of the canine cervical vertebrae. (**A,** Courtesy Seneca College of Applied Arts and Technology, King City, Ontario.)

Ventrodorsal View of the Cervical Vertebrae—cont'd

1. Left occipital condyle
2. Dens of axis
3. Atlantoaxial joint
4. Spinous process of axis
5. Left thyrohyoid bone
6. Left transverse process of axis
7. Tracheal cartilages
8. Left transverse process of C3
9. Left caudal articular process of C3
10. Left cranial articular process of C4
11. Left transverse process of C4
12. Left transverse process of C5
13. Left transverse process of C6
14. Left transverse process of C7
15. Spinous process of T1
16. Spinous process of C7
17. Spinous process of C6
18. Spinous process of C5
19. Spinous process of C4
20. Intervertebral disk space between C3 and C4
21. Right wing of atlas
22. Right atlanto-occipital joint

FIG. 20.4, cont'd C, Ventrodorsal radiograph of the cervical vertebrae. (**C**, From Thrall DE. *Textbook of Veterinary Diagnostic Radiology.* 7th ed. St. Louis: Elsevier; 2017.)

Hyperextended Lateral View of the Cervical Vertebrae—Ancillary

The hyperextended and hyperflexed views are referred to as *dynamic views* and are usually completed after myelography to note any spinal cord impingement due to extradural changes associated with vertebral instability.[2] These procedures should only be completed by the veterinarian because of the possibility of atlantoaxial lunation and further instability, causing subsequent death. Always have emergency drugs/intubation supplies readily available.

Positioning

Place In: Lateral recumbency.

Hindlimbs: Superimpose and place the pelvic limbs caudally; secure with Velcro/sandbag.

Forelimbs: Position and superimpose the forelimbs caudally; secure with Velcro/sandbag.

A small foam pad may be placed between the limbs.

Head/Neck/Sternum: Elevate and keep the nose level to the table, using a foam pad.

To see if the head is in a true lateral, draw an imaginary line between the medial canthi and make sure this line is perpendicular to the table.

Hyperextend the neck and head dorsally and caudally until resistance is met.

Support the cranial area of the head with a sandbag, or secure with tape/Velcro strapping. Place foam pads under the sternum to achieve true alignment with the vertebrae.

Vertebrae: Use a foam pad or cotton beneath the cervical vertebrae as needed to keep each vertebra parallel to the table (Fig. 20.5).

Comments and Tips

- For true hyperextension, all cervical vertebrae need to be extended dorsally.
- Keep the head and entire body in a true lateral position using proper padding. Do not overextend the limbs.
- Collimate tightly to obtain a coned-down view.
- If an endotracheal tube is present, be careful that the patient's breathing is not restricted at any point.
- The hyperextended view is usually completed before the hyperflexion to determine if the latter is required.

MEASURE: C3 to C4 intervertebral space across the neck.

CENTRAL RAY: C3 to C4 intervertebral space.

BORDERS: *Cranial*: Base of the skull.

Caudal: Spine of the scapula (just past the shoulder joint).

Dorsally and Ventrally: Collimate tightly to the edge of the wings of the atlas and the center of the spine of the scapula.

FIG. 20.5 A, Positioning for the lateral hyperextended cervical vertebrae. B, Left-to-right lateral anatomy of the hyperextended cervical vertebrae. C, Lateral radiograph of the hyperextended cervical vertebrae. (C, Courtesy Joshua Schlote, BS, LVT, Northeast Community College.)

Hyperflexed Lateral View of the Cervical Vertebrae—Ancillary

Positioning

Place In: Lateral recumbency.

Hindlimbs: Superimpose and position the pelvic limbs caudally; secure with Velcro/sandbags.

Forelimbs: Position and superimpose the forelimbs ventrally and caudally, and secure with Velcro/sandbag. A small foam pad can be placed between the limbs.

Head/Neck/Sternum: Place tape, Velcro, or thin rope around the nose and gently apply traction on the end so the neck and head are flexed.

Pull the tape caudally between the forelimbs close to the body and secure to a sandbag.

If needed, elevate the nose using a sponge so the head is in true lateral.

Draw an imaginary line between the medial canthi and make sure this line is perpendicular to the table.

A sandbag can be placed dorsal to the nose to maintain the hyperflexed position.

Place sponges under the sternum to achieve true alignment with the vertebrae.

Vertebrae: If needed, use sponges beneath the cervical vertebrae to keep the spine parallel to the table and at the same plane as the thoracic vertebrae (Fig. 20.6).

Comments and Tips

- Collimate tightly so that a coned-down view is obtained for less distortion and better contrast.
- As with other cervical laterals, the head must be in a true lateral position; keep true lateral positioning of the entire body using proper padding, and do not overextend the limbs.
- The flexed lateral dynamic view is generally used to assess small-breed dogs with suspected subluxation.[2]
- The radiographs should only be completed by a veterinarian and taken with the patient under general anesthesia and placement of an endotracheal tube. Be careful with hyperflexing the neck so as not to cause tracheal trauma or constriction of the endotracheal tube. Begin with the mildest extension that will demonstrate instability, as marked flexion may further damage the spinal cord.

MEASURE: C3 to C4 intervertebral space across the neck.

CENTRAL RAY: C3 to C4 intervertebral space.

BORDERS: *Cranial*: Base of the skull.

Caudal: Spine of the scapula (just past the shoulder joint, ~T2).

Dorsally and ventrally: Collimate tightly to the edge of the wings of the atlas and the center of the scapular spine.

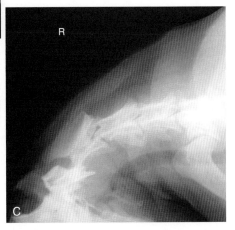

FIG. 20.6 A, Positioning for the lateral flexed cervical vertebrae. B, Lateral anatomy of the flexed cervical vertebrae. C, Lateral radiograph of the flexed cervical vertebrae. (C, Courtesy Joshua Schlote, BS, LVT, Northeast Community College.)

Lateral Oblique View for the Odontoid Process—Ancillary

Positioning

Place In: Lateral recumbency.

Hindlimbs: Superimpose and place the pelvic limbs caudally; secure with sandbag.

Forelimbs: Position and superimpose the forelimbs caudally; secure with sandbag.

A small foam pad can be placed between the limbs.

Head/Neck/Sternum: Use tape/Velcro strapping to keep the head in its natural oblique position.

Place sponges under the sternum so it is on the same plane as the thoracic vertebrae.

Vertebrae: Use padding to keep the cervical vertebrae lateral. Keep the head and C1 oblique (Fig. 20.7).

Comments and Tips

• Position the ear pinnae laterally and pull the tongue to avoid shadows on the radiograph.

• Lateral oblique views of C1 to C2 are used to demonstrate the dens.

MEASURE: C1 (for odontoid process).

CENTRAL RAY: C1 (for odontoid process).

BORDERS: *Cranially*: Midskull.

Caudally: C4.

Dorsally and Ventrally: Collimate tightly.

FIG. 20.7 **A,** Positioning for the lateral oblique view of the cervical vertebrae. The head is kept in a natural oblique position and a wedge is placed under the sternum. **B,** A lateral oblique view of the cervical vertebrae. **C,** Lateral oblique radiograph of all the cervical vertebrae. For the odontoid process, center at C1 and include from the midskull to C4.

Thoracic Vertebrae

Lateral View of the Thoracic Vertebrae—Routine

Positioning

Place In: Lateral recumbency with pelvis moved ventrally to straighten the thoracic spine.

Hindlimbs: Superimpose and place the pelvic limbs caudally; secure with Velcro/sandbag.

A small foam pad can be placed between the limbs.

Forelimbs: Superimpose and cranially position the forelimbs slightly; secure with Velcro/sandbag. A small foam pad can be placed between the limbs.

Head/Neck/Sternum: Keep the head in a natural position, and support the neck with a sandbag.

If needed, use sponges under the sternum and between the limbs to achieve true alignment of the sternum and vertebrae.

Vertebrae: Use padding if needed to keep each thoracic vertebra on the same horizontal plane as the sternum.

Using tape as in Fig. 20.1 can assist with proper alignment (Figs. 20.8 and 20.9).

Comments and Tips

- Try to keep lateral positioning of the entire body even if radiographing only the thoracic area.
- In the mid-to-caudal thoracic vertebrae region, dogs and cats have a natural area of kyphosis.[1]
- Superimpose the ribs to better view the intervertebral spaces. Keep the sternum on the same plane as the vertebrae. Use foam pads appropriately.
- Large dogs may require two separate views.
- Placing a lead mask or saline bag dorsal to the thoracic spine helps prevent scattered/secondary radiation from darkening the spinous processes in large dogs.

MEASURE: Highest point of sternum.

CENTRAL RAY: T6 to T7 or the caudal border of the scapula.

BORDERS: *Cranial:* Include C7 (shoulder joint)

Caudal: L1 (past the origin of the last rib).

Dorsally and Ventrally: Tightly collimate

TECHNICIAN NOTES For all lateral positions: place padding under the nose, the natural curvatures of the spine (neck and lumbar regions), and between the limbs. This will keep the spine parallel and horizontal with the table/image receptor and perpendicular to the center ray.

Visualize and palpate to keep a true lateral position of the entire body for each view so the sternum and vertebrae are on the same plane, parallel to the table and perpendicular to the x-ray beam and receptor.

Lateral View of the Thoracic Vertebrae—Routine—cont'd

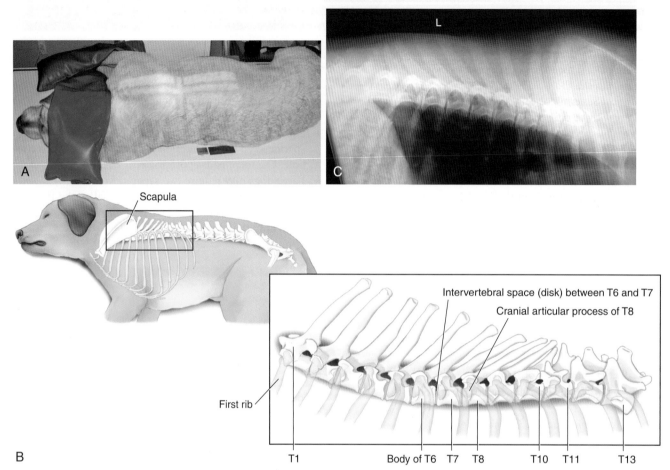

FIG. 20.8 A, Positioning for the lateral view of the thoracic vertebrae. B, Left-to-right lateral anatomy of the thoracic vertebrae. C, Lateral radiograph of the thoracic vertebrae. (C, Courtesy Joshua Schlote, BS, LVT, Northeast Community College.)

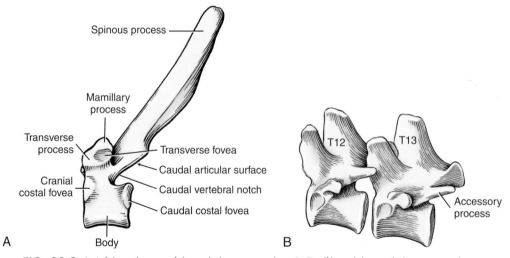

FIG. 20.9 A, Left lateral views of the sixth thoracic vertebra. B, Twelfth and thirteenth thoracic vertebrae.

Ventrodorsal View of the Thoracic Vertebrae—Routine

Positioning

Place In: Dorsal recumbency in a V-trough or use sandbags, if needed, to prevent rotation.

Hindlimbs: Equally place the pelvic limbs in a neutral position; secure with Velcro/sandbags.

Forelimbs: Equally position the forelimbs cranially and tie or secure with Velcro/sandbags.

Head/Neck/Sternum: Position the head and neck with the nose equidistant between the limbs.

Support with Velcro or a sandbag, being careful not to restrict breathing.

Vertebrae: Superimpose the sternum and vertebrae to minimize any rotation (Fig. 20.10).

Comments and Tips

- Ensure that there is a straight line from the tip of the nose to the base of the tail to achieve rib symmetry on the image.
- Large dogs may require two separate views.
- The symmetry of the normal patient is noted on an image when the spinous processes are evident on the midvertebral body and the sternum is superimposed over the vertebrae.

MEASURE: T6 to T7 or xiphoid midpoint (highest part of sternum).

CENTRAL RAY: T6 to T7 or midpoint xiphoid.

BORDERS: *Cranial:* C7 (shoulder joint).

Caudal: L1 (past the origin of the last rib).

Laterally: Tightly collimate.

✎ TECHNICIAN NOTES Image fewer vertebrae to prevent distortion due to the divergence of the x-ray beam.

FIG. 20.10 A, Positioning for the ventrodorsal view of the thoracic vertebrae. **B,** Overlay of the ventrodorsal view of the thoracic vertebrae. **C,** Ventrodorsal radiograph of the thoracic vertebrae. (C, Courtesy Veterinary Teaching Hospital, Diagnostic Imaging at the University of Guelph.)

Thoracolumbar Vertebrae

Lateral View of the Thoracolumbar Vertebrae—Routine

Positioning

Place In: Lateral recumbency.

Hindlimbs: Superimpose and place the pelvic limbs caudally; secure with Velcro/sandbag.

A small foam pad can be placed between the limbs.

Forelimbs: Superimpose and cranially position the forelimbs slightly; secure with Velcro/sandbag. A small foam pad can be placed between the limbs.

Head/Neck/Sternum: If needed, use foam pads under the sternum to achieve true alignment with the vertebrae.

Keep the head in a natural position and support the neck with a sandbag, being careful not to restrict breathing.

Vertebrae: Keep the thoracolumbar vertebrae on the same plane as the sternum (Fig. 20.11).

Using tape as in Fig. 20.1 can assist with proper alignment.

Comments and Tips

- Try to maintain true lateral positioning of the entire body even if radiographing only the thoracolumbar area.
- Collimate tightly. The vertebrae should be limited to four on either side of the thoracolumbar junction. If interested in both the thoracic and lumbar vertebrae, each area should be radiographed separately so that the number of vertebrae is limited.
- The ribs should be superimposed over each other so that the intervertebral spaces are better viewed. The sternum should be at the same distance from the table as the vertebrae.
- On the image, the intervertebral foramina should be superimposed. They should be of equal sizes from the thoracolumbar junction toward the sacrum.

MEASURE: Highest point of the ribs.

CENTRAL RAY: T13 to L1 intervertebral space.

BORDERS: *Cranial:* Xiphoid.

Caudal: Most caudal portion of the last rib.

Dorsally and Ventrally: Tightly collimate.

> **TECHNICIAN NOTES**   Keep these practical landmarks in mind as a general basis for the borders of all vertebrae:
> - Base of the skull
> - Shoulder
> - Origin of the last rib
> - Greater trochanter

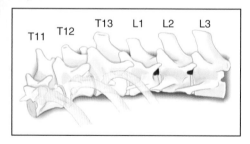

FIG. 20.11 **A,** Positioning for the lateral view of the thoracolumbar vertebrae. **B,** Right-to-left lateral radiographic anatomy of the thoracolumbar vertebrae. **C,** Lateral radiograph of the thoracolumbar vertebrae. Limit the number of vertebrae on either side of the thoracolumbar junction. (**C,** Courtesy Mount Pleasant Veterinary Hospital, Toronto, ON)

Ventrodorsal View of the Thoracolumbar Vertebrae—Routine

Positioning

Place In: Dorsal recumbency in a V-trough or use sandbags, if needed, to prevent rotation.

Hindlimbs: Place the pelvic limbs in a neutral position; secure with Velcro/sandbags if needed.

Forelimbs: Position the forelimbs cranially; tie or secure with Velcro/sandbags.

Head/Neck/Sternum: The head and neck can be in a natural position.

If needed, support with a sandbag, being careful not to restrict breathing.

The nose should be equidistant between both front limbs.

Vertebrae: Superimpose the sternum and vertebrae to minimize any rotation (Fig. 20.12).

Comments and Tips

- Ensure that there is a straight line from the tip of the nose to the base of the tail.
- Collimate tightly. If interested in both the thoracic and lumbar vertebrae, each area should be radographed separately so that the number of vertebrae is limited.
- See Box 20.1 to ensure you have proper symmetry on the image.

MEASURE: Highest point of the midthorax.

CENTRAL RAY: T13 to L1 intervertebral space.

BORDERS: *Cranial*: Xiphoid.
Caudal: Caudal portion of last rib.
Laterally: Tightly collimate.

FIG. 20.12 A, Positioning for the ventrodorsal view of the thoracolumbar vertebrae. B, Overlay of the ventrodorsal thoracolumbar vertebrae. C, Ventrodorsal radiograph of the thoracolumbar vertebrae. (C, Courtesy Joshua Schlote, BS, LVT, Northeast Community College.)

Ventrodorsal View of the Thoracolumbar Vertebrae—Routine—cont'd

✎ TECHNICIAN NOTES   Provide enough support with a V-trough, foam pads, Velcro, or sandbags to prevent any axial rotation.

Ventrodorsal views: Superimpose the spine and sternum and keep perpendicular to the table and receptor.

Lateral views: Keep the spine and sternum on the same horizontal plane, parallel to the table and receptor.

✎ TECHNICIAN NOTES   Collimate tightly to include the transverse process and muscle mass, but do not include the fat and skin.

BOX 20.1   Assessing Correct Positioning on a Vertebral Image

To assess correct positioning on a finished image[1-3]:

Cervical and thoracic vertebrae:
- Lateral view:
  - The wings of the atlas and individual transverse processes and rib heads are superimposed.
  - The articular processes are parallel.
  - The intervertebral disks are of even thickness and regular shape.
- Ventrodorsal view:
  - Equivalent anatomical features are symmetrical.
  - Spinous processes are on midvertebral body.

Thoracolumbar vertebrae:
- Lateral view:
  - The intervertebral foramina should be superimposed and should be of equal size and shape from the thoracolumbar junction toward the sacrum.

Lumbar and sacral vertebrae:
- Lateral view:
  - Transverse processes and wings of the ilia are superimposed.
  - The lumbar transverse process superimposition has been described as a "Nike swoosh."[1]
  - The intervertebral foramina should be superimposed and of equal size and shape from the thoracolumbar junction to the sacrum.
- Ventrodorsal view:
  - Spinous processes are superimposed on the midvertebral body.
  - Sacroiliac joints and equivalent anatomical features are symmetrical.

Lumbar Vertebrae

Lateral View of the Lumbar Vertebrae—Routine

Positioning

Place In: Lateral recumbency.

Hindlimbs: Superimpose and place the pelvic limbs slightly caudally; secure with Velcro/sandbag.

A small foam pad can be placed between the limbs.

Forelimbs: Superimpose and position the forelimbs slightly cranially; secure with Velcro/sandbag.

A small foam pad can be placed between the limbs.

Head/Neck/Sternum: If needed, use foam pads under the sternum to achieve true alignment with the vertebrae.

Keep the head in a natural position; support the neck with a sandbag, being careful not to restrict breathing.

Vertebrae: Keep each lumbar vertebra parallel to the table and image receptor, and on the same horizontal plane as the sternum.

Using tape as in Fig. 20.1 can assist with proper alignment (Figs. 20.13, 20.15A).

Comments and Tips

- Maintain true lateral positioning of the entire body, even if radiographing only the lumbar area.
- Collimate tightly.
- See Box 20.1 to ensure you have proper symmetry on the image.

MEASURE: Level of L1.

CENTRAL RAY: L3 to L4 (palpate).

BORDERS: *Cranial*: T12 (to origin of last rib).

Caudal: S1 (just before the greater trochanter).

Dorsally and Ventrally: Tightly collimate.

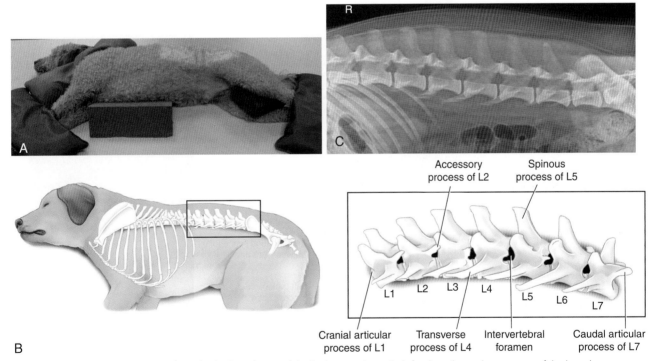

FIG. 20.13 A, Positioning for the lateral view of the lumbar vertebrae. **B,** Left-right radiographic anatomy of the lateral lumbar vertebrae. **C,** Lateral radiograph of the lumbar vertebrae of a 19-year-old male neutered French Bulldog. Note the calcification at T12 to T13, L1 to L2, and L3 to L4. The transverse processes should be superimposed at their origins from the vertebral bodies, with each pair appearing as one. This appearance has been described as a "Nike swoosh." (**A,** Courtesy Seneca College of Applied Arts and Technology, King City, ON; (**B,** from Evans H, de Lahunta A. *Guide to the Dissection of the Dog.* 7th ed. St Louis: Saunders; 2010; **C,** Courtesy Jennifer White, Mississauga Oakville Veterinary Emergency Hospital and Referral Group, Oakville, ON.)

Ventrodorsal View of the Lumbar Vertebrae—Routine

Positioning

Place In: Dorsal recumbency in a V-trough or use sandbags, if needed, to prevent rotation.

Hindlimbs: Place the pelvic limbs in a neutral position; secure with Velcro/sandbags if needed.

Forelimbs: Position the forelimbs cranially and secure with Velcro/sandbag if needed.

Head/Neck/Sternum: The head can be in a natural position. Support with a sandbag, being careful not to restrict breathing.

Position the nose equidistant between the forelimbs.

Vertebrae: Superimpose the sternum and vertebrae to prevent any rotation (Fig. 20.14).

See Figs. 20.15 through 20.17 for further vertebral anatomy.

Comments and Tips

- Ensure that there is a straight line from the tip of the nose to the base of the tail.
- The transverse processes should be present and symmetrical on the image.
- A cleansing enema 1 to 2 hours before radiography should be considered to remove any feces in the colon that could obscure spinal lesions.

MEASURE: Level of L1.

CENTRAL RAY: Level of L4 (palpate).

BORDERS: *Cranial*: T12 (origin of the last rib)
Caudal: S1 (greater trochanter).
Laterally: Tightly collimate.

TECHNICIAN NOTES   To avoid rotation of the spine in the VD position, extend the forelimbs and hindlimbs and secure them to provide further support.

T13
L1

Intervertebral space (disk) between T13 and L1

Left transverse process of L4

L7

Left sacroiliac joint

A   B   C

FIG. 20.14 A, Positioning for the ventrodorsal view of the lumbar vertebrae. **B,** Overlay of the ventrodorsal lumbar vertebrae. **C,** Ventrodorsal radiograph of the lumbar vertebrae.

Lumbar, Sacral and Caudal Vertebrae

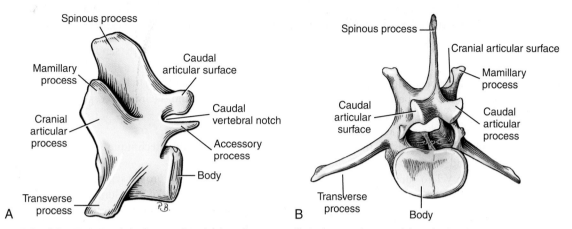

FIG. 20.15 A, Fourth lumbar vertebra, left lateral view. **B,** Fifth lumbar vertebra, caudolateral view. (From Evans H, de Lahunta A. *Guide to the Dissection of the Dog.* 8th ed. St Louis: Saunders; 2017.)

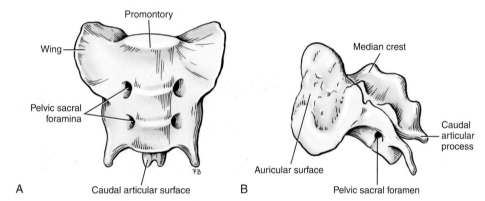

FIG. 20.16 Sacrum. **A,** Ventral view. **B,** Left lateral view. (From Evans H, de Lahunta A. *Guide to the Dissection of the Dog.* 8th ed. St Louis: Saunders; 2017.)

FIG. 20.17 A, Third caudal vertebrae, dorsal view. **B,** Fourth caudal vertebrae, cranial view. **C,** Sixth caudal vertebra, dorsal *(left)* and lateral *(right)* views. (From Evans H, de Lahunta A. *Guide to the Dissection of the Dog,* 8th ed. St Louis: Saunders; 2017.)

Lumbosacral Vertebrae

Lateral View of the Lumbosacral Vertebrae—Natural Positioning—Routine

Positioning

Place In: Lateral recumbency.

Hindlimbs: Superimpose and position the pelvic limbs slightly caudally, with a foam pad between them; secure with Velcro/sandbags.

Superimpose the wings of the ilia and keep parallel to the image receptor by placing padding under the upper limb.

Forelimbs: Superimpose and cranially position the forelimbs slightly; secure with Velcro/sandbag.

A small foam pad can be placed between the limbs.

Head/Neck/Sternum: Use foam pads under the sternum to achieve true alignment with the vertebrae.

Keep the head in a natural position.

Support the neck with sandbag, being careful not to restrict breathing.

Vertebrae: Use padding to keep each lumbar vertebra parallel to the table and the image receptor (Fig. 20.18).

Comments and Tips

- Use the pelvis technique chart to ensure adequate penetration.
- See Box 20.1 for proper symmetry on the image.
- Ancillary views of the lumbosacral include hyperextended and hyperflexed views of the vertebrae.

MEASURE: Wings of the ilia.

CENTRAL RAY: Level of the lumbosacral junction (just caudal to the wings of the ilia).

BORDERS: *Cranial:* L4 (cranial wings of the ilia).
Caudal: Femoral head.
Dorsally and ventrally: Tightly collimate.

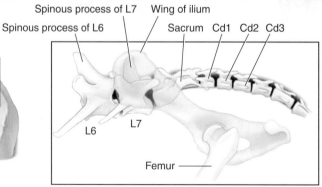

Spinous process of L7 Wing of ilium
Spinous process of L6 Sacrum Cd1 Cd2 Cd3
Pelvis
L6 L7
Femur

FIG. 20.18 A, Positioning for the lateral view of the lumbosacral vertebrae. B, Overlay and radiographic anatomy of the lateral lumbosacral vertebrae. C, Radiograph of the lateral lumbosacral vertebrae. (C *Courtesy Joshua Schlote, BS, LVT, Northeast Community College.*)

Lateral View of the Lumbosacral Vertebrae—Ancillary

Comments and Tips

- These views are used to demonstrate lumbosacral instability.
- The measuring, centering, borders, and positioning is exactly the same as for the lateral view except for positioning of the hindlimbs:
  - For the hyperextended view (Fig. 20.19A): hyperextend the superimposed hindlimbs as far caudally as possible, placing Velcro/sandbag over them to hold in position.
  - For the hyperflexed view (Fig. 20.19B): position the superimposed hindlimbs as far cranially as possible, placing Velcro/sandbag over them to hold in position.

> ✎ **TECHNICIAN NOTES** Collimate, ensuring that labels/markers are included and that borders are visible for every image.

FIG. 20.19 A, Positioning for the lateral view of the lumbosacral vertebrae—hyperextended view. B, Positioning for the lateral view of the lumbosacral vertebrae—hyperflexed view.

Ventrodorsal View of the Lumbosacral Vertebrae—Routine

Positioning

Place In: Dorsal recumbency in a V-trough or use sandbags if needed.

Hindlimbs: Partially extend the pelvic limbs equally in a normal position, and secure with Velcro/sandbags if needed. The pelvic limbs may be externally rotated.

Forelimbs: Position the forelimbs cranially and secure with Velcro/sandbag.

Head/Neck/Sternum: The head can be in a natural position. Support with a sandbag, being careful not to restrict breathing.

Vertebrae: Maintain the sternum and vertebrae in the same vertical plane (Fig. 20.20).

Comments and Tips

- Ensure that the wings of the ilia are parallel to the table.
- A cleansing enema 1 to 2 hours before radiography should be considered to remove any feces in the colon that could obscure spinal lesions.

MEASURE: Wings of the ilia.

CENTRAL RAY: On the lumbosacral junction, caudal to the wings of the ilia, at an angle of 20 to 30 degrees in a caudocranial direction.

BORDERS: *Cranial:* Cranial wings of the ilia.
Caudal: Femoral heads.
Laterally: Tightly collimate.

FIG. 20.20 A, Positioning for the ventrodorsal view of the lumbosacral vertebrae. **B,** Radiographic anatomy of the ventrodorsal lumbosacral vertebrae. **C,** Ventrodorsal radiograph of the lumbosacral vertebrae. (**C** *Courtesy Jennifer White, Mississauga Oakville Veterinary Emergency Hospital and Referral Group, Oakville, Ontario.*

Caudal Vertebrae

Lateral View of the Caudal Vertebrae—Routine

Positioning

Place In: Lateral recumbency.

Hindlimbs: Superimpose and pull the pelvic limbs in a neutral position; secure with Velcro/sandbag.

Forelimbs: Superimpose and cranially position the forelimbs slightly; secure with Velcro/sandbag if needed.

Head and Neck: Keep the head in a natural position; support with a sandbag if needed.

Vertebrae: Place a foam pad to keep the vertebrae parallel to the table.

A receptor can be placed on the foam pad under the tail. Secure the tail if needed (Fig. 20.21).

Comments and Tips

• If the film cassette can be placed on the tabletop, split the plate so that both views are on one cassette.

MEASURE: Thickest part of the tail.

CENTRAL RAY: Area of interest.

BORDERS: Four or five vertebrae on either side of the area of interest, or the full tail.

FIG. 20.21 A, Positioning of the lateral caudal (coccygeal) vertebrae. B, Radiographic anatomy of the lateral caudal vertebrae. C, Lateral radiograph of the caudal vertebrae that are fractured near the tip. (C, Courtesy Mount Pleasant Veterinary Hospital, Toronto, ON.)

Ventrodorsal View of the Caudal Vertebrae—Routine

Positioning

Place In: Dorsal recumbency in a V-trough or supported by tape/Velcro strapping or sandbag if needed.

Hindlimbs: Extend the pelvic limbs; secure with Velcro/sandbags if needed.

Forelimbs: Position the forelimbs cranially; secure with Velcro/sandbags if needed.

Head/Neck/Sternum: The head can be in a natural position. Secure if needed.

Vertebrae: Secure the tail with tape, if required, and keep it in a straight line with the body (Fig. 20.22).

MEASURE: Thickest part of the tail.

CENTRAL RAY: Area of interest.

BORDERS: Four or five vertebrae on either side of the area of interest, or the full tail.

FIG. 20.22 A, Positioning for the ventrodorsal view of the caudal (coccygeal) vertebrae. B, Ventrodorsal radiograph of the caudal vertebrae.

Further Ancillary Views

- Oblique view, lateral decubitus view, and a DV view are alternatives if a routine VD view of the spinal column using a vertical beam is not feasible due to patient injury or other concerns.
- Apply the principles of measuring, centering, and borders for each of the positions described here.
- Center the beam on the area of interest and collimate.

Lateral Decubitus View of the Vertebrae (Ventrodorsal View with a Horizontal Beam)—Ancillary

- The VD view can also be achieved using a horizontal beam (Fig. 20.23A) with the dog in lateral recumbency, as described for the thoracic and abdominal views in Chapters 16 and 17.

Dorsoventral View of the Vertebrae—Ancillary

- A DV view with the dog in sternal recumbency (Fig. 20.23B) can also be completed if the patient is compromised in a VD position or if the machine does not allow a lateral decubitus view.
- It is more difficult to maintain the vertebrae parallel to the table for a DV. Additionally, the OFD is increased, which means increased magnification.
- For completion of this view, keep a pad under the head so that all the vertebrae are parallel to the table (Fig. 20.23B).
- Fig. 20.24 is a mystery radiograph. Review it and answer the question presented with it.

Oblique View of the Vertebrae—Ancillary

- To help localize a lesion identified on the lateral or VD views that requires further examination, an oblique view may be requested.
- Place the patient in dorsal recumbency and rotate the body either to the right or to the left.
- Use padding under the mandible, cranial sternum, and pelvis to obtain a 30- to 45-degree oblique projection.
- Both the right and left oblique views should be compared.

FIG. 20.23 A, Positioning for ventrodorsal view of the vertebrae with a horizontal beam. Tightly collimate the beam on the area of interest. **B,** A dorsoventral view can be obtained if it is difficult to obtain a ventrodorsal view. Object-film distance and magnification will be increased with the dorsoventral view, and the vertebrae are more difficult to keep parallel. Collimate the beam in tightly for spinal radiographs.

FIG. 20.24 Mystery Radiographs. Compare the two images of the cervical lateral spine of the same patient. What is the problem with image A and how was it solved in image B?

✳ KEY POINTS

1. General anesthesia or sedation allows for more accurate positioning.
2. Lateral and VD views of each spinal area are routine. Ancillary views may further assist diagnosis.
3. Each imaged vertebra must be parallel to the table/image receptor. The central ray is perpendicular to both. This minimizes distortion that could lead to misdiagnosis.
4. Measure at the thickest part of the area of interest.
5. Collimate tightly to the vertebrae, being conscious of the placement of the labels and markers.
6. Multiple views are recommended. Limit the number of vertebrae on an image to avoid the optical illusion of x-ray beam divergence.
7. Manipulation of the limbs and spine of patients with spinal column injury may be contraindicated.

REVIEW QUESTIONS

1. The ventrodorsal cervical vertebrae of a Doberman are to be radiographed. It is best to measure:
   a. And center at C6
   b. At C6 and center at C3–C4
   c. At C1 and center at C3–C4
   d. And center at C3–C4

2. For a radiograph of the lateral cervical vertebrae of the Doberman, foam pads can be used to help ensure proper patient positioning. A foam pad is not likely needed:
   a. Under the sternum
   b. Beneath the cervical vertebrae
   c. Between the rear limbs
   d. Under the nose

3. The front limbs of the Doberman for the lateral cervical vertebrae should be:
   a. Superimposed and positioned slightly caudally
   b. Superimposed and positioned slightly cranially
   c. Scissored and positioned slightly caudally
   d. Scissored and positioned slightly cranially

4. A flexed lateral view is required for the cervical vertebrae of this Doberman. The cervical vertebrae should be flexed, and:
   a. The head should be in a natural oblique position
   b. The head should be in a true lateral position
   c. The limbs should be extended as far cranial as possible
   d. No padding is required under the cervical vertebrae

5. A lateral view of the thoracolumbar vertebrae is required of a Dachshund. You should measure at the:
   a. T13 to L1 intervertebral space
   b. Cranial border of the scapula
   c. Highest point of the ribs
   d. Level of L4

6. The borders for this lateral view of the Dachshund thoracolumbar vertebrae should be at:
   a. The xiphoid to the most caudal portion of the last rib
   b. The cranial portion of C1 to T6
   c. T13 to caudal portion of L1
   d. T1 to just past L7

7. To ensure proper positioning for a ventrodorsal thoracolumbar view:
   a. Superimpose the ribs so that the intervertebral spaces are better viewed
   b. Place padding under the cervical vertebrae and sternum
   c. Place the pelvic limbs over each other in a neutral position and secure with sandbags
   d. Superimpose the sternum over the vertebrae

8. In the lateral view of the TL junction, the label and positional markers should be placed:
   a. Ventral to the vertebrae being imaged
   b. Dorsal to the vertebrae being imaged
   c. At the cranial aspect of the vertebrae being imaged
   d. At the caudal aspect of the vertebrae being imaged

9. The veterinarian suspects compression fracture of an Irish Setter and requires perpendicular views of the thorax and lumbar vertebrae but is concerned about causing further injury. With film radiography and if the x-ray unit allows, you should complete a:
   a. Right lateral and right lateral decubitus view
   b. Right lateral only
   c. Right lateral and VD view
   d. Right and left lateral and DV view

10. In radiographing an Irish Wolfhound's thoracic and lumbar vertebrae for lateral and orthogonal views, you should measure and center at:
    a. T6/T7 and L4 to obtain four radiographs total
    b. T6/T7, TL junction, and L4 to obtain six radiographs total
    c. T6/T7 and L4 to obtain two radiographs total
    d. T6/T7, TL junction, and L4 to obtain three radiographs total

11. In radiographing the Irish Wolfhound's thoracolumbar vertebrae, you should include from:
    a. T1 to L3 on one image
    b. T4 to L3 on one image
    c. T10 to L3
    d. T1 to L7

12. You are checking the lateral lumbar radiographs of the Irish Wolfhound's vertebrae to ensure that you are giving the veterinarian properly positioned radiographs. On the lateral image, you are looking for:
    a. Superimposed intervertebral foramina and transverse processes
    b. Equal symmetry of the transverse processes
    c. A colon that does not contain any stool
    d. Spinous processes that are evident on the midvertebral body

13. To note symmetry on the VD lumbar radiograph of the Irish Wolfhound, you are looking for:
    a. Superimposed intervertebral foramina that are of equal size
    b. Superimposed pelvic limbs that are slightly positioned caudally
    c. Spinous processes that are evident on the midvertebral body
    d. A "Nike swoosh" created by the superimposition of transfer processes

14. A cleansing enema performed 1 to 2 hours before exposure is recommended for:
    a. The ventrodorsal lumbar and lumbosacral views
    b. Lateral and ventrodorsal lumbar and lumbosacral vertebrae views
    c. All ventrodorsal vertebrae views
    d. All ventrodorsal and lateral vertebrae views

15. Lumbosacral instability is suspected in a Greyhound. Along with the regular lateral, the veterinarian will complete dynamic studies after a myelography study. The dynamic study is in reference to:
    a. VD and DV views
    b. Hyperextended only
    c. Hyperflexed only
    d. Both hyperextended and hyperflexed views

16. For a hyperextended lumbosacral view, a German Shepherd will be positioned in:
    a. Ventral recumbency with a horizontal beam aimed at the lumbosacral junction
    b. Lateral recumbency with the hindlimbs superimposed and extended quite caudally
    c. Lateral recumbency with the hindlimbs superimposed and extended quite cranially
    d. Dorsal recumbency with the hindlimbs superimposed and extended quite cranially

17. If oblique views are to be taken of the vertebrae, the patient should be placed in:
    a. Lateral recumbency with 30 to 45 degrees rotation
    b. Sternal recumbency with 30 to 45 degrees rotation
    c. Dorsal recumbency with 30 to 45 degrees rotation
    d. Dorsal recumbency with 15 to 25 degrees rotation

18. A stabilized and paralyzed feline patient had been HBC (hit by car). The veterinarian suspects a complete fracture in the thoracic and lumbar region but wishes to take an initial radiograph to assist the owners to determine if treatment is an option. The veterinarian suggests that for now, she would like you to obtain:
    a. Right and left lateral radiographs from C1 to S1
    b. Right lateral and VD radiographs from C1 to S1
    c. Three right lateral radiographs: C1 to L1, T10 to L3, and T12 to S1
    d. A right lateral radiograph from C7 to S1

Chapter Review Question answers are located in the Instructor Resources on Evolve and can be provided to students at the discretion of the instructor.

References

1. Thrall DE. *Textbook of Veterinary Diagnostic Radiology*. 7th ed. St. Louis: Elsevier; 2017.
2. Holloway A. *BSAVA Manual of Canine and Feline Radiography and Radiology: A Foundation Manual*. Suffolk: BSAVA; 2014.
3. Muhlbauer MC, Kneller SK. *Radiography of the Dog and Cat: Guide to Making and Interpreting Radiographs*. Oxford: Wiley-Blackwell; 2013.

Bibliography

Ayers S. *Small Animal Radiographic Techniques and Positioning*. Oxford: Wiley-Blackwell; 2013.

Colville T, Bassert J. *Clinical Anatomy and Physiology for Veterinary Technicians*. 3rd ed. St. Louis: Mosby; 2016.

Done SH, Goody PC, Evans S, Stickland NC. *Color Atlas of Veterinary Anatomy, the Dog and Cat*. London: Mosby; 2009.

Evans H, de Lahunta A. *Guide to the Dissection of the Dog*. 7th ed. St. Louis: Saunders; 2010.

Singh B. *Dyce, Sack and Wensing's Textbook of Veterinary Anatomy*. 5th ed. St. Louis: Elsevier; 2018.

Sirois M, Schlote J. *Diagnostic Imaging for Veterinary Technicians*. Minneapolis, MN: Bluedoor, LLC; 2017.

Tighe M, Brown M. *Mosby's Comprehensive Review for Veterinary Technicians*. 5th ed. St. Louis: Mosby; 2019.

CHAPTER 21

Small Animal Skull

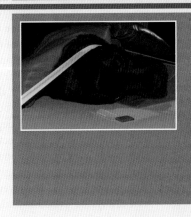

Marg Brown, RVT, BEd Ad Ed

"Nothing is tough but your skull, so think out of the skull box and let the thoughts fly."
—Vikram Verma (1944), author of *10 Golden Steps of Life*

OUTLINE

LEARNING OBJECTIVES

When you have finished this chapter, you will be able to:

1. Identify common positions and principles used to radiograph the small-animal skull.
2. Properly and safely position a dog or cat for the various common positions of the skull with an emphasis on non-manual restraint.
3. Correctly measure and center the patient to include the peripheral borders.
4. Ensure that the body part is parallel to the image receptor and the central ray is perpendicular to both the field of view (FOV) and detector.
5. Recognize other views that may need to be completed as an alternative.
6. Identify normal skull anatomy found on a radiograph.

KEY TERMS

Key terms are defined in the Glossary on the Evolve website.

Brachycephalic
Canthi
Commissure
Dolichocephalic
Dorsal

Lateral oblique
Mesaticephalic
Positional terminology
Quadrant
Rostral

Rostrocaudal
Rostrodorsal-caudoventral oblique
Rostroventral-caudodorsal oblique

Skyline
Ventral

TECHNICAL NOTE: To preserve space, the radiographic images presented in this chapter do not show collimation. For safety, always collimate so that the beam is limited to within the image receptor edges. In film radiography, you should see a clear border of collimation (frame) on every radiograph. In some jurisdictions, evidence of collimation is required by law. In digital imaging, the algorithm depends on proper collimation.

The skull, along with the spine, makes up the axial skeleton. Proper imaging of the skull can be challenging because of complicated anatomy, superimposition of many of the structures, and the variation in size and shape of the various breeds. Images of the skull (Table 21.1) are often taken to evaluate trauma, congenital abnormalities, inflammatory lesions, tumors, or degenerative changes. Radiography may be inaccurate for detecting certain diseases and not as diagnostic as cross-sectional imaging modalities such as magnetic resonance imaging (MRI) and computerized tomography (CT). However, alternative modalities might not always be available and are expensive, so radiography remains a primary diagnostic tool.[1]

> ✐ **TECHNICIAN NOTES** To be more efficient for any view, ensure that the body parts that are not in the beam are positioned and secured first. Position the area of interest last.

Radiographic Concerns and Anatomy

1. Symmetrical positioning of the skull is essential, especially in lateral and dorsoventral/ventrodorsal (DV/VD) views, to help identify asymmetrical structures and opacities. Most disease processes of the skull are not bilateral.[1]
2. Fortunately, the skull is relatively symmetrical and, in most small animals, approximately the same width in lateral and DV/VD dimensions. Both positions are measured at the widest area of the cranium. If air-filled sinus cavities are to be radiographed, measure just rostral to the thickest part of the cranium to avoid overexposure. Fig. 21.1 indicates the different skull types of canines.
3. Heavy sedation or general anesthesia will be required for most patients for views other than the routine lateral and dorsoventral survey to ensure that proper symmetry will be maintained. Consult an anesthesia text for suggested protocols and considerations.

TABLE 21.1	Protocol for Skull Radiography
ANATOMICAL LOCATION	**VIEW(S)**
Routine Views	
Skull: routine or survey	Lateral (affected side down)
	Dorsoventral (DV) or Ventrodorsal (VD)
Ancillary Views	
Routine views for other areas of interest *(In addition to routine skull survey)*	
Frontal sinuses	Rostrocaudal frontal sinus view—frontal 90-degree, rostrocaudal closed-mouth
	Lateral Oblique View (LeD-RtVO or RtD-LeVO) (Ancillary)
	Opposite lateral (L)
Nasal cavity	Intraoral dorsoventral
	Ventrodorsal open-mouth—Ventral 20–30-degrees Rostral-Dorsocaudal Oblique (V20–30°R-DCdO) open-mouth
	Closed-mouth caudoventral-rostrodorsal oblique (CdV-RDO)—for brachycephalic breeds
Foramen magnum	Rostrocaudal closed-mouth view—Rostral 20–30-degree Ventral-Caudodorsal oblique (R20–30°V-CdO)
Frontal sinus	Rostrocaudal—90-degree closed-mouth (for those breeds with frontal sinus)
Tympanic bullae	Open-mouth Rostrocaudal (Rostral 10–30-degree Ventral-Caudodorsal Oblique) (R10–30°V-CdDO)
	Feline and brachycephalic dogs: Closed-mouth Rostral 10-degree Ventral-Caudodorsal Oblique (R10° V-CdDO)
	Lateral oblique views: LeD-RtVO or RtD-LeVO, affected side up
	Lateral oblique (LeV-RtDO or RtV-LeDO), affected side down
Temporomandibular joint	Lateral oblique (LeV-RtDO or RtV-LeDO), affected side down
	Lateral oblique (LeD-RtVO or RtD-LeVO), affected side up
Zygomatic bone and orbit	Rostrocaudal—90-degree closed-mouth
Maxilla and dental extraoral studies*	Right or left open-mouth lateral
	Intraoral dorsoventral
	Lateral oblique (LeV-RtDO or RtV-LeDO)
Mandible and dental extraoral studies*	Right or left open-mouth lateral
	Intraoral ventrodorsal
	Lateral oblique views with affected side down (Le-20° D-RtVO or Rt-20° D-LeVO)

*For extraoral views, please see Chapter 22.

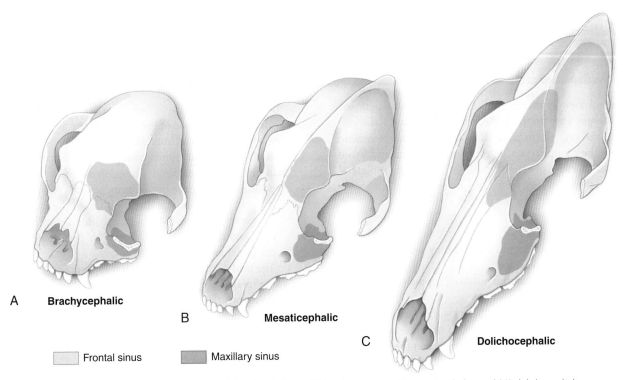

FIG. 21.1 The three basic shapes of the dog skull are **(A)** brachycephalic, **(B)** mesaticephalic, and **(C)** dolichocephalic. The positions of the maxillary and frontal sinus on half of the skull are also shown. (From Aspinall V, Cappello M. *Introduction to Veterinary Anatomy.* London: Butterworth-Heineman, Elsevier; 2009.)

4. Recognize that the endotracheal tube, tongue, and pinnae could all cause artifacts that may interfere with diagnosis, so they should be repositioned or removed from the field of view when possible.

5. High-contrast exposure is recommended. Use a grid for measurements over 10 cm in film radiography. Use high milliampere-seconds (mAs) with a longer time station so that the lowest mA can be used that allows a small focal spot to improve geometric sharpness. When possible, the radiograph should be tightly collimated to the primary area of interest to reduce secondary radiation and to improve image quality. Keep the thickest part of the skull toward the cathode.

6. No special preparation is required other than brushing the hair coat and removing any collars or devices.

7. Various-sized radiolucent wedges are required to properly and consistently position for extraoral oblique radiographs of the mandible and maxilla.

8. Place the appropriate marker toward the nose. Correctly identifying the anatomy with right and left markers is essential, especially for any oblique views. Both markers should be placed on the image detector for oblique images so that there is no confusion as to which is the dependent jaw. The markers also help identify the different quadrants of the teeth.

9. The oblique mandible and maxilla views are further discussed in Chapter 22.

✎ TECHNICIAN NOTES Use positioning aids strategically to give the patient the illusion that it is being held. A sandbag over the neck and limbs, and Velcro/tape are essential if not properly sedated. Keep talking to your patient in a calm, low voice.

Routine Views

Lateral View of the Skull

The lateral view evaluates the nasal cavity, frontal sinuses, nasal margin and frontal bones, dorsal margin of the calvarium, and cribriform plate. The lateral is the best view to examine the nasopharynx, retropharyngeal area, and hyoid apparatus. Because of superimposition, significant unilateral disease of the nasal cavity and bony margins may be missed.[1] Place the affected side on the table.

Positioning (Fig. 21.2)

Place In: Right or left lateral recumbency with the affected side to the image receptor.

Hindlimbs: Leave in a natural position; support with a sandbag or ties if needed.

Forelimbs: Pull caudally, and support with a sandbag or ties.

Head and Neck: Position the head so that the mandible is parallel to the long edge of the image receptor.

Put padding under the cranioventral cervical region. Place a foam pad under the ramus of the mandible to superimpose the rami and to prevent rotation of the skull.

Tape the head or use Velcro straps over the nose and neck area so that the tape is extended across the table. A sandbag may be placed over the neck and against a foam pad at the dorsal aspect of the head to keep the head in position.

Comments and Tips

- Ensure that the pinnae of the ears and tape are not superimposed over areas of interest.
- Pulling the pectoral limbs caudally may help keep the skull in a true lateral position.
- To ensure that you have proper symmetry, as you position:
  - View in a rostrocaudal direction (from the front). An imaginary line drawn through the medial canthi of the eyes and the hard palate should be perpendicular to the tabletop.
  - The midsagittal plane and nasal septum are parallel to the image receptor.
  - If you position your hand under the ventral mandible, it should be perpendicular to the table.
- The rami of the mandible and the tympanic bullae should be superimposed on the image.
- Because the skull in a brachycephalic breed is wider, geometrical distortion due to the divergent nature of the beam may not allow the appearance of symmetry of all structures.
- If either the mandible or maxilla are of particular interest, it may be beneficial to keep the mouth open with a speculum to minimize superimposition.

MEASURING, CENTERING, BORDERS: **See Table 21.2.**

✏️ **TECHNICIAN NOTES**   Pads under the nose and neck will help keep the skull in a horizontal plane to minimize rotation. The wings of the atlas and all aspects of the skull should be even and superimposed on the image.

✏️ **TECHNICIAN NOTES**   Prior to positioning the patient:

- Turn on the machine, set the main voltage calibration if required, have proper source image distance, measure the skull in the correct position, and set the exposures. Have the image receptors ready. Positioning devices should be close at hand.
- Place your patient. Ensure proper location of markers and identification (if using at this stage); correct body part and view; properly centered; borders correct and collimated.
- To minimize scattered radiation, remove any objects or distractions not utilized. There should be no artifacts in the area of interest, and the patient should be chemically restrained if possible.
- Lastly, position and quickly go through your mental checklist to make sure everything is completed prior to pushing the exposure button.

✏️ **TECHNICIAN NOTES**

- True symmetry in a lateral view of a normal patient has been achieved if there appears to be only one structure on the image—the two sides are superimposed.
- True symmetry in a DV/VD view of a normal patient has been achieved if the left and right sides are mirror images.

FIG. 21.2 A, Positioning for the lateral skull view.

Lateral View of the Skull—cont'd

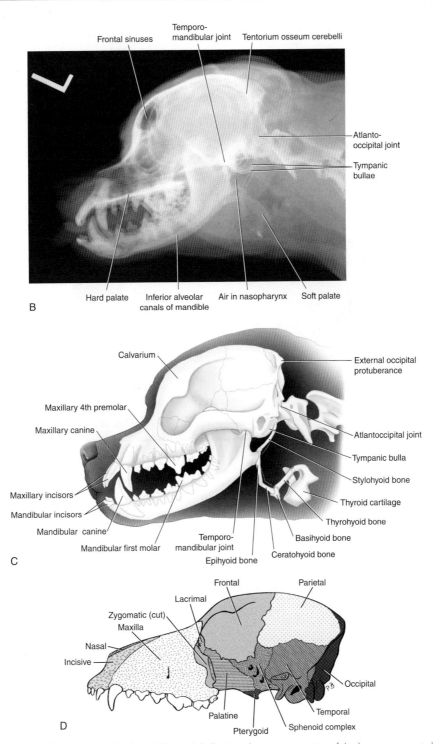

FIG. 21.2, cont'd B, Radiograph of the left lateral skull. Note the superimposition of the bones, tympanic bullae, and teeth in a true lateral view. C, Lateral left-to-right radiographic anatomy of the canine skull. D, Bones of the skull, lateral aspect (zygomatic arch and mandible removed).

Lateral View of the Skull—cont'd

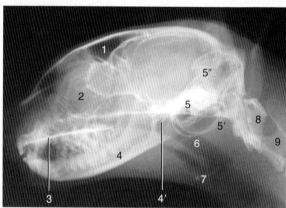

FIG. 21.2, cont'd E, Lateral left-to-right radiographic anatomy of the feline skull. **F**, Radiograph of a feline lateral. *1*, Frontal sinus; *2*, cribriform plate and ethmoidal conchae; *3*, hard palate; *4*, mandible; *4'*, temporomandibular joint; *5*, petrous temporal bone; *5'*, tympanic bullae; *5"*, tentorium cerebelli; *6*, nasopharynx; *7*, basihyoid; *8*, atlas; *9*, axis. (D, From Hermanson J, de Lahunta A. *Miller's Anatomy of the Dog*. 5th ed. St Louis: Elsevier; 2019; **F**, From Singh B. *Dyce, Sack and Wensing's Textbook of Veterinary Anatomy*. 5th ed. St Louis: Elsevier; 2018.)

TABLE 21.2	Lateral View of the Skull			
	SURVEY	**TEMPOROMANDIBULAR JOINT**	**TYMPANIC BULLAE**	**NARES/TEETH**
Measure (on the area of interest)	Highest point of the zygomatic arch at the center of the cranium.	Highest point of the zygomatic arch over the joint.	Highest point of the zygomatic arch over the bullae.	Highest point of the zygomatic arch just rostral to the medial canthi.
Central ray (on the area of interest)	Lateral canthus of eye, midway between the eye and ear, or on area of interest.	Center just rostral to the ears.	Palpate and center on the base of the ear.	Just rostral to the lateral canthus.
Borders (depends on the area of interest)	Full skull: tip of the nose to the occipital protuberance.	Cranial and caudal to the joint.	Cranial and caudal to the ear.	Tip of the nose to the lateral canthi.

Dorsoventral View of the Skull

The DV is used for routine skull images and preferred over the VD, as it is easier to obtain true symmetry due to greater stability and less rotation when resting on the mandibles. The area of interest is close to the image receptor, geometrical distortion is reduced, and the image indicates right and left symmetry.

Both DV and VD views assess lateral and caudal aspects of the skull, external ear canal and middle ear, and the temporomandibular joints (TMJs). In the DV, there will be superimposition by the mandibles on the lateral nasal cavities and frontal sinuses.[2]

Positioning (Fig. 21.3)

Place In: Sternal recumbency.

Hindlimbs: Place in a natural position and support with a sandbag or ties.

Forelimbs: Pull caudally or leave in a natural position alongside the head, out of the field of view; support them with a sandbag or ties.

Head and Neck: Extend the neck and head.

Place a sandbag over the neck for support, being careful not to restrict breathing.

Tape/Velcro across the nasal septum and the cranium to keep the sagittal plane of the head perpendicular to the image receptor.

Make sure the ears are positioned laterally, equidistant from the head.

Comments and Tips

- To ensure symmetry during positioning: Look at the skull in a rostrocaudal direction and draw an imaginary line between the medial canthi. This line should be parallel to the table.
- Symmetrical mandibles will provide a flat and stable surface to support the head. Slight downward pressure applied with positioning aids will facilitate a perfect DV image.[2] Make sure the hard palate is parallel to the image receptor.
- To prevent unwanted artifacts, minimize the use of tape/ Velcro over the area of interest when lower exposure factors are used. Have the thickest part of the skull toward the cathode to minimize opacity changes.
- Place the marker on either side of the nose.
- Endotracheal tubes may have to be removed for the exposures if safe to do so.

Intraoral Dorsoventral—Ancillary

- With the patient positioned as in the DV view, the image receptor is positioned in the mouth between the maxilla and endotracheal tube for the nasal cavity. The beam is centered on the dorsal aspect on the hard palate between the nasal planum and right and left orbits. This will be further described in Chapter 22.

MEASURING, CENTERING, BORDERS: **See Table 21.3.**

> **TECHNICIAN NOTES** To maintain symmetry for the DV view, ensure that an imaginary line drawn between the medial canthi is parallel to the table. Look from the rostrocaudal direction. Keep the hard palate parallel to the table and image receptor.

FIG. 21.3 A, Positioning for the dorsoventral skull view. B, DV skull radiograph of a dog. Note the symmetry of left and right sides and superimposition of the mandibular symphysis on the vomer bone.

Dorsoventral View of the Skull—cont'd

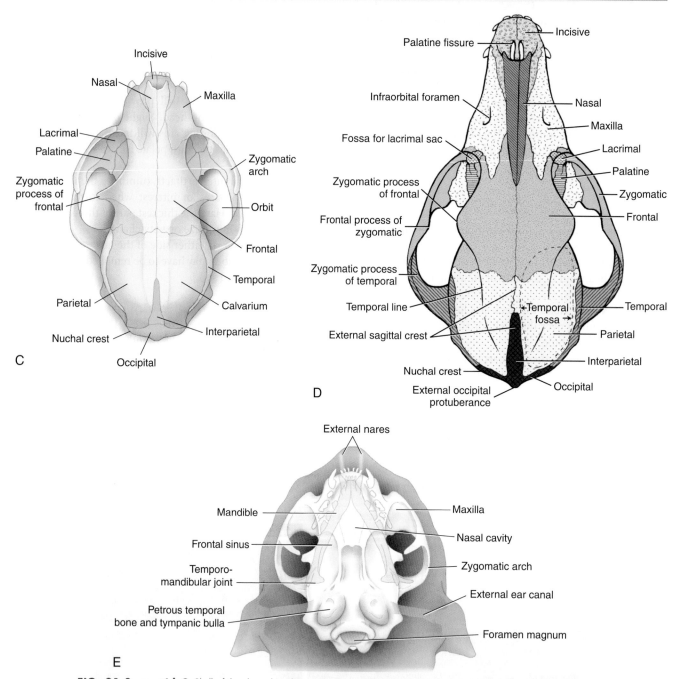

C, Skull of the dog, dorsal view. D, Bones of the skull dorsal aspect. E, Overlay and radiographic anatomy of the ventrodorsal feline skull.

FIG. 21.3, cont'd C, Skull of the dog, dorsal view. D, Bones of the skull dorsal aspect. E, Overlay and radiographic anatomy of the ventrodorsal feline skull. (B, From Thrall DE. *Textbook of Veterinary Diagnostic Radiology.* 7th ed. St. Louis: Elsevier; 2018; D, Hermanson J, de Lahunta A. *Miller's Anatomy of the Dog.* 5th ed. St Louis: Elsevier; 2019; E, From Singh B. *Dyce, Sack and Wensing's Textbook of Veterinary Anatomy.* 5th ed. St Louis: Elsevier; 2018.)

TABLE 21.3	Dorsoventral and Ventrodorsal Views of the Skull			
	SURVEY	**TEMPOROMANDIBULAR JOINT**	**TYMPANIC BULLAE**	**NARES/TEETH**
Measure (on the area of interest)	Highest point of the cranium just caudal to the lateral canthi.	Rostral to the ears on the dorsal (DV)/ventral (VD) midline of the skull.	Highest point of the cranium just caudal to the lateral canthi.	Rostral to the medial canthi.
Central ray (on the area of interest)	Between the two lateral canthi of the eyes on the sagittal crest (DV)/ventral midline (VD) or on the area of interest.	Center just rostral to the ears on the dorsal/ventral midline of the skull.	Palpate the base of the ear and center on the dorsal/ventral midline between the ears.	Center more rostral.
Borders (depends on the area of interest):	Full skull: tip of the nose to the occipital protuberance.	Cranial and caudal to the joint.	Cranial and caudal to the ear.	Tip of the nose to the lateral canthi.

Ventrodorsal View of the Skull

Because the dorsal surface of the canine or feline head is not generally flat, it is more difficult to symmetrically position the head in a VD view; however, this view can be used for a routine skull, particularly for evaluation of the nasal sinus as the nasal passages are located dorsally.

Positioning (Fig. 21.4)

Place In: Dorsal recumbency in a V-trough, if required, and support with sandbags.

Hindlimbs: Leave the hindlimbs in a natural position, and support with sandbags or ties.

Forelimbs: Pull the front limbs caudally, lateral to the chest, and support with sandbags or ties.

Head and Neck: Position a foam pad or sandbag under the neck so that the hard palate is parallel with the image receptor. Place a small foam pad under the nose and tape/Velcro across the mandible to keep the head aligned with the table.

Comments and Tips

- Make sure the nose is parallel with the table and the head is symmetrical.
- To ensure proper positioning, place your hands on either side of the skull, feeling for symmetry of the mandible and/or zygomatic arches. Your hands should be equidistant from the table on both sides.
- Move the tongue and endotracheal tube (if present) to minimize artifacts on the area of interest. The endotracheal tube may have to be removed to prevent midline structures from being obscured.
- A VD for a deep-chested dog may be easier to maintain proper skull symmetry rather than a DV view. See Fig. 21.1 for comparisons of the different skull types.

MEASURING, CENTERING, BORDERS: **See Table 21.3.**

TECHNICIAN NOTES   For the VD view, extend the neck so that the nose/hard palate are parallel with the table.

A

FIG. 21.4 A, Positioning for the ventrodorsal skull view.

Ventrodorsal View of the Skull—cont'd

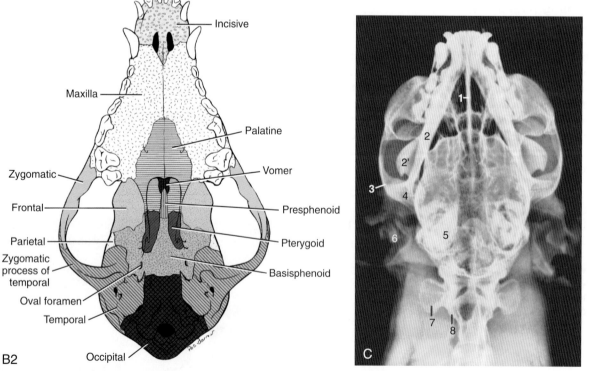

FIG. 21.4, cont'd B, Overlay and radiographic anatomy and bones of the ventrodorsal skull. C, Radiographs of a feline ventrodorsal skull. *1,* Nasal septum; *1',* infraorbital foramen; *2,* mandible; *2',* coronoid process; *3,* zygomatic arch; *4,* temporomandibular joint; *5,* petrous temporal bone; *6,* external ear; *7,* wing of atlas; *7',* atlanto-occipital joint; *8,* axis (B, Hermanson, J, de Lahunta A. *Miller's Anatomy of the Dog.* 5th ed. St Louis: Elsevier; 2019; **C,** From Singh B. *Dyce, Sack and Wensing's Textbook of Veterinary Anatomy.* 5th ed. St Louis: Elsevier; 2018.)

Ancillary Views

Because of the complexity of the skull, ancillary projections may assist in diagnosis and are chosen based on the study required. Some of these views may be routine requirements depending on the area of interest. Generally, either the area of interest is at an angle to the primary beam or the x-ray beam is angled to the table. If available, it is best to rotate the x-ray tube. For any oblique views, proper identification, often with both the L and R markers, is essential.[3]

Ventrodorsal Open-Mouth—(V20–30°R-DCdO open-mouth)

- The ventrodorsal open-mouth view (ventral 20–30-degree rostral-dorsocaudal oblique) images the nasal sinus and ethmoid regions without superimposition of the mandible.[1-3]
- The patient is in a VD position with the mouth open and the tube angled (generally 20 to 30 degrees), depending on the breed. This position can be used only if the x-ray tube is movable or can rotate.

> **✎ TECHNICIAN NOTES** "Ventrorostral-caudodorsal oblique–(V20-30°R-CdDO) (open-mouth)" means that the central ray enters the body ventrally, from the nose (rostral) at an angle of 20 to 30 degrees and then exits obliquely toward the patient's back in a caudal direction. The patient is thus lying on its back in a VD position, with the nose almost parallel to the table, with its mouth open. The detector is under the dorsal aspect of the head.

Positioning (Fig. 21.5)

Place In: Dorsal recumbency in a V-trough or support with sandbags.

Hindlimbs: Leave in a natural position and sandbag or secure them to the table with ties.

Forelimbs: Pull the front limbs caudally, lateral to the chest, and support them with sandbags or ties.

Head and Neck: Place a small foam pad under the nose.

Have the hard palate parallel to the table and the pinnae equally lateral to the head.

Position a strip of tape inside the mouth and carefully adhere the ends to the table in a cranial direction so the maxilla is parallel to the table.

Open the mouth wide by securing tape or gauze around the mandible and gently secure the head caudally and ventrally, being careful to avoid injury.

Depending on how wide the mouth is opened, the beam should be directed at 20 to 30 degrees from the vertical into the mouth and parallel to the mandible.[1,2,4]

Brief Overview

- Place patient in dorsal recumbency. Support the maxilla against the x-ray table so the hard palate is parallel to tabletop. Gently open the mouth widely with speculum gauze traction on mandible. Angle the x-ray beam 20 degrees rostrally and center the x-ray beam on hard palate (Fig. 21.5).

Comments and Tips

- In film radiography, decrease the kilovoltage (kV) slightly from that on the skull chart to account for decreased tissue density to be penetrated.
- Keep the hard palate parallel to the cassette.
- The mouth can also be propped open with a modified tongue depressor, plastic speculum, or 1-mL syringe barrel placed between or over the canine teeth. Be careful to avoid any injury, especially if the patient is compromised.
- If possible, move positioning devices, tongue, and endotracheal tube away from the area of interest to prevent artifacts.
- On a normal healthy patient, the nasal opacity and turbinate detail should be equal on both sides of the head.
- Feline patients will not likely require angulation of the beam.

Brachycephalic Breeds

- A better projection to image the nasal cavity of these breeds is a closed-mouth caudoventral-to-rostrodorsal oblique (CdV-RDO) projection with the nose (hard palate) tipped down toward the film approximately 30 degrees and the vertical beam centered 2 to 3 cm rostral to the angular processes of the mandible (Fig. 21.6).[2,3]
- See Fig. 21.1 for a comparison of the different skull types.

MEASURE: At the thickest area near the commissure of the lip (over the level of the third maxillary premolar).

CENTRAL RAY: On the nasal cavity—at the back of the palate about the level of the third premolar. Angle the x-ray tube rostrocaudally 20 to 30 degrees.

BORDERS: Tip of the maxilla to the pharyngeal region (all of the upper palate).

> **✎ TECHNICIAN NOTES** If the machine allows the tube to be tilted for the nasal sinuses, have the patient in a VD position with an open mouth. Keep the maxilla parallel to the table and tilt the x-ray tube. The collimator light should be on the hard palate back to the rear molars, and the image receptor must capture the primary beam at this area.

Ventrodorsal Open-Mouth—(V20–30°R-DCdO open-mouth)—cont'd

FIG. 21.5 A, Positioning for the ventrodorsal open mouth (Ventral 20–30° Rostral-Dorsocaudal Oblique [V20-30°R-DCdO] open-mouth) for the nasal sinuses. B, Overlay and radiographic anatomy of the ventrodorsal open-mouth view. Tilt the x-ray tube about 20 to 30 degrees in relation to the table in a rostrocaudal direction as in D. C, V20°R-DCdO open-mouth view of the nasal cavity of an 8-month-old mixed breed dog. Beam angulation will cause some distortion of the nasal cavity. Note the tape used to hold the maxilla. *Solid black arrow,* frontal process of the zygomatic bone; *solid black arrowhead,* rostral aspect of the cranial vault; *hollow black arrowhead,* lateral margin of the frontal sinus; *white arrow,* nasal septum. D, Diagram of patient positioning. (C and D, From Thrall DE. *Textbook of Veterinary Diagnostic Radiology.* 7th ed. St. Louis: Elsevier; 2018.)

Ventrodorsal Open-Mouth — (V20–30°R-DCdO open-mouth) — cont'd

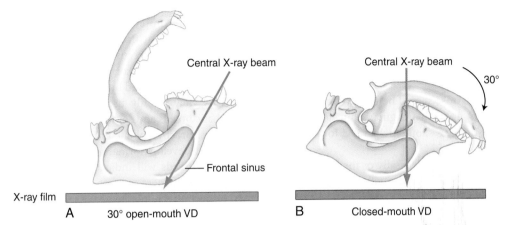

Central X-ray beam

Central X-ray beam

30°

Frontal sinus

X-ray film

A   30° open-mouth VD

B   Closed-mouth VD

FIG. 21.6 A, The ventrodorsal open-mouth view (rostroventral-caudodorsal oblique) is not as effective at imaging the nasal cavity in brachycephalic breeds. **B,** The closed-mouth caudoventral-rostrodorsal oblique (CdV-RDO) projection is more satisfactory. The nose (hard palate) is tipped down toward the film about 30 degrees with the central beam 2 to 3 cm rostral to the angular processes of the mandible.

Rostrocaudal Views

- Remember proper nomenclature rules.[1,4] The central ray enters the body part closest to the x-ray tube and exits the body part closest to the table or image receptor.
  - Thus, a true rostrocaudal view means that the beam enters at the nose and exits at the back of the head. "Rostro" is derived from the Latin word "rostrum," which means beak, or emitting from the head. To make it easier to remember, just think rostrocaudal means the nose is pointing up in some degree, so the dorsum (caudal) is down.
  - The descriptions are more accurate if the angle of either the beam or the position of the head away from the vertical

plane is also included. Thus, an open-mouth, rostral, 10-degree, ventral-caudodorsal oblique (R10°V-CdDO) means that the patient is lying on its back with its mouth open and pointing to the x-ray tube:

- The head is positioned so that the central ray enters from the front of the patient inside the mouth (RV).
- The beam exits toward the back of the mouth and head (CdD) at a 10-degree angle (O) ventral from the plane of the hard palate.
- The mouth can be open or closed in an oblique view.

Rostrocaudal Frontal Sinus View (Rostrocaudal—90-Degree, Closed-Mouth)

This frontal sinus view images the frontal sinuses, zygomatic bone, and orbits. The patient is in the VD position with the nose straight up and mouth closed. Another term for this view is *skyline view.*

Positioning (Fig. 21.7)

Place In: Dorsal recumbency in a V-trough if required; support with sandbags.

Hindlimbs: Leave in a natural position and secure with a sandbag or ties.

Forelimbs: Pull the front limbs caudally, lateral to the chest, and support with a sandbag or ties.

Head and Neck: If needed, position a foam pad or sandbag under the neck so that the hard palate is perpendicular to the image receptor.

Point the nose up, keeping it perpendicular to the image receptor and the long axis of the body.

Keep in position by placing tape, tubing, Velcro, or gauze around the nose.

Secure caudally, keeping the nose pointed up.

Rostrocaudal Frontal Sinus View *(Rostrocaudal—90-Degree, Closed-Mouth)—cont'd*

Brief Overview

- Patient in dorsal recumbency. Head flexed 90 degrees to spine so the nose points directly at x-ray tube. Center x-ray beam on frontal sinuses (Fig. 21.7).

Comments and Tips

- The hard palate and nose should be perpendicular to the table (nose points up). An imaginary line joining the medial canthi of the eyes should be parallel to the image receptor.
- If the nose is rotated too far dorsally or the beam is centered too far ventrally, the nasal cavity will be superimposed over the frontal sinus.

- Be careful that the endotracheal tube is not kinked at the level of the oropharynx or that the tongue does not create objectionable artifacts on the area of interest.
- Reduce the kV because there is minimal tissue to penetrate.
- When positioned correctly, you should see two "bumps" (Fig. 21.7C) created by the shadow of the collimator light.
- This view is only useful in mesaticephalic, dolichocephalic breeds and some cats with a well-developed frontal sinus. Brachycephalic breeds and some cats do not commonly develop normal frontal sinuses. The lateral view of these breeds will indicate if there are gas filled sinuses present. If there are not, this rostrocaudal-frontal sinus projection will not be useful.[1,2]

MEASURE: Over the site of the nasal sinuses (nasal stop), from medial canthus of eye to caudal part of the head.

CENTRAL RAY: Between the eyes (on the frontal sinuses).

BORDERS: Occipital crest to the dorsal aspect of the nasal planum (tip of nose).

🖉 **TECHNICIAN NOTES**   Keep the nose straight up and pointed at the x-ray tube for the frontal sinuses in medium- (mesaticephalic) and long-nosed (dolichocephalic) dogs in the 90-degree, closed-mouth rostrocaudal frontal sinus view.

🖉 **TECHNICIAN NOTES**   For any of the rostrocaudal ventrodorsal views, the patient will be in dorsal recumbency with the nose pointing at some angle toward the x-ray beam. The angle will depend on what is being imaged. The mouth may be open or closed.

A

FIG. 21.7 A, Positioning for the frontal 90-degree rostrocaudal closed-mouth view of the skull for the frontal sinuses. The nose is pointing straight up, and the beam is centered between the eyes.

Rostrocaudal Frontal Sinus View (Rostrocaudal–90-Degree, Closed-Mouth)—cont'd

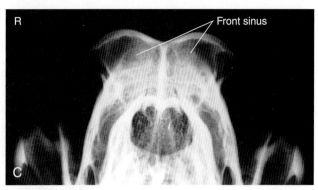

FIG. 21.7, cont'd B, Overlay and radiographic anatomy of the frontal 90-degree rostrocaudal closed-mouth view of the skull. **C,** A frontal 90-degree rostrocaudal closed-mouth radiograph to show the frontal sinus. The nose is pointing straight up. (Courtesy Susan McNeil, RVT, Georgian College.)

Rostrocaudal Closed-Mouth View (R20–30°V-CdO)

The rostrocaudal closed-mouth (rostral 20–30-degrees, ventral-caudodorsal oblique) or fronto-occipital view demonstrates the foramen magnum, cranial vault, calvarium, and sagittal crest. This position is the same as the rostrocaudal frontal sinus view except that the nose is positioned caudally.

Positioning (Fig. 21.8)
Place In: Dorsal recumbency in a V-trough, if required, and support with sandbags.
Hindlimbs: Leave in a natural position; support with sandbags or ties if needed.
Forelimbs: Pull caudally, lateral to the chest; support with sandbags or ties.
Head and Neck: Point the nose upward and apply a long strip of tape or tubing to the nose. Angle the hard palate in a caudal direction toward the chest by pulling on the strip and securing it caudally (about 20 to 30 degrees).

Brief Overview (Fig. 21.8)
• Patient in dorsal recumbency. Nose pointed up, secured and pulled caudally 20 to 30 degrees. Center midway between the eyes.

Comments and Tips
• The central ray should intersect the bridge of the nose at an angle of 20 to 30 degrees to the dorsum of the nose or at an angle of 45 degrees to the hard palate.[1–3] The actual angle depends on the type of skull.
• The tongue and endotracheal tube may cause artifacts. Try to keep the pinnae equally lateral to the head.
• The difference with this view from the regular rostrocaudal view is that the nose points caudally 20 to 30 degrees to view the foramen magnum.
• Some sources suggest that the nose should be positioned down for an occipitofrontal projection with the beam centered at the junction of the right and left frontonasal sutures for dolichocephalic and mesaticephalic breeds, and about the top of the nasal fold for brachycephalic breeds.[4]

MEASURE: At the site of the frontal sinuses (from medial canthus of eye to caudal part of the head).
CENTRAL RAY: Midway between the eyes so that the cranium is centered, and the beam intersects the bridge of the nose.
BORDERS: Entire cranium.

TECHNICIAN NOTES The eyes are looking up at the x-ray tube for both the frontal sinuses and foramen magnum in the rostrocaudal views. The difference is that the nose points straight up for the frontal sinus and points caudally 20 to 30 degrees for the foramen magnum.

Rostrocaudal Closed-Mouth View *(R20–30°V-CdO)—cont'd*

A

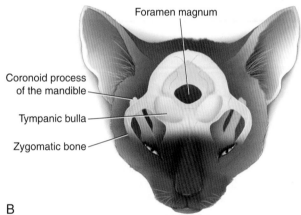

Foramen magnum

Coronoid process
of the mandible

Tympanic bulla

Zygomatic bone

B

R

C

FIG. 21.8 **A,** Positioning for the rostrocaudal or fronto-occipital (rostral 30-degree dorsal-caudoventral) view of the skull to image the foramen magnum, cranial vault, calvarium, and sagittal crest. The nose is pulled more caudally than for the frontal 90-degree view. **B,** Overlay and radiographic anatomy of the rostrocaudal view (R30°D-CdV) or fronto-occipital of the feline skull to view the foramen magnum. **C,** A skull radiograph of the rostrocaudal (R30°D-CdV) or fronto-occipital view. Another term for when the nose points up is *rostrocaudal tangential*. (Courtesy Susan McNeil, RVT, Georgian College.)

Rostrocaudal Open-Mouth View (R10–30°V-CdDO)

The rostrocaudal open-mouth view (rostral 10–30-degrees ventral-caudodorsal oblique) demonstrates the tympanic bullae, the base of the skull, and the odontoid process. This position is similar to the frontal sinus view, except that the mouth is opened for dogs. There is minimal superimposition of the petrous temporal bone. This view is often referred to as the basilar view.

Positioning (Fig. 21.9)

Place In: Dorsal recumbency in a V-trough, if required, and support with sandbags.

Hindlimbs: Leave in a natural position; support with sandbags or ties if needed.

Forelimbs: Pull caudally, lateral to the chest, and support with sandbags or ties.

Head and Neck: A small amount of padding under the neck may help keep the head pointing up and cervical spine parallel to the tabletop. Avoid rotation. Try to keep the pinnae equilateral to the head.

Point the nose upward and apply a long strip of tape or gauze just below the maxillary canines.

The commissures of the lip should be over C2.

Gently retract the nose about 10 degrees cranially and secure, being careful to avoid injury.

Apply tape or gauze to the mandibular canines, encompassing the endotracheal tube if used. Gently retract and secure the tape so that the mandible is about 10 degrees caudal from the perpendicular being careful to avoid injury.

Brief Overview (Fig. 21.9)

- Patient in dorsal recumbency. Head flexed 90 degrees to spine such that nose points directly at x-ray tube. Gently open mouth by retracting maxilla and mandible equally with gauze or tape so the nose is displaced 10 to 30 degrees cranially, depending on the breed. Center x-ray beam through the mouth.

Comments and Tips

- The hard palate should be at about a 10-degree angle from the vertical for mesaticephalic breeds.[1,2,5] The beam should bisect the angle of the open mouth or at the junction of the hard palate and the horizontal rami of the mandible, allowing the bullae to project freely.
- The mouth can also be propped open with a tongue depressor, plastic speculum, or 1-mL syringe barrel placed between or over the canine teeth, being careful not to cause injury. The tongue and positioning devices may cause artifacts.
- The angle of the beam varies with the patient and with how wide the mouth can be opened. Brachycephalic breeds likely require a larger palatial angle (21 degrees) and dolichocephalic breeds a smaller angle (4 degrees).[1]
- Brachycephalic breeds are often better imaged by keeping the mouth closed and positioning as for a cat by having the hard palate at a 10-degree angle from the perpendicular (Fig. 21.10).[1]
- Slightly less kV is required because there is less tissue to penetrate.

MEASURE: At the commissure of the lips (level of maxillary third premolar).

CENTRAL RAY: At the commissure of the mouth just dorsal to the tongue from a rostroventral direction.

BORDERS: Entire nasopharyngeal region of the cranium.

> ✎ **TECHNICIAN NOTES** To evaluate the tympanic bullae of dogs in the rostrocaudal open-mouth view, point the nose to the x-ray tube, open the mouth, and separate the mandible and maxilla, securing them slightly in each direction, being careful to avoid injury. Secure the tongue and endotracheal tube to the mandible or remove the endotracheal tube.

> ✎ **TECHNICIAN NOTES** Collimate, ensuring that labels/markers are included, and borders are visible for every image.

Rostrocaudal Open-Mouth View *(R10–30°V-CdDO)*—cont'd

A

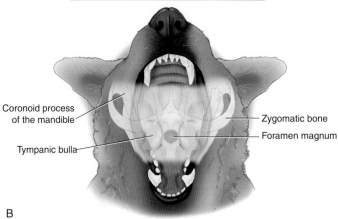

Coronoid process
of the mandible

Zygomatic bone

Foramen magnum

Tympanic bulla

B

Plane of hard palate   RV-CdDO

10°

C

D

FIG. 21.9 A, Positioning for the rostrocaudal open-mouth (rostral 10- to 30-degree ventral-caudodorsal oblique) view. This rostrocaudal view demonstrates the tympanic bullae, the base of the skull, and the odontoid process. Measure and center at the level of the commissure of the lips. **B,** Overlay and radiographic anatomy of the rostrocaudal open-mouth (RV-CdDO) view of the skull. **C,** Open-mouth rostrocaudal view providing a relatively unobstructed view of the tympanic bullae in a dog *(black arrows).* **D,** RV-CdDO Open-Mouth: Rostroventral-caudodorsal oblique view. The central ray enters from inside the mouth or the front and ventral aspect of the head (RV) and exits toward the back and top of the head (CdD) at an angle (O) 10 degrees ventral from the plane of the hard palate. (**C,** From Thrall DE. *Textbook of Veterinary Diagnostic Radiology.* 7th ed. St. Louis: Elsevier; 2018.)

Cat and Brachycephalic Dog Tympanic Bullae Closed-Mouth View (R10°V-CdDO)

Comments and Tips

- Because the cat tympanic bullae are positioned anatomically more caudally than in a dog, the cat's mouth is kept closed to view the tympanic bullae and odontoid process.
- Rest the dorsal aspect of the head on an angled foam wedge so that the hard palate is at an angle of 10 degrees from the vertical.
- Apply tape over the maxilla to secure.
- Center the beam at the level of the base of the mandibular body at the commissure of the mouth about 1 cm ventral to the external nares[5] (level of ears).

Brief Overview of Closed-Mouth Rostral 10-Degree Ventral-Caudodorsal Oblique

- Patient in dorsal recumbency. Head flexed 90 degrees to spine so nose points directly at x-ray tube. Keep mouth closed and angle head/neck 10 degrees caudally. Center x-ray beam at base of skull (Fig. 21.10).

> **TECHNICIAN NOTES** Point the nose to the x-ray tube, keep the mouth closed, and pull slightly cranially for evaluation of the tympanic bullae of feline patients and possibly for brachycephalic breeds.

> **TECHNICIAN NOTES** Remember to apply the label appropriately in each image and to collimate the beam as tightly as possible.

FIG. 21.10 A, Positioning for the rostrocaudal closed-mouth (rostral 10-degree ventral-caudodorsal) view of the skull for the feline tympanic bullae. The patient is in dorsal recumbency, with nose pointing directly at the x-ray tube, the mouth closed, and both mandible and maxilla displaced dorsally 10 degrees. **B,** Rostral 10-degree ventral–caudodorsal view of the tympanic bullae in a feline. (From Thrall DE. *Textbook of Veterinary Diagnostic Radiology.* 6th ed. St Louis: Saunders; 2018.)

Lateral Oblique Views

Lateral oblique views isolate the tympanic bulla, TMJs, frontal sinus, and maxillary or mandibular dentition depending on the rotation of the skull. The patient is lying in lateral recumbency, and the jaw is either pointed up or down.

To understand oblique terminology using the LeD-RtVO (left dorsal-right ventral oblique) view as an example:

1. Le**D**—the beam enters the head from the patient's left side toward the dorsal aspect of the head.
2. Rt**V**—the right side is closest to the table; the beam exits from the ventral part of the head.
3. O—indicates an angle.
4. Thus, the patient is lying in right lateral recumbency with the head in a dorsoventral oblique position.

5. To help remember, temporarily ignore the left and right. A Le**D**-Rt**VO** means the beam is coming from the top of the head. The jaw is pointing down in a modified dorsoventral oblique position ("dorsoventral down"—note the alliteration) (see Fig. 21.11C). The short form would be Right DVO.
6. Except for tympanic bullae, TMJ, and mandibular dentition, the unaffected side is usually up. If a patient is positioned in right lateral recumbency, the right marker (unaffected bulla) will be dorsal to the skull and the left marker (affected bulla) ventral to the skull.

Lateral Oblique View for the Tympanic Bullae, Frontal Sinus (LeD-RtVO/RtD-LeVO)

The lateral oblique or LeD-RtVO (modified dorsoventral oblique) view with the head lying in a natural position isolates the tympanic bullae. The view can also be used for mandibular dentition, frontal sinus, and an oblique view of the TMJ.

Positioning (Fig. 21.11)

Place In: Right or left lateral recumbency with the unaffected side to the image receptor:
  • Right lateral—to view the left oblique tympanic bulla
  • Left lateral—to view the right oblique tympanic bulla

Hindlimbs: Leave the hindlimbs in a natural position; support with sandbags or ties if needed.

Forelimbs: Position caudally and support with sandbags or ties.

Head and Neck: Position the head so that the mandible is initially parallel to the long edge of the table.

Allow the head to lie oblique naturally, with the jaw pointing to the table.

If needed, tape/Velcro the head over the nose and neck area, extending the tape across the table.

Comments and Tips

  • Both labels are used. For right lateral recumbency, the right marker (unaffected bulla) will be dorsal and the left marker (affected bulla) ventral.
  • The degree of rotation from the true lateral depends on the species and type of skull. Generally, wider skulls require less rotation and narrower skulls require more.
  • Allow enough rotation to isolate each tympanic bulla.

MEASURE: At the base of the ear over the tympanic bullae at the widest part of the cranium.

CENTRAL RAY: At the base of the ear over the tympanic bullae.

BORDERS: Cranial and caudal to the ear.

🖉 **TECHNICIAN NOTES** For the tympanic bullae or frontal sinus, have the patient lie in a natural oblique lateral position with the affected tympanic bulla up. This is also referred to as a modified DV oblique view (the jaw is "down in a DV").

Lateral Oblique View for the Tympanic Bullae, Frontal Sinus (LeD-RtVO/RtD-LeVO)—cont'd

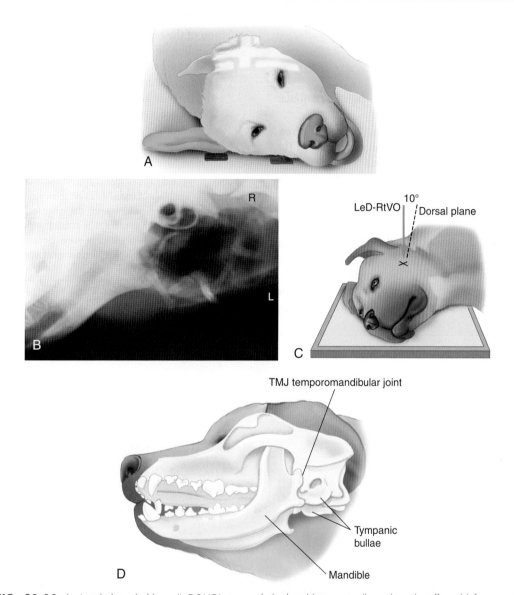

FIG. 21.11 A, A right lateral oblique (LeD-RtVO) view with the head lying naturally to show the affected left tympanic bullae in isolation. The unaffected right tympanic bullae is closer to the film. The dependent-side marker is placed dorsally, and the marker for the upper side is placed ventrally. **B,** Radiograph of the lateral oblique view of the tympanic bullae. The affected bulla is magnified and positioned ventrally. **C,** LeD-RtVO: Left dorsal–right ventral oblique view. The central beam enters the skull dorsally (from the top of the head) on the patient's left side (LeD) and exits the skull ventrally (toward the chin) on the patient's right side (RtV). Because the skull is not in a true lateral position, it is an oblique (O). The most accurate description is Le10°D-RtVO. This locates the entrance angle at 10 degrees dorsal to the dorsal plane through the area of interest such as for the left temporomandibular joint. **D,** Overlay and radiographic anatomy of the lateral oblique or dorso-ventral oblique view to visualize the tympanic bullae, temporomandibular joints, and maxilla.

Lateral Oblique View for the Mandible *(LeD-RtVO/RtD-LeVO)*

This lateral oblique view (modified dorsoventral oblique) for the mandible is used to radiograph the lower dental arcade or bony lesions of the nondependent mandible. The affected side will be down (Fig. 21.12).

Comments and Tips

- The right side is down to visualize the right mandibular teeth.
- A foam pad under the maxilla, creating a 20- to 45-degrees angle of the mandible with the table, is required. (The affected mandible is closest to the table.)
- The actual angle depends on the breed and how wide the mouth is open. There should be no superimposition of the affected mandibular premolars and molars by the other teeth or quadrant.
- The mouth is widely opened, with the central ray over the fourth premolar.
- The endotracheal tube is tied to the maxilla.
- Label the teeth with both positional markers so that the dependent marker is placed dorsally and the upper side

marker is ventral. Note that on the image, the dependent teeth will be grayer because there is minimal superimposition of the rami of the mandibles.

- Depending on the angle, this view is referred to as:
  - Right side down: Le20–45 degrees D-RtVO: left 20 to 45 degrees dorsal, right ventral oblique (beam enters the left side and exits on the right).
  - Left side down: Rt20–45 degrees D-LeVO: right 20 to 45 degrees dorsal, left ventral oblique (beam enters right side and exits on the left.

> ✐ **TECHNICIAN NOTES**   For the lateral oblique view of the mandibular teeth, the affected mandible is on the table and the maxilla is raised with a foam wedge. This is a modified DV oblique view because the beam enters at the top of the head and exits ventrally. The jaw is pointing down (DV is down).

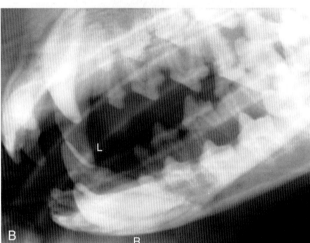

FIG. 21.12 A, Lateral oblique or dorsoventral oblique (Rt20D-LeVO) positioning for viewing the left mandibular dental arcade. The maxilla is raised from 20 to 45 degrees, depending on how wide the mouth is open or on the breed of the patient. **B,** Lateral oblique (or modified DVO, specifically the RtD-LeVO) view for the left mandibular arcade. Note that the left mandibular teeth appear grayer because there is no superimposition with the mandible. The head angle also causes elongation, making the affected mandibular teeth appear more magnified. If the mouth is opened wider, there is less overlapping by the maxillary teeth.

Lateral Oblique View for the Maxilla, TMJ, and Tympanic Bullae *(LeV-RtDO/RtV-LeDO)*

1. This lateral oblique or modified ventrodorsal oblique (jaw up) view can be used for the tympanic bullae, TMJ, and maxillary teeth.
2. This provides a different view of the mandibular condyle than is projected on the lateral and DV/VD views.
3. Another way to describe the view is laterorostral-laterocaudal oblique.

Positioning (Fig. 21.13)

Place In: Right or left lateral recumbency with the affected side down on the image receptor.

Hindlimbs: Leave the hindlimbs in a natural position; support with sandbags or ties if needed.

Forelimbs: Position caudally and support with sandbags or ties.

Head and Neck: Start by positioning the head with the mandible parallel to the long edge of the image receptor.

Keep the skull in a straight lateral position.

Place a foam pad under the mandible to raise the jaw from 10 to 30 degrees, depending on the breed of dog. The mouth can be partially opened.

If needed, Velcro/tape the head over the nose and neck area, extending the tie across the table.

A sandbag may be placed over the neck and against a foam pad at the dorsal aspect of the head.

Brief Overview

- Patient in lateral recumbency affected side down with mouth secured open. Position a foam wedge under the mandible to raise it 10 to 30 degrees, depending on the breed. Center the beam on the affected maxillary arcade or the tympanic bullae (Fig. 21.13).

Comments and Tips

- This position displaces the nondependent bulla (upper) caudally and the dependent (down) bulla rostrally.
- The distance the mandible is raised depends on the breed. Dolichocephalic breeds require an angle of about 10 degrees, and mesaticephalic breeds about 15 degrees. Brachycephalic breeds generally require an angle of 25 to 30 degrees from the table.[1,4]
- Both right and left lateral oblique views should be taken for comparison.
- Ensure that the pinnae, tongue, and endotracheal tubes will not create objectionable artifacts.
- Place the marker indicating the dependent side ventrally near the joint and the nondependent side marker dorsal to the nares. This indicates that the raised joint is dorsal to the joint on the table.
- Use the skull technique chart, as more exposure is required to penetrate the cranium.

Upper Dental Arcade

1. This view can also be used to radiograph the upper dental arcade or bony lesions of the nondependent maxilla.
2. Place a foam pad under the mandible to create a 30- to 45-degree angle of the mandible with the table (Fig. 21.13A). The mouth should be widely opened, with the central ray over the fourth premolar. The endotracheal tube should be tied to the mandible.
3. To image the teeth, keep the affected maxilla closer to the table.
4. The teeth should be marked with both positional markers—the dependent marker placed ventrally and the upper side marker dorsally. (The dependent teeth will be grayer because there is some superimposition of the palate.)

Fig. 21.14 is a mystery radiograph. Review it and answer the question presented with it.

MEASURE: Just caudal to the lateral canthus over the joint.

CENTRAL RAY: Between the caudal mandibular ramus and the base of the ear.

BORDERS: Cranial and caudal to the joint.

✎ **TECHNICIAN NOTES** For a lateral oblique view of the TMJ or maxillary teeth, position the jaw up on a foam with the affected joint or teeth closer to the table *(LeD-RtVO/RtD-LeVO).*

✎ **TECHNICIAN NOTES** This view could also be called a *modified ventrodorsal oblique view* because the jaw is tipped up at an angle and the beam enters the head more from the ventrodorsal aspect. The maxilla is closer to the table than the mandible (jaw up)—LeD-RtVO (left dorsal-right ventral oblique).

✎ **TECHNICIAN NOTES** When placing the positional markers for an oblique view, consider the following:
1. What quadrant are you attempting to image?
   a. When that quadrant is in the correct position, look at which part of the jaw is touching the table.
   b. Will it appear more ventral, or will it be displaced dorsally in relation to the opposite side of the jaw?
2. If imaging the right mandible, the patient is lying on its right side and the jaw is pointed down.
   a. The sponge under the maxilla tips the left, or upper, side of the mandible more ventrally than the right mandible, which is displaced dorsally.
   b. Place the R marker near the tips of the right premolars and the L marker at the ramus of the left mandible.
3. In these views, the markers do not indicate which side the patient is lying on, but rather the specific quadrant.[2]

Lateral Oblique View for the Maxilla, TMJ, and Tympanic Bullae (*LeV-RtDO/RtV-LeDO*)—cont'd

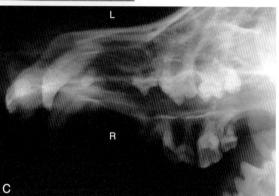

FIG. 21.13 A, Positioning for the lateral oblique (specifically LeV-RtDO) view of the skull for the maxillary teeth. The affected side is against the table. A smaller angle is used to visualize the tympanic bullae and temporomandibular joints. The left marker indicates that the left or nondependent side will be positioned more dorsally than the right maxilla when the head is rotated from the table. The R marker shows that the side closest to the film will be more ventral. It is under the foam pad nearer the right maxilla. The R and L marker in oblique cases do not show the side the animal is lying on. The markers only show the position of the jaws relative to each other. **B,** Left 20-degree rostral–right caudal projection of the right temporomandibular joint *(single white arrow)* and right tympanic bulla *(double white arrows)* in a dog. Elevating the nose positions the upper left nondependent tympanic bulla *(single black arrow),* caudal to the lower right dependent tympanic bulla *(double white arrows).* **C,** Centering on the maxilla and opening the mouth wider in the open-mouth lateral oblique (LeV-RtDO open-mouth) radiograph provides this image of the maxillary dental arcade. (From Thrall DE. *Textbook of Veterinary Diagnostic Radiology.* 7th ed. St Louis: Saunders; 2018)

FIG. 21.14 Mystery Radiograph. What would the correct terminology be for this view?

✳ **KEY POINTS**

1. General anesthesia or sedation is required for accurate positioning for all skull views.
2. In order to achieve symmetry of the skull to minimize distortion and possibly misdiagnosis, the anatomical structures being examined must be parallel to the table/image receptor and perpendicular to the central ray:
   a. To help maintain symmetry for a lateral view, draw an imaginary line between the medial canthi. This line should be perpendicular to the table.
   b. To help maintain symmetry for a dorsoventral view, draw an imaginary line between the medial canthi. This imaginary line should be parallel to the table.
3. Collimate tightly to the area of interest, carefully placing the labels and markers.
4. Views imaged will depend on the suspected pathology.
5. In rostrocaudal projections, the angle of the central ray with the head varies because of breed variations. The patient will be in a VD position with the nose pointing to the x-ray beam with some angle variation.
6. To label oblique views, think of which part of the jaw is against the film and how the opposite side is positioned.

REVIEW QUESTIONS

1. A Rottweiler requires a lateral survey radiograph of the skull. You should measure at the highest point of the:
   a. Zygomatic arch just rostral to the lateral canthi of the eyes
   b. Zygomatic arch at the center of the cranium
   c. Cranium just caudal to the lateral canthi
   d. Occipital protuberance
2. In the lateral survey of the Rottweiler, peripheral borders are:
   a. From the tip of the nose to the occipital protuberance
   b. The rostral and caudal calvarium borders
   c. Cranial and caudal to the ears
   d. From the tip of the nose to the lateral canthi
3. You are also completing a survey dorsoventral radiograph of the Rottweiler. The central ray will be:
   a. Just rostral to the ears on the dorsal midline of the skull
   b. On the dorsal midline between the ears on the sagittal crest
   c. On the dorsal midline between the lateral canthi on the sagittal crest
   d. More rostral for this head type
4. In the survey dorsoventral radiograph of the Rottweiler, there will likely be:
   a. Even opacity of all of the tissues
   b. Overexposure of the cranium
   c. Overexposure of the nasal passages
   d. No overexposure of any part if the thickest part is toward the cathode
5. How can you determine whether there is likely to be symmetry on the final image of this dorsoventral skull of the Rottweiler as you are positioning the patient?
   a. The nasal septum is parallel with the image receptor.
   b. An imaginary line drawn between the medial canthi should be perpendicular to the table.
   c. An imaginary line drawn between the medial canthi should be parallel to the table.
   d. The tongue will not obliterate any of the essential anatomy.

6. A Collie is to be imaged for frontal sinus view, and the veterinarian wishes a rostrocaudal position. This means that the patient is lying in:
   a. Ventral recumbency and the head is parallel to the table
   b. Ventral recumbency with the nose pointing to the x-ray tube and the mouth open
   c. Dorsal recumbency with the nose pointing to the x-ray tube and the mouth closed
   d. Dorsal recumbency with the nose pointing to the x-ray tube and the mouth open
7. The x-ray beam for the frontal view of the sinus in the Collie will be positioned:
   a. At the nasal cavity at the back of the palate
   b. At the lateral canthi of the eyes
   c. Rostral to the lateral canthi of the eyes
   d. Midway between the eyes so the cranium is centered
8. The veterinarian also requires a ventrodorsal open-mouth view of the nasal sinuses for the Collie. This is correctly referred to as:
   a. Open-mouth ventral 20–30° rostral-dorsocaudal oblique
   b. Caudoventral-rostrodorsal oblique view
   c. 90-degree-rostrocaudal open-mouth view
   d. LeD-RtVO or RtD-LeVO depending on the side the patient is lying on
9. To position the VD open-mouth of the nasal sinuses of the Collie and if the machine allows:
   a. The nose is parallel to the table and the beam directed 90 degrees inside the mouth
   b. The nose is pointed upward with the hard palate angled in a caudal direction
   c. The mouth is opened wide and the x-ray tube tilted about 20 to 30 degrees in a rostrocaudal direction inside the mouth
   d. The mouth is opened wide and the x-ray tube tilted about 20 to 30 degrees to the table in a rostrocaudal direction on the mandible

10. The veterinarian would also like a foramen magnum view of the Collie. The patient is lying in dorsal recumbency and the nose is:
    a. Parallel to the table with the x-ray tube angled in a rostrocaudal direction
    b. Perpendicular to the table with the beam tilted 20 to 30 degrees
    c. Perpendicular to the table and the long axis of the body
    d. Pointed upward and pulled caudally 20 to 30 degrees

11. A complete evaluation of the tympanic bullae for a Boxer includes a lateral, DV/VD, and:
    a. Frontal 90-degree and two lateral oblique views
    b. Open-mouth rostrocaudal and two lateral oblique views
    c. Open- and closed-mouth rostrocaudal and two lateral oblique views
    d. Both dorsoventral oblique views

12. A LeD-RtVO radiograph is required for the tympanic bullae of the Boxer. This means that the patient is lying on its:
    a. Right side with the jaw pointing down
    b. Right side with the jaw pointing up
    c. Left side with the jaw pointing down
    d. Left side with the jaw pointing up

13. For this LeD-RtVO radiograph, the left marker should be placed:
    a. Dorsally with no right marker
    b. Dorsally alongside the right marker
    c. Ventrally and the right marker dorsally
    d. Ventrally with no right marker

14. The borders for the LeD-RtVO of the tympanic bullae radiograph should include:
    a. The tip of the nose to the occipital-atlas junction
    b. Cranial and caudal to the ear
    c. The full cranium
    d. The occipital crest to the dorsal aspect of the nasal planum

15. The veterinarian requires a rostrocaudal view of a feline patient. Unlike in positioning for a normal canine skull, the mouth should be:
    a. Closed with the hard palate at 10° from the vertical
    b. Open with the hard palate at 10° from the vertical
    c. Closed and parallel to the table
    d. Closed and pulled caudally

Chapter Review Question answers are located in the Instructor Resources on Evolve and can be provided to students at the discretion of the instructor.

References

1. Holloway A. *BSAVA Manual of Canine and Feline Radiography and Radiology: a Foundation Manual.* Suffolk: BSAVA; 2013.
2. Thrall DE. *Textbook of Veterinary Diagnostic Radiology.* 7th ed. St. Louis: Elsevier; 2018.
3. Smallwood JE, Shively MJ, Rendano VT, Habel RE. A standardized nomenclature for radiographic projections used in veterinary medicine. *Vet Radiol.* 1985;26:2-9.
4. Kus S, Morgan J. Radiography of the canine head: optimal positioning with respect to skull type. *Vet Radiol.* 1985;26:196-202.
5. Hammond Gawain J, Sullivan M, Weinrauch S, King AM. A comparison of the rostrocaudal open mouth and rostro 10 degrees ventro-caudodorsal oblique radiographic views for imaging fluid in the feline tympanic bulla. *Vet Radiol Ultrasound.* 2005;46: 205-209.

Bibliography

Aspinall V, Cappello M. *Introduction to Veterinary Anatomy.* London: Butterworth-Heinemann; 2009.

Ayers S. *Small Animal Radiographic Techniques and Positioning.* Oxford: Wiley-Blackwell; 2013.

Colville T, Bassert J. *Clinical Anatomy and Physiology for Veterinary Technicians.* 3rd ed. St. Louis: Mosby; 2016.

Done SH, Goody PC, Evans S, Stickland NC. *Color Atlas of Veterinary Anatomy, the Dog and Cat.* London: Mosby; 2009.

Evans H, de Lahunta A. *Guide to the Dissection of the Dog.* 8th ed. St. Louis: Saunders; 2017.

Fauber TL. *Radiographic Imaging and Exposure.* 5th ed. St. Louis: Elsevier; 2017.

Hermanson, J, de Lahunta A. *Miller's Anatomy of the Dog.* 5th ed. St. Louis: Elsevier; 2019.

Muhlbauer MC, Kneller SK. *Radiography of the Dog and Cat: Guide to Making and Interpreting Radiographs.* Oxford: Wiley-Blackwell; 2013.

Owens JM. *Radiographic Interpretation for the Small Animal Clinician.* St. Louis: Ralston Purina; 1999.

Singh B. *Dyce, Sack and Wensing's Textbook of Veterinary Anatomy.* 5th ed. St. Louis: Elsevier; 2018.

Sirois M, Schlote J. *Diagnostic Imaging for Veterinary Technicians.* Minneapolis: Bluedoor, LLC; 2017.

Smallwood JE, Shively MJ, Rendano VT, Habel RE. A standardized nomenclature for radiographic projections used in veterinary medicine. *Vet Radiol.* 1985;26:2-9.

Tighe M, Brown M. *Mosby's Comprehensive Review for Veterinary Technicians.* 5th ed. St. Louis: Mosby; 2019.

Wilson M, Mauragis D, Berry C. Small animal skull & nasofacial radiography including the nasal cavity & frontal sinuses. *Todays Vet Pract.* 2014;4(2):47-51.

CHAPTER 22
Dental Imaging and Radiography

Susan MacNeal, RVT, CVDT, BSc

A man begins cutting his wisdom teeth the first time he bites off more than he can chew.
—Herb Caen, San Francisco Chronicle, 1916–1997

OUTLINE

LEARNING OBJECTIVES

When you have finished this chapter, you will be able to:

1. Describe the dental x-ray unit and discuss its unique qualities.
2. Process dental x-ray film.
3. Understand dental radiography using film or digital systems, discussing the merits of each system.
4. Accurately identify dental anatomy, terminology, nomenclature, and formulas.
5. Produce diagnostic high-quality extraoral and intraoral dental radiographs of the dog and cat by properly centering, collimating, and positioning using either the parallel or bisecting angle with CR digital systems/film or DR sensors
6. Correctly view dental films.
7. Identify further concerns and idiosyncrasies, including the variations between dogs and cats.

KEY TERMS

Key terms are defined in the Glossary on the Evolve website.

Alveolar bone
Apical
Arch
Bisecting angle
Buccal
Carnassial tooth
Caudal
Cementoenamel junction
 (CEJ)
Chairside darkroom
Computed radiography
Concave
Contralateral
Convex

Coronal surface
Cusp
Direct digital radiography
Distal
Distolateral oblique
Dorsal
Elongation
Enamel bulge
Extraoral
Extension arm
Facial
Foreshortening
Frenulum
Furcation

Incisal
Intraoral
Ipsilateral
Labial
Lamina dura
Lateral (side)
Lingual
Malocclusion
Mental foramina
Mesial
Mesiobuccal
Mesiolateral oblique
Mesiolingual
Occlusion

Palatal surface
Parallel technique
Periapical
Position indicating device
Processing chemicals
Radicular groove
Rostral
Rostrocaudal oblique
Scissor arm
SLOB rule
Stationary anode
Source-image distance
 (SID)
Ventral

Dental radiography has become a significant diagnostic tool in the veterinary clinic. Once the basic anatomy, terminology, and positioning principles are understood, dental radiographs are readily completed.

For true diagnostic radiographs of the canine and feline mouth, a dental x-ray machine should be used. The articulating arm on a dental x-ray machine enables one to obtain quality radiographs quickly and easily with minimal maneuvering of the patient. If there is no access to a dental x-ray unit, extraoral and intraoral radiographs can still be taken with a regular x-ray machine, though the resulting images will not be as easily obtained or detailed, depending on the position.

The Dental X-Ray Unit

Dental x-ray units used in veterinary practices are designed based on the similar technology used in human dental x-ray units. Many veterinary practices use refurbished human dental x-ray units, but a separate technique chart needs to be designed. To determine the settings in newer veterinary dental x-ray units, you simply press the selection button that applies to the tooth you are going to radiograph (Fig. 22.1).

Dental x-ray units all consist of the same parts: generator, extension arm, scissor arm, and the x-ray tube, which has the collimator cone (Fig. 22.2). The generator is a small box that is located on the wall of the dental operatory room and requires a standard 110-volt power outlet without any special wiring. Most dental x-ray units are preset with a kilovoltage (kV) of 70 or 80 and a milliampere (mA) of

either 7 or 8, so the only variable is seconds. Some of the newer dental x-ray units have the ability to vary the kV.

The extension arm extends from the generator. It swings 180 degrees and is available in variable lengths. At the end of the extension arm is the scissor arm. The scissor arm and extension arm allow the dental x-ray machine to maneuver about the patient to allow ease of positioning.

The x-ray tube is a stationary anode tube (see Chapter 2) that is encased in the tube housing at the end of the scissor arm and will rotate around that stem. Because it is a stationary anode, there is no rotor noise. The collimator cone or positioning indicator device (PID) is a projection from the

FIG. 22.1 Dental X-Ray Control Panel.

FIG. 22.2 A Dental X-Ray Machine.

Labels: Scissor arm; Main extension arm; Tube housing; Control panel; Extension cone

FIG. 22.3 A and B, Two examples of collimator cones on dental x-ray machines. The length of the cones, as well as the diameter of the cone, varies between machines.

FIG. 22.4 The angle meter on the side of the dental x-ray tube. The angle meter is used for imaging canine teeth when the beam direction needs to be adjusted.

tube housing. Cones are not interchangeable and are available in variable lengths and diameters depending on the manufacturer (Fig. 22.3). Most presets on the unit are based on a distance of 2 inches or 5 cm from the tooth. Any variation does require a change in settings as based on the inverse square law stated in Chapter 5. There is no collimator light; thus the operator must view the cone from different perspectives to best estimate the center of the beam.

Every dental cone has an angle meter with indentations up to 90 degrees around the cone (Fig. 22.4). The angle meter is useful for setting up some dental x-ray views, depending on what technique is used. The angle meter is especially helpful for imaging canine teeth, as a "tilt" in the cone is required to prevent superimposition on the premolars distal to it.

Dental X-Ray Imaging

Three imaging choices are available. One is nonscreen dental film and the other two are digital systems. The digital systems are divided into computed radiography (CR), available as photostimulable plates (PSP), and direct digital receptors (DDR or DR).

Film

The kV required for imaging teeth is generally much higher than imaging a cat abdomen with a cassette-screen system because there are no intensifying screens.

Dental film is available in different speeds and brands. The common speed of film used in veterinary practice is D-speed (Fig. 22.5). An F-speed film is also available, under the brand name Insight, which is a faster-speed film, allowing for a decreased radiation dose. It is not practical to switch between film speeds once the technique chart has been established. Film is available in four sizes (Table 22.1). The most common sizes used are 2 and 4, as well as the 0 for small dogs and cats (Fig. 22.6).

FIG. 22.5 Dental film, D-speed. This is the most common speed of film used in veterinary practice.

TABLE 22.1	Dental X-Ray Film Sizes
FILM SIZE	**FILM DIMENSIONS**
0	1⅜ × ⅞ in 35 mm × 22 mm
1	19/16 in × 15/16 in 40 mm × 24 mm
2	1⅝ in × 1¼ in 40.5 mm × 30.5 mm
4	3 in × 2¼ in 57 mm × 76 mm

FIG. 22.7 An Opened Dental Film Packet.

FIG. 22.6 Size 0, 2, and 4 dental x-ray film. These are the most common sizes used for imaging dog and cat teeth.

FIG. 22.8 The reverse side of a dental film packet. The reverse side should face away from the x-ray tube. It is a different color and has a tab used to open the film packet during processing.

The film packet has several layers (Fig. 22.7). The film is wrapped in a paper layer with a thin lead foil layer at the back of the packet, all enclosed in a plastic outer covering. The back of the film packet is clearly identified with a green or purple color, as well as a small tab for opening the packet (Fig. 22.8). The purpose of the lead layer in the film packet is to prevent x-rays from continuing through the packet, causing extra radiation exposure to the patient (Fig. 22.9). In many municipalities, the lead is considered a hazardous substance and must be disposed of through an environmental control company or a lead recycling program.

On the front of the film packet is a convex dot with the same raised dot on the film inside the packet (Fig. 22.10). On the opposite side of the film, the dot is concave. The purpose of the "dot" is to help determine left or right once the film is developed, as dental films are too small to put a left/right marker on them. The film is always positioned with the convex dot facing the tube and at the front of the mouth. If the dot is consistently kept toward the front of the mouth, it is easy to determine left or right based on the orientation of the teeth.

An easy way to ensure that the dot is toward the front of the mouth is to always hold the packet by the dot. Keeping your fingers on the dot will ensure that you know where the dot is positioned once the film is processed.

FIG. 22.9 The thin lead sheet enclosed in the dental film packet. The lead sheet should be disposed of with an environmental control company.

FIG. 22.11 A Chairside Darkroom.

FIG. 22.10 The convex dot on the dental film. The convex side of the film should face the tube head, and the dot should be placed rostrally.

FIG. 22.12 The Inside of the Chairside Darkroom. From left to right: developer, water, fixer, water.

Manual Film Processing

Manual processing is the most common way to process films in a veterinary hospital. This can be accomplished by using a chairside darkroom (Fig. 22.11) or by setting up four small jars with sealed lids in the regular darkroom. The chairside darkroom allows the operator to process the films in close proximity to where they are being exposed. The chairside darkroom has a red translucent cover and light-tight arm holes. Inside the chairside darkroom are four jars containing (left to right) developer, water (stop bath), fixer, and water (Fig. 22.12). The solutions should be at room temperature (70–76°F [21–24°C]).

Once the film is exposed, the technician takes the film to the chairside darkroom and inserts both hands into the light-tight sleeves, holding the film packet in one hand. The packet is opened and a film clip is attached to the film. The film clip allows the operator to move the film through the chemicals safely while keeping his or her hands out of the liquids (Fig. 22.13). The red translucent cover allows the technician to view the process without light fogging the film.

The times for processing vary with the brand of chemicals used, and it is best to consult the manufacturer's instructions. Kodak Rapid Access Dental Developer and Fixer by Carestream (Fig. 22.14) are examples of rapid dental processing solutions that are available. The instructions for these solutions state that their system is compatible with both Ultraspeed and Insight dental films. Ready-to-read radiographs are available by immersing for 15 seconds in developer, rinsing in water, then immersing for 15 seconds in fixer, followed by a thorough rinse in water. If the films appear to have a yellow discoloration after drying, this indicates they were not thoroughly rinsed. If the radiographs are to be kept as part of the patient's record, they should be developed, put in the stop bath for 15 seconds (agitating constantly), then fixed for 2 to 4 minutes, and then washed in running water for 10 minutes.

FIG. 22.13 A film clip attached to a dental film. The film clip is attached in the chairside darkroom to move the film through the processing chemicals.

FIG. 22.15 A Dental Film Mount. Dental radiographs are arranged as if you are looking at the animal.

FIG. 22.14 An Example of Rapid Dental X-Ray Processing Chemicals.

Ideally, the solutions should be used for the dental session and then disposed of. Watch for signs of chemical deterioration.

Labeling, Mounting, and Storing the Images

Each clinic should develop their own system for storing dental radiographs. Some veterinary governing bodies require the films to be permanently labeled. This can be accomplished by writing on the film with a fine-point permanent marker or using a film mount (Fig. 22.15), which is also considered acceptable. The film mount allows the films to be organized in a prearranged layout and filed for future reference. Digital systems also have templates built into the software to mount the digital radiographs.

A full-mouth set of dental radiographs should always be mounted as if you were looking directly at the animal's mouth. The animal's right side of the mouth should be on your left when viewing the full set of radiographs (Fig. 22.16).

Dental radiographs can be attached in an envelope to the dental chart, or if in a paperless clinic, a separate filing system can be used. The radiographs are part of the patient's medical record and must be saved for future reference.

Digital Dental Radiography

The advantage of any digital dental imaging system is the ease with which images can be processed, manipulated, and stored. Dental radiography is generally said to have a "steep learning curve," and if films need to be manually processed, it can become a very time-intensive procedure. Digital systems also allow the image to be easily manipulated with annotation tools (Fig. 22.17). For example, magnification, windowing and leveling for optimizing the image, labeling of the exact tooth, and emailing the image with the press of a button are all advantages of digital systems. The dental x-rays can easily be attached to the patient's file and incorporated into a discharge summary.

Computed Radiography

The computed radiography (CR) dental processor (Fig. 22.18) is similar in design to the standard CR unit used in whole-body radiographs described in Chapter 8.

Photostimulable phosphor (PSP) plates are used as image receptors. They are thin and flexible and are available in sizes 0, 1, 2, 3, and 4 (Fig. 22.19). Each plate has a small "a," which replaces the "dot" used in regular dental film. The PSP plates are light sensitive and must be protected from light. They are sealed in a barrier envelope for patient use (Fig. 22.20). The active side of the plate is light blue with the rear side of the plate containing the writing; it is easily viewed through the window of the barrier envelope. Once exposed, the PSP plate is removed from the barrier envelope and put through the scanner, which converts it into an image viewed on the computer. As the plate is scanned, the plate is erased and is ready to use again once the scanning is complete.

Direct Digital Imaging

The image receptor for DR is a size 2 sensor (Fig. 22.21). Smaller sensors are available, but are not practical for

FIG. 22.16 A Full Set of Dental X-Ray Films on a Cat. The maxillary views are on the top and the mandibular views on the bottom. The cat's right is on your left and vice versa.

FIG. 22.17 Annotation Tools on a Digital X-Ray System. The colors in this image have been inverted.

veterinary use. The sensor is attached directly to the computer's universal serial bus (USB) port. Once the sensor is exposed, the software program immediately converts the information into an image. DR sensors have an inactive area around the perimeter of the sensor.

A size 2 sensor is typically 30 by 43 mm, but has an active area of 26 by 36 mm (Fig. 22.22). Table 22.2 lists the advantages and disadvantages of the different types of image receptors.

Digital Sensor Safety Information

The sensor should be protected from fluids by using a barrier sleeve. The digital sensor supplier usually supplies sleeves for the sensor. Once these are finished, the fingers cut off a latex rubber glove work very well. A thin layer of plain vet wrap around the sensor, once covered with the plastic sleeve, enables the sensor to stay in place without slipping. DR sensors can be permanently damaged if dropped and are costly to replace. When the sensor is to be used, the cord should be

FIG. 22.18 An Example of a Computed Radiography (CR) Digital Dental X-Ray Unit.

FIG. 22.20 CR plates are light sensitive and need to be protected from light and moisture. **A,** A size 2 plate enclosed in a barrier envelope, showing the reverse side of the plate. **B,** This is the side of the CR plate that needs to face the x-ray tube.

FIG. 22.19 CR PSP Plates. Sizes 0, 1, 2, 3, and 4 are available. Shown here is the reverse side of the plate. Note the "a" acts as the dot in regular film and should be placed rostrally.

FIG. 22.21 An Example of a Direct Digital Radiography (DR) Sensor. The sizes of the sensor are only available as size 1 or 2 (most common).

taped to the table with enough slack to allow the sensor to be moved but short enough so that if it is inadvertently brushed off the table, it will not land on the floor.

Dental Exposures

For most dental x-ray machines, the choice of settings is simple because most of the machines have presets based on the tooth to be x-rayed. The majority of dental x-ray machines have a preset mA and kV, so the only variable is seconds, although newer machines also have variable kV. If using an older machine or a refurbished human dental x-ray

FIG. 22.22 A DR Sensor. The active portion of the sensor is smaller than the dimensions of the sensor. The active portion of the sensor is outlined in red.

machine, you will need to create your own technique chart. Table 22.3 is a suggested chart for imaging teeth.

Radiography Log

It is essential that all dental x-ray exposures are recorded in a log designated for your dental x-ray machine. If the dental x-ray machine has a preset mA and kV, you will need a column to record only seconds for each exposure as long as there is a statement at the beginning of the log stating the presets. The log requires an entry for each exposure, including patient, client, date, area imaged, and settings as discussed. This is a legal requirement from various radiation protection agencies.

> ✎ **TECHNICIAN NOTES** In this chapter, the term *film* is used with the understanding that in digital radiography, the digital sensor or PSP plate is substituted for the film.

Indications for Dental Radiography

In veterinary medicine, it is essential to have dental radiographs as part of a comprehensive oral health examination. The visual inspection and tactile examination (probing) of the tooth is only a small part of the information required to

TABLE 22.2	A Comparison of Dental Image Receptors' Advantages and Disadvantages	
DENTAL RECEPTOR	**ADVANTAGES**	**DISADVANTAGES**
Film	Inexpensive for initial setup in comparison to digital systems Easy to use and store Different film sizes available: size 0, 1, 2, and 4 Switching between sizes is easily done Exceptionally high resolution	Time consuming—film must be manually processed Individual storage means that films can be lost or damaged Processing adds time and ongoing cost Must be viewed on a viewing box Radiation amounts may be higher as compared to digital systems (varies among dental x-ray machines)
Computed radiography (CR)	Different receptor sizes available: size 0, 1, 2, 3, and 4 Photostimulable plates (PSP) are thin and flexible, similar to regular film Scanning time is approximately 30 seconds Plates can be imaged hundreds of times and are inexpensive to replace	More expensive than digital receptor (DR) systems Ongoing costs for barrier envelopes Intermediate step for processing takes time Plates can be damaged (scratched or bent) if used carelessly "Plate" is removed for processing, so it cannot be repositioned according to its previous position
Direct digital radiography	Less expensive than CR systems Sensor remains in position while radiograph is reviewed so adjustments are simplified if positioning is incorrect No intermediate step—image is displayed within seconds of the exposure	Size of the sensor is limited to #1 or #2, which necessitates multiple exposures for full-mouth radiographs The sensor is thick and inflexible, making sensor placement difficult for trickier areas; alternative techniques must be used Larger teeth must be imaged with two exposures after repositioning of sensor The sensor may be damaged by rough handling and is very expensive to replace Inactive area on sensor makes sensor smaller than it appears

TABLE 22.3	Suggested Exposure of Dental Equipment Supplied Without a Technique Chart	
	EXPOSURE(S) BASED ON 70-kV, 8-mA DENTAL X-RAY MACHINE REDUCE EXPOSURE BY 40% FOR DIGITAL	
	DOG (S)	**DOG (M)**
Maxillary PM/M	0.33	0.40
Maxillary canine tooth	0.41	0.50
Maxillary incisor	0.20	0.23
Mandibular PM/M	0.27	0.30
Mandibular canine tooth	0.33	0.40
Mandibular incisor	0.18	0.20
	CAT	
Maxillary teeth	0.30	
Mandibular teeth	0.20	

PM/M, Premolar/molar.

make informed treatment decisions. Dental radiography is an essential component of a proper diagnosis, treatment planning, and monitoring.

Oral disease is common in dogs and cats. A particular challenge with these patients is their inability to communicate pain and discomfort until oral disease is well advanced. Even then, isolating the exact origin and extent of the disease is difficult. Dental radiographs enable us to thoroughly evaluate the entire tooth and surrounding tissues, including bone.

Full-mouth radiographs should be taken as part of a complete oral examination. Specific indications for radiographs include but are not limited to periodontal disease, missing teeth, resorptive lesions, oral tumors and gingival inflammation, malformed teeth, discolored teeth, dental extractions, and dental trauma.

Positional Terminology

Some of the terms you should be familiar with are those associated with the direction of the beam and the intraoral terminology (Fig. 22.23).

Tooth Anatomy and Dental Formula

Tooth Anatomy

In Fig. 22.24, the crown is above the gums (supragingival) and the root below the gums (subgingival). The apex is the tip of the root. At the tip of the root, there are small openings to allow the blood supply and nerves to enter the tooth; these openings are referred to as the *apical delta.*

On a radiograph, the pulp chamber is the darker inner content of the tooth extending throughout the crown and the root. The root portion of the pulp chamber is generally referred to as the *root canal.*

The dentin constitutes the bulk of the tooth and appears lighter than the pulp chamber on a radiograph. As a patient ages, secondary dentin is continuously produced. Over time, the pulp chamber decreases in size because of the secondary dentin. Fig. 22.25 illustrates how the size of the pulp chamber evident on a radiograph of the lower first molar can help with aging of an animal.

The enamel is the outer covering of the crown, and the cementum is the outer covering of the root. The area where they meet is termed *the cementoenamel junction* (CEJ). The enamel and cementum are difficult to distinguish from the dentin.

The periodontal ligament forms the attachment of the cementum to the alveolar bone. It appears as a thin gray line surrounding the roots.

The lamina dura is the wall of the alveolar socket that surrounds the tooth. It appears as a dense white line adjacent to the periodontal ligament space.

The four basic tooth types in dogs and cats are as follows:
1. Incisors (I or i) are used for grooming as well as grasping and cutting food. All incisor teeth are single rooted.
2. Canine teeth (C or c) are single-rooted teeth that are used for grasping and holding prey. The structure of feline canine teeth supports that cats are true carnivores. There are shallow longitudinal groves on the buccal surfaces of the canine teeth. These grooves "wick" away blood from held prey.
3. Premolar teeth (P or p) are designed for cutting and shearing meat. Premolar teeth have prominent sharp cusps and have one to three roots.
4. Molar teeth (M or m) generally have flattened occlusal surfaces with the exception of the mandibular first molar tooth in dogs, which does have a cutting edge on the mesial cusp. The first mandibular molar tooth in cats has no flattened occlusal table; instead, it has two cutting edges. Molar teeth have two or three roots, but some roots appear to be fused together to give the appearance of being single rooted (feline maxillary first molar). Molar teeth in dogs are used for grinding food.

Dental Formula

The *dental formula* illustrates how many of each tooth type are present in half of a dog's and cat's mouth. The short form for the type of tooth is followed by the number of that particular type. The formula is presented in a "fraction," with maxillary teeth shown above the teeth in the mandible, using the following conventions:

Tooth type: Refer to description given in former discussion of tooth anatomy
Permanent: Uppercase (I, C, P, M)
Deciduous: Lowercase (i, c, p, m)

Canine Dental Formula

Fig. 22.26 illustrates the canine dental formula, which is as follows:

$$\text{Deciduous teeth: } 2 \times \left(\frac{\text{i3c1p3m0}}{\text{i3c1p3m0}} \right) = 28 \text{ in total}$$

A shortened version to remember is 313/313.

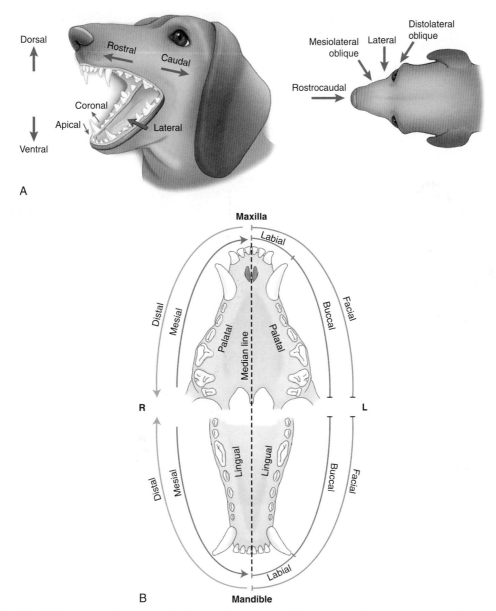

FIG. 22.23 A, Anatomical directions. B, Directional terminology of the oral cavity. Directions and terminology apply to both sides of the mouth.

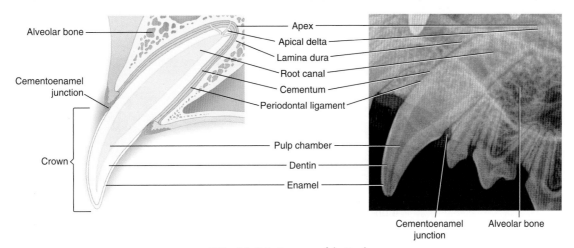

FIG. 22.24 Anatomy of the Tooth.

FIG. 22.25 A–I, Radiographs show how the pulp chamber decreases in size as animals age (youngest, A; oldest, I). A, 6 months, open apex (*arrowheads*); B, 9 months, apical closure; C, 16 months; D, 2 years; E, 3 years; F, 4 years; G, 6 years; H, 8 years; I, 12 years. (From Tutt C, Deeprose J, Crossley DA. *BSAVA Manual of Canine and Feline Dentistry.* 3rd ed. Gloucester, UK: British Small Animal Veterinary Association; 2007.)

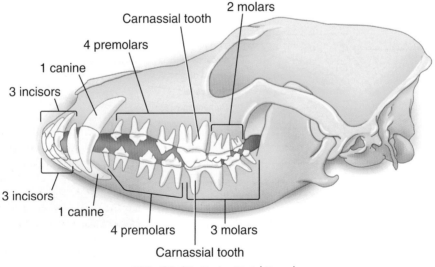

FIG. 22.26 Canine Dental Formula.

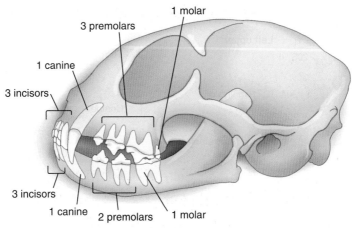

3 premolars
1 molar
1 canine
3 incisors
3 incisors
1 canine
2 premolars
1 molar

FIG. 22.27 Feline Dental Formula.

Permanent teeth: $2 \times \left(\dfrac{I3C1P4M2}{I3C1P4M3} \right) = 42$ in total

A shortened version to remember is 3142/3143.

Feline Dental Formula

Fig. 22.27 illustrates the feline dental formula, which is as follows:

Deciduous teeth: $2 \times \left(\dfrac{i3c1p3m0}{i3c1p3m0} \right) = 24$ in total

A shortened version to remember is 313/312.

Permanent teeth: $2 \times \left(\dfrac{I3C1P3M1}{I3C1P2M1} \right) = 30$ in total

A shortened version to remember is 3131/3121.

> ✏ **TECHNICIAN NOTES** There are no deciduous precursors for the first premolar of the adult dog. Cat and dog molar teeth never have deciduous precursors.

Nomenclature

Two types of numbering systems are used in veterinary medicine for identifying teeth. The anatomical system is an older system but is still used in veterinary clinics. The modified Triadan system is the current numbering system of choice. It is easily integrated into paperless records, and it is much faster to use than the anatomical system once it has been learned. Fig. 22.28 illustrates the anatomical orientation and structure of the teeth with each system illustrated.

Anatomical System for Notation

The anatomical system uses a combination of short forms for tooth type (I, C, P, M for permanent teeth or i, c, p, m for deciduous teeth) and the numbers of those teeth in their group (i.e., premolars 1–4) to designate a specific tooth. The number of the tooth is placed on the left for a left-sided tooth and the right for a right-sided tooth; the number is superscript for a maxillary tooth and subscript for a mandibular tooth. For example, I^2 designates the right maxillary second incisor (intermediate incisor).

Modified Triadan System

The modified Triadan system labels each tooth with a code of three numbers, starting at the midpoint of the arch in each quadrant. The first number designates the quadrant. The upper-right quadrant uses the number 1 as the quadrant designation, the upper-left quadrant uses 2, the lower-left quadrant uses 3, and the lower-right quadrant uses 4. Deciduous teeth use the series 5 through 8 for the quadrants.

The second two numbers are determined by the tooth position, counting back from the midline of the arch in each quadrant. Incisors are numbered 01, 02, and 03; the canine tooth is 04; premolars are 05, 06, 07, and 08; and the molars are 09, 10, and 11. So, for example, the Triadan number for ^3I is 203.

The Triadan system is adaptable to any species regardless of how many teeth are normally present for that species. However, in order to assign the Triadan numbers to species that are normally missing teeth in the dental formula, you need to know the anatomical number designations, especially for the premolars. Because the cat is missing the upper first premolar, there is no 105 or 205 tooth in a cat. Likewise, for the mandibular premolars, because the cat is missing the first and second premolars, the numbers 305, 306, 405, and 406 are not used.

> ✏ **TECHNICIAN NOTES** The canine tooth always ends in a 04, and the first molar always ends in a 09. From there, you can count forward or backward in the dental arch as needed.

Roots of the Various Teeth

It is very important to appreciate the structure and number of tooth roots (Fig. 22.29). The appreciation of this anatomy

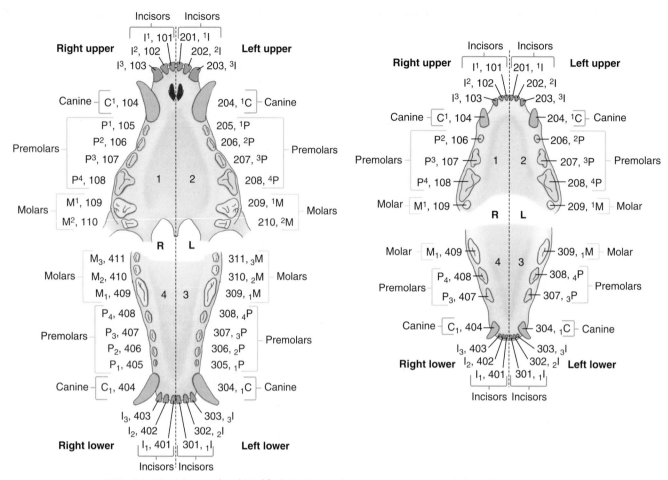

FIG. 22.28 Anatomical and Modified. Triadan numbering systems in canine (*left*) and feline (*right*) teeth.

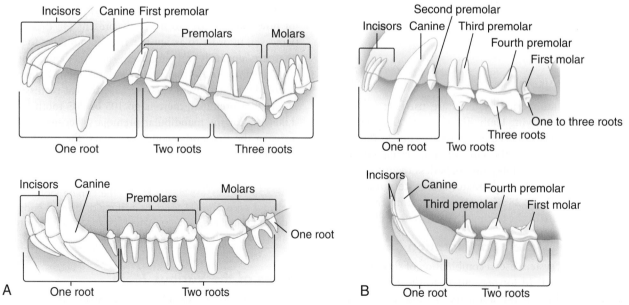

FIG. 22.29 A, Roots of the permanent teeth of a canine. **B,** Roots of the permanent teeth of a feline.

is vital to determine tooth angle and to decide when to change the direction of the x-ray beam to isolate the roots. It is also important in the interpretation of radiographs to recognize extra or malformed roots.

Normal Radiographic Anatomy in Dogs and Cats

The following radiographs illustrate normal findings of the areas listed here. It is important to be able to distinguish between the mandible and the maxilla when viewing radiographs. It is also important to become familiar with the orientation of the teeth and the anatomical differences in root and crown structure. The more familiar you are with these areas, the easier it will be to distinguish between teeth on a radiograph.

1. Normal adult maxillary incisors: Look for white space distal to incisors, with two oval (dark) spaces, which are the palatine fissures (Fig. 22.30).
2. Normal adult mandibular incisors: Look for a dark black line distal to incisors that separates mandibular rami (mandibular symphysis) (Fig. 22.31).
3. Normal adult maxillary premolars and molars: Look for the fine white line representing the maxillary recess apical to the roots (Fig. 22.32).
4. Normal adult mandibular premolars and molars: Look for dark black areas above and below the mandible (Fig. 22.33).

FIG. 22.30 Normal Radiographic Anatomy of the Canine Adult Maxillary Incisors. *1*, 203; *2*, 202; *3*, 201; *4*, 101; *5*, 102; *6*, 103; *7*, incisive canal; *8*, interincisive suture; *9*, palatine fissure.

FIG. 22.31 Normal Radiograph Anatomy of the Canine Adult Mandibular Incisors. *1*, 403; *2*, 402; *3*, 401; *4*, 301; *5*, 302; *6*, 303; *7*, mandibular symphysis.

FIG. 22.32 Normal Radiograph Anatomy of the Canine Maxillary Premolars and Molars. *1*, 105; *2*, 106; *3*, 107; *4*, 108; *5*, 109; *6*, 110; *7*, nasal surface of the alveolar process of maxilla; *8*, nasal cavity; *9*, infraorbital canal; *10*, infraorbital foramen; *11*, palatine canal; *12*, palatal marginal enamel; *13*, mesiopalatal root; *14*, mesiobuccal root; *15*, radicular groove on distal root; *16*, palatal root; *17*, distobuccal root; *18*, mesiobuccal root.

FIG. 22.33 Normal Radiograph Anatomy of the Canine Mandibular Premolars and Molars. *1*, 405; *2*, 406; *3*, 407; *4*, 408; *5*, 409; *6*, 410; *7*, 411; *8*, alveolar margin; *9*, mandibular canal; *10*, middle mental foramen; *11*, overlap of enamel; *12*, radicular groove; *13*, ventral mandibular cortex.

> ✎ **TECHNICIAN NOTES** The same parallel and bisecting angle techniques are used for digital radiography as for the film system. The digital sensor or plate replaces the film.

Viewing Dental Radiographs

Film is always exposed with the convex dot at the rostral end of the mouth; therefore, views on the right side have the dot in a different location from those on the left side. Fig. 22.34

Right maxilla   Left maxilla

Right mandible   Left mandible

FIG. 22.34 A–D, Digital films showing how placement of dot (a) differs.

demonstrates with digital films how the locations of the dot ("a" on digital plates) differ.

Once the film has been developed, hold it so the convex dot is raised toward you (as it was placed in the mouth). Determine whether you are looking at a maxilla or a mandible (see earlier discussions of tooth anatomy and normal anatomy radiographs).

Orient the radiograph so the cusps of the maxillary teeth are pointing down toward the floor and the cusps of the mandibular teeth are pointing up toward the ceiling (Fig. 22.35). Look at the film as if you were looking at the animal with the film positioned in its mouth. The anatomical structures and orientation of the teeth will allow you to determine if it is a maxilla or mandible and left or right (Fig. 22.36).

⏻ FIGURE IT OUT Several films were imaged on a canine patient. When viewing one of the radiographs, the vet was unsure as to which teeth he was viewing. The technician says: "If the dot was placed toward the front of the mouth, then it makes sense for this to be a right maxillary premolar." Upon further explanation she says: "We are viewing it with the convex side of the dot facing us as it was placed in the mouth. The smaller teeth are at the rostral end of the mouth, which is where we placed the 'dot,' and this radiograph agrees with our film placement, so this must be a right maxillary premolar."

FIG. 22.35 Proper Viewing of a Radiograph. Note that the maxillary cusps are pointing down and the mandibular cusps are pointing up.

FIG. 22.36 Proper Film Placement in Mouth and Accompanying Radiograph (Right Maxilla). Note the convex dot in the upper-right corner of the film.

> **✎ TECHNICIAN NOTES** With the convex dot facing you, visualize the film inside the patient's mouth to determine whether the film is showing the left or right side.

Projection Geometry

Parallel Technique

The parallel technique involves placing the dental film directly behind and parallel to the tooth and then directing the x-ray beam perpendicular to the film (Fig. 22.37A). The anatomy of dog and cat mouths allows the parallel technique to be used in only one area. This area encompasses the teeth distal to and including the mandibular third premolars ($_3P_3$ or 307/407).

Bisecting Angle Technique

Because of the anatomical structure of the mouths of dogs and cats, film cannot be placed directly behind most teeth. The bisecting angle technique is used to image these teeth. This technique is used on all maxillary teeth, all incisors and canines, and mandibular premolars 1 and 2.

FIG. 22.37 A, Parallel technique. **B,** Bisecting angle.

FIG. 22.38 Bisecting angle; the bisecting angle is shown in red. Note the x-ray beam is perpendicular to the bisecting angle. **A,** Radiograph setup for maxillary premolars (lateral recumbency). *Note:* You must be at the front of the patient to appreciate the angle where the tooth enters the skull. **B,** Radiograph setup for mandibular incisors (lateral recumbency). *Note:* You must be at the side of the patient (looking from overhead if patient is in lateral recumbency) to appreciate the angle where the tooth enters the skull.

The bisecting angle is formed by the intersection of the plane of the film and the long axis of the tooth. If the central ray is perpendicular to a line that bisects this angle, the resulting image is as accurate as possible (Fig. 22.37B).

In order to accurately visualize the long axis of the tooth, you should stand at the patient's front (premolar teeth) or the patient' side (incisor and canine teeth) to find the bisecting angle (Fig. 22.38).

> ✎ **TECHNICIAN NOTES** Another way to think of the bisecting angle is to split the difference between pointing the beam at the tooth angle and the film angle. Simply speaking, the bisecting angle is aiming the cone halfway between the tooth and film.

Foreshortening and Elongation

If the x-ray beam is not aimed directly at the bisecting angle, the image will not be a true representation of the tooth. An artifact—elongation or foreshortening—will result.

The analogy of using the shadows created by the position of the sun overhead is one way to explain elongation and foreshortening. If you were standing in the middle of a field, the shadow created on the ground by the sun coming up on the horizon would create quite different shadows from those created by the sun directly overhead. When the sun is coming up on the horizon, a very long shadow is created; this effect is elongation. At noon, the sun is overhead, and your shadow is smaller than you are; this effect is foreshortening.

Elongation results when the x-ray beam is aimed too directly at the long axis of the tooth instead of at the bisecting angle (the sun is lower on the horizon). Because the beam is directed at the angle of the tooth, the image will appear "stretched out," and the entire tooth may not have been captured on the film (Fig. 22.39).

Foreshortening results when the x-ray beam is aimed too directly at the film instead of at the bisecting angle (the sun is directly overhead). Because the beam is directed at the angle of the film, the tooth will appear to have the crown overlapping on the root (Fig. 22.40).

> ✎ **TECHNICIAN NOTES** If the beam is perpendicular to the film, the image is foreshortened. If the beam is perpendicular to the tooth, the image is elongated. If you split the difference, the image is truer. The bisecting angle is splitting the difference.

FIG. 22.39 Elongation. **A,** Radiograph setup. **B,** Resulting radiograph demonstrating elongation. The red line is the bisecting angle that the x-ray beam should be perpendicular to. In this setup, the x-ray beam is focused too much on the tooth angle.

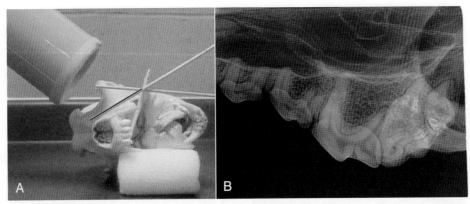

FIG. 22.40 Foreshortening. **A,** Radiograph setup. **B,** Resulting radiograph demonstrating foreshortening. The red line is the bisecting angle that the x-ray beam should be perpendicular to. In this setup, the x-ray beam is focused too much on the film angle.

Intraoral Dental Radiography with a Dental X-Ray Machine

The size of CR plate/film chosen for each view depends on the size of the animal and the tooth to be radiographed. The largest DR sensor is a size 2, which often means multiple exposures are required for larger teeth. In general, when choosing a CR plate/film size for incisors and canine teeth, pick a film size where both of the patient's canine teeth can occlude with the film. This allows the film to sit evenly in the mouth and provides ample room for imaging the teeth. In many cases, size 4 films are used for canine patients, except for small dogs. If performing full-mouth radiographs, choose a size 4 film, which allows multiple teeth to be taken with one exposure. Most views in cats utilize size 2 films, with the exception of the mandibular premolars and molar, where a size 0 works best.

The following views are demonstrated with the patient in lateral recumbency. This is the recommended patient position because it greatly reduces moving the patient during anesthesia. The mandible and maxilla should be kept parallel with the tabletop. A small roll or foam wedge can be used to accomplish this goal. The source of many issues with non-diagnostic radiographs is that the patient was not in true lateral, especially with views that require a degree of angulation of the cone (imaging the canine tooth). If maxillary views are taken, the endotracheal tube should be tied to the mandible. If views of mandibular teeth are to be taken, the endotracheal tube should be tied to the maxilla. A paper towel should be used to position the film in the mouth.

The distance between the cone and film depends on the size of film that is used. If using small film (sizes 0, 1, or 2), the standard SID of 2 inches will provide optimal density. If size 4 film is used, the SID should be increased to 4 to 6 inches to allow for a wider area of x-rays (Fig. 22.41). If any change in density is noted, alter the settings based on the SID changes suggested in Chapter 5.

The exposure will have to be increased if the SID is increased beyond 4 inches. Each machine varies, but generally, if the distance is approximately 6 inches from the film, the

FIG. 22.41 Field of View Illustrated as Focal Film Distance Differs.

exposure will have to be increased by 1.5 times the normal exposure for that area. Remember the inverse square law from Chapter 5. Digital systems may not need an increase in exposure because of the greater sensitivity of digital plates.

Always center the cone on the tooth in question. This is often the source of many nondiagnostic radiographs. Dental x-ray machines have no collimator light; therefore, you must view the cone from different perspectives to ensure the "imaginary crosshairs" are centered on the tooth in question (Fig. 22.42). Remember that once the beam leaves the collimator cone, it gets wider the farther it must travel.

Also remember in film imaging that the "dot" should be placed rostrally with the convex side of the film (white side) facing the tube head ("a" on digital plates).

> **✎ TECHNICIAN NOTES** To find the bisecting angle: If the cone is coming from the side (premolars), you should be standing at the patient's front (kneel down at the nose level to visualize the tooth angle). If the cone is coming from the patient's front (incisors and canines), you should be standing at the patient's side (look from overhead when the patient is in lateral). This gives you the "bird's-eye view" to visualize the edge of the film and best estimate the tooth angle you should use when determining the bisecting angle.

FIG. 22.42 The center of the cone must be visualized from the side **(A)** and the front **(B)** to accurately determine where the beam is directed.

Dental X-Ray Techniques

The techniques in the following sections described detailing approaches with CR and standard dental film as well as approaches with DR systems. The techniques can vary slightly between these two groups, as the properties of the imaging receptor differ.

Dental Radiographs of Dogs

Familiarity with tooth anatomy is essential when taking dental radiographs. The canine and incisor teeth have long roots that curve distally. When estimating tooth angle, it is essential that the root of the tooth is used. The variation in head types can make dental radiography difficult especially in brachycephalic breeds. The patient should be positioned in true lateral for all views; this is especially important in images that require a tilt of the x-ray cone.

Dental Radiographs of Cats

Anatomical differences between dogs and cats allow for some modifications to the views. Maxillary canine and incisor teeth are more upright in cats than in dogs. This is important when estimating the long axis of the tooth for the bisecting angle technique. Follow the crown when estimating the long axis of the tooth, as the root follows the same angle. Mandibular canine teeth in cats do curve distally, and the curvature of the root should be used when estimating the long axis of the tooth. Cats are missing mandibular premolars 1 and 2, which allows the mandibular incisors and canine teeth to be imaged together.

Maxillary premolars and molars in cats are the most difficult area to image due to a very prominent zygomatic arch. If a standard bisecting angle technique is used, the zygomatic arch will superimpose over the teeth, negating any diagnostic value to the radiograph. The cat should be positioned in true lateral for all views. It is often difficult to get the cone low enough to the table to image the incisors and canines due to the design of the tube head. In order to avoid this, raise the cat's head up on a small towel.

Canine Radiographs with Dental X-Ray Units

The techniques described in this section are used with a dental x-ray machine. The techniques for CR plates and standard film are the same because CR and film share similar characteristics such as the availability of the same sizes (0, 1, 2, and 4) and CR plates are thin and flexible. There are often slight modifications when using a DR sensor, especially in large dogs. The modifications are due to the smaller size of the sensor and the inactive area around the perimeter. DR sensors are also rigid and bulky making positioning difficult in some areas.

> ✎ **TECHNICIAN NOTES** Although some authors use the angle meter at predetermined angle settings with sternal or lateral patient positioning, it this author's experience to learn one technique: bisecting angle. This technique can be easily applied to any head type. The variation in canine head types especially makes the aforementioned technique impractical.

Canine Maxillary Premolars and Molars

The techniques described are used for premolars and molars in dogs. The 4th premolar and molars present additional challenges due to location and tooth anatomy; additional radiographs may be necessary. If using a size 4 CR plate or film to image this area, it is recommended to use the 4th premolar to estimate tooth angle. If using a DR sensor, the 4th premolar may have to be imaged in two separate radiographs, as the tooth can be too large to capture in entirety with one radiograph.

CR PLATE/FILM: The opposite edge of the film should be touching the hard palate; if a size 4 film is used, the opposite edge will be resting against the palatal surface of the contralateral teeth. The tips of the premolar/molar should be at the edge of the film closest to the cone to allow ample space for the roots of the tooth to "fall onto" the film. A size 0 or 2 film is likely necessary to capture distal molars because of anatomical space constraints (Fig. 22.43).

DR SENSOR: Same approach as described for CR Plate/Film. In larger dogs, the root tips may need to captured in an additional exposure. Keep everything the same, except push the DR sensor into the mouth (towards palate).

The plate will not be touching the crown for the second exposure (Fig. 22.44).

CENTRAL RAY: The cone is directed laterally and centered over the tooth in question. The SID depends on the size of film. For a size 4 film, the SID is 4 to 6 inches.

ANGLE: The bisecting angle is found by standing at the patient's front rostral aspect.

> ✎ **TECHNICIAN NOTES** Superimposition of multirooted teeth is always a concern. Multiple radiographs may be necessary to isolate specific roots if required (see later).

Canine Maxillary Premolars and Molars—cont'd

FIG. 22.43 Canine Maxillary Premolars and Molars: CR/Film. **A,** Setup viewed from front. **B,** Final setup. **C,** Radiograph.

Canine Maxillary Premolars and Molars—cont'd

FIG. 22.44 Canine Maxillary Premolars and Molars: DR Sensor. A, Setup viewed from front. B, Final setup viewed from front. C, Sensor is pushed distal to capture apex.

Canine Maxillary Premolars and Molars—cont'd

Canine Molars

Capturing distal molars may be difficult due to space constraints with film placement, especially in brachycephalic dogs. If the technique described for maxillary premolars and molars does not capture the distal molar(s), then a modification of the technique can be used. The CR plate, film, or sensor can be twisted slightly to enable it to be positioned more distally in the mouth (Fig. 22.45). If difficulty is still experienced, use the distolateral beam direction with the bisecting angle. Difficulty is generally experienced in small breeds and brachycephalics.

CR PLATE/FILM: Size 2 film or smaller (depending on the breed). Film should be pushed as far distal in the mouth as possible. A slight "twist" in the plate will allow the corner of the plate to rest against the softer tissue of the soft palate (Fig. 22.46).

DR SENSOR: Same approach as described for CR plate/film (Fig. 22.47).

CENTRAL RAY: The cone is directed laterally and centered over the tooth in question. To separate the roots, or if there is limited space for film placement and the roots are cut off, use a distolateral beam direction

ANGLE: The bisecting angle is found by standing at the patient's front rostral aspect.

FIG. 22.45 Canine Molars. Sensor placement on a skull showing the slight twist of the plate.

FIG. 22.46 Canine Molars: CR/Film. **A,** Final setup using a size 2 CR plate with a distolateral beam direction. **B,** Radiograph.

Canine Maxillary Premolars and Molars—cont'd

FIG. 22.47 Canine Molars: DR Sensor. Final setup using a size DR sensor with a distolateral beam direction.

FIG. 22.48 SLOB Rule. Left hand used to demonstrate root isolation of 208 by changing x-ray beam direction. The second image depicts beam direction from the distal aspect and the ability to visualize all roots.

Maxillary 4th Premolar: SLOB Rule

The maxillary fourth premolar (108 [P⁴] or 208 [⁴P]) is a triple-rooted tooth that has one large distal root and two smaller mesial roots. The mesial roots superimpose over each other if the beam is directed from the lateral aspect. If a desired root needs to be isolated, the direction of the beam can be directed from the mesial or the distal aspect to "split" the roots on the film. This view is necessary if endodontics are to be performed and the diseased root needs to be isolated. The distolateral beam direction can also be used for capturing distal molars in patients where film placement is difficult.

The SLOB rule stands for "same lingual opposite buccal." This term is used to help identify the particular root when the beam is directed from the mesial or distal aspect. "Same lingual" means that the lingual-mesial root (which is actually the palatal root-maxilla) appears to move in the same direction as where the x-ray beam is being directed from. "Opposite buccal" means that the buccal-mesial root appears to move in the opposite direction from where the x-ray beam is coming from.

The SLOB rule can be illustrated using your hands as shown in Fig. 22.48. In this diagram, the root structure of 208 or ⁴P is depicted. In the first diagram, you can see the thumb and one finger. In the second diagram, you can see an additional finger. If the direction the beam is coming from is changed, you will be able to see objects that were superimposed on the initial view. In the second diagram, you can see that if the beam (your eyes) is directed from the distal aspect, the palatal root appears to move in the same direction as where the beam is being directed.

If the beam is directed from the distal aspect, the palatal root will appear as the middle of the three roots on the radiograph. If the beam is directed from the mesial aspect, the buccal root will appear as the middle of the three roots on the radiograph.

Technique

The same setup for the film, cone, and bisecting angle as described previously for maxillary premolars and molars is used as the starting point. Once the bisecting angle is found and the cone is aimed perpendicular to it from the lateral aspect, the cone can be directed from the mesial or distal aspect (Fig. 22.49).

Mesiolateral Oblique View

For the mesiolateral oblique view, the cone is directed from the mesial aspect (mesial to distal), approximately 30 degrees from the initial position. Fig. 22.50 shows the mesial roots isolated on the radiograph. However, the distal root will superimpose over the first maxillary molar tooth.

Distolateral Oblique View

For the distolateral oblique view, the cone is directed from the distal aspect (distal to mesial), approximately 30 degrees from the initial position. Fig. 22.51 shows the mesial roots separated on the radiograph. However, the mesial roots may superimpose over the third maxillary premolar tooth.

> **✎ TECHNICIAN NOTES**   The SLOB rule states that if the beam is directed from the distal aspect, the palatal root will appear as the middle of the three roots on the radiograph. If the beam is directed from the mesial aspect, the buccal root will appear as the middle of the three roots on the radiograph.

Canine Maxillary Premolars and Molars—cont'd

FIG. 22.49 Oblique Angles for Imaging Maxillary Fourth Premolar. **A,** Initial setup for imaging the fourth maxillary premolar as viewed from the patient's side. **B,** Mesiolateral oblique radiograph setup of maxillary fourth premolar (lateral recumbency) showing final oblique x-ray cone with the beam 30 degrees from the initial setup. **C,** Distolateral oblique radiograph setup of maxillary fourth premolar (lateral recumbency) showing final oblique x-ray cone with the beam 30 degrees from the initial setup. **D,** Distolateral as viewed from front. **E,** Final preparation for distolateral on canine patient as viewed from front. **F,** Final preparation for distolateral on canine patient as viewed from side.

Canine Maxillary Premolars and Molars—cont'd

FIG. 22.50 Mesiolateral oblique radiograph; the central root is the mesial-buccal root *(arrow).*

FIG. 22.51 Distolateral oblique radiograph; the central root is the mesial-palatal root *(arrow).*

Maxillary Canine Teeth

The radiograph of the maxillary canine tooth is set up using the long axis of the tooth, which can be visualized from the side of the patient while the x-ray cone is tilted at 30 degrees (use the angle meter on the tube head). This change in beam angle helps prevent superimposition of the canine tooth over the premolar teeth. The 30-degree tilt only works if the animal is in true lateral. The canine tooth curves distally, with its apex typically over the root of the second premolar. Canine teeth in larger dogs will likely require two exposures due to the size of the tooth and the size limitation of the size 2 sensor.

CR PLATE/FILM: Choose a film size where both canine teeth are touching the film ("biting on it"). Size 4 is used for most dogs. The film should be placed sufficiently rostral to evaluate the ipsilateral incisors as well (Fig. 22.52).

DR SENSOR: Place the tip of the canine tooth on the outside corner (nearest you) of the sensor and push the sensor into the mouth so the same edge is up against the palate. If the apex of the tooth is missing, then reposition the sensor until the sensor is flat on the palate behind the canine tooth (the sensor will not be touching any teeth). Move the cone distal to center over apex while maintaining a 30-degree tilt and angle (Fig. 22.53).

CENTRAL RAY: Ensure the animal is in true lateral and adjust the cone until the angle meter reads 30 degrees. Center the middle of the cone on the maxillary canine tooth.

ANGLE: The bisecting angle of the tooth is found by standing at the patient's side using the long axis of the tooth. Canine teeth curve distally. Visualize the curvature of the root to accurately reflect the long axis of the tooth.

Maxillary Canine Teeth—cont'd

FIG. 22.52 Canine Maxillary Canine Tooth: CR/Film. **A,** View from the patient's side to aim at the bisecting angle. **B,** View from the front while finding the bisecting angle (angle meter should be at 30 degrees). **C,** Final preparation for view from patient's side on a canine patient. **D,** View from patient's front on a canine patient, demonstrating 30-degree tilt. **E,** Radiograph of the maxillary canine tooth. Note: Ipsilateral incisors can be imaged as well.

Maxillary Canine Teeth—cont'd

FIG. 22.53 Canine Maxillary Canine Tooth: DR Sensor. **A,** The crown is on the corner of the sensor, and the rest of the sensor is against the palate. **B,** View from the patient's side to aim at the bisecting angle. **C,** View from the front while finding the bisecting angle (angle meter should be at 30 degrees). **D,** Final preparation for view from patient's side on a canine patient. **E,** View from patient's front on a canine patient, demonstrating 30-degree tilt.

Maxillary Canine Teeth—cont'd

FIG. 22.53, cont'd   F, Repositioning of the sensor flat against the palate to image the apex. G, Final setup on canine patient. The bisecting angle and 30-degree tilt are maintained while centering over the apex. H, Radiograph of crown and apex in separate radiographs.

Maxillary Incisors

The typical rostrocaudal view can capture all the incisors on one film when using a CR plate or film. This view is not necessary if the technique for imaging the canine tooth provides a suitable radiograph for ipsilateral incisors. Dog incisors have long roots that curve distally, like the root(s) of a canine tooth. When using a DR sensor, the technique may vary depending on the size of dog. If both canine teeth can bite down on the sensor, then you can be assured all six incisors will be captured in one image. If the sensor rests between the canine teeth, there will likely be cutoff of 103 and 203 (due to the inactive perimeter of the sensor). If this is the case, then the teeth will need to be imaged three at a time (see Maxillary Incisors–Large Dog Technique with DR Sensor).

CR PLATE/FILM: The tips of the incisor teeth should be at the rostral edge of the film to allow ample space for the roots of the incisors. Choose a film size where both canine teeth are touching the film ("biting on it"). Size 4 film is used for most medium to large dogs (Fig. 22.54).

DR SENSOR: If both canine teeth can touch the sensor at the same time, then the same technique is used as described for CR plate/film (Fig. 22.55). If the sensor fits evenly between the canine teeth, use the large dog technique with DR sensor (next).

CONE: The cone is directed in a rostrocaudal direction and centered between all six incisors. If the patient is in true lateral, the angle meter is at 0. It is imperative that the cone is centered between all six incisors (Fig. 22.56).

ANGLE: The bisecting angle is found by standing at the patient's side. Remember that the incisor teeth in dogs curve distally.

FIG. 22.54 Canine Maxillary Incisors: CR/Film. **A,** Skull setup showing the bisecting angle viewed from the patient's side. **B,** Canine patient as viewed from the front. Note: The cone is low enough to be centered between all six incisors. **C,** Canine patient as viewed from the side prior to taking the image. **D,** Radiograph of the maxillary incisors.

Maxillary Incisors—cont'd

FIG. 22.55 Canine Maxillary Incisors: DR Sensor. **A,** Setup showing the bisecting angle viewed from the patient's side. **B,** Setup as viewed from the front. Note: The cone is low enough to be centered between all six incisors.

FIG. 22.56 The Cone is Centered Between the Maxillary Incisors.

Maxillary Incisors—cont'd

Maxillary Incisors—Large Dog Technique with DR Sensor

If the sensor rests between the canine teeth, there will likely be cutoff of 103 and 203 (due to the inactive perimeter of the sensor). If this is the case, then the teeth will need to be imaged three at a time.

DR SENSOR: The sensor is positioned with a slight tilt toward the ipsilateral canine tooth.

CENTRAL RAY: Have the cone at 15 degrees (patient in true lateral). Ensure the cone is centered on the three ipsilateral incisors.

ANGLE: The bisecting angle is found by standing at the patient's side. Remember that the incisor teeth in dogs curve distally (Fig. 22.57).

FIG. 22.57 Canine Maxillary Incisors—Large Dog Technique: DR Sensor. **A,** The sensor is angled toward the canine. **B,** The bisecting angle is visualized from the side. **C,** View from the front showing the 15-degree tilt with the cone centered on the three incisors that are up. **D,** Maxillary incisors (large dog) technique on a canine patient, view from the front. **E,** View from the side on a canine patient. **F,** Radiograph 201—203.

Mandibular Incisors

The typical rostrocaudal view can capture all the incisors on one film when using a CR plate or film. This view is not necessary if the technique for imaging the canine tooth provides a suitable radiograph for ipsilateral incisors. Because the mandibular incisors converge at the midline, the roots cannot always be isolated, as they will overlap slightly. In some instances, if a specific incisor needs to be isolated, the x-ray cone can be directed obliquely from the left or right side so its root is more isolated (see the technique used to image incisors with the DR sensor in large dogs). Dog incisors have long roots that curve distally, like the root(s) of a canine tooth. When using a DR sensor, the technique may vary depending on the size of dog. If both canine teeth can bite down on the sensor, then you can be assured all six incisors will be captured in one image. If the sensor rests between the canine teeth, there may be cutoff of 303 and 403 (due to the inactive perimeter of the sensor). If this is the case, then the teeth will need to be imaged three at a time (see Mandibular Incisors–Large Dog Technique with DR Sensor).

CR PLATE/FILM: The tips of the incisor teeth should be at the rostral edge of the film to allow ample space for the roots of the incisors. Choose a film size where both canine teeth are touching the film ("biting on it"). Size 4 film is used for most medium to large dogs (Fig. 22.58).

DR SENSOR: If both canine teeth can touch the sensor at the same time, then the same technique is used as described for CR plate/film (Fig. 22.59). If the sensor fits evenly between the canine teeth, use the large dog technique with DR sensor (next).

CENTRAL RAY: The cone is directed in a rostrocaudal direction and centered between all six incisors. If the patient is in true lateral, the angle meter is at 0. It is imperative that the cone is centered between all six incisors (Fig. 22.60).

ANGLE: The bisecting angle is found by standing at the patient's side. Remember that the incisor teeth in dogs curve distally.

FIG. 22.58 Canine Mandibular Incisors: CR/Film. **A,** Setup showing the bisecting angle viewed from the patient's side. **B,** Canine patient as viewed from the front. Note: The cone is low enough to be centered between all six incisors. **C,** Canine patient as viewed from the side prior to taking the image. **D,** Radiograph of the mandibular incisors.

Mandibular Incisors—cont'd

FIG. 22.59 Canine Mandibular Incisors: DR Sensor. **A,** Setup showing the bisecting angle viewed from the patient's side. **B,** Setup as viewed from the front. Note: The cone is low enough to be centered between all six incisors.

FIG. 22.60 The Cone is Centered Between the Mandibular Incisors.

Mandibular Incisors—cont'd

Mandibular Incisors—Large Dog Technique with DR Sensor

For larger dogs, incisors should be imaged three at a time. If the patient's size allows the sensor to fit evenly between the canine teeth, the lateral edge of 303 and 403 may be cut off.

This is due to the inactive perimeter on the sensor. It is less likely that this will happen with mandibular incisors because they naturally converge towards the midline. To avoid this, image three incisors at a time.

DR SENSOR: The sensor is positioned with a slight tilt toward the ipsilateral canine tooth.

CENTRAL RAY: Have the cone at 15 degrees (patient in true lateral). Ensure the cone is centered on the three ipsilateral incisors.

ANGLE: The bisecting angle is found by standing at the patient's side. Remember that the incisor teeth in dogs curve distally (Fig. 22.61).

FIG. 22.61 Canine Mandibular Incisors—Large Dog Technique: DR Sensor. **A,** The sensor is angled toward the canine. **B,** The bisecting angle is visualized from the side. **C,** View from the front showing the 15-degree tilt with the cone centered on the three incisors that are up. **D,** View from the front on a canine patient. **E,** View from the side on a canine patient. **F,** Radiograph of 301–303.

Mandibular Canine Teeth

The radiograph of the mandibular canine tooth is set up using the long axis of the tooth, which can be visualized from the side of the patient while the x-ray cone is tilted at 15 degrees (use the angle meter on the tube head). This change in beam angle helps prevent superimposition of the canine tooth over the premolar teeth. The 15-degree tilt only works if the animal is in true lateral. The canine tooth curves distally, with its apex typically over the root of the second premolar. Canine teeth in larger dogs will likely require two exposures due to the size of the tooth and the size limitation of the size 2 sensor.

CR PLATE/FILM: Choose a film size where both canine teeth are touching the film ("biting on it"). Size 4 is used for most dogs. The film should be placed sufficiently rostral to evaluate the ipsilateral incisors as well (Fig. 22.62).

DR SENSOR: Place the tip of the canine tooth on the outside corner (nearest you) of the sensor and push the sensor into the mouth so the same edge is on the floor of the mandible. If the apex of the tooth is missing, then reposition the sensor until the sensor is flat on the floor of the mandible behind the canine tooth (the sensor will not be touching any teeth). Move the cone distal to center over the apex while maintaining a 15-degree tilt and angle (Fig. 22.63).

FIG. 22.62 Canine Mandibular Canine: CR/Film. **A,** View from the patient's side to aim at the bisecting angle. **B,** View from the front while finding the bisecting angle (angle meter should be at 15 degrees). **C,** Final preparation for view from patient's side on a canine patient. **D,** View from patient's front on a canine patient, demonstrating 15-degree tilt. **E,** Radiograph of the mandibular canine tooth. Note: Ipsilateral incisors can be imaged as well.

Mandibular Canine Teeth—cont'd

FIG. 22.63 Canine Mandibular Canine: DR Sensor. **A,** The crown is on the corner of the sensor, and the rest of the sensor is on the floor of the mandible. **B,** View from the patient's side to aim at the bisecting angle. **C,** View from the front while finding the bisecting angle (angle meter should be at 15 degrees). **D,** Final preparation for view from patient's side on a canine patient. **E,** View from patient's front on a canine patient, demonstrating 15-degree tilt. **F,** Repositioning of the sensor flat against the floor of the mandible to image the apex. **G,** Final setup on canine patient; the bisecting angle and 15-degree tilt are maintained while centering over the apex.

Mandibular Premolars 1 and 2

The parallel technique cannot be used on mandibular premolars 1 and 2. Dogs have an elongated mandibular symphysis, which makes correct film placement impossible. The bisecting angle technique must be used on these teeth.

CR PLATE/FILM: The film (size 2) should be resting on both first and second premolars (left and right), behind the canine teeth, facing the floor of the mandible. The tips of the premolars to be radiographed should be at the edge of film closest to you (lateral) to allow ample space for the roots of the tooth to "fall onto" the film. The film can be lengthwise or widthwise depending on the size of the patient (Fig. 22.64).

DR SENSOR: Same approach as described for CR plate/film (Fig. 22.65).
CENTRAL RAY: The cone is directed laterally and centered at the tooth to be radiographed.
ANGLE: The bisecting angle is found by standing at the patient's front.

FIG. 22.64 Canine Mandibular Premolar 1 and 2: CR/Film. **A,** Setup with the bisecting angle viewed from the front. **B,** Canine patient showing final setup. **C,** Radiograph of mandibular premolars 1, 2, and 3.

Mandibular Premolars 1 and 2—cont'd

FIG. 22.65 Canine Mandibular Premolars 1 and 2: DR Sensor. A, Setup with the bisecting angle viewed from the front. B, Canine patient showing final setup.

Mandibular Premolars 3 and 4 and Molars

The parallel technique can be used for the mandibular premolars 3 and 4 and the mandibular molars because there is no hard palate to interfere with film placement behind the roots of these teeth.

CR PLATE/FILM: The film is placed between the tongue and the mandible, parallel to the long axis of the teeth. It is necessary to push the film down until you can feel the film pop out under the ventral mandible. This maneuver ensures that the entire tooth is captured. A paper towel can be used to keep the film pushed down. The film can be gently bent to accommodate placement, and if a larger film is used, it can be placed behind the tooth diagonally so it fits (Fig. 22.66).

DR SENSOR: Same approach as described for CR plate/film. For larger teeth, multiple exposures may be necessary to capture the entire crown and root. This is due to size limitations of the sensor. The 1st molar is an example of a tooth that may need an additional exposure. Push the sensor apically to ensure the roots are captured and repeat exposure (Fig. 22.67).

CENTRAL RAY: The cone is directed laterally and centered on the tooth to be radiographed, perpendicular to the film.

ANGLE: Parallel technique.

Mandibular Premolars 3 and 4 and Molars—cont'd

FIG. 22.66 Canine Mandibular Premolars 3, 4, and Molars: CR/Film. **A,** Setup with size 4 film; the beam is directed perpendicular to the film. **B,** Setup with size 2 film. **C,** Canine patient showing final setup with a size 2 plate. **D,** Radiograph of mandibular premolars 3, 4, and molars. Note: 411 is missing.

Mandibular Premolars 3 and 4 and Molars—cont'd

FIG. 22.67 Canine Mandibular Premolars 3, 4, and Molars: DR Sensor. **A,** Setup with the beam directed perpendicular to the sensor. **B,** Canine patient showing final setup from the front. **C,** Sensor pushed apically to capture distal roots. Note: Paper towel keeps sensor pushed towards apex.

Feline Radiographs with Dental X-Ray Units

> **✏ TECHNICIAN NOTES** CR plates are enclosed in a barrier envelope. For some views, it is necessary to tape the excess envelope behind the plate to ensure the actual plate is as close as possible to the desired area. This approach is necessary for imaging maxillary premolars and molars (intraoral technique: tape edge that will be against the palate) as well as mandibular premolars and molars (parallel technique: tape edge closest to the mandibular symphysis).

Feline Maxillary Premolars: Intraoral Technique with CR/Film

The standard bisecting angle that is traditionally used for maxillary premolars in a dog cannot be used for feline teeth because the zygomatic arch will be superimposed on these teeth. A "modified parallel technique" is used to minimize this superimposition.

CR PLATE/FILM: The endotracheal tube should be carefully repositioned for this view. Untie the tube from behind the cat's ears, leaving the top tie loose and secure the other side to the cat's fur with a hemostat (Fig. 22.68). The top edge of the film (size 2) is resting against the palatal aspect of the maxillary premolar teeth on the side of the mouth opposite to the teeth you are imaging (tape excess envelope behind the plate if using CR plates). The bottom edge of the film rests against the lingual aspect of the tip of the mandibular canine tooth on the side of the mouth you are radiographing. The tongue and tube should be behind the film on the mandible. The maxillary arcade should be parallel to the tabletop.

CENTRAL RAY: The x-ray cone is directed perpendicular to the film visualized from the front and ventral aspect of the patient. The center of the cone should be on the roots.

ANGLE: The angle is referred to as a *modified parallel technique*. It is very important that the beam is perpendicular to the film from the front and side. Note: If root cutoff occurs, the beam must be centered more on the roots of the teeth (Fig. 22.69). If there is too much zygomatic interference, center more on the crown.

FIG. 22.68 Positioning of endotracheal tube and adjustment to ties for feline maxillary premolars (intraoral technique). *Arrow* points to untied tie; other tie is secured to hair with hemostats.

Feline Maxillary Premolars: Intraoral Technique with CR/Film—cont'd

FIG. 22.69 Feline Maxillary Premolars and Molar (Intraoral Technique): CR/Film. **A,** Setup showing film placement. Top edge of film is against palatal aspect of teeth on opposite side; bottom edge of film is resting against lingual aspect of the mandibular canine on the same side. The beam is directed perpendicular to the film. **B,** Feline patient showing final setup as viewed from the front. **C,** Radiograph of feline maxillary premolars and molar. Note: The zygomatic arch is present but the teeth can still be assessed.

Feline Maxillary Premolars Extraoral Technique When Using a DR Sensor

The extraoral technique is preferred for imaging this area. The inactive area of the DR sensor as well as the bulkiness of the sensor make imaging this area problematic with an intraoral approach. The cat should be positioned in lateral recumbency with the mouth propped open with a radiolucent mouth gag. A 1-mL syringe (cut down to a 0.4-mL measurement) can be used to prop the mouth open. The endotracheal tube should be gently pulled ventrally so it is not superimposed over the premolars. NOTE: The mouth should only be propped open for a very short time and not to maximum exertion due to concern of impeding the blood flow through the maxillary artery.

DR SENSOR: The sensor is placed extraorally under the side to be radiographed. The cusps of the premolars should be at the edge of the sensor, with most of the sensor under the cat's maxilla.

CENTRAL RAY: As a starting point, with the patient in lateral recumbency, the cone is aimed at both maxillary arcades as if to superimpose them on the radiograph. Then the cone is directed toward the film, centering at the roots of the premolars near the film and bypassing the opposite arcade.

ANGLE: The beam is aimed at the film in a "near-parallel" technique. From near-parallel, it is approximately a 20- to 25-degree tilt *from the starting point* to bypass the opposite arcade (Fig. 22.70).

Note: On the radiograph, you will see the premolars on the opposite side, but they should not be superimposing on the maxillary premolars in question. If the arcades are superimposed, a greater tilt in the cone is required. If there is too much zygomatic interference, there was too much of a tilt with the cone.

The film will need to be identified properly because the extraoral technique was used.

FIG. 22.70 Feline Maxillary Premolars and Molar (Extraoral Technique): Preferred for DR Sensor. **A,** Labeled extraoral sketch for imaging maxillary premolars and molar in a cat. **B,** Setup showing sensor placement under maxilla with beam directed at arcade that is closest to the table. **C,** Feline patient showing final setup. **D,** Radiograph. Note the contralateral premolars at the top of the film edge (*arrow*).

Feline Maxillary Canine Teeth

The radiograph of a maxillary canine tooth in a cat is set up using the long axis of the tooth, which can be visualized from the side of the patient while the x-ray cone is tilted 30 degrees (use the angle meter on the tube head). This change in beam angle helps prevent superimposition of the canine tooth over the premolar teeth. The 30-degree tilt only works if the animal is in true lateral. The canine tooth tilts distally but not in as pronounced a way as the same tooth in a dog.

Comments and Tips

The ipsilateral maxillary incisors cannot be captured in one image as those of dogs can because of anatomical differences between these species in tooth placement and the rostral maxilla.

CR PLATE/FILM: Size 2 film is used. Both canine teeth should be touching the film ("biting on it"). The tip of the canine tooth desired should be at the lateral edge of the film to allow ample space for the root of the canine tooth (Fig. 22.71).

DR SENSOR: The same approach as described for CR/film is used (Fig. 22.72).

CENTRAL RAY: The tube head is tilted 30 degrees so that the canine tooth does not superimpose over the premolars distal to it. Center the beam on the canine tooth.

ANGLE: The bisecting angle of the tooth is found by standing at the patient's side using the long axis of the tooth (follow the crown, as the root follows the same axis).

FIG. 22.71 Feline Maxillary Canine Tooth: CR/Film. **A,** Setup showing bisecting angle from the side. **B,** Setup showing 30-degree tilt from the front. **C,** Feline patient showing final setup from the side. **D,** Feline patient showing final setup with 30-degree tilt from the front.

FIG. 22.71, cont'd   E, Radiograph of maxillary canine tooth.

FIG. 22.72 Feline Maxillary Canine Tooth: DR Sensor. **A,** Setup showing bisecting angle from the side. **B,** Setup showing 30-degree tilt from the front. **C,** Feline patient showing final setup from the side. **D,** Feline patient showing final setup with 30-degree tilt from the front.

Feline Maxillary Canine Teeth—cont'd

Feline Maxillary Incisors

CR PLATE/FILM: Size 2 film is used for the maxillary incisors. The tips of the incisor teeth should be at the edge of the film closest to you (rostral) to allow ample space for the roots of the incisors to "fall onto" the film (Fig. 22.73).

DR SENSOR: The same approach as described for CR/film is used (Fig. 22.74).

CENTRAL RAY: The cone is directed in a rostrocaudal direction and centered between all six incisors.

ANGLE: The bisecting angle is found by standing at the patient's side.

FIG. 22.73 Feline Maxillary Incisors: CR/Film. **A,** Setup showing bisecting angle from the side. **B,** Setup showing the cone centered between all six incisors. **C,** Final setup on a feline patient as viewed from the side. **D,** Final setup on a feline patient as viewed from the front. **E,** Radiograph of maxillary incisors.

Feline Maxillary Canine Teeth—cont'd

FIG. 22.74 Feline Maxillary Incisors: DR Sensor. **A,** Setup showing bisecting angle from the side. **B,** Setup showing the cone centered between all six incisors. **C,** Final setup on a feline patient as viewed from the side. **D,** Final setup on a feline patient as viewed from the front.

Feline Mandibular Canines and Incisors

Both mandibular canines and all incisors of the cat can be imaged in one view. The reason is that cats are missing premolars 1 and 2, thus allowing for a rostrocaudal beam without superimposition on other teeth. If positioning the film distal in the mouth is problematic due to interference of the lingual frenulum, you can place the tongue between the film and mandible. The x-ray beam can easily penetrate the tongue before the film with minimal interference.

CR PLATE/FILM: Size 2 film is used. Both canine teeth should be touching the film ("biting on it"). The tongue should be pushed out of the way, ideally on the opposite side of the film (Fig. 22.75).

DR SENSOR: The same approach as described for CR/film is used (Fig. 22.76).

CENTRAL RAY: The cone is directed in a rostrocaudal direction and centered between all six incisors. If the patient is in true lateral, the angle meter is at 0. It is imperative that the cone is centered between all six incisors.

ANGLE: The bisecting angle is found by standing at the patient's side. The long axis of the canine tooth, not the incisors, should be used to find the bisecting angle. Remember that the canine tooth has a large root that curves in distally.

FIG. 22.75 Feline Mandibular Incisors and Canines: CR/Film. **A,** Setup showing bisecting angle from the side. **B,** Setup showing the cone centered between all six incisors and canines. **C,** Final setup on a feline patient as viewed from the side. **D,** Final setup on a feline patient as viewed from the front. **E,** Radiograph of mandibular incisors and canines.

Feline Mandibular Canines and Incisors—cont'd

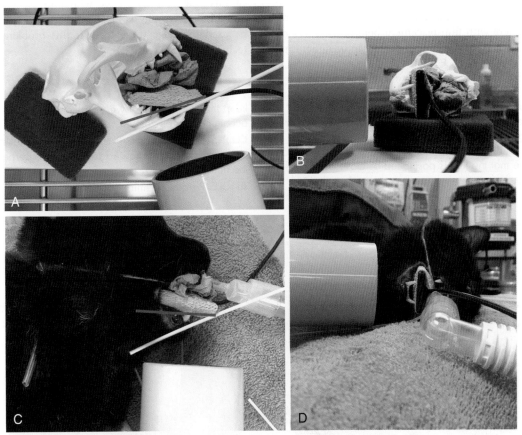

FIG. 22.76 Feline Mandibular Incisors and Canines: DR Sensor. **A,** Setup showing bisecting angle from the side. **B,** Setup showing the cone centered between all six incisors and canines. **C,** Final setup on a feline patient as viewed from the side. **D,** Final setup on a feline patient as viewed from the front.

Feline Mandibular Premolars and Molars: Parallel Technique for CR/Film

The parallel technique can be used to image the mandibular premolars and molars of the cat because there is no hard palate to interfere with film placement behind the roots of these teeth. The mesial root of premolar 3 can be difficult to capture due to interference with film placement and the mandibular symphysis. A bisecting angle technique can be used to image these teeth if this problem occurs (see technique in DR section).

CR PLATE/FILM: The film (size 0) is placed behind the teeth parallel to the long axis of the teeth and in line with the border of the mandible. It is necessary to push the film down until you can feel it pop out under the ventral mandible, and it is imperative that the film is positioned as close as possible to the mandibular symphysis (tape excess envelope behind plate if using CR PSP plates). A paper towel can be used to keep the film pushed down. The film can be gently bent to accommodate placement.

CENTRAL RAY: The cone is directed in a lateral direction and centered at the tooth to be radiographed, perpendicular to the film (Fig. 22.77).

ANGLE: Parallel technique.

FIG. 22.77 Feline Mandibular Premolars and Molar (Parallel Technique). **A,** Setup showing parallel technique. The x-ray cone is perpendicular to the film (size 0). **B,** Final setup showing correct placement of plate. **C,** Final setup on a feline patient as viewed from the front. **D.** Radiograph of mandibular premolars 3, 4, and molar.

Feline Mandibular Premolar and Molar: Bisecting Angle Technique for DR Sensors

This is the preferred technique when using a DR sensor because sensor placement using parallel technique often results in root cutoff of the third premolar. The parallel technique can be used to image the mandibular molar of the cat if the bisecting angle technique for this area is unsuccessful in capturing the molar. This does occur, as it can be difficult positioning the sensor distal in the mouth.

DR SENSOR: The sensor should be pushed as far distal as possible in the mouth, preferably with the tongue on the opposite side of the film. If this is not possible, the tongue can be left between the sensor and the teeth. If the sensor is not pushed far enough back in the mouth, the molar will be cut off (use the parallel technique for the molar if this is problematic). When using parallel technique for the molar, the sensor will be placed diagonal behind the teeth.

CENTRAL RAY: The cone is directed in a lateral direction at the tooth to be radiographed.

ANGLE: The bisecting angle is found by standing at the patient's front (Fig. 22.78).

FIG. 22.78 Feline Mandibular Premolars and Molar (Bisecting Angle Technique). **A,** Setup showing bisecting angle technique as viewed from the front. **B,** Final setup on a feline patient as viewed from the front. **C,** Sensor placement for parallel technique of molar if needed. **D,** Radiograph of mandibular premolars 3, 4, and molar.

Canine and Feline Nasal Sinus Radiographs

Indications for radiographs of the nasal sinus cavity in either the dog or cat include evaluation of disease, such as neoplasia, as well as the detection of foreign bodies.

Examples

POSITION: The patient should be in sternal recumbency with the maxilla parallel to the tabletop.

CR PLATE/FILM: For dogs, size 4 film is inserted as far as possible into the patient's mouth between the maxilla and the endotracheal tube. For cats, the film may need to be placed in on an angle, or a size 2 film may be used.

DR SENSOR: For dogs, the sensor is inserted as above. Two exposures may have to be taken to view the entire sinuses on dogs, particularly large dogs.

CENTRAL RAY: The cone is 6 to 8 inches away from the film and centered on the nasal cavity. Use settings for a maxillary canine tooth, and adjust for the distance from the film.

ANGLE: The cone is directed perpendicular to the film (Fig. 22.79).

FIG. 22.79 Setup for Radiograph of Nasal Sinus. A, Skull setup. B, Radiograph.

Dental Radiography with Conventional Cassette: Common Views

The use of conventional cassettes is not the ideal way to image teeth, but if there is no dental x-ray machine or nonscreen film, it is the only option. Screened cassettes and radiolucent positioning devices are required.

Difficulties expected include positioning of the cassettes in the mouth because of the general characteristics of cassettes (size, thickness, and weight). Teeth in the distal aspect of the mouth may be difficult to image due to superimposition of the contralateral arch.

See further discussion of intraoral radiography with a conventional machine elsewhere in this chapter.

Maxillary Premolars and Molars: Ventrodorsal Oblique Extraoral Views

Positioning

Position the patient in lateral (side) recumbency with a foam roll under the nose, affected side down, on the cassette. Once in this position, rotate the patient so it is placed midway onto its back, in an oblique between the lateral and ventral-dorsal (ventrodorsal [VD]) positions. Place the mandible on a foam wedge, rotating the mandible at a 45-degree angle to the table surface. The mouth should be propped wide open with a radiolucent mouth gag in place (Fig. 22.80).

Comments and Tips

- Make sure the contralateral maxillary teeth and roots do not superimpose against interested maxilla premolars and molars.

Examples

MEASURE: Caudal hard palate at commissure of lips.
CENTRAL RAY: Maxillary third premolar.
INCLUDE: Maxillary premolars and molars.

> **✐ TECHNICIAN NOTES** The contralateral maxillary premolars and molars appear whiter because of bone superimposition. The affected side's premolars and molars appear magnified because of the angle of the head, causing elongation.

FIG. 22.80 Extraoral Technique of Maxillary Premolars and Molars. A, Setup. B, Radiograph.

Mandibular Premolars and Molars: Dorsoventral Oblique Extraoral Views

Positioning

Position the patient in lateral recumbency with the affected side down on the cassette.

Place the maxilla on a foam wedge, raising the maxilla to a 20-degree angle to the table surface. The mouth should be propped wide open with a radiolucent mouth gag (Fig. 22.81).

Comments and Tips

• Make sure the contralateral mandibular teeth and roots do not superimpose over the areas of interest, which are the mandibular premolars and molars.

• The contralateral mandibular premolars and molars appear whiter because of the bone superimposition.

• The affected side's premolars and molars appear magnified because of the angle of the head, causing elongation.

Examples

MEASURE: Thickness of mandible at the commissure of lips.
CENTRAL RAY: Site of interest.
INCLUDE: Mandibular premolars and molars.

 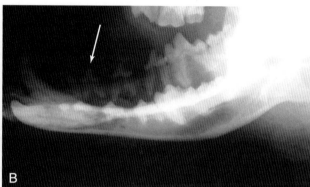

FIG. 22.81 Extraoral Technique of Mandibular Premolars and Molars. A, Setup. B, Radiograph.

Maxilla Incisors and Canine: Dorsoventral Intraoral/Occlusal View

Positioning
Position the patient in sternal recumbency. A foam sponge should be placed under the mandible and cassette to keep it parallel to the tabletop. Place one corner of the film cassette into the mouth as far as possible (Fig. 22.82).

Comments and Tips
- Source-image distance (SID) will have to be adjusted because of the raised cassette.

- The roots of the canine teeth will be superimposed over the premolars distal to the canine tooth.
- The rostral nasal sinus cavity can be assessed with this view.

Examples
MEASURE: At the level of the commissure of the lips (maxilla thickness).
CENTRAL RAY: Site of interest.
INCLUDE: All incisors and canines, including roots.

FIG. 22.82 Intraoral Technique with Cassette of Maxillary Incisors and Canine. A, Setup. B, Radiograph.

Mandibular Incisors and Canine: Ventrodorsal Intraoral/Occlusal View

Positioning

The patient should be positioned in dorsal recumbency with a foam sponge placed under the nose and cervical spine to keep the mandible and cassette parallel to the tabletop. Place one corner of the film cassette into the mouth as far as possible (Fig. 22.83).

Comments and Tips

- Raise the tube head because the SID has decreased.
- The mandibular canine tooth will be slightly superimposed over the first premolar.

Examples

MEASURE: At the level of the commissure of the lips (mandible thickness, which is $_1M_1$ in dogs).

CENTRAL RAY: Site of interest.

INCLUDE: All incisors and canines, including roots.

 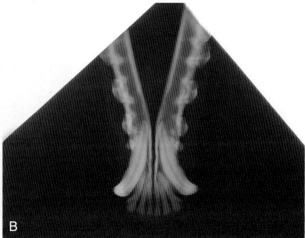

FIG. 22.83 Intraoral Technique with Cassette of Mandibular Incisors and Canine. A, Setup. B, Radiograph.

Intraoral Dental Radiography with a Conventional Machine

If a dental radiography machine is not available, the intraoral radiographs previously described can be accomplished with a conventional machine. In the descriptions of the intraoral views, the x-ray cone was maneuvered to focus on the bisecting angle or film where indicated. With use of a conventional x-ray machine, the patient's body position and skull must be rotated so the previously described angles will line up with the vertical central ray.

The following procedure and supplies are used with this technique:

- Nonscreen dental film
- Foam wedges or rolls (assortment of sizes)
- SID should be 15 inches from the tabletop
- Settings: 60 to 70 kilovolts (kV), 100 milliamperage (mA), 1.6 milliamperes-seconds (mAs)
- If SID cannot be reduced, the following settings should be used: 40 inches SID, 60 to 70 kV, 100 mA, 3.2 mAs

Any of the previously described views can be accomplished with this technique, as illustrated by two examples. Fig. 22.84 shows a radiographic setup for imaging the maxillary premolars with a conventional machine. The bisecting angle is found as previously described (see Fig. 22.43), but note that in the setup shown, the skull is rotated ventrally so that the vertical central ray is aimed at the bisecting angle. In Fig. 22.85, the mandibular incisors are imaged with a conventional machine. The patient is in dorsal recumbency with a small foam wedge placed under the nose. This positioning allows the central ray to be directed at the bisecting angle.

Errors in Film Placement and Artifacts

Some common errors in film placement (not including previously described elongation and foreshortening) are as follows:
a. Not pushing film in far enough (root cut off) (Fig. 22.86A)
b. Cone not centered on tooth (cone cut off) (Fig. 22.86B)

FIG. 22.84 Setup for a radiograph of the canine maxillary premolars using a conventional x-ray machine. Note: The beam comes from straight above.

FIG. 22.85 Setup for a radiograph of the canine mandibular incisors using a conventional x-ray machine. Note: beam comes from straight above.

c. Light exposure in darkroom (Fig. 22.86C)
d. Processing errors (Fig. 22.86D)
e. Fingerprints and scratches on film (Fig. 22.86E)
f. Bent film (crescent line) (Fig. 22.86F)
g. Double exposure (Fig. 22.86G)
h. X-ray taken through back of film (Fig. 22.86H)
i. Light exposure on CR PSP plate (haze on top half of image) (Fig. 22.86I)

Radiographs of Abnormal Dental Pathology

Examples of common abnormal pathology found in dogs or cats include the following:
a. Horizontal bone loss (Fig. 22.87A)
b. Vertical bone loss (Fig. 22.87B)
c. Periapical lucency (Fig. 22.87C)
d. Resorptive lesions (Fig. 22.87D)
e. Ankylosis (Fig. 22.87E)
f. Missing teeth (Fig. 22.87F)
g. Unerupted teeth (Fig. 22.87G)
h. Supernumerary teeth (Fig. 22.87H)
i. Complete extraction (Fig. 22.87I)
j. Retained root tip (Fig. 22.87J)

> ### ✳ KEY POINTS
> 1. Dental radiography is essential for a proper assessment of the oral cavity in dog and cat mouths.
> 2. Dental radiographs can be accomplished in any veterinary hospital, even those without a dental x-ray unit.
> 3. The bisecting angle technique is used in most areas of dog and cat mouths.
> 4. Manual processing of films can be a source of many errors.
> 5. The SLOB rule helps identify specific roots when the x-ray cone is directed obliquely.

FIG. 22.86 A, Root cut off because of improper film placement (film not pushed in far enough). B, Cone cut off. C, Light exposure in chairside darkroom. D, Film processing error; fixer not rinsed off film. E, Black fingerprints and scratches on film. F, Bent film (crescent line). G, Double exposure.

FIG. 22.86, cont'd H, X-ray taken through back of film (note faint checkerboard pattern on left side). I, Light exposure on CR PSP plate (gray haze).

FIG. 22.87 A, Horizontal bone loss evident on 106. B, Vertical bone loss (*arrows*). C, Periapical lucency on 410. D, Feline resorptive lesion 407. E, Ankylosis of canine mandibular premolar and molars. F, Congenitally missing tooth 406. G, Unerupted canine tooth 304. H, Supernumerary 105. I, Complete extraction of 103. J, Retained root tip 305. (Courtesy Dental Vet, Weston, Florida.)

REVIEW QUESTIONS

1. If one used a conventional unit to image a mandible, the kV is likely 45 to 50, yet when using the dental unit for mandibular teeth, the settings are generally preset at 70 or 80. More exposure is required:
   a. Because dental units are high-frequency units
   b. For teeth as compared to the mandible itself
   c. Because there are no intensifying screens in dental film
   d. Because the SID is increased in dental radiography

2. Your clinic has ordered a dental radiography unit, and the veterinarian wishes you to investigate what extra electricity is required. You report that the dental unit requires:
   a. A 110-volt line with no special wiring
   b. A 110-volt line with special grounding
   c. A 220-volt line with a ground wire
   d. A 220-volt line without special wiring

3. Which part of your new dental x-ray machine can swing 180 degrees?
   a. Scissor arm
   b. X-ray tube
   c. Extension arm
   d. Control panel

4. Direct digital dental radiography in dentistry:
   a. Requires an intermediate step for processing
   b. Is more expensive to buy compared with the other digital system
   c. Generally utilizes a smaller sensor
   d. Utilizes thin and flexible plates similar to regular film

5. CR PSP plates are available in the following size, which is not available in film:
   a. 0
   b. 2
   c. 3
   d. 4

6. You are getting a patient file for the veterinarian to review about a month after dental films were processed. You notice that the films, which were perfectly diagnostic at the time, now appear foggy and have a coffee-color appearance with poor density and contrast. You realized that you:
   a. Fixed the film for 15 seconds and dabbed the film in the water jar
   b. Fixed the film for 2 to 4 minutes and washed in running water
   c. Developed for 15 seconds and fixed for 2 to 4 minutes
   d. Used fresh chemicals for processing these films

7. The dental formula for the permanent teeth in the cat is:
   a. (3121/3131) = 30
   b. (3131/3121) = 30
   c. (3133/3142) = 42
   d. (3142/3143) = 42

8. A dog has the following three rooted teeth:
   a. 108, 109, 110, 208, 209, 210
   b. 308, 309, 310, 408, 409, 410
   c. $_4^4P_4^4$, $_{1,2}^{1,2}M_{1,2}^{1,2}$
   d. 208 and 108 only

9. The area on the periphery of the tooth where the crown and root meet is the:
   a. Dentin
   b. Enamodental junction
   c. Cementoenamel junction
   d. Cementum

10. When x-raying a maxillary canine tooth, what is the angle in which the tube head is moved up vertically to prevent superimposition of the canine tooth over the premolars distal to it?
    a. 20
    b. 30
    c. 15
    d. 45

11. The bisecting angle technique in a dog is used on all of the following areas except:
    a. 303
    b. 409
    c. 204
    d. 105

12. The veterinarian suspects damage of tooth 104 in a Border Collie. You are best to position the patient in:
    a. Right lateral recumbency
    b. Left lateral recumbency
    c. Dorsal recumbency
    d. Ventral recumbency

13. You should utilize the bisecting angle with the long axis of the maxillary canine tooth. This is best visualized from the:
    a. Side of the patient with a 30-degree tilt of the x-ray cone
    b. Side of the patient with a 45-degree tilt of the x-ray cone
    c. Front of the patient with a 30-degree tilt of the x-ray cone
    d. Front of the patient with a 45-degree tilt of the x-ray cone

14. The tips of the teeth should be situated on this size 4 film on the:
    a. Center of the film
    b. Convex side of the film
    c. Away from the convex dot side of the film
    d. Concave side of the film

15. As you are setting up for tooth 104, you notice that the central ray is angled more on the film instead of the bisecting angle. You alter the angle because otherwise you will have:
    a. Foreshortening
    b. Elongation
    c. Magnification
    d. A blurred image

16. You are using the extraoral technique for a mandible of a Lhasa Apso. To isolate the maxillary premolars, you will need to angle the mandible:
    a. 60 degrees
    b. 40 degrees
    c. 20 degrees
    d. 45 degrees

17. A modified x-ray technique is used to x-ray the maxillary premolars in a cat because of interference of which structure?
    a. Palatine fissure
    b. Mandibular symphysis
    c. Zygomatic arch
    d. Nasal sinus

18. The extraoral x-ray technique for a feline's patient tooth 208 (left maxillary premolar) that is preferred is with the patient lying in lateral recumbency and the DR sensor placed:
    a. In the mouth under the right maxillary premolar
    b. In the mouth under the left maxillary premolar
    c. Under the right side of the patient because it is in right lateral recumbency
    d. Under the left side of the patient because it is in left lateral recumbency

19. The beam for this modified x-ray technique of the maxillary premolar should be aimed:
    a. In a parallel technique with the beam 90 degrees to the film
    b. Perpendicular to the film visualized from the front and ventral aspect of the patient
    c. Laterally and the bisecting angle found by standing at the patient's front
    d. In a near-parallel technique with a 20- to 25-degree tilt to bypass the opposite arcade

20. If the x-ray cone is directed from the distal aspect of tooth 108, the root that will appear in the middle on the radiograph is:
    a. The distal root
    b. The mesial-palatal root
    c. The mesial-buccal root
    d. Neither, as they will be superimposed

Chapter Review Question answers are located in the Instructor Resources on Evolve and can be provided to students at the discretion of the instructor.

Bibliography

Bellows J. *The Practice of Veterinary Dentistry: A Team Effort.* Iowa City: Iowa State Press; 1999.

Bellows J. *Small Animal Dental Equipment, Materials and Techniques: A Primer.* Iowa City: Blackwell Publishing; 2004.

Derbyshire G. *Veterinary Dentistry for the Nurse and Technician.* St. Louis: Elsevier; 2005.

Hale F. *Veterinary Dentistry.* July 2020. Available at: http://www.toothvet.ca/Old%20CUSP%20Articles.htm#INTRA-ORAL%20DENTAL%20RADIOLOGY.

Han C, Hurd C. *Practical Diagnostic Imaging for the Veterinary Technician.* 3rd ed. St. Louis: Mosby; 2005.

Holmstrom SE. *Veterinary Dentistry: A Team Approach.* 3rd ed, St. Louis: Elsevier; 2019.

Iannucci J, Howerton LJ. *Dental Radiography: Principles and Techniques.* St. Louis: Saunders; 2012.

Lobprise HB, Dodd JR. *Wiggs's Veterinary Dentistry: Principles and Practice.* 2nd ed. New Jersey: John Wiley & Sons Inc; 2019.

Mulligan TA. *Atlas of Canine and Dental Radiography in Dogs and Cats.* United Kingdom: Elsevier Health Science; 2008.

Niemic BA. *A Color Handbook of Small Animal Dental, Oral and Maxillofacial Disease.* London, UK: Manson Publishing; 2010.

Tutt D. *BSAVA Manual of Canine and Feline Dentistry.* 3rd ed. Gloucester, UK: British Small Animal Veterinary Association; 2007.

(Courtesy Rosedale Animal Hospital, Toronto, ON.)

CHAPTER 23
Small Animal Special Procedures

Marg Brown, RVT, BEd Ad Ed

We are so constituted that we can gain intense pleasure only from the contrast, and only very little from the condition itself.
—Sigmund Freud, 1856–1939, *Civilization and Its Discontents*, written 1929

OUTLINE

LEARNING OBJECTIVES

When you have finished this chapter, you will be able to:

1. Recognize the types of contrast media, including the differences between positive- and negative-contrast media, the physiological effects, the appearances on an image, the indications, and the contraindications.
2. Comprehend the value of proper survey images and patient preparation before the performance of contrast studies.
3. Summarize the procedures and protocols for common contrast studies.

4. Explain other radiographic contrast studies that may be used in practice.
5. Appreciate the other modalities used in addition to or in lieu of contrast studies.
6. Identify normal contrast study anatomy found on a radiographic image.

KEY TERMS

Key terms are defined in the Glossary on the Evolve website.

Angiocardiography
Angiography
Antegrade
Arthrography
Barium sulfate
BIPS
Cathartic
Celiography
Contrast medium

Cystography
Dimer
Double contrast
Dyschezia
Esophagography
Excretory urography
Filling defects
Fistulography
Functional study

Gastrography
Granuloma
Iatrogenesis
Inert
Ionic iodine
Lower gastrointestinal (LGI) study
Monomer
Morphological studies

Myelography
Negative-contrast agents
Nephrogram
Nonionic iodine
Osmolality
Parasympatholytic agents
Pneumocystogram
Pneumoperitoneography
Positive-contrast agents

TECHNICAL NOTE: To preserve space, the radiographs presented in this chapter do not show collimation. For safety, always collimate so that the beam is limited to within the image receptor edges. In film radiography, you should see a clear border of collimation (frame) on every radiograph. In some jurisdictions, evidence of collimation is required by law. In digital imaging, the algorithm depends on proper collimation.

Overview

Organs or soft tissue structures are often difficult or impossible to identify on plain or survey abdominal images because the tissue densities of many organs are similar without inherent contrast. The introduction of negative-contrast or positive-contrast media differentiates these structures from the surrounding tissues by enhancing the tissue density with a medium that absorbs the radiation and outlines the anatomy/pathology within the structure. In normal radiographic imaging, positive-contrast agents appear white, or radiopaque, on the completed image, whereas negative-contrast agents appear black, or radiolucent.

The agents are administered so that they will either demonstrate the anatomy or the physiology. They can be useful in determining the anatomy, such as size, shape, location, position, and contour; defects in the mucosal surface of an organ; the luminal contents; or the presence of extramural lesions. Physiology or functional assessment of the organ can be obtained through determining transit time after giving a contrast meal or by injecting a water-soluble organic iodide; however, this is more time consuming and detailed.

The desired effect of any contrast substance injected into the body is to change density and organ visibility yet still be harmless to the patient. With any procedure, there are contraindications. To minimize risks, certain questions must be asked before administration of a contrast agent to determine whether the procedure should be completed. Depending on the procedure, the veterinarian needs to determine whether the contrast study will be useful, whether it is the best diagnostic tool, and whether it will furnish sufficient information to be worthwhile. The patient may not tolerate fasting, which is usually required, or may not be a good anesthetic risk if anesthesia is recommended. Also, because of the time and costs involved, other diagnostic procedures may be more useful. Patient preparation, equipment, and technique vary, depending on the special procedure.

A contrast study should never replace routine survey images. Survey images performed before the contrast study help determine proper exposure and patient preparation for the contrast study. The need for contrast media may also be eliminated if a diagnosis can be achieved with a survey image.

These special contrast studies are used to provide information that might not otherwise be available to make a diagnosis, further evaluate the character of a suspected lesion, or determine appropriate treatment.

Endoscopy, ultrasound, and other imaging modalities, when available and feasible, have replaced contrast radiography for many evaluations. Some of these modalities use similar contrast agents.

> **TECHNICIAN NOTES** Strategically used positioning aids give the patient the *illusion* that it is being held. A sandbag over the neck and limbs and/or the use of tape/Velcro/ties is essential if the patient is not sedated. Keep talking to your patient while taking the images, gradually stepping back from the primary beam. Be safety conscious at all times and apply the three tenets of safety—time, distance, and shielding.

> **TECHNICIAN NOTES** Quickly go through a mental checklist such as this one before pushing the exposure button:
> - Are the settings correct?
> - Is the plate/cassette/machine/grid in position?
> - Is the thickest part toward the cathode, if applicable?
> - Are the markers and ID (if using) in the proper location and not obstructing relevant anatomy?
> - Do you have the correct body part and view?
> - Is the patient properly centered? Are the peripheral borders correct?
> - Is the x-ray beam correctly collimated?
> - Is the patient properly prepared, positioned, and restrained so that the body part is parallel to the image receptor and the central ray is perpendicular to both?
> - If applicable, is the patient in the correct phase of respiration?

Contrast Media Used for Radiographic Imaging

Positive-Contrast Media

- Barium sulfate and water-soluble organic iodides (Fig. 23.1)—both ionic and nonionic—produce a positive-contrast or a radiopaque image (Table 23.1).

FIG. 23.1 Positive Contrast Media. A, Ionic iodine. B, Nonionic iodine. C, Barium paste. D, Barium suspension E, Barium-impregnated polyurethane spheres (BIPS).

- The atomic numbers of barium (56) and iodine (53) are higher than that of tissues and bones, which is why the media is even "whiter" than bone on an image. Calcium, an element of bone, has an atomic number of 20.
- Barium sulfate is used exclusively for radiographic examination of the gastrointestinal (GI) tract and can be administered orally or rectally. It is chemically inert and is an insoluble, white, crystalline substance that is available commercially as a powder, colloid suspension, or paste, with each molecule covered with a wetting agent to keep the barium in suspension. Proper viscosity is required for the specific area being studied. Esophageal studies require a paste, whereas a thin mixture is needed for a single-contrast enema.
- If there is a suspected bowel perforation, barium should not be used (see Table 23.1). It resists dilution in the peritoneal cavity and is completely insoluble. If it is leaked into the peritoneal cavity, a granuloma or adhesions may occur. Barium should never be injected intravenously.
- Also, be very careful that barium is not accidentally aspirated into the lungs.

TABLE 23.1	Positive Contrast Agents for Gastrointestinal (GI) Studies in Animals[4-7]		
CONTRAST AGENT*	**USES**	**ADVANTAGES**	**DISADVANTAGES**
Barium Sulfate Suspensions			
Trade name(s): • Liquid Polibar Plus • Esobar esophageal cream (60% w/w)	Routine GI contrast studies—use only rectally or orally. Do not use if a GI perforation is suspected.	Low cost Palatable Delineates the mucosal walls well Excellent opacity Remains in suspension Does not become diluted with secretions Not absorbed through the intestines Good density	Slow to be transmitted Insoluble—cannot use with perforation Aspiration in lung can be fatal, although small amounts are usually benign Very irritating to the peritoneum Can hide mucosal surfaces during surgical or endoscopic procedures Blocks ultrasound waves
Characteristics of or Concerns or Comments About Barium			
• Radiodense • Physiologically inert • Resists dilution • Completely insoluble • If leaked into peritoneal cavity, may induce granulomas or adhesions • Hygroscopic nature absorbs water from the bowel, so may cause a bowel obstruction from barium impaction in debilitated patients			
Radiopaque Markers			
Trade name • BIPS	Determine orocolic transit rate Note obstructive disease	Easy to administer Not likely to be aspirated or to cause peritonitis Can be given with food Time frame for images not as important Do not obscure abdominal detail More likely to detect motility disorders	Cannot visualize mucosal detail or luminal margins Expensive in comparison with barium suspension Studies can take longer
Ionic Iodine			
Oral Organic Iodine—Ionic Solution			
Type, trade name(s) • Common oral forms: meglumine diatrizoate and sodium diatrizoate (Gastrografin)	Suspected intestinal perforation or obstructions	Rapid transit time Nonirritating to serosal surfaces and peritoneum Readily absorbed from peritoneal cavity if leakage Can be absorbed across the mucosa and excreted by the urinary tract	Has a bitter taste Expensive in comparison with barium suspension Hypertonicity can cause: • Fluid movement into the lumen (osmotic diarrhea) • Dilution of the contrast medium • Electrolyte imbalance • Dehydration • Nausea, vomiting • Decreased blood pressure

Continued

TABLE 23.1	Positive Contrast Agents for Gastrointestinal (GI) Studies in Animals—cont'd		
CONTRAST AGENT*	**USES**	**ADVANTAGES**	**DISADVANTAGES**

Injectable Organic Iodine—Ionic Solution

| Type, trade name(s)
 • IV: Sodium diatrizoate (Hypaque); meglumine diatrizoate (Hypaque M)
 • Iothalamate meglumine (Conray) | Intravenous (IV) injections for urinary radiography, infusion in hollow organs | Less viscous | The hypertonicity effects listed earlier are more likely to occur after rapid IV bolus, causing peripheral vasodilation and bradycardia due to increased parasympathetic activity
 Irritating to the brain and spinal cord
 Can cause toxicity and tissue irritability (e.g., in kidney, bladder) |

Characteristics of or Concerns or Comments About Ionic Iodine

- Diatrizoates provide opacification for excretory urography. Because the ions dissociate when absorbed into the bloodstream, hypertonicity is a real concern, especially with sodium diatrizoate. They cannot be used for pyelography. Hypaque is not commonly used anymore due to these side effects.
- Rapid IV administration is more likely to initiate the vasovagal response that can cause nausea and brief retching or vomiting.[5]

Injectable Organic Iodine—Nonionic Solution

| Type, trade name(s)
 • Iohexol (Omnipaque)
 • Iopamidol (Isovue)
 • Ioversol (Optiray)
 • Iopromide (Ultravist)
 • Iotrolan (Isovist, Osmovist)
 • Ioxilan (Oxilan)
 • Nonionic dimer iodixanol (Visipaque) | Myelography.
 Can be used IV, especially for young or debilitated patient | Fewer side effects than with ionic form—rapid transit time
 Nonirritating
 Resorbed after extraluminal leakage
 Does not become increasingly dilute
 Endoscopy and ultrasonography will not be impaired if a contrast study is first completed | Expensive |

Characteristics of or Concerns or Comments About Nonionic Iodine

- Low osmolarity and chemical nature
- Nonionic dimer contrast media is virtually isotonic with blood and cerebrospinal fluid

Characteristics of or Concerns or Comments About BIPS

- If delayed emptying occurs, the cause will not be known.
- Do not use barium-impregnated spheres (BIPS) for 24–48 hours after barium suspension.

*Note: Depending on availability or your region, not all products listed may be available or produced after publication.

TECHNICIAN NOTES

- Osmosis is the movement of water through a semipermeable membrane from a liquid of low concentration to one of a higher concentration until the two concentrations are equal.
- Osmotic pressure is the pressure of a solution against a semipermeable membrane to prevent water from flowing inward across that membrane. It is determined solely by the concentration of dissolved particles.
- An osmole is the unit of measurement that refers to the number of moles of a compound that contributes to the osmotic pressure of a solution.
- Osmolality is the number of osmoles of solute per kilogram of solvent and is usually expressed as mOsmol/kg (milliosmoles/kg). (Osmolarity is the concentration of the osmotic solution and is expressed as mOsm/L.)

- Tonicity is the measure of this osmotic pressure.
- An isosmolar solution has the same osmolality as the plasma. There is no osmosis between the blood vessels and the surrounding fluids and thus no water exchange.
- A hyperosmolar or hypertonic fluid will have a higher osmolality than the plasma, and thus liquid will be pulled into the plasma.
- A hypotonic or hyposmolar fluid will have a lower osmotic pressure than plasma, so water will leave the plasma.
- A centipoise (cPs) is the unit used to describe the viscosity of a solution. It is one-hundredth of a poise and is the amount of force needed to move one layer of liquid in relation to another liquid.

- Water-soluble organic iodides are generally used in intravascular studies or injected into other body cavities. Iodides mix readily with blood or other body fluids and are excreted through the kidneys. The iodine atoms in the contrast medium molecule are the primary attenuators of the x-ray beam, so the concentration of the iodine in the contrast agent is important. A higher iodine concentration shows more contrast on an image.

- The two major types of iodinated contrast media are ionic and nonionic. The media whose molecules dissociate and cause changes in osmolality are termed *ionic,* and the media whose molecules remain whole in solution are termed *nonionic.*[1]

- Water-soluble organic ionic iodides are triiodinated compounds derived from the benzoic acid ring structure (Fig. 23.2). These compounds are called *ionic* because an anion (negative) and cation (positive) make up each compound; when they dissociate, the ions are dispersed, changing the osmolality of the solution they are in.

- The cation is a salt, usually sodium (Hypaque) or meglumine (Conray), or a combination of the two. Sodium is slightly more toxic than either the meglumine or the combination. The salts increase the solubility of the compound.

- The cation is combined with a negatively charged component called an *anion.* The benzene ring with

CLASSIFICATION OF CONTRAST MEDIA (CM) FOR RADIOGRAPHY

FIG 23.2 A, Chart of classification of contrast media (CM) for radiography.

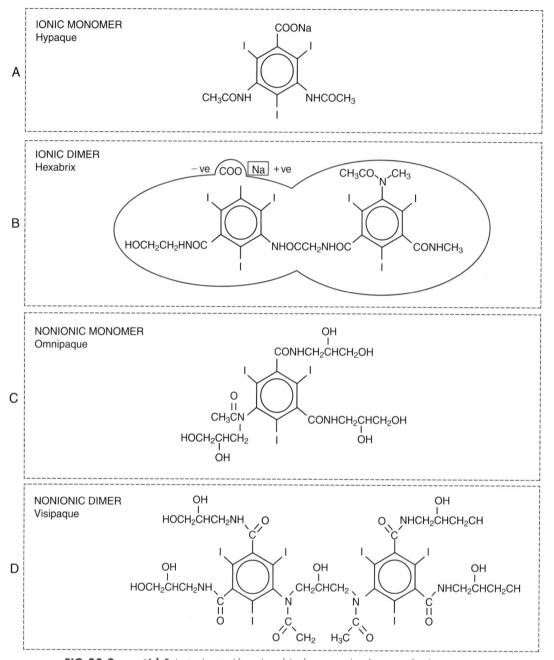

FIG 23.2, cont'd B, Ionic chemical formulae of the four main classifications of iodine contrast.

three iodine atoms attached, plus other chemical components (side chains), makes up the anion. Diatrizoate and iothalamate are common anions.

- In an ionic contrast medium, there are three iodine atoms to two particles in the solution, which will give a 3:2 ratio (3 components of the iodine: 1 positive cation + 1 negative ion), resulting in higher osmolality. These are referred to as *high-osmolar contrast agents* (HOCAs). The higher the osmolality, the greater the risk of anaphylactic reactions. These contrast agents can have an osmolality above 2000 mOsm/kg water, whereas normal serum or plasma osmolality is around 300 mOsm/kg water.

- In the water-soluble organic *nonionic* iodide contrast agent, the ionizing carboxyl group is replaced with a group such as amide or glucose that does not dissociate into ions, so the molecule remains whole, which means fewer reactions in the body. This lack of dissociation differentiates ionic from nonionic iodide contrast agents.
- When dissolved in water, a single nonionic compound forms, with each molecule containing three iodine atoms, for a ratio of 3:1 (3 iodine: 1 nondissociating molecule).
- Due to their nonionizing nature, these contrast media are referred to as *low-osmolality contrast agents* (LOCAs), and therefore they do not increase the osmolality of the blood plasma.

- The nonionic contrast agent is closer to being isotonic and is therefore better tolerated by the body, causing fewer anaphylactic reactions. The downside is that it is more viscous and more expensive to purchase.
- Intravascular contrast media molecules are also classified according to a second characteristic—monomer versus dimer.
  - Both ionic and nonionic contrast agents come in a monomer form (one benzene ring) and a dimer form (two benzene rings). The osmolality is reduced when there are more iodine molecules.
  - The ionic monomer has the highest osmolality, and the nonionic dimer has the lowest osmolality.
  - When low-osmolar agents or nonionic dimers are administered intravenously (IV), they cannot cross an intact blood–brain barrier. Instead, they are directly excreted via glomerular filtration through the kidneys, causing fewer side effects.[2] Fewer side effects mean greater patient comfort. In addition, these compounds also have a high contrast agent ratio (CAR), which, mean they have increased opacity without increasing the dose.
- See Table 23.2 and Fig. 23.2 for further comparisons among positive-contrast media used for radiographic imaging. Trade names and concentrations constantly change.

> ✎ **TECHNICIAN NOTES** The iodine contrast media currently on the market that are the safest and causes fewer side effects are the water-soluble organic nonionic dimers.

Physiological Effects of Intravenous Contrast Media

- Injecting a solution into the body with a higher osmolality than blood (hyperosmolar) will cause water to move into the vessels, both from the extravascular tissues and from the red blood cells. The red blood cells begin to shrink, or crenate. With crenation, circulating blood volume and peripheral blood flow increase; systemic vascular resistance and blood pressure decrease.
  - Peripheral vasodilation due to increased parasympathetic activity, produced by the injection of a contrast medium, is thought to be the primary cause of the accompanying pain, discomfort, and flushing.
- Many of the side effects of using ionic and nonionic contrast media have been alleviated with the introduction of the ionic and nonionic dimers, which have lowered the osmolality of contrast media to an almost isosmolar level. When an isotonic contrast agent is used, the discomfort and flushing are reduced. *Isotonic* means that the osmolalities or concentrations of the two fluids (contrast media and blood) are the same relative to each other.
- There are other factors to consider as well, such as viscosity and contrast agent ratio.
  - *Viscosity* refers to the resistance of fluid to flow. This influences the injectability or delivery of the contrast agent.
  - Nonionic dimers such as iodixanol (Visipaque) have the lowest osmolality but the highest viscosity of the water-soluble organic iodides due to their large molecular size. This means that the solution will pass slowly through the syringe. Warming the solution decreases the viscosity. The thinner the liquid, the lower the viscosity and cPs (water at 21°C [70°F] is about 1 cPs), whereas the cPs for a nonionic dimer is 27 at 20°C but 12 at body temperature (see Table 23.2).
  - In addition to osmolality and viscosity, iodinated contrast media can also be differentiated by the iodine to solute particle ratio, known as the contrast agent ratio (CAR). Contrast agent ratio = number of iodine atoms/number of particles in solution. Ionic monomers have a CAR of 1.5, whereas the CAR nonionic dimer is 6. The higher the ratio, the better the radiopacity without having to increase the dose[3] (see Table 23.2 and Fig. 23.2).

TABLE 23.2	Chemical Structure and Physiochemical Properties of Iodine-Based Contrast Agents[3]					
CHEMICAL STRUCTURE	**OSMOTIC CLASS**	**REPRESENTATIVE COMPOUNDS**	**CONCENTRATION**	**OSMOLALITY (MOSM/KG)**	**CONTRAST AGENT RATIO**	**VISCOSITY* (CPS AT 37°C/98°F)**
Ionic						
Monomer	High osmolality	Diatrizoate (Renografin, Hypaque), metrizoate (Isopaque), iothalamate (Conray), ioxithalamate (Telebrix)	~350–400	~2000	1.5	4
Dimer	Low osmolality	Ioxaglate (Hexabrix)	320	600	3	8
Nonionic						
Monomer	Low osmolality	Iohexol (Omnipaque), iopamidol (Isovue), ioversol (Optiray), iopromide (Ultravist)	240–350	600–850	3	5–10
Dimer	Iso-osmolality	Iodixanol (Visipaque)	270–320	290	6	12

*cPS, Centipoise is a unit to describe the viscosity of a solution.
Note: The listed trade names may not be available in all areas or after time of printing.

- The clearance or elimination of the molecules of injectable contrast media occurs primarily by glomerular filtration and renal clearance. The speed of elimination depends on the glomerular filtration rate, but virtually 100% of the contrast agent will be out of the body in 24 hours. None of the molecules are reabsorbed or secreted by the renal tubules.
- In the case of complete cessation of renal function, breakdown and elimination take place through the liver and gut at a much slower rate. The thyroid and liver retain about 1.5% of the contrast media, which can result in elevation of blood values after a procedure.
- Nuclear medicine scans of the thyroid should not be attempted after a contrast medium injection because the results will be inaccurate.

Negative-Contrast Media

- Negative-contrast media are the low–atomic number or low-density agents such as air, nitrous oxide, oxygen, and carbon dioxide. These substances absorb fewer x-rays than soft tissue and appear dark or radiolucent on the radiograph. This effect enhances the contrast between the soft tissues. There is less mucosal detail with the use of negative-contrast than with positive-contrast media, but double-contrast media does assist in mucosal detail.
- Oxygen and carbon dioxide are more soluble than water. Be careful not to overinflate organs such as the bladder, especially if using room air, because air embolism leading to cardiac arrest can result if an organ ruptures or if there are ulcerative lesions.[2,3] Symptoms will develop immediately, and severity depends on volume and extent of embolism.
- If any unexplained symptoms are noted, place the patient in left lateral recumbency and elevate the caudal portion of the body immediately to trap the gas in the right ventricle. Further treatments will likely be required.

Double-Contrast Procedures

- Double-contrast procedures employ both positive-contrast and negative-contrast agents to image an organ, commonly the urinary bladder, stomach, or colon. To avoid air bubbles in an organ such as the bladder, which can be misinterpreted as lesions, the negative-contrast medium is generally administered first, followed by the positive-contrast agent.

Gastrointestinal Tract Studies

Patient and Other Preparation

1. Patient preparation is essential.
2. Actual preparation does vary slightly according to the procedure, but generally the area that is being radiographed should not have any radiodense artifacts, such as food, bowel contents, and gas that could be misdiagnosed as lesions or abnormalities.
   a. The patient should be fasted so that the GI tract is emptied.

b. A cathartic or enema should be administered in a timely manner to minimize gas production.
3. Make sure the hair coat is clean and dry, with no mats.
4. If transit time for the contrast agent through the GI tract is of concern, sedation or anesthetics may change the outcome. Anticholinergics such as atropine slow down the GI tract.
5. Survey images are required before giving contrast media to validate the procedure and determine proper radiation techniques.
6. Along with proper preparation of the patient, it is important to give the correct amount of contrast medium to properly coat or distend the organ.
7. It is essential to take enough images in the proper sequence. Imagine judging a book by reading the front and back covers and perhaps a few pages in the middle. For accurate diagnosis of the stomach, all four views (ventrodorsal [VD], dorsoventral [DV], and right and left lateral views) should be imaged. Depending on the study, oblique views or abdominal compression may be required. The views must be properly positioned and centered, and must include the appropriate landmarks. See Chapter 16 to review the positions of the abdomen and common anatomy.

Indications for Gastrointestinal Studies

Special studies of the GI tract are usually completed when there are concerns about vomiting, diarrhea, constipation, hematochezia, melena, abdominal mass, abdominal pain, foreign bodies, or postabdominal trauma. In the study, the barium is administered, and the GI tract is generally evaluated for morphological changes, blockages, and functional changes such as the rate of gastric emptying or small bowel transit time.

Contraindications

Special studies should not be completed if the patient has a fluid-filled distended esophagus (Fig. 23.3A) or stomach, or

FIG. 23.3 Lateral Thorax Showing Megaesophagus. If megaesophagus is to be evaluated, the esophagus should be emptied before administration of a contrast agent. (Courtesy Mount Pleasant Veterinary Hospital, Toronto, ON.)

FIG. 23.4 Gastric Torsion. Note the characteristic double bubble. **A,** Right lateral abdomen. **B,** Ventrodorsal abdomen. (Courtesy Secord Animal Hospital, Toronto, ON.)

if the bowel is atonic. Patients with ileus due to torsion (Fig. 23.4) or other conditions are not good candidates.

Contrast Agents

- Barium sulfate suspension does settle upon standing, so shake before using. Barium is not sterilely produced, and once the container is open, there is a possibility for contamination to occur. Any equipment that is reused, such as a reservoir-type container, enema tube, or syringes, must be thoroughly cleaned and sterilized before use.
- Barium sulfate is not hypertonic and does not increase the intraluminal fluid.
- A disadvantage is the slow transit time through the small bowel. Chilling the barium sulfate for an upper gastrointestinal (UGI) study does speed up the transit time; however, for a lower gastrointestinal (LGI) study, it is more comfortable for the patient if barium temperature is between room and body temperature.
- If there is a perforation of the bowel, a combination of diatrizoate meglumine and diatrizoate sodium (Gastrografin) iodinated water-soluble organic iodine can be used. The hyperosmolality of the solution and the resulting complications that could arise with use in dehydrated patients or those with severe electrolyte imbalance need to be considered. Safer yet are the more isosmolar nonionic compounds which draw less fluid into the bowel with minimal dilution of the contrast agents, but the high

cost of nonionic compounds limits their use to mostly small patients.

> **TECHNICIAN NOTES**
> - To decrease the viscosity of organic nonionic dimer iodine solutions such as iodixanol, warm the solution before use.
> - Chill barium to quicken the transit time in UGI studies.
> - For LGI studies, have the solution at room to body temperature for patient comfort.

Esophagram

Contrast radiography of the esophagus, or esophagography, is best used to evaluate morphological or structural alterations of the esophagus and is often needed to accurately identify lesions or further characterize survey radiographic findings (Box 23.1 and eFig. 23.1). Dynamic imaging such as fluoroscopy is recommended for specific evaluation of functional abnormalities (Fig. 23.5). The esophagus is best evaluated on a lateral image of the neck and on lateral and DV views of the thorax.

> **TECHNICIAN NOTES** To convert kg to lb, multiply by 2.2; thus 10 kg is basically 22 lb. To convert lb to kg, divide by 2.2; thus 88 lb would be 40 kg.

BOX 23.1 | Esophagram Contrast Study Procedure

Indications

- Dysphagia, regurgitation of undigested food, acute gagging or retching, excessive salivation, megaesophagus (see Fig. 23.3), abnormal swallowing, esophageal dysfunction, and foreign bodies are all indications for esophagography.
- The double-contrast study evaluates morphological abnormalities such as mucosal abnormalities, intraluminal foreign bodies, and partial strictures or stenosis.

Precautions or Contraindications

- Patients with dysphagia may aspirate the contrast agent.
- It may not be necessary to add contrast media to a dilated, fluid-filled, or food-filled esophagus as there may be sufficient visualization of lesions or abnormalities.
- If asphyxiation is a concern, barium sulfate paste should not be used.
  - Consider the use of organic iodine preparation in cases of perforation.
  - Do not use if there is a known allergy or sensitivity to contrast agents.

Contrast Media and Dosage

- The dosage is 5–20 mL 60% weight/volume (w/v) barium sulfate suspension liquid or paste (preferred), depending on the size of the patient, to induce several swallows.[3]
- A barium meal can be used by mixing 1 cup dry kibble with 20 mL barium sulfate suspension for dog and half of each for cats.[3]
- For oral aqueous iodine solution (Gastrografin): mix 1:2 and give 5–15 mL, depending on the patient's size.

Equipment and Supplies

- Large-dose syringe
- Optional—canned food or kibble

Patient Preparation

- Remove collar; clean hair coat.
- Fast if further GI studies are to be completed.

Positions

- Generally lateral, pulling downward limb more cranial and upper limb caudal (minimize brachium musculature over thoracic inlet).
- VD or VD oblique optional.

Borders

- Full length of esophagus: atlantooccipital junction (oropharynx) to T12 (cranial portion of stomach).

Procedure for Positive-Contrast Esophagram

1. Expose survey images—lateral and VD.
2. Position the patient in lateral recumbency on the x-ray table.
3. Place paper towels on tabletop or towels around the patient's mouth and neck.
4. Slowly infuse the barium into the buccal pouch. Close the mouth and wait for the patient to swallow.
5. Take serial images of the patient in lateral recumbency—the right is usually easier for the positioner.
6. Administer additional barium or barium-soaked kibble in the buccal pouch. Close the mouth and wait for the patient to swallow.
7. Obtain further lateral images if required, or place the patient in ventral recumbency for VD or oblique views as required. The oblique projections avoid superimposition of the esophagus over the spine (see Chapter 16 for positioning).
8. If a lesion has been noted by esophagoscope or with the passage of a tube, a partial esophagram can be made. Gently pass the tube until the point of the abnormality, and administer barium sulfate at the site.

Procedure for Double-Contrast Study Esophagram

1. Obtain survey images and perform an esophageal study using liquid barium suspension as described previously.
2. Pass a stomach tube through an oral speculum if required. Avoid forcing the tube through partial obstructions.
3. Take a lateral image to confirm the placement of the tube in case the tip of the tube needs to be readjusted for study of a specific portion of the esophagus.
4. Attach a syringe and inject barium sulfate, 3–5 mL for a small dog or cat and 8–10 mL for a large dog.
5. Keeping the patient in lateral recumbency, attach an air syringe and inject 20–30 mL of air for a small dog or cat and 40–50 mL of air for a large dog.
6. Immediately image the dorsal thorax.
7. Reposition the patient in sternal recumbency. Repeat the air injection and image immediately.

Comments and Tips

- Avoid getting contrast medium on the patient, image receptor, and table, as artifacts may interfere with the diagnosis.
- Iodine should be used if endoscopy is to follow, because barium will obscure the mucosa.
- The patient is usually sedated or anesthetized for the double-contrast study.
- Esophagram is usually completed after gastrography, when the stomach tube is retracted to the esophagus.
- If there is gastroesophageal reflux, further barium sulfate suspension is not needed. Administer only the air.
- A very small amount of aspirated barium sulfate is generally well tolerated in healthy lungs and cleared from the airways within 24 hours.[3]
- Oropharyngeal issues are best evaluated in the midst of a swallow and during a pause after completion of the swallow.
- Oblique views may eliminate superimposition of the spine and sternum for better visualization of the esophagus.

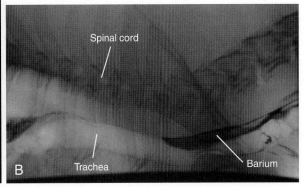

FIG 23.5 A, Fluoroscopy in right lateral recumbency without any contrast study. Note that the trachea is white and the bones are dark. **B,** Fluoroscopy of the esophagus in right lateral recumbency with barium. (Ontario Veterinary College, University of Guelph, ON.)

✎ TECHNICIAN NOTES To calculate dilution, use either ratio and proportion, proportional sets, or a fraction method.

For example: You need to use 120 mL of a final dilution of 20% barium. The initial barium sulfate comes as a 60% concentrated solution. How much of the concentrated barium will you use, and how much diluent will you need?

1) Ratio and proportion method:
   Final diluted percentage: Initial concentration = volume needed: Final volume administered
   20%:60% = ×:120 mL

2) Proportional sets $C_1 \times V_1 = C_2 \times V_2$

   Concentration$_1$ (start) × Volume$_1$ (start) = Concentration$_2$ (final) × Volume$_2$ (final)
   60% × X mL = 20% × 120 mL

3) Fraction method:

$$\frac{\text{Final diluted percentage}}{\text{Initial concentration}} = \frac{\text{Volume needed}}{\text{Final volume administered}}$$

$$\frac{20\%}{60\%} = \frac{X}{120 \text{ mL}}$$

For dilution of contrast medium, saline is best, especially for barium studies.

In all cases, now continue as:

$$(20)(120) = X(60)$$
$$60X = 2400$$
$$X = 40 \text{ mL of the concentrated barium needed}$$

If 120 mL total volume is required and you will use 40 mL of the 60% solution, this means you need 80 mL of diluent (120 mL − 40 mL = 80 mL). Saline is the best diluent for barium.

Upper Gastrointestinal Study

- Contrast medium is administered orally. Then images are taken during the transit of the contrast medium through the stomach, small bowel, and colon as required.
- See Box 23.2 and Table 23.3 for the full procedure, although actual timing and centering depend on the patient's condition.
- Morphological studies of the stomach and intestines are made to examine (1) the size, shape, and position of the organs; (2) the character of the stomach wall and the stomach contents; or (3) extramural, mural, or intramural lesions of the GI tract. Gastric motility and pyloric and intestinal function can be determined by noting gastric and intestinal emptying, keeping in mind that the times vary, depending on the size and nature of the test meal. Functional studies are performed slightly differently from morphological ones. Sedation or anesthesia affects transit time in functional studies.
- Barium food mixture studies have also been completed to further evaluate gastric function. There appears to be evidence that there is a wide range of normal gastric emptying times. Unless there are gross abnormalities, a barium solid food meal is not useful. Barium-impregnated polyethylene spheres (BIPS, Chemstock Animal Health Ltd., Christchurch, New Zealand) have been used as an alternative to evaluate the emptying of solids in dogs and cats (see Fig. 23.1E), but their usefulness is limited.
- Endoscopy is an alternative modality that can be used, although it is difficult to adequately access the mesenteric small intestine with the endoscope. Ultrasonography can often provide small bowel diagnostic information, negating the need for a contrast radiographic study.

BOX 23.2 | Upper Gastrointestinal Study Procedures[2,3]

Indications
- Recurrent unresponsive vomiting, diarrhea, hematemesis, anorexia, melena, mass lesions, suspected foreign body or obstruction, wall distortions, wall lesions, abdominal organ displacement, chronic weight loss, persistent abdominal pain, and inconclusive results on a survey radiograph.[2,3]

Precautions or Contraindications
- If rupture or perforation is suspected, use water-soluble organic iodides. In dehydrated patients, avoid the use of such agents.
- Endoscopy or ultrasonography should be considered if available or feasible, especially in compromised patients. Avoid barium if endoscopy or surgery is anticipated.
- Delay the study if the stomach is filled with ingesta.
- The use of barium in gastric dilatation/volvulus, chronic obstructive bowel disease, and paralytic ileus cases is complicating (see Fig. 23.4).
- Gastric distention is not recommended immediately after gastric surgery or deep biopsy.
- Prior use of tranquilizers or other drugs affects the transit time.
  - Avoid parasympatholytic agents and drugs used for treatment in gastrointestinal disorders, which may cause gaseous distention or decrease motility before the contrast study.
  - Use of anticholinergics should be suspended at least 24 hours but preferably 48–72 hours before the administration of contrast media.[3]

Contrast Media and Dosage
- Barium sulfate suspension, 60%: dosages vary depending on source. The following tends to be common[2,3]:
  - 8–10 mL/kg for dogs less than 10 kg and cats
  - 5–7 mL/kg for medium-sized dogs, 10–40 kg
  - 3–5 mL/kg for dogs heavier than 40 kg
- Iodine (less than 300 mg/mL)[2]:
  - Dogs 2.0–3.0 mL/kg
  - Cats 1.0–2.0 mL/kg
- For double-contrast or negative-contrast study:
  - 20 mL/kg via orogastric tube[2]
- Effervescent granules (Baros, E-Z-Gas II)

Equipment/Supplies
- Gastric tube
- Oral speculum
- 50-mL syringe
- Towels

Patient Preparation
- The gastrointestinal tract should be empty so there is no interference with interpretation of transit time.
  - Ingesta may obscure foreign bodies or small gastric and intestinal lesions.
  - Fast at least 12 hours before administration of the contrast media unless the patient is anorectic or vomiting.
  - Twenty-four-hour fasting is best if mucosal disease of the small intestine is being evaluated.
- Take lateral and VD images before the administration of an enema.

- If an enema is required, as indicated by the survey image, administer at least 2–4 hours before the procedure to minimize gas artifacts.
- If the patient has severe abdominal stress, fasting, enemas, or laxatives are not suggested.
- Perform without sedation, if possible, as motility-altering drugs may affect interpretation.
  - If sedation is required, consider acepromazine in dogs and ketamine/diazepam in cats.[3]

Measure, Center, and Peripheral Borders
- Measure at the thickest part (liver) at the thoracolumbar (TL) junction.
- Center over caudal aspect of 13th rib at level of L2–L3 or over umbilicus for the canine and two to three finger widths caudal to 13th rib for the feline.
- Include about an inch cranial to xiphoid and caudally to the acetabulum.
  - For gastrography and cranial abdomen, just include to L5–L6 distally.

Procedure for Positive-Contrast Upper Gastrointestinal Study (Figs. 23.6 and 23.7)
1. Using either the buccal pouch and syringe or a gastric tube, administer barium sulfate.
   a. An orogastric tube is preferred, with the patient lying on the x-ray table ready for exposure (especially for gastrogram).
2. If completing a gastrogram, immediately take four images centering over the cranial abdomen: ventrodorsal, right and left lateral, and dorsoventral views.
3. Fifteen minutes after administration: ventrodorsal and right lateral views.
4. Thirty minutes after administration: ventrodorsal and right lateral views.
5. Sixty minutes after administration: ventrodorsal and right lateral views.
6. Hourly after administration: ventrodorsal and right lateral views until the study is completed (see Fig. 23.8 for feline images and eFigs. 23.2 to 23.9 for further canine images demonstrating 15 minutes to 6.5 hours post administration of barium).
7. See Table 23.3 for barium GI times.

Comments and Tips
- A gastrogram may not be required, or the 15-minute images may be eliminated in dogs, depending on the nature of the study, but are highly recommended in cats because of the rapid GI transit time. An extra image at 90 minutes may also reveal further information for the cat.
- If gastric and intestinal emptying time is of concern, perform the study early enough in the day to be able to properly complete the procedure.
- It is important to give sufficient volume of barium sulfate suspension to optimally distend the stomach, and in as much of a bolus as possible. An orogastric tube minimizes barium leaving the stomach before all the agent is administered.

BOX 23.2	Upper Gastrointestinal Study Procedures[2,3]

- The gastrogram is finished when the majority of the barium is no longer visible in the stomach, whereas a small bowel study ends when there is little evidence of barium left in the small intestine. The rugal folds are best seen on gastric emptying.
- If the pylorus is of interest, oblique views may be required.

Procedure for Double-Contrast Upper Gastrointestinal Study

1. Double-contrast imaging may provide further information primarily for the stomach wall and further visualization of extramural lesion, as well as mural and intraluminal gastric lesions. A double-contrast study does not evaluate motility or emptying.
2. It should not be performed if the patient is not fasted.
3. The patient is best chemically restrained.
4. Complete a routine noncontrast survey.
5. Administer barium sulfate using a gastric tube.
   a. For small dogs, use 2 mL/kg; large dogs 1 mL/kg, and cats 6 mL/kg.[3]
6. Attach an air-filled syringe, and administer air until the stomach is distended.
7. Withdraw the tip of the tube into the caudal esophagus or remove completely.
8. Gently rotate the patient to coat the gastric mucosa.
9. Immediately take required views of the stomach: right and left laterals, ventrodorsal, and dorsoventral if gastrogram is desired; otherwise, a right lateral and VD.
10. Center the beam over the cranial abdomen. (Fig. 23.9)

11. Administer further negative-contrast medium if air has been lost by regurgitation or has passed into the small bowel, and repeat the images.

Comments and Tips

- It is difficult to determine the exact dosage. Judge the amount required by noting the resistance to injection of air as well as palpating for the distended stomach. Make sure stomach is distended so that the gastric wall will appear thin and uniform, but be careful.
- Negative-contrast gastrography or a pneumogastrogram can be substituted for a positive-contrast study or a double-contrast study.
  - Follow the same procedure as for the double-contrast study, omitting the barium sulfate.
- If required, the study can be continued as a double-contrast or negative-contrast morphological study of the small intestine:
  - Take lateral and ventrodorsal images at 15 minutes, 30 minutes, 60 minutes, and hourly as required.
- If inserting a gastric tube is not practical, carbon dioxide–producing granules or spansules that cause effervescence, such as Baros or E-Z-Gas II, can be substituted for the air in both the double-contrast and negative-contrast studies.
  - Place the granules/spansules in the patient's buccal pouch and close the mouth to prevent foam from dissipating before it reaches the stomach.
  - Radiograph immediately because the gas produced may be belched.[2,3]

TABLE 23.3	Upper Gastrointestinal Tract Positive-Contrast Film Sequence and Typical Structures in Normal Canine and Feline[2,3]	
BARIUM	**IONIC AND NONIONIC ORGANIC IODINE**	**STRUCTURES TYPICALLY OPACIFIED IN NORMAL ANIMALS***
Dog		
Immediate	Immediate	Stomach
15 minutes		Stomach begins to empty, duodenum fills
30 minutes	15 minutes	Stomach small amount, duodenum, jejunum
1 hour		Stomach vestigial, duodenum, jejunum filled and reaches ileum
1.5–2 hours	30 minutes	Stomach mostly empty, complete small intestine, ileocecal junction
4 hours	1 hour	Small and large intestine
1–4 hours		Stomach empty
3–5 hours		Small intestines empty
Cat		
Immediate	Immediate	Stomach
5–10 minutes	5 minutes	Stomach empties, duodenum fills
15–20 min		Reach jejunum
30–60 minutes	30–60 minutes	Complete small intestine, cecum fills
1 hour	1 hour	Small and large intestine
30–60 minutes		Stomach empty
1–3 hours		Small intestines empty

*Individual transit times vary greatly based on various factors. Times are approximations only.

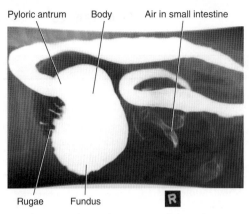

Pyloric antrum　Body　Air in small intestine

Rugae　Fundus

R

FIG. 23.6 An upper gastrointestinal image taken within minutes of the administration of barium. This is an inverted fluoroscopic image. (Courtesy Ontario Veterinary College, University of Guelph, ON.)

↓ Left lateral　　↓ Right lateral　　↓ Ventrodorsal　　↓ Dorsoventral
Immediately post oral barium sulfate suspension administration

15 min post oral contrast administration

60 min post oral contrast administration

FIG 23.7 Positive-Contrast Barium Gastrography in a Dog in Different Positions and with Various Time Delays After Contrast Medium Administration. Immediately (A–D), 15 minutes (E–H), and 60 minutes (I–L) after contrast medium administration. Continuous emptying of the stomach is noted with increasing time after contrast medium administration. **A, E, I,** Left lateral views. Most of the contrast medium is initially present in the gastric body and fundus. A small amount of gas is noted in the pylorus in the initial images, which is increasing 15 minutes after contrast medium administration and decreasing at 60 minutes with continuous emptying of the stomach. The pylorus is in part located cranial to the body of the stomach. **B, F, J,** Right lateral views. In the immediate image, the entire stomach is filled with contrast medium. In later images, gas is present in the fundus of the stomach and fluid is predominantly present in the pylorus. The pylorus is summating ventrally with the body of the stomach. **C, G, F,** Ventrodorsal views. Most of the contrast medium in the stomach is in the fundus. A gas bubble is present in the body of the stomach. **D, H, L,** Dorsoventral views. Most of the contrast medium is in the body to pylorus of the stomach. Gas is present in the fundus of the stomach. (From Thrall DE. *Textbook of Veterinary Diagnostic Radiology.* 7th ed. St. Louis: Elsevier; 2018.)

FIG. 23.8 Normal Feline Upper Gastrointestinal Series. Note the "string-of-pearls" appearance of the duodenum, which is not uncommon in cats. **A** and **B,** Lateral views made 15 minutes after barium administration. **C** and **D,** Ventrodorsal views made 3 hours after barium administration. (From Han C, Hurd C. *Practical Diagnostic Imaging for the Veterinary Technician.* 3rd ed. St Louis: Mosby; 2005.)

FIG. 23.9 Double-Contrast Gastrogram. **A,** Lateral view. **B,** Ventrodorsal view.

✎ **TECHNICIAN NOTES**

- In order for the barium study to be diagnostic, give the complete volume to properly distend the lumen.
- To minimize artifacts, always make sure that the patient has a clean, dry hair coat, with no traces of contrast medium. Remove the collar if cranial body radiographic views are to be taken.
- Before administering the barium, have everything ready, such as the image receptors in position, technique set, protective gear, patient near the table, etc. Make sure to minimize barium spillage, and thus artifacts, if administering the barium with the patient on the table.
- To avoid technical errors, make sure you take survey images, properly prepare the patient, use the correct exposures, center the beam correctly, place the tube in the stomach, use the correct volume, and take the required number and proper sequence of images.
- When using an orogastric tube, always verify correct placement in the esophagus prior to administration. Before removing the tube, clear it with a small amount of air, and kink the tube to minimize aspiration into the lungs.
- The UGI is complete when the barium is in the colon.

Lower Gastrointestinal Study

- This procedure is less common due to other modalities such as endoscopy in addition to the low yield of diagnostic information with contrast enema (Box 23.3). The radiographic examination of the cecum, colon, and rectum through retrograde administration of contrast medium generally evaluates extramural masses, mural or larger mucosal lesions, and intraluminal lesions. Smaller mucosal lesions are better determined endoscopically. Disease in the area of the ileocolic valves and the ascending and transverse processes is better examined with contrast studies.[3]
- For visualization of the entire large bowel and small lesions such as mucosal irregularities, full distention of the area and removal of feces are required. Oral administration of a positive-contrast medium does not fully distend the large bowel, so rectal administration of contrast media is required for certain procedures. Chemical restraint is usually needed, as many patients will not otherwise tolerate rectal infusion.

Use of Barium-Impregnated Polyethylene Spheres

- Barium-impregnated polyethylene spheres (BIPS) are inert, low-density, radiopaque spheres designed for evaluation of gastric dysmotility and intestinal transit time in dogs and cats (Box 23.4). The spheres are a mixture of plastic and barium sulfate and come in two diameters: 5-mm spheres to evaluate partial and complete obstruction and 1.5-mm spheres meant to mimic food passage. The number and size of the spheres, fasting period, and type and amount of food will affect the gastric emptying time and orocolic transit. Strict adherence to the manufacturer's suggestions should be followed for a proper functional study. See advantages and disadvantages in comparison with barium suspension in Table 23.1.

BOX 23.3 | Lower Gastrointestinal Study Procedures[2,3]

Indications

- Abnormal defecation, especially in combination with excessive mucus or bright red stool, stricture, tenesmus, colonic obstruction, dyschezia, colonic or rectal neoplasia, colitis, and ileocolic intussusception are all indications to complete a barium enema study (Fig. 23.10).
- The barium enema is especially indicated when narrowing of the lumen prevents passage of an endoscope, a mural or extramural lesion is suspected, or the mucus is found to be normal endoscopically.

Precautions

- Transient spasm may occur if the agent is cold, the wall is irritated by the tube, or narcotic premedication is used.
- Do not complete a retrograde administration or barium enema if perforation or a known allergy is suspected. Barium enemas are not recommended if the patient has had proctoscopy within 12 hours due to a possible weakened wall.
- Reflux into the distal small bowel may occur without overdistention.

Contrast Media and Dosage

- 20% barium sulfate brought between room and body temperature.

- Approximate dosage to fill the large intestine administered rectally[2]:
  - 10–20 mL total in a small dog or cat; 30 mL in medium-sized dogs (10–40 kg); 60 mL for dogs heavier than 40 kg. (Another source quotes 7–15 mL/kg.[3])
  - Use half the dosage to evaluate the rectum or to partially fill the colon.
- Dosage for double-contrast technique:
  - Dog: 5–10 mL of barium sulfate and 50–200 mL of air.
  - Cat: 2–3 mL of barium sulfate suspension and 25–50 mL of air.
- Dosage for negative-contrast technique:
  - Dog: 60–100 mL of air; cat: 20–30 mL of air.

Equipment/Supplies

- Bardex or Foley catheter for the inflatable cuff
- Syringe/enema bag/can/commercial enema set
- Three-way stopcock valve
- Lubricant
- Compression paddle

Patient Preparation

- The colon should be absent of fecal material if mucosal disease is being studied.
  - No food for 24–36 hours.

BOX 23.3 Lower Gastrointestinal Study Procedures—cont'd

- Water up to 4 hours before the procedure, but make sure the patient is properly hydrated.
- Administer both cathartic and warm-water enemas the previous evening if the disease process has not emptied the gastrointestinal tract. Consider using a low nonsoap enema to stimulate defecation if stool is present. Just before the study, confirm with a warm-water enema that the effluent is clear. Unlike for endoscopy, the colon does not need to be washed clean, but any feces or ingesta in the colon could create confusing artifacts.
- Take survey lateral and VD images of the abdomen if not done previously. This is best completed 2–4 hours before the procedure.
- Sedate or anesthetize the patient.
- For patients with acute abdominal pain, acute persistent vomiting, or palpable, enlarged, fluid- or gas-filled bowels, no preparation is needed. The gas or fluid may be helpful in diagnosis.
- Endoscopy will likely be more diagnostic than radiographic contrast for this study.

Measure, Center, and Include
- Measure, center, and include as for the small intestinal study.

Procedure for Positive Contrast Barium Enema for Both Dogs and Cats
1. Place the sedated or anesthetized patient on the table.
2. Insert the Foley catheter rectally and inflate the cuff to prevent leakage.
3. Keep the reservoir bag slightly above the tabletop to maximize gravity or use minimum pressure with a syringe.
4. Clamp the tube, stopping the infusion if there is resistance to the flow of the contrast agent.
5. Close off the three-way stopcock.
6. Take ventrodorsal and both right and left lateral images.
7. Oblique views may be required, especially in males (see Chapter 16 for technique).
8. Examine the images, and if no additional contrast agent or images are required, remove as much of the contrast medium as possible before removal of the catheter.
   a. Placing the patient in left lateral recumbency, raising the cranial part of the body, and allowing the barium to drain into the bag placed on the floor, may assist in barium removal.
9. Further images may be obtained if desired once the barium is removed.

Comments and Tips
- The catheter should be removed from the rectum away from the x-ray table, preferably above a container near a floor drain.
- Compression of the large bowel may further show the presence of a lesion.

- It is best to give small increments of the barium until the desired effect is seen on the images.
- Soapy water enemas too close to time of imaging could irritate the large bowel mucosa, leading to spasms or gas accumulations that could cause radiographic artifacts during a barium enema study.

Procedure for Double-Contrast Large Intestinal Study for Both Dogs and Cats
1. Place the sedated or anesthetized patient on the table.
2. Insert the rectal catheter and inflate the cuff to prevent leakage. Place a three-way stopcock valve at the end of the catheter.
3. Infuse the barium sulfate suspension (2–10 mL; see dosages listed earlier) through the three-way stopcock valve and close the valve.
4. Open the valve, infuse the air, and close the valve.
5. Take ventrodorsal and right and left lateral images.
6. View the images and determine whether additional contrast agents or images are required.
7. Release the stopcock valve. Gently remove as much air and barium as possible before removing the catheter.
   a. Place the patient in left lateral recumbency to minimize effects of air embolism.
   b. Gentle massage of abdomen with catheter in place may aid in removing air from colon.
8. Further images may be obtained if desired once the barium is removed.

Comments and Tips
- Move the patient to an appropriate location to defecate.
- The amount of air infused can be decreased if distention is not required.

Pneumocolon
- This large intestine negative-contrast study can be used if the colon is not emptied.
- The same procedure is followed as for the double-contrast large intestinal study without barium sulfate.
- Infuse 20–100 mL of air according to the weight of the patient as previously outlined.

Double-Contrast Technique of Ileocecum in Connection With UGI
1. Indicated if the patient is unable to tolerate a conventional barium enema study or if a view of the ileocecal region is required.
2. When the swallowed barium reaches the right ileocolic junction, insufflate the calculated amount of air through a small rectal catheter.
3. Inflate the cuff and use a three-way stopcock valve to infuse the air so it remains in the colon.
4. Take the images, open the stopcock valve and remove the catheter.
5. Continue the study if required.

FIG. 23.10 Barium Enema. **A,** Lateral view. **B,** Ventrodorsal view.

BOX 23.4	Use of BIPS[3,5]

Dosage

- The inert spheres are available in capsules of two sizes that can be purchased as 5- or 10-dose packs (contains 10 large spheres and 30 small spheres).
- Give either 1 large orange capsule or 4 small blue capsules (see Fig. 23.1E).

Patient Preparation

- Do not feed if gastrointestinal obstruction is suspected or there are acute gastrointestinal concerns.
- For chronic gastric emptying or orocolic transit problems, feed with an intestinal diet following the BIPS package insert.
- Sedatives and drugs influence gastrointestinal motility.

Procedure for Use of BIPS

1. Obtain a right lateral and ventrodorsal simultaneously at each time period, using proper positioning techniques for the full abdomen.
2. To rule out pyloric and small intestinal blockage, give the capsules on an empty stomach. Image generally from 6–24 hours after administration, noting the time taken (Fig. 23.11).
3. To detect delayed gastric emptying or if there is chronic vomiting or diarrhea, administer the capsules with food and image about 8 hours later.
4. It is essential to note on the image the actual time elapsed post administration of the spheres so the reference can be properly consulted.
5. If gastric dumping is suspected, take one set of images within 1–2 hours after BIPS administration.[5]
6. Continue the study until the BIPS are in the colon.
7. Large bowel transit can be assessed:
   a. An enema or cathartic should be given to remove the retained feces.
   b. Give the BIPS with recommended diet, and radiograph at 24, 48, and 72 hours.

Comments and Tips

- A separate reference interval for gastric transit if acetylpromazine is administered is provided. Check the reference intervals to make sure to follow the time suggestions.[5]
- The gastric emptying rate and orocolic transit rate are determined by applying a formula separately to the large and small spheres (see Technician Note).
- Generally, small BIPS are used to determine the gastric emptying for motility disorders, as they more closely mimic food.
- The gastric emptying rate of the large BIPS is best considered for partial obstructions of the pylorus or intestine.[5]
- Compare the results based on the size of the sphere, whether food is given, or the type of food eaten, with a standardized chart indicating average and mean emptying rate/transit times probable at that time after administration.
- Times are quicker if the capsules are given without food.
- The total number seen on the image will be a maximum of 10 large or 30 small spheres.
- If the location of a sphere cannot be accurately determined, it is not included in the formula calculation.
- If obstruction is noted, it is not necessary to calculate the formula, as the large spheres are trapped at the orad aspect of an obstructing lesion, giving the appearance of dumping.
- Both views are required to determine exactly where the spheres are located. In the VD view, parts of the large intestine are superimposed over the cardia of the stomach, just caudal to the left crus of the diaphragm in some animals, whereas in the lateral views, BIPS in the transverse colon can be mistaken as being bunched in the small intestine.
- Because of the limited use of BIPS, the procedure is not common.

FIG. 23.11 A, Ventrodorsal abdomen 4 hours after administration of barium-impregnated polyethylene spheres (BIPS). All of the small BIPS have left the stomach, but the majority of large BIPS are still present. **B,** Right lateral abdomen BIPS study 4 hours after administration. None of the BIPS are in the colon, so the orocolic rate is 0% for both the small and large BIPS. Both views are required to determine the actual location of the BIPS.

TECHNICIAN NOTES

Formula for gastric emptying with use of BIPS:
1. Count the number of BIPS that have left the stomach.
2. Calculate as follows:

$$\frac{\text{Number of BIPS that have left stomach}}{\text{Total number of BIPS seen on image}} \times 100 = \text{\% of BIPS that have left stomach}$$

Formula for orocolic transit rate:
1. Count the number of BIPS that are in the colon and calculate as follows:

$$\frac{\text{Number of BIPS in colon}}{\text{Total number of BIPS seen on radiograph}} \times 100 = \text{\% of BIPS in the colon}$$

Normal Radiographic Anatomical Considerations of the Gastrointestinal Tract

- Please review the anatomy in Chapter 16 and Appendix A on the Evolve website to view what is generally visualized on a survey image as well as normal canine and feline stomach diagram. Table 16.1, Figs. 16.3, 16.5, 16.6, 16.9, and 16.10 give an overview of the anatomy in the various positions. Figs. 16.10, 16.11, and 23.7 shows normal variations in fluid and gas distribution depending on patient position. Box 23.1 indicates the image sequence for the positive-contrast UGI study. See the table in the Technician Notes box for a simplified version of where gas and fluid can be found as the position of the patient changes.
  - The rugal folds are best seen at the periphery as the stomach begins to empty (see Fig. 23.7 and eFigs. 23.6 to 23.9). They are also more evident with negative contrast, but if the stomach is too distended in a double-contrast study, the folds may disappear.
- The gastric emptying time of normal animals varies greatly. Factors such as the effect of medication and the type or volume of meal given also alter times. Low dosages of barium may delay emptying and transit time because the stomach empties more slowly when there is less volume in it. Delay may also occur in nervous animals or in a stressful environment.
- Delayed gastric or intestinal emptying can be evaluated by means of a simple or double-contrast radiographic study, BIPS, scintigraphy, ultrasonography, or endoscopy. In some cases, gastric outflow obstruction may be documented only with food or with BIPS. Scintigraphy using a radioactive meal is the ideal modality to study gastric emptying because it is very close to natural conditions and gives a quantitative index.[2,3] Scintigraphic evaluation of gastric emptying can be completed in 4 to 5 hours and is more consistent than gastric emptying times as measured by BIPS.[3] Magnetic resonance imaging (MRI) has not yet been applied for assessment of gastric emptying in small animals. Ultrasonography for determining gastric emptying can be subjective. Further methods are not practical outside the laboratory.[3]
- In about a third of cats, the duodenum has a "string-of-pearls" appearance during a positive-contrast study (see Fig. 23.8). This is due to the peristaltic contractions.[3]
- The cecum in a cat appears pointed, whereas in a dog it has a corkscrew appearance. On VD or DV views, the cecum appears just to the right of midline in both species.

🖉 **TECHNICIAN NOTES** The following box summarizes how positioning with the use of a vertical beam affects the distribution of gas and liquid[3]:

View	Location of Gas	Location of Fluid
Dorsoventral	Fundus	Body/pylorus
Ventrodorsal	Body (± pylorus)	Fundus
Left lateral	Pylorus (± body)	Fundus
Right lateral	Fundus dorsal body	Pylorus

- Upon removal of the positive-contrast medium, longitudinal folds of the colon are visible that are made more detailed with the infusion of air. The VD or DV view of the colon shows a question-mark configuration.

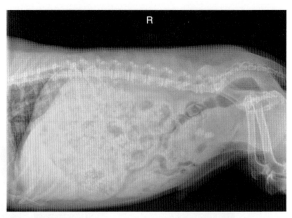

FIG. 23.13 Lateral Survey of the Abdomen of a Diabetic Patient. Positive-contrast studies would hide the presence of bladder stones. (Courtesy Secord Animal Hospital Toronto, ON.)

Contrast Studies of the Urinary System

Contrast studies of the urinary system evaluate the kidneys, urinary bladder, ureters, prostate gland, and urethra. Survey images of the kidneys may provide external anatomical information such as size, shape, and radiographic opacity if existing radiographic contrast is adequate. However, when kidneys cannot be assessed by survey images or when qualitative functional urography is needed, excretory urography or ultrasonography may provide better information than survey images.[3] Survey images may also indicate if contrast studies are not necessary or if lesions would be obliterated (Figs. 23.12 and 23.13).

There are different ways of evaluating the urinary system, as well as different dosages and techniques. The method chosen is dictated by the clinical signs of the patient and the clinician.

Studies performed through contrast radiography have limitations, and with the advent of ultrasonography, a safer and more accurate method for evaluating the kidneys and prostate is available; however, the combination of the two methods may provide the greatest information.

🖉 **TECHNICIAN NOTES** Never use barium for any urinary studies, including cystography.

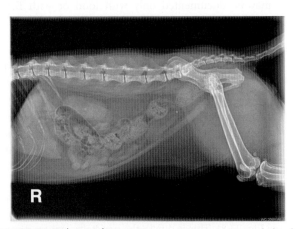

FIG. 23.12 Right Lateral Survey Prior to a Cystogram. Note calculi in the bladder and in the ureter close to the kidney. The stool could be obliterating other calculi. Also note right kidney enlargement (due to hydronephrosis).

Retrograde Cystography

Cystography is the study of the bladder and retrograde cystography is via the retrograde infusion of contrast media through a urinary catheter. Positive-, negative-, or double-contrast studies can be performed, with or without an excretory urogram. The actual study used is dictated by clinical history, clinical signs, radiographic signs, and character of the urine obtained with bladder catheterization (Box 23.5). Ultrasonography, if available and feasible, is preferred.

🖉 **TECHNICIAN NOTES** While inserting contrast medium into the bladder, stop the infusion when external palpation of the bladder shows that it is moderately distended, if reflux occurs around the catheter, or if you feel back pressure on the syringe.

🖉 **TECHNICIAN NOTES** To calculate the concentration of contrast medium needed, use one of the following formulae for this example:

A 15-kg dog requires 60 mL of a 10% iodinated contrast medium for a urinary study. If the stock bottle is 50%, what is the amount in mL taken from the bottle?

1) $\dfrac{\text{Final diluted percentage}}{\text{Initial concentration}} = \dfrac{\text{Volume needed}}{\text{Final volume administered}}$

$$\dfrac{10\%}{50\%} = \dfrac{X}{60\,\text{mL}} \quad \left(\dfrac{1}{5}\right)(60\,\text{mL}) = X\,\text{mL}$$

2) $C_1 \times V_1 = C_2 \times V_2$ Concentration (start) × Volume (start) = Concentration (final) × Volume (final)

$$50\% \times X\,\text{mL} = 10\% \times 60\,\text{mL}$$
$$50X = 600$$
$$X = 12\,\text{mL that should be taken from the bottle}$$

Note: The sterile diluent required will be total volume of 60 mL required − 12 mL of the concentrate, which will be 48 mL of diluent.

BOX 23.5 Retrograde Cystography[2,3]

Indications

- Clinical indications for retrograde cystography include unresponsive clinical signs due to abnormal urine (hematuria, crystalluria, and bacteriuria), abnormal urination (dysuria, pollakiuria), trauma, and abnormalities noted on survey images such as abdominal masses, a change in bladder opacity or wall, or a change in location[2,3]
- Retrograde positive-contrast cystography is used to evaluate the bladder wall character in a trauma patient or to locate the bladder after trauma or herniation.
- Retrograde negative-contrast cystography (pneumocystogram) is used to identify the integrity of the bladder wall after trauma or to locate the bladder. A pneumocystogram is best for cystic calculi.
- Double-contrast cystography is best for assessing bladder wall lesions and intraluminal filling defects.
- In the absence of ultrasound, the studies can help determine caudal abdominal masses.

Precautions

- Iatrogenesis due to catheterization and cystographic procedures—trauma, bacterial infections, kinked or knotted urethral catheters—can occur.
- Intramural or subserosal accumulation of contrast media occurs more frequently in cats and usually does not cause a clinical problem.
- Mucosal ulceration, inflammation, and granulomata reactions are usually transitory with no serious clinical problems.
- Fatal, although rare, complications can occur with the introduction of a gas embolism after administration of negative-contrast media.
  - Nitrous oxide or carbon dioxide should be used, especially in patients with hematuria, because blood in the urine may be evidence of communication between the bladder lumen and vascular system. Nitrous oxide or carbon dioxide is 20 times more soluble in serum than air or oxygen.
  - Left lateral recumbency may lessen the chances for emboli to reach the lungs.[3]

Contrast Media and Dosage

- Volume depends on body weight, species, and pathological process.
- Positive-contrast media:
  - Water-soluble nonionic organic iodide: 240 mg/mL or 300 mg/mL
  - Dogs 5–10 mL/kg; cats 2–5 mL/kg (maximum 25 mL in cats)[6]
- Negative-contrast media:
  - Nitrous oxide, carbon dioxide, air
  - Volume varies: 3–12 mL/kg.
- Double-contrast media:
  - Total: Positive nonionic contrast media: 0.5–6 mL, depending on species and weight.

Equipment/Supplies

- Sterile male or female urinary catheter.
- Vaginal speculum or adapted otoscope for female dogs.
- Skin prep, gauze, sterile gloves, sterile lubricating jelly.
- Light source.
- 20- to 50-mL syringe.
- 2% lidocaine jelly.
- Three-way stopcock.
- Source to deposit urine.
- 2–5 mL total of 2% lidocaine without epinephrine (optional).
- Broad-spectrum antibiotics (optional).

Patient Preparation

- Sedation is suggested, as urinary bladder distention can be uncomfortable, especially in patients with cystitis.
- Withhold food for 24 hours if possible, and administer an enema 4 hours before the study to avoid superimposition of fecal matter and to minimize gas artifacts (Fig. 23.12)
- Take survey images (Fig. 23.13).
- Proper sterile technique is required.
- Collect any urine samples prior to infusion of the agent. Contrast agents increase specific gravity, cause a false-positive increase in protein as detected by sulfosalicylic acid, and may inhibit bacterial growth.

Measure and Center

- Measure and center over the bladder (cranial to the crest of the ilium).

Procedure for Negative-Contrast Study (Pneumocystogram) or Positive-Contrast Cystography

1. Take ventrodorsal and lateral survey images of the full urinary tract.
2. Apply sterile 2% lidocaine jelly on the tip of a premeasured urethral catheter and aseptically and atraumatically insert until the catheter tip is within the urinary bladder.
3. Gently empty the bladder, and note the volume of urine removed.
4. Apply a syringe and three-way stopcock, and infuse with 2–5 mL total of 2% lidocaine without epinephrine to reduce bladder pain and spasm.
5. Carefully infuse the medium; stop when bladder feels firm and adequately distended through external palpation or back pressure of syringe plunger.
6. Close the stopcock valve when adequate distention is reached.
7. Take images: right and left laterals and ventrodorsal views.
8. An oblique view is optional but is suggested for evaluation of prostate or urethral pathology in a male.
9. If further distention of the bladder is required, inject additional contrast agent and repeat the images.
10. Carefully remove the contrast medium.
11. Flush with a broad-spectrum antibiotic if the patient is not receiving systemic antibiotics as per the veterinarian.
12. Remove the catheter.

Procedure for Double-Contrast Retrograde Cystography

1. Follow the preparation and procedures, infusing the negative-contrast medium first.
2. Take the required images. (Figs. 23.14 and 23.15).

Continued

BOX 23.5 | Retrograde Cystography—cont'd

3. Infuse the organic water-soluble iodine into the bladder, gently rotating the patient from side to side to coat the bladder wall with iodine.
4. Take the required images as noted earlier.
5. Complete the process as noted earlier.

Comments and Tips

- Both lateral views are suggested because a change in position may define a lesion more accurately; an oblique may also be suggested.
- Ensure that the catheter has been premeasured to just within the urinary bladder.
- Infusing the same amount of contrast medium as the amount of urine removed from a relatively full bladder is a good guide.
- It is best if the small bowel is empty and the colon is void of fecal material.
- Using lidocaine without epinephrine helps decrease the possibility of spasm and helps obtain complete bladder distention.
- Moderate distention is preferred because full distention may hide subtle mucosal and mural lesions if the bladder wall is stretched.
- A diseased bladder may only hold a fraction of the anticipated volume (as little as 1 mL/kg)[3] of air or positive-contrast medium. Palpate carefully, note resistance in the syringe, and watch for leakage.
- If the catheter has an inflatable cuff, deflate after the images have been taken.
- Any urine leakage with positive-contrast medium should be cleaned from the table, image receptor, or patient to minimize artifacts on the image.

- A decrease in exposure factors may be required for the pneumocystogram because of inherent contrast.
- Compression through the use of a paddle will help move the contrast pool for better evaluation of the integrity of the bladder wall.
- After taking the positive-contrast cystography images, the catheter tip can be repositioned into the urethra to perform a urethrogram. This will better evaluate the bladder neck.
- Urethral reflux of positive-contrast agent may be a normal finding.
- If a ruptured bladder is suspected, contrast agent can be used without dilution to better visualize the agent in the peritoneal cavity. Extravasation of the positive-contrast agent in the extraperitoneal soft tissues or peritoneal cavity is well tolerated.[2,3]

Cystography via Cystocentesis in the Dog and Cat

1. Manually palpate the urinary bladder, immobilizing it with your fingers against the ventral or lateral abdomen.
2. Aseptically introduce a 1-inch, 22-gauge needle in a cat or a 2-inch, 22-gauge needle in the dog through the midline abdominal wall.
3. Extract the urine, noting the volume.
4. Infuse positive-contrast media or air so that there is minimal bladder distention.
5. Remove the needle.
6. Take lateral and ventrodorsal or oblique images.

Comments and Tips

- There will likely be minimal leakage into the peritoneal cavity.
- Do not apply any bladder compression after injection to minimize possible leakage.

FIG. 23.14 A, Catheter injected with iodine before a cystogram. B, Lateral positive-contrast cystogram. (Courtesy Ontario Veterinary College, University of Guelph, ON.)

FIG. 23.15 Double-Contrast Cystogram. Note the bubble of air at the tip of the urinary catheter. (Courtesy Ontario Veterinary College, University of Guelph, ON.)

Excretory Urography[2,3,5]

Excretory urography is primarily used to determine the size, shape, location, and integrity of the kidneys, as well as the size, shape, and appearance of the collecting systems (Box 23.6). Although excretory urography is not a quantitative measurement of renal function, it can be used to assess the relative function of the kidneys and, indirectly, the pathophysical mechanism of renal failure.[3] The principle of the study is that sterile, water-soluble, iodinated contrast medium is injected intravenously. The iodine is concentrated and excreted in the kidney, outlining the kidneys, ureters, and urinary bladder. The study was formerly called an *intravenous pyelogram* (IVP) or an *intravenous urogram* (IVU).

Ultrasound images the anatomy without using contrast media and when available, is preferred.

TECHNICIAN NOTES Some suggestions for minimizing reactions to contrast media injections are as follows[1]:
- Before the injection, check that the solution is clear and colorless.
- Check the expiration date and discard outdated contrast material.
- Keep the contrast medium out of direct light for storage.
- There are no preservatives, so immediately use the bottle once it is opened, and discard the remainder.
- Keep the agent close to body temperature. The warmed solution decreases the viscosity for easier injection and reduces the potential for cardiovascular collapse.
- Use the minimum effective dose.
- To prevent incompatibility, do not administer other medications in the same syringe or IV administration set.
- Ensure patency of the catheter before the injection.
- If a contrast medium needs to be injected into a line, use normal saline (NS), dextrose and water (D/W), or lactated Ringer's solution (R/L). Potassium chloride (KCl) added to the IV is the *only* compatible medication. However, fluids dilute the concentration, lessening the contrast noted on an image.
- If a reaction occurs, stop injecting immediately and leave the catheter in the vein.
- Monitor carefully throughout.

BOX 23.6	Excretory Urography[2–4]

Indications for Excretory Urography
- Specific indications include abnormal urine or urination, suspected renal or urethral calculi, dysuria, pyuria, or intraabdominal mass that may involve or displace the kidney.
- Excretory urography can be used in both azotemic and nonazotemic patients provided there is adequate hydration.
- Various image sequences are listed in the literature. Alternative modalities if available should be used.

Precautions
- Avoid the study if anuria, severe dehydration, severe uremia, or urethral obstruction is present.
- Use proper technique to minimize iatrogenesis that may be caused by placement of the catheter.
- A temporary decrease in renal function may occur after excretory urography.
- Dehydration can result in kidney damage, so a dehydrated patient should be rehydrated before the procedure. It is important that the patient's hydration status be determined and corrected before administration of the agent. Kidney function parameters such as blood urea nitrogen (BUN) and serum creatinine levels should be checked before the start of the procedure.

- Abdominal compression may have to be modified because of precluded conditions.
- Even though the incidence of reaction to contrast media is low, especially with the use of low-osmolar, nonionic contrast media, it is imperative to be prepared and not to become complacent. An emergency resuscitation kit should be on hand before the injection.
  - Monitor vital signs before, during, and after the procedure to observe for adverse reactions which can occur quickly and without warning. The most severe acute reactions occur within the first 1–5 minutes after administration.
  - Signs can range from mild to fatal. The most common signs tend to be vomiting, defecation, urination, urticaria, tachycardia, and hypotension with or without collapse.
  - Most reactions can be reversed with immediate and proper intervention.

Contrast Media and Dosage
- Water-soluble organic iodide, 600–700 mg/kg up to 880 mg/kg body weight.[2,3,6]
- A maximum dose of 90 mL in dogs and 15 mL in cats is suggested.

Continued

BOX 23.6 | Excretory Urography—cont'd

- A concentration of 300–400 mg iodine per mL is the suggested dilution if uremia is present.[3]
- Nonionic compounds are highly recommended (see Tables 23.2 and 23.3).

Equipment/Supplies

- Indwelling intravenous catheter, syringe, and system for abdominal compression.
- Urethral catheter if continuing the study.
- Emergency resuscitation kit and oxygen.
- Markers to identify exposure time.

Patient Preparation

- No food for 24 hours before the study; water ad libitum.
- Perform a cleansing enema the previous evening if possible or at least 2 hours before (best if 4 hours to minimize gas artifacts).
- Collected urine samples before infusion of the medium. Contrast agents increase specific gravity, cause a false-positive increase in urinary protein as detected by sulfosalicylic acid, and may inhibit bacterial growth.
- Assess patient hydration, and proceed only if normal.
- Remove the urine so the contrast medium will not be diluted.
- Have image receptors, settings, markers, timers, protective gear, etc., ready so that upon administration of the contrast agent, the image can be taken immediately.
- Aseptically insert an indwelling catheter.
- Proper patient preparation is essential to ensure quality images.

Measure, Center, and Include

- As for the full abdomen, measure over the thickest part, center midabdomen and include an inch cranial to xiphoid and caudally to the acetabulum.
- The cranial pole of the right kidney of a dog is generally found at T13.
- Place time markers at the cranial aspect for VD views and at the ventral cranial abdomen for lateral views.

Procedure for Excretory Urography

1. The patient is best sedated or anesthetized to minimize discomfort.
2. Obtain survey images.
3. Place the patient in ventrodorsal recumbency with a patent intravenous indwelling catheter.
4. Inject the calculated warmed solution quickly as a bolus—within 2 minutes.
5. Flush the catheter with heparinized saline after the solution is administered.
6. Sequence the images as follows after injection (Fig. 23.16):
   a. Immediately—within 5–20 seconds: ventrodorsal (arteriogram and nephrogram).
   b. 5 minutes: ventrodorsal and right lateral (pyelogram phase).
   c. If there is evidence of contrast agent within both kidneys, compression may be applied.
   d. 15–20 minutes: ventrodorsal—both collecting systems should be filled with contrast medium (view ureters and urinary bladder).
   e. If compression has been applied, remove the compression band.
   f. 30–40 minutes or until a diagnosis is reached: right lateral and ventrodorsal oblique to view the bladder (optional if retrograde cystography is contraindicated).
   g. Further contrast study of the bladder can be completed:
7. Positive-contrast retrograde cystography: Infuse positive-contrast medium solution retrogradely via the urethral catheter. The amount would be determined by pressure and what is noted on the previous image.
8. Double-contrast retrograde cystography can be completed by infusing negative-contrast medium via the urethral catheter.

Comments and Tips

- Diagnostically, the bolus is best administered fairly quickly. Watch patient for nauseousness and vomiting if it is given too rapidly.
- Right lateral positioning is suggested to show greater longitudinal separation of the right and left kidneys.
- For better visualization of the ureters, obtain an oblique after 5 minutes.
- Apply compression over the bladder for better visualization of the renal collecting system by delaying the drainage of the contrast media. Compression of the urinary bladder increases intraluminal pressure and prevents drainage through the ureters.
- Compression can be applied by placing a flat radiolucent sponge on the central abdomen and securing it with elastic bandage. Commercially available compression devices can also be used.
- In ureter examination, the agent can be administered more slowly and the sequence delayed.
- A negative contrast cystogram is performed to diagnose ectopic ureters rather than abdominal compression.
- IV fluids administered during the sequence will reduce the concentration of the iodine and subsequent image intensity.
- Contrast media may be noted in the liver if the kidneys are highly compromised.
- The excretory urogram consists of the vascular (arteriogram), nephrogram, pyelogram, ureteral, and drainage:
  - During the vascular phase, which is seen with rapid bolus infusion, the aorta and renal arteries are seen.
  - Opacification of the functional renal parenchyma (nephrons) occurs almost immediately and is known as the nephrographic phase.
    - The vascular supply and perfusion of the kidney help differentiate the cortex from the medulla.
    - Absence in both kidneys may indicate disease or insufficient contrast media.
- The pyelographic phase shows the renal pelvis, pelvic recesses, and ureters.
  - The renal collecting channels extend into the medulla from the pelvis of the kidneys.
  - A compression band slows the drainage from the pyelogram.
- The ureteral and drainage phases occur when the agent is in the ureter and bladder.

BOX 23.6 | Excretory Urography—cont'd

- Proper distention of the urinary bladder cannot be achieved solely with an excretory urogram study—retrograde cystography is required.[4] However, it may be difficult to position a urethral catheter in traumatized female cats.
- The status of patient hydration, dosage rate, and renal function all affect the concentration, excretion, and opacification of the positive-contrast medium.

- Opaque material in the intestinal lumen, intestinal gas over the urinary bladder or urethra, and nipples can be mistaken for uroliths or filling defects.
  - Gas bubbles in the bladder or urethra introduced by urinary catheterization may appear as mineralized lesions in the tissues of the bladder wall.
- Additional views can be decided on the basis of individual findings.

TECHNICIAN NOTES

Measure, Center, and Include
- Remember that for the full abdomen, you are generally:
  - Measuring at the thickest part (liver), at the TL junction.
  - Centering over caudal aspect of 13th rib at level of L2–L3, or over umbilicus for the canine and two to three finger widths caudal to 13th rib for the feline.
  - Including about an inch cranial to xiphoid and caudally to the acetabulum.

FIG. 23.16 Ventrodorsal views of a normal cat after intravenous administration of 400 mg iodine per pound of body weight in the form of sodium iothalamate. **A**, 10 seconds after injection; **B**, 5 minutes; **C**, 20 minutes; **D**, 40 minutes. (From Thrall DE. *Textbook of Veterinary Diagnostic Radiology*. 5th ed. St. Louis: Elsevier; 2007.)

Further Urinary Tract Contrast Procedures

Box 23.7 includes further urinary tract contrast procedures.

Complete Urinary Tract Examination

Box 23.8 gives a summary of a complete urinary tract examination.

> **✎ TECHNICIAN NOTES**
>
> - Properly prepare the patient.
> - Obtain survey images.
> - Give the correct dose.
> - Follow proper procedure; set the correct technical factors.
> - Properly center, and include peripheral borders and position accurately.
> - Monitor, monitor, monitor.

BOX 23.7	Further Urinary Tract Contrast Procedures

Urethrography[2,3]

Indications

- Urethrography is indicated to determine the abnormal passage of urine due to urethral trauma, stricture, obstruction, or other pathological disturbances.

Overview

- Urethrography consists of filling the urethra with contrast medium for evaluation (Fig. 23.17). The actual technique varies with the sex and species of the patient.
- Can be accomplished in either a retrograde manner with a positive-, negative-, or double-contrast medium, or by applying compression on a positive-contrast–filled bladder to cause a voiding urethrogram.
- Often performed after completion of a retrograde cystogram merely by repositioning the catheter tip more caudally.
- Most often performed in male dogs for evaluation of the urethra and suspected prostatic disease. Only indirect evidence of prostatic disease is provided, however.
- In females, a combination vaginourethrogram can be completed (Fig. 23.18).

Precautions

- If injury results upon catheterization, injected air may enter the venous system, leading to fatal venous air embolism.
- Compression for a voiding urethrogram is contraindicated if the bladder is diseased because of the greater possibility of rupture.

Contrast Media and Dosage

- Positive-contrast organic ionic or nonionic agent (diluted to 150–200 mg of iodine/mL):
  - Dogs: 10–15 mL volume.
  - Cats: 5–10 mL volume.

Equipment/Supplies

- Sterile catheter with inflatable bulb if possible (Foley, Swan-Ganz).
- Skin prep solution, gauze, sterile gloves, sterile lubricating jelly.
- Catheter adapter/three-way stopcock.
- Large syringe.
- Sterile saline solution.
- 2% lidocaine jelly and lidocaine solution.
- Vaginal speculum or adapted otoscope for female dogs.

Measure and Center

- Measure and center at the crest of the ilium.

Patient Preparation

- Sedation is suggested, as the procedure may cause discomfort.
- Give a cleansing enema to remove fecal matter from the descending colon and rectum.
- Proper sterile technique is required. If the catheter was used for cystography, leave it aseptically inserted.
- If urine samples are required for examination, they should be collected before infusion of contrast media.

Procedure for Retrograde Positive-Contrast Urethrography

1. If not previously imaged, take ventrodorsal and lateral survey images of the full urinary tract.
2. If the catheter is not yet inserted, fill the lumen of the catheter with contrast medium.
3. Insert the lubricated tip about 1–3 cm into the urethral orifice, and inflate the balloon.
   a. For prostatic urethra, advance catheter to the level of ischial arch.[2]
4. Depending on the size of the patient, inject the warmed contrast medium until you feel back pressure.
5. Take lateral images toward the end of the infusion, repeating the administration if needed.
   a. Pull pelvic limbs cranially for a flexed lateral in males for a better view of the urethra (see Fig. 16.8).
6. A ventrodorsal oblique image may be helpful.
7. Remove the catheter.

Comments and Tips

- If the catheter does not have a cuff, use a larger catheter to limit leakage of the contrast medium. Place a towel to absorb leaking contrast agent.
- Avoid using a stiff catheter to minimize iatrogenesis.
- Avoid the use of sterile lubricating jelly with a positive-contrast agent to prevent filling defects and false-positive diagnosis.
- Minimize the length of time the catheter balloon is inflated to avoid mild reversible inflammatory reaction.
- A fully distended urinary bladder with urine, contrast medium, or sterile saline during urethrography allows better distention of the urethra, especially the prostatic urethra.

BOX 23.7 Further Urinary Tract Contrast Procedures—cont'd

- Vesicoureteral reflux and urethroprostatic reflux occur frequently in mature, healthy dogs undergoing maximum distention urethrocystography.
- Left lateral recumbency minimizes air embolus development and assists patient recovery if the bladder is distended with air/gas. Some radiographers prefer the typical right lateral position because it helps decrease renal overlap on images. If you suspect that an air embolus has developed during the procedure, immediately deflate the bladder and place the patient in left lateral recumbency.

Antegrade or Voiding Urethrogram
Procedure for Antegrade or Voiding Urethrogram
Because it is harder to catheterize female dogs and cats, the antegrade or voiding urethrogram is easier to complete than the retrograde study.
1. Apply gentle pressure on the positive-contrast–filled, distended bladder with a paddle or wooden spoon. Place a towel under the patient to absorb any leakage.
2. Take a lateral image when urine is noted at the urethral orifice.

Vaginocystourethrography[3]
Procedure for Vaginocystourethrography
Vaginocystourethrography is another method of evaluating the urethra in female dogs.
1. If not previously imaged, take ventrodorsal and lateral survey images of the full urinary tract.

2. Patients should be given general anesthesia.
3. If the catheter is not yet inserted, fill the lumen of the catheter with contrast medium (estimated dose: dogs 10–30 mL and cats 5–10 mL).[2]
4. Insert the lubricated tip into the vestibule and inflate the balloon to occlude outflow. The tip of the catheter distal to the balloon should be as short as possible to prevent it from entering the vagina.
5. It may be necessary to clamp the vulvar lips tightly to prevent reflux.
6. Inject amount of positive-contrast media for the size of the patient. The vagina will fill preferentially.
7. Infuse so the contrast medium will reflux into the urethra and bladder. Overdistention may result in expulsion of the contrast medium.[3] Take lateral images (optional VD and VD oblique) at the end of the infusion. The catheter can removed at the same time.
   Note: To avoid air bubbles that may be mistaken for calculi, prefill the catheter.

BOX 23.8 Summary of Complete Urinary Tract Examination[4]

Preparation
- No food for 12–24 hours. Give water ad libitum.
- Withhold water at least 1–2 hours or as required before sedation or anesthesia.
- Give an enema at least 4 hours previously to lessen the chance of gas artifacts.
- Assess patient hydration and proceed only if normal.
- Have receptors, settings, markers, protective apparel, etc., ready.
- Sedate patient and obtain survey images—right lateral and ventrodorsal (VD).
- Aseptically place intravenous (IV) catheter in vein and urethral catheter in bladder.
- Place a three-way stopcock valve on the urethral catheter.
- Remove any urine from the bladder.
- Place the patient in dorsal recumbency.

Excretory Urography/Double-Contrast Cystogram/Urethrogram
- Inject nonionic iodinated contrast medium as a bolus within 2 minutes. Note maximum limits.

- Flush catheter with heparinized saline after the solution is administered.
- Take VD image within 20–40 seconds of completing injection (vascular and nephrogram).
- Distend bladder with negative contrast media at about 1–2 mL/kg to keep iodine in kidney.
- Take VD and right lateral images of the kidneys 5 minutes after IV injection (pyelogram).
- Gently palpate the bladder and determine whether more negative-contrast agent should be administered.
- At 20 minutes after IV injection, obtain VD, lateral, and oblique images (optional) of kidneys, ureters, bladder (drainage and cystogram).
- Inject iodinated medium (5–15 mL) into the urethra as you withdraw the catheter.
- Take lateral image as soon as you see contrast agent leaking from the external orifice of the urethra.

FIG. 23.17 Urethrogram with Fluoroscopy of a Dog Positioned in Right Lateral Recumbency. Iodine has been injected retrograde via a catheter. Some of the iodine has dispersed in the bladder. (Courtesy Ontario Veterinary College, University of Guelph, ON.)

FIG. 23.18 Fluoroscopy of a Vaginogram Iodine Study with the Patient Positioned In Lateral Recumbency. (Courtesy Ontario Veterinary College, University of Guelph, ON.)

Normal Radiographic Anatomy of the Urinary Tract

Review the anatomy of the kidneys, bladder, urethra, and prostate found in Chapter 16 and Appendix A on the Evolve website.

Excretory urograms allow further quantitative measurements of the kidney and proximal ureters. The cortex is more radiopaque than the medulla in the early nephrogram phase. Generally, the pyelogram is more radiopaque than the nephrogram. The normal nephrogram is most radiopaque within 10 to 30 seconds after administration of a bolus injection of contrast medium.[6] The pyelogram should be consistently opaque.

The ureter width varies because of peristalsis. The normal bladder wall is about 1 mm thick, regardless of the amount of distention.[6]

Additional Techniques

Myelography[2,3]

Myelography (Fig. 23.19 and Box 23.9) is the placement of radiopaque contrast agent into the subarachnoid space in either the cerebellomedullary cistern or the lumbar region for evaluation of the spinal cord. Computerized tomography (CT) and MRI are replacing the use of myelography for spinal evaluation in many practices because they are quicker and noninvasive.

Further Contrast Studies

Box 23.10 gives a brief overview of additional contrast radiography techniques, many of which have been replaced by ultrasound or other modalities. See other sources for more complete information.

Box 23.11 provides a quick review of the contrast studies explained in this chapter.

Contrast Agents Used for Other Modalities

Ultrasound

Many substances may act as contrast agents in ultrasonography. Orally ingested fluid may expel gas from the stomach and create an acoustic window to the pancreas. Echo-free fluids such as water and saline may distend body cavities to improve visualization of the luminal walls. Contrast media for intravenous use have been limited to encapsulated microbubbles, which may produce up to a 25-dB increase in echo strength. They are generally used in Doppler ultrasonography of the heart. See Chapter 10 for ultrasound techniques.

Computerized Tomography

Generally, the nonionic contrast agents used in radiographic contrast studies are used in CT. See Chapter 12 for information on computerized tomography.

Magnetic Resonance Imaging

Most MRI contrast media contain the heavy metal gadolinium encapsulated in a chelate that makes it less toxic. These contrasts are called Gadolinium, Based Contrast Agents (GBCA). Gadolinium contrast is often given midway through the MRI session by injection into a vein to enhance tumors, blood vessels, or infection. GBCAs should only be administered intravenously. The contrast enhancement is best seen on T1 weighted and FLAIR images. Each injection of gadolinium is followed by a saline flush. Gadolinium is best injected slowly except for bolus vascular studies. See Chapter 13 for more specifics.

FIG. 23.19 **A,** Lateral projection during myelography study. **B,** Ventrodorsal view during a myelography study. (Courtesy Ontario Veterinary College, University of Guelph, ON.)

BOX 23.9	Myelography

Indications

- Myelography helps localize and identify the cause of suspected transverse spinal myelopathy, such as the size of the lesion or the extent of cord compression.
- The location helps determine prognosis and course of treatment.
- Specific indications for myelography include paresis, paralysis, proprioceptive or sensory deficit, and spinal pain thought to be due to a transverse myelopathy.

Precautions

- General anesthesia is required; any contraindications need to be evaluated.
- The cerebrospinal fluid (CSF) should be examined to check that there is no systemic or local infection such as myelitis or meningitis.
- The needle must be aseptically placed.
- The anesthetic regimen should not include a phenothiazine derivative, which might lower the seizure threshold.

- Corticosteroids should not be administered intrathecally with the contrast agent.
- The patient should be adequately hydrated to help minimize side effects and complications due to delayed elimination of contrast medium from the subarachnoid space.
- Incorrect procedure can cause trauma and have fatal consequences.
- Myelography may also cause intensification of preexisting neurological signs.

Contrast Media and Dosage

- Organic nonionic positive-contrast iodine: iopamidol (Isovue), 200–300 mg/mL, or iohexol (Omnipaque), 240 mg/mL.
- Dosage for the dog[2,3]:
  - Cisternal injection: cervical spine: 0.3 mL/kg; TL spine: 0.45 mL/kg
  - Lumbar injection: cervical spine: 0.45 mL/kg; TL spine: 0.3 mL/kg.

Continued

BOX 23.9   Myelography—cont'd

Equipment/Supplies

- Clippers, scrub solutions, drape, sterile gloves.
- Dog: 20-gauge spinal needle with a flat bevel, 2–4 inches in length; two 10-mL syringes.
- Cat: 22-gauge spinal needle with a flat bevel, 1.5 inches in length; two 5-mL syringes.
- Two 10 mL syringes for the dog and two 5 mL syringes for the cat; 18-gauge 1-inch needle, 3-mL syringe to collect cerebrospinal fluid.
- CSF collection tube, extension set, 0.22-μ nucleopore (millipore) filter.

Patient Preparation

- Use general anesthetic without a phenothiazine derivative.
- Shave the hair caudal to the skull (for cisternal) or over the lumbar spine (lumbar), and complete three scrubs.

General Procedure

For actual needle placement, consult more complete references. The veterinarian performs the injection and administers the agent.

1. After obtaining the survey images of the appropriate areas and anesthetizing the patient, aseptically prepare the region by shaving a 4-inch (10-cm) square; complete a surgical scrub and drape as follows.
2. Position the patient in perfect lateral recumbency with the aid of sandbags or foam sponges. See Chapter 20 for specific positioning.
3. Withdraw CSF in a volume that is at least equal to the volume of contrast agent to be injected.
4. Slowly inject the contrast medium.
5. Rotate the patient to ensure equal mixing of contrast agent and CSF.
6. Keeping the patient under general anesthesia for about an hour after injection lessens the frequency of postmyelography convulsions.
   a. Keep the head raised during recovery to prevent contrast medium from flowing into the ventricles of the brain, which may increase the pressure and risk of convulsions.

Further Specifics for Cervical Myelography

1. Obtain surveys, shave, scrub, and place drape caudal to external occipital protuberance.
2. Position so that the head is in maximum ventral flexion (chin touching the sternum) with the aid of sandbags or foam pads, and the midline of the head and neck is parallel to the table. The table can be tilted at 10 degrees with the patient's head at the raised end.
3. With the stylet in place, insert the needle into the cerebellomedullary cistern through the atlantooccipital space.
4. After withdrawing the CSF, inject the contrast medium over 3–4 minutes, and remove the needle.
5. Rotate the patient.
6. Keep the head elevated for a few minutes to allow contrast medium to flow caudally. The head may also need to be massaged.
7. A lateral image can confirm the location of the contrast volumes. Take lateral views beginning at the site of injection and move caudally.
8. Once contrast medium reaches the area of interest, further lateral, ventrodorsal, and oblique images accurately identify and locate lesions.

Further Specifics for Lumbar Myelography

1. Obtain surveys, shave, scrub, and place drape over L5–L6.
2. Position the patient flexing the pelvic limbs forward so the feet are along the abdomen. Sandbag in place.
3. With the stylet in place, insert the needle into the subarachnoid space.
4. Collect the CSF and slowly inject agent over 5 minutes. Keep the capped needle in place. This prevents the contrast from leaking into the needle tract and the epidural space
5. Rotate the patient.
6. Upon completion of the lateral view, remove the needle and immediately take the ventrodorsal view[2,6] (Fig. 23.19).

Comments and Tips

- There must be no patient movement during the placement of the spinal needle and injection. The veterinarian will perform the procedure.
- The patient can remain in sternal recumbency for either injection. This position makes it more difficult to determine the depth of the needle, which is better evaluated and radiographed in the lateral position.
- Cautions for positioning of the needle for the cerebellomedullary cistern through the atlantooccipital space:
  - Incorrect lateral positioning would puncture the vertebral sinus and cause bleeding.
  - Incorrect cranial positioning may put the tip in the hind brain, causing respiratory collapse and death.
  - Any movement during positioning may lacerate the spinal cord or medulla.
- If the needle position is accurate for the cervical injection, the most common problem is that the contrast medium does not flow caudally to fully visualize the lesion:
  - The contrast medium flows rostrally into the ventricular system when resistance to caudal flow is met, so only the cranial margin of a compressive lesion may be identified.
  - Positioning the head up during the injection or after removal of the spinal needle and massaging the neck may assist in the flow.
- Cervical myelography is not likely diagnostic if there is severe thoracolumbar cord swelling.
- There is less danger in incorrect positioning of the needle for lumbar myelography but keep in mind the following:
  - If the venous sinuses are punctured, creating a bloody tap, the interpretation of the CSF will be compromised.
  - The most common problem with lumbar punctures is the injection of the contrast agent into the epidural space and/or into the venous sinuses.
  - Extradural passage of contrast agent decreases the amount available in the subarachnoid space.
- If there is a bloody tap, do not inject the contrast agent because the mixture of blood and contrast agent is highly irritative in the subarachnoid space.
- If postmyelography convulsions occur, intravenous diazepam in therapeutic doses is recommended. If this is not effective, intravenous barbiturates are suggested.
- Keep in mind the suggestions for minimizing reactions to contrast media injections as described in the Technician Notes box for excretory urography.

BOX 23.10	Additional Contrast Radiography Techniques		
STUDY	**AGENT(S) USED**	**INDICATION/PROCEDURE**	**COMMENTS**
Angiocardiography— nonselective (selective study is direct injection into the right ventricle)	Water-soluble organic iodide.	Inject into the cephalic or jugular vein to obtain information on cardiac abnormalities such as occlusion of a particular blood vessel, to demonstrate pathological lesions of the vascular system, or to provide evidence of a tumor noted on the survey. Use when echocardiography is unavailable.	Sedation or anesthesia is usually required. Fluoroscopy or a method of rapidly exposing multiple images is recommended because a series of radiographs is to be taken every second.
Arthrography	Water-soluble organic iodide— nonionic low-osmolar agent. Pneumoarthrogram can be completed with carbon dioxide or nitrous oxide, which is preferred to air. Carbon dioxide is resorbed much more quickly than other gases.	Injection into the synovial fluid to contrast the articular surfaces and joint capsule. An arthrogram can be used to evaluate a ruptured joint capsule, the presence of a cartilaginous flap, meniscal injuries, or the necessity for surgery.	Dilute with sterile saline to a concentration of 20%–40%. General anesthesia and a surgically prepared 8- × 8-cm area are required. Contraindicated if there is infection of surrounding soft tissues.
Bronchography	Nonionic water-soluble iodine.	Tracheobronchial lesions that cause coughing or dyspnea.	CT and MRI have displaced this procedure.
Celiography—positive-contrast	Water-soluble organic iodide.	Evaluates the abdominal cavity and the integrity of the diaphragm often to determine a diaphragmatic hernia.	Surgical preparation of the site just caudal to the umbilicus.
Fistulography	Water-soluble organic iodide (nonionic preferred) or negative contrast media.	Evaluates the extent of fistulous tracts, sinus cavities, or draining wounds. Will detect radiolucent foreign bodies. Infuse into the fistulous tract with a syringe and flexible catheter, preferably one with a balloon tip.	Infection in the area may disseminate into the site. Often, the site of the wound is distant from the site of drainage.
Pneumoperitoneography, peritoneography, and herniography. (These are generally replaced by CT, MRI, or ultrasound.)	Negative-contrast media with carbon dioxide and nitrous oxide are preferred gases due to more rapid absorption in the body and less chance of air embolism.	Evaluates the abdominal cavity and integrity of the diaphragm. Often used to determine a diaphragmatic hernia. A horizontal beam should be used. The gas does not need to be removed.	Sedation is usually required. Surgical preparation caudal to the umbilicus is required. Use a stylet and syringe. Fasting and a full bladder are suggested.

Positron Emission Tomography and Nuclear Medicine Imaging Agents

Nuclear imaging (or scintigraphy) requires use of radioactive contrast agents (called *radiopharmaceuticals*) to obtain images. Some agents used for positron emission tomography (PET) provide information about tissue metabolism or some other specific molecular activity. The most commonly used agent in veterinary medicine is technetium-99mTc, which is used to radiolabel many different common radiopharmaceuticals. It is used most often in bone and heart scans. See Chapter 14 for further information.

Fig. 23.20 is a mystery radiograph. Review it and answer the question presented with it.

FIG. 23.20 Mystery Radiograph. What contrast study is this an image of and why is there a difference in density on the lower portion of the radiograph?

BOX 23.11 | Overview of Gastrointestinal, Urinary, and Spinal Contrast Studies

Esophagus Contrast Study:
1. Prepare the patient, including survey images.
2. Administer the barium, and immediately expose images with the patient in lateral position.
3. Administer more barium, and take further positions as required.

UGI Study
1. Prepare the patient, including fasting, an enema, survey images.
2. Make sure everything is ready so the exposure can be made immediately.
3. Administer the barium antegrade.
4. Place the patient in position, and follow the required sequence for times and positioning for proper completion of positive-contrast UGI study.
5. Follow up with a negative-contrast study if required.

Use of BIPS
1. Prepare the patient, including fasting or feeding as required and survey images.
2. Administer the capsules.
3. Expose lateral and VD views at the suggested time, depending on the condition. Repeat images if required.
4. Follow up with barium study or negative-contrast study if required.

LGI Contrast Study
1. Prepare the patient, including fasting, enema, sedation, and survey images.
2. Make sure everything is ready.
3. Administer the barium.
4. Place the patient in position and follow the required sequence for times and positioning for proper completion of a positive-contrast LGI.
5. Follow up with a negative-contrast study if required.

Retrograde Cystography
1. Prepare the patient, including fasting, enema, emptying of the bladder, insertion of the urinary catheter, survey images, and sedation/anesthesia. Follow proper aseptic technique.
2. Have everything ready before administering the contrast media.
3. Administer the required solution—warmed positive-contrast water-soluble organic iodide and/or negative-contrast medium.

4. Obtain the required images shortly after administration.
5. If required, follow up with the opposite-contrast media for the bladder or urethra.
6. Remove contrast medium; insert antibiotic if required; remove the catheter, and recover the patient.

Retrograde Urethrography and Vaginocystourethrography
1. Prepare the patient, including fasting, enema, emptying of the bladder, insertion of the urinary catheter, survey images, and sedation/anesthesia. Follow proper aseptic technique.
2. Have everything ready prior to administration of the contrast medium.
3. Administer the warmed positive-contrast water-soluble organic iodide via the catheter.
4. Obtain the required images shortly after administration.
5. Remove the contrast medium; insert antibiotic if required; remove the catheter; and recover the patient.

Excretory Urography
1. Prepare the patient, including fasting, enema, emptying of the bladder, insertion of IV line and urinary catheters, survey images, and sedation/anesthesia. Follow proper aseptic technique.
2. Have everything ready so exposures can be made immediately post administration of contrast medium.
3. Administer the warmed contrast water-soluble organic iodide IV as a quick bolus.
4. Expose the required images in the correct time sequence.
5. Apply compression if required, and continue the sequence of exposure.
6. Follow up with a positive or negative retrograde contrast medium if required for the bladder or urethra.
7. Remove the contrast medium, insert an antibiotic if required, remove the catheter, and recover the patient.

Myelography
1. Prepare the patient, including fasting, enema (if required), survey images, general anesthesia, and shaving and scrubbing of the site. Follow proper aseptic technique.
2. Have everything ready.
3. Place the needle; remove CSF, and slowly inject warmed organic nonionic positive-contrast iodine.
4. Obtain the required lateral, VD, and oblique images.
5. Recover the patient when appropriate.

✴ KEY POINTS

1. Contrast medium enhances the surrounding tissue or organ to make it more visible radiographically.
2. Positive-contrast medium is denser and has a greater atomic number than the elements of soft tissue and bone. Thus, agents such as barium (atomic number 56) attenuate the x-rays to a greater degree, absorb more x-rays, and create a more radiopaque image on the image than bone or tissues.
3. Negative-contrast media have lower atomic numbers and are less dense than soft tissue, so the x-rays will not be attenuated. X-rays pass through more easily, causing a black image to appear on the radiograph. According to the literature, carbon dioxide and nitrous oxide are the negative-contrast agents of choice because room air can create air emboli.
4. Double-contrast studies utilize both positive- and negative-contrast agents. Depending on the study, the negative-contrast medium is often administered first and the positive-contrast agent second.
5. A contrast study is generally more effective for determining the change in morphology than for determining the function of an organ.
6. There is a risk involved in any contrast study. The benefits and contraindications need to be weighed by the veterinarian.
7. Various dilutions of barium sulfate suspension are the most commonly used positive-contrast agent for GI studies.
8. Barium should not be used if there is a suspected perforation and should never be injected intravenously.
9. Water-soluble organic iodides can be used if there is suspected intestinal perforation. They have a rapid transit time, are readily absorbed from the peritoneal cavity across the mucosa, and are excreted by the kidney.
10. Water-soluble organic ionic iodine is hypertonic and can cause electrolyte imbalance, dehydration, nausea, vomiting, decreased blood pressure, and other physiological problems.
11. Water-soluble organic nonionic iodine with a dimer chemical structure is almost isotonic to blood and cerebral fluid; thus it has fewer side effects than ionic iodine.
12. Patient and other preparation are essential for the full benefit of the contrast study to be obtained. Depending on the study, this could include fasting, enema administration, and/or sedation. Make sure that the correct concentration in sufficient amount is given and that enough images are made at the appropriate times. Have image receptors, markers, timers, protective apparel, etc., ready before the administration of the contrast agent.
13. Survey images before the administration of the contrast agent are essential for ensuring that the correct exposure is made, that patient preparation is adequate, and that the contrast study still needs to be completed.
14. The actual procedure and images taken are dictated by the clinical signs in the patient and by the veterinarian's assessment. Only one area may need to be evaluated, or a full-system contrast study may be required.
15. Ultrasound and other imaging modalities, when available, have replaced contrast radiography for many evaluations.
16. The nonionic contrast agents used for radiography are generally used for CT. Gadolinium can be used for MRI, and radiopharmaceuticals are used for PET or nuclear medicine imaging.

REVIEW QUESTIONS

1. A contrast agent solution is completely insoluble, radiopaque, and physiologically inert. This would be in reference to:
   a. Barium
   b. Iodine
   c. Air
   d. BIPS

2. To increase the viscosity of organic nonionic dimer solutions, it is best to:
   a. Chill the solution
   b. Warm the solution
   c. Keep the solution at room temperature
   d. Add saline to the solution

3. To increase the transit time of barium for a UGI study, it is best to:
   a. Chill the solution
   b. Warm the solution
   c. Keep the solution at room temperature
   d. Add saline to the solution

4. Vomiting, defecation, urination, urticaria, tachycardia, and hypotension with or without collapse are more likely to occur when administrating a/an:
   a. Nonionic monomer contrast agent
   b. Nonionic dimer contrast agent
   c. Ionic monomer contrast agent
   d. Ionic dimer contrast agent

5. Urinary samples are best collected _____ administration of the contrast agents because:
   a. after; bacterial growth is not inhibited by contrast media
   b. after; there will not be a false positive in urinary protein
   c. before; bacterial growth is inhibited by contrast media
   d. either before or after; there will be no change in either urinary protein or bacterial growth

6. A nonionic dimer, iodine-based contrast agent is almost isotonic because:
   a. The ionizing carboxyl group is replaced with a group that does not dissociate
   b. The cations separate when injected into the blood or given orally
   c. There are three iodine atoms to every two particles in solution
   d. It has a low viscosity

7. A hypertonic contrast agent is likely to cause:
   a. Water to move from the vessels into the extravascular tissues and red blood cells
   b. Minimal side effects as the plasma and the agent have almost the same osmolality
   c. Crenation, vasodilation, and decreased blood pressure
   d. Elimination to take place through the liver and not the kidney

8. You have just administered barium via gastric gavage to a cat. For a full study, it is best to take the images:
   a. At 15, 30, 60, and 90 minutes and then hourly until completed
   b. Immediately; at 5, 10, 20, and 60 minutes; and then hourly
   c. Immediately; at 15, 30, 60, and 90 minutes; and then hourly until completed
   d. Immediately; at 30, 60, and 90 minutes; and then hourly until completed

9. You are looking at an image of a terrier in right lateral recumbency. Barium has just reached the cecum. The time of the image, assuming average filling, is probably:
   a. 15 minutes
   b. 30 minutes
   c. 1 hour
   d. 2 hours

10. Five small BIPS and two large BIPS are still remaining in the stomach of a Doberman. In the large intestine, there are 15 small BIPS and 3 large BIPS. The rest of the BIPS are all accounted for in the small intestine. The orocolic transit time for the large BIPS is:
    a. 20%
    b. 30%
    c. 50%
    d. 70%

11. The primary function of the large barium-impregnated polyethylene spheres is to:
    a. Determine extramural, mural, or intramural lesions
    b. Mimic the passage of food and calculate transit times
    c. Detect gastrointestinal tract obstructions
    d. Visualize the mucosal irregularities of the large intestine

12. A retrograde double-contrast cystogram is to be performed. The patient is best fasted:
    a. 12 to 24 hours
    b. 4 to 12 hours
    c. 1 to 4 hours
    d. Not at all, as fasting is not needed for this study

13. An esophagogram is to be completed. An enema should be given how many hours before?
    a. 1 to 4 hours
    b. 4 to 12 hours
    c. 12 to 24 hours
    d. Not at all, as an enema is not needed for this study

14. The best radiograph contrast procedure to assess the urinary bladder mucosa is:
    a. Excretory urography
    b. Double-contrast cystography
    c. Positive-contrast cystography
    d. Negative-contrast cystography (pneumocystogram)

15. The nephrogram phase of an excretory urogram shows the:
    a. Vascular supply and perfusion of the kidneys and should be taken immediately
    b. Vascular supply and perfusion of the kidneys and should be taken at 5 minutes
    c. Renal collection system and should be taken immediately
    d. Renal collection system and should be taken at 5 minutes

16. The most appropriate contrast medium for a positive-contrast cystography in dogs is:
    a. Barium sulfate paste
    b. Barium sulfate solution
    c. Carbon dioxide
    d. Iodinated water-soluble liquid

17. You are going to perform a positive-contrast retrograde cystography on a 35-kg male Retriever. If the total dose is 240 mL of a 10% diluted iothalamate (Conray), how much diluent will you add if the original Conray solution is 60%?
    a. 40 mL
    b. 160 mL
    c. 200 mL
    d. 280 mL

18. When radiographing for a double-contrast cystogram of a large dog, the central ray should be at:
    a. The umbilicus
    b. L2 or L3
    c. The caudal portion of the wings of the ilia
    d. The cranial portion of the wings of the ilia

19. The peripheral borders for a double-contrast cystogram for a large dog will likely be:
    a. T13 to the caudal portion of the ischium
    b. T8 to the caudal portion of the ischium
    c. L2 to the cranial portion of the ischium
    d. L2 to the caudal portion of the ischium

20. For a double-contrast cystogram of a male Retriever, it is best to obtain right lateral:
    a. left lateral, VD (optional), and DV
    b. left lateral, and oblique (VD optional)
    c. and VD
    d. VD, and oblique (optional)

Chapter Review Question answers are located in the Instructor Resources on Evolve and can be provided to students at the discretion of the instructor.

References

1. Kelly EA. Ontario Association of Medical Radiation Technologists (OAMRT): Intravenous contrast injection for medical radiation technologists & related allied health professionals, revised November 2010. File No: 4010-4036. Ontario Association of Medical Radiation Technologists.

2. Muhlbauer MC, Kneller SK. *Radiography of the Dog and Cat*: Guide to Making and Interpreting Radiographs. Oxford: Wiley-Blackwell; 2013 [chapter 3].

3. Thrall DE. *Textbook of Veterinary Diagnostic Radiology*. 7th ed. St. Louis: Elsevier; 2018.

4. Rendano V. UGI-stomach-ohiostate.htm/veterinary radiography. In: *Proceedings of the Ontario Association of Veterinary Technician Conference*. Toronto: OAVT; February 2005.

5. Medical ID Systems, Inc. BIPS Manual. Available at: http://www.medid.com/manual_bipers.pdf.

6. Ayers S. *Small Animal Radiographic Techniques and Positioning*. Oxford: Wiley-Blackwell; 2013.

Bibliography

Colville T, Bassert J. *Clinical Anatomy and Physiology for Veterinary Technicians*. 3rd ed. St. Louis: Mosby; 2016.

Done SH, Goody PC, Evans S, Stickland NC. *Color Atlas of Veterinary Anatomy, the Dog and Cat*. London: Mosby; 2009.

Evans H, de Lahunta A. *Guide to the Dissection of the Dog*. 8th ed. St. Louis: Saunders; 2017.

Owens JM, Biery DN. *Radiographic Interpretation for the Small Animal Clinician*. 2nd ed. Baltimore: Williams & Wilkins; 1999.

Singh B. *Dyce, Sack and Wensing's Textbook of Veterinary Anatomy*. 5th ed. St. Louis: Elsevier; 2018.

Sirois M. *Principles and Practice of Veterinary Technology*. 4th ed. St. Louis: Mosby; 2017.

Tighe M, Brown M. *Mosby's Comprehensive Review for Veterinary Technicians*. 5th ed. St. Louis: Mosby; 2019.

(Courtesy Epona Tech LLC, Paso Robles, California.)

CHAPTER 24
Equine and Large Animal Radiography*

Marg Brown, RVT, BEd Ad Ed

Strength does not come from physical capacity. It comes from an indomitable will.
—Mahatma Gandhi, Indian lawyer, politician, social activist, and writer, 1869–1948

OUTLINE

LEARNING OBJECTIVES

When you have finished this chapter, you will be able to:

1. Understand equine and large-animal radiography terminology.
2. Produce a diagnostic radiograph for common radiographic procedures of the equine/large-animal patient, using proper safety and positioning techniques.
3. Identify the less common views.
4. Identify skeletal and normal equine and large-animal anatomy found on a radiograph.

KEY TERMS

Key terms are defined in the Glossary on the Evolve website.

Caudoproximal-craniodistal (CdPr-CrDi)
Cranioproximal-caudodistal (CrPr-CdDi)
Crena
Dorsolateral-palmaromedial oblique (DLPMO)
Dorsolateral-ventrolateral oblique (DLVLO)

Dorsomedial-palmarolateral oblique (DMPLO)
Dorsoproximal-dorsodistal oblique (DPr-DDi)
Dorsoproximal-palmarodistal (DPr-PaDi)
Flexor view
High coronary view
Lateromedial (LaM)

Midsagittal plane
Occlusal
Palmaroproximal-palmarodistal oblique (PaPr-PaDi)
Plantaroproximal-plantarodistal (PlPr-PlDi)
Positional terminology
Skyline

Sulcus
Tangential
Ungular or collateral cartilages
Upright pedal route
Ventrolateral–dorsolateral oblique
Weight bearing

*Special thanks to Shannon T. Brownrigg, RVT, who co-wrote this chapter for the previous edition, and to Shana Lemmenes, CVT, VTS-EVN

TECHNICAL NOTE: To preserve space, the radiographic images presented in this chapter do not show collimation. For safety, always collimate so that the beam is limited to within the image receptor edges. In film radiography, you should see a clear border of collimation (frame) on every radiograph. In some jurisdictions, evidence of collimation is required by law. In digital imaging, the algorithm depends on proper collimation.

Special Considerations

Imaging large animals requires good planning, good teamwork, lots of patience, and being prepared to expect the unexpected. The common principles of radiography that apply to small animals also apply to large animals, with the major differences due to patient size and posture, which necessitate special consideration for areas of patient restraint, equipment, preparation, radiation safety, and positioning devices. Safety of personnel and patient is critical.

Compare the large-animal anatomy with human and small-animal anatomy (Fig. 24.1). The technical terms are similar, but common terms differ.

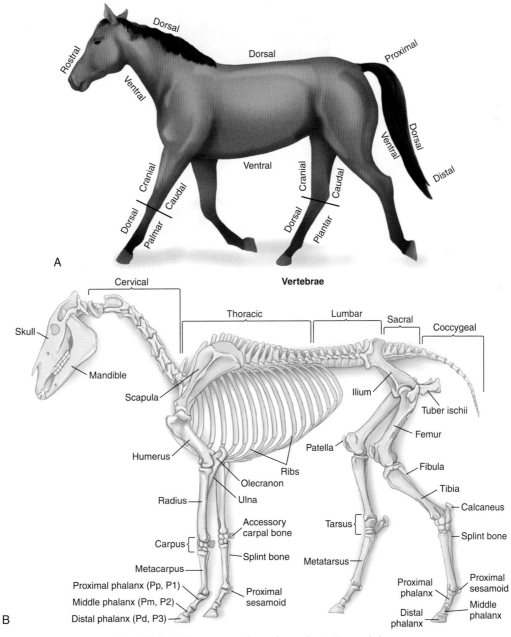

FIG. 24.1 A, Key terms used in radiography. B, Equine skeleton.

Continued

Radius

Accessory carpal bone

Carpal bones

Splint bone

Metacarpus

Proximal phalanx (Pp, P1)

Proximal sesamoids

Middle phalanx (Pm, P2)

Metacarpophalangeal joint (Fetlock joint)

Distal phalanx (Pd, P3)

Proximal interphalangeal joint (Pastern joint)

Distal interphalangeal joint (Coffin joint)

C

Distal sesamoid (navicular bone)

Radius

Accessory carpal bone

Carpus

Splint bones
Second (medial) or fourth (lateral) metacarpus

Third metacarpal
Cannon bone

Proximal phalanx
Long pastern

Proximal sesamoids

Fetlock joint

Middle phalanx
Short pastern

Pastern joint

Distal phalanx
Coffin bone

Navicular bone

Coffin joint

D

FIG. 24.1, cont'd C and D, Radiographic anatomy of the left lateral forelimb, which is technically referred to as a lateromedial view.

Restraint and Patient Preparation

- Large animals in the standing position are minimally restrained, which is a concern for both human and machine safety. Large animals can easily become startled when confronted with unfamiliar objects, so it is important to minimize sudden movements and loud noises. Keep the behavior of the particular patient in mind, and modify your restraint to take advantage of that behavior, being aware that any sights or sounds such as uncoiling electrical cords or moving positioning devices can startle a typically quiet horse.

- Ensure there is a solid ground surface that is level, clean, and nonslippery. The area should be quiet, free of obstacles, and large enough for personnel to move around the horse safely. Sedation may calm the patient and curtail startling that can cause movement blur on the image. Depending on the patient, consider various strategies such as raising the opposite limb, using a twitch, offering food, or using stocks. A competent handler is essential if the horse is being difficult or sedation is not an option.

- Movement artifacts, poor positioning of the patient or the x-ray beam, and inadequate exposure are the most common reasons that images must be repeated. Among other inconveniences, any repetition means further radiation dose for the restrainer or the patient.

  - To help minimize repeat radiographs, take the time to properly position the patient and the image receptor, and correctly direct the central ray.

Ulna

Radius

Radial carpal bone

Second carpal bone (C2)

Third carpal bone (C3)

Third metacarpal bone
Cannon bone

Proximal sesamoids

Proximal phalanx (Pp, P1)
(Long pastern)

Middle phalanx (Pm, P2)
(Short pastern)

Distal phalanx (Pd, P3)
(Coffin bone)

Intermediate carpal bone

Ulnar carpal bone

Fourth carpal bone (C4)

Splint bones
Second (medial)
or fourth (lateral)
metacarpus

Metacarpophalangeal
joint (Fetlock joint)

Proximal interphalangeal
joint (Pastern joint)

Distal interphalangeal
joint (Coffin joint)

Navicular bone

E

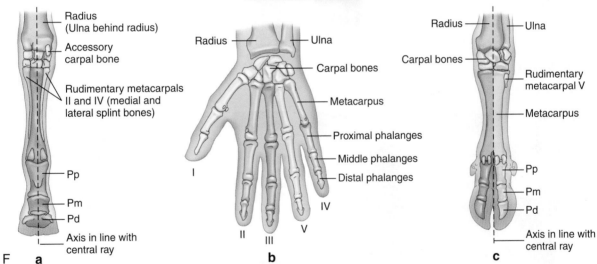

Radius
(Ulna behind radius)

Accessory
carpal bone

Rudimentary metacarpals
II and IV (medial and
lateral splint bones)

Pp

Pm
Pd

Axis in line with
central ray

F   a

Radius   Ulna

Carpal bones

Metacarpus

Proximal phalanges

Middle phalanges

Distal phalanges

I

II   III   V

IV

b

Radius   Ulna

Carpal bones

Rudimentary
metacarpal V

Metacarpus

Pp

Pm

Pd

Axis in line with
central ray

c

FIG. 24.1, cont'd E, Radiographic anatomy of the DP or dorsopalmar (dorsoproximal-palmarodistal) of left forelimb. F, Comparison of the palmar views of the (a) horse's limb, (b) human hand, and (c) ruminant's limb. (C and E courtesy Vetel Diagnostics, San Luis Obispo, CA, and Seth Wallack, DVM, DACVR, AAVR, director and CEO of Veterinary Imaging Centrer of San Diego.)

- Proper patient preparation is essential to obtain high-quality radiographs and to minimize radiation exposure. The hair coat should be dry, brushed, and cleared of dirt or other debris.
  - If the navicular bone is being radiographed, it is important to prevent overlying shadows superimposed on the field of view. This is especially true of dorsopalmar/dorsoplantar and oblique views. Remove the shoe and trim back any overgrown portions of the foot. Pick and thoroughly clean the sole and clefts, and then pack the sulci adjacent to and in the center of the frog

with a substance of similar radiographic opacity, such as Play-Doh, methylcellulose, or softened soap, to eliminate gas shadows due to the grooves of the frog (Fig. 24.2). Shoe removal, sole cleaning, and foot trimming are not essential if only the lateromedial view of the digit is needed.

- Double-check that you have all proper equipment and supplies with you, including foot blocks and other devices to permit personnel to be as far from the primary beam as possible. Proper personal protective equipment (PPE) is essential. If film cassettes are used and radiographs are being taken off site, make sure to take enough cassettes and film to the facility to allow for "repeats" and unexpected views.

- For digital radiography, make sure that all required equipment such as spare cords, hand switches, or required batteries is on hand.

✏ **TECHNICIAN NOTES** Debris such as shavings, mud, sand, small stones, and manure may cause radiographic artifacts. Sweep the area you are working in to keep the packing clean and minimize artifacts. Visually inspect well and clean the legs and hooves before taking images of the area. Depending on the size of the foot, try brown paper bags, kraft paper, sandwich bags, plastic wrap, paper towel, or dry gauze to keep the packing material from picking up particles.

FIG. 24.2 For diagnostic radiographs of the distal foot, the shoe should be removed and the sole cleaned **(A)** then packed with a radiolucent material **(B)**. **(A** courtesy Shannon Brownrigg.)

Radiation Safety and Positioning Devices

- All of the radiation safety principles applied to small animals equally apply to large animals. When working with large animals, concern for physical safety often supersedes radiation safety. Thus, it is essential to constantly keep the three tenets of radiation safety in mind (shielding, distance, and time).
- Portable machines can be particularly dangerous with regard to radiation exposure as they can be aimed in any direction and, due to limited machine power, they use longer exposure times than stationary units to produce diagnostic images. It is critical for all individuals who will be in the path of the beam, near the beam, or holding the portable x-ray unit to have appropriate and proper fitting protective lead attire, thyroid collars, and a monitoring badge (see Chapter 3).
- All PPE must undergo a routine maintenance schedule to evaluate weaknesses and breakage (see Chapters 3 and 9). Proper storage of PPE is important; avoid folding gowns and gloves. The most significant safety action is to increase one's distance from the primary beam through the use of a cassette holder (Fig. 24.3) and the use of a

FIG. 24.3 A and B, Commercial cassette holders used for equine positioning.

tripod to hold the x-ray unit if space and circumstances allow. Because the construction of x-ray machines does not allow the primary beam to be centered less than about 10 cm (4 inches) from the ground, a positioning block is needed to raise the affected foot (Fig. 24.4) for most views of the foot and pastern.

• Always collimate. The primary beam should only include the area of interest so that all margins of the primary beam are visible on the processed film. Stand out of direct or bright light to see the collimator guidelight. Always be conscious of where the horizontal beam is directed and where individuals are standing; a cassette holder should be used when possible. To help decrease exposure time, use a fast combination of film and screen if using this system and keep in mind that in digital imaging, the algorithm depends on proper collimation.

FIG. 24.4 An Example of Positioning Devices Used to Hold the Cassette. **A,** Used for the upright pedal route dorsopalmar (DP) positions. **B,** Redden navicular x-ray block. **C,** Ideal for lateral views of the metacarpus. **D,** Use for the lateral phalanx and sesamoids. The block can be rotated for a DP weight bearing view so the beam is parallel to the ground. **E,** EZ Blox Strap-On X-ray blocks.

Continued

FIG. 24.4, cont'd F, Use of a radiolucent cassette tunnel for the digital plate. **G,** Homemade cassette tunnel for film cassette. **H,** Redden offset lateral and DP x-ray positioning block. (**B** and **H** courtesy NANRIC, www.nanric.com; **E** courtesy Equine Digit Support System, Inc., www.ezxrayblox.com.)

- The source-image distance (SID) is generally less for large animals, with the common SID being 26 to 30 inches (66 to 76.2 cm), compared with 40 inches (100 cm) in radiography of small animals. Always use the retractable tape measure to determine the proper SID based on the technique chart. Do not guess! Some units have two small laser pointers at precise angles that merge at the correct distance when the collimator light is on. A shorter SID also helps decrease the exposure time. If the SID changes from what is suggested on the technique chart, keep this formula in mind to change the milliampere-seconds (mAs):

$$\text{Old mAs} \times \frac{(\text{New SID})^2}{(\text{Old SID})^2} = \text{New mAs}$$

- Review Chapters 5 and 6 if you need to adjust the image technique.
    - A cassette tunnel is also useful for digital images to protect the image receptor for dorsopalmar/dorsoplantar and oblique views of the foot (Fig. 24.5).
    - A cassette tunnel can be purchased or can be manufactured out of radiolucent wood (avoid use of nails) or hard plastic durable enough to withstand the weight of the horse. If using a cassette tunnel, make sure it is strong enough to support the weight of the horse and is translucent to minimize artifacts on the film (Fig. 24.4F,G). To minimize a slippery surface, cover with duct tape or use a mouse pad or section of yoga mat between the hoof and tunnel.

- A foot block needs to be high enough so that when the hoof is placed on it, the beam can be directed in a horizontal plane on the area of interest. Ideally, the block should have a slot to support the cassette close to the limb to minimize distortion (Fig. 24.4D). For equal weight bearing, both front feet should be on a foot block. If only the affected foot is placed on the block, improper pressure of the distal limb joints may affect the accuracy of the diagnosis. The opposite limb may need to be lifted to ensure full weight bearing and to prevent motion if equal weight bearing is not required.
- Keep the image receptor as close and parallel to the limb as possible to minimize object-film distance (OFD) and distortion. The suggested angle with the ground may change depending on the limb confirmation of the patient. Always aim the central ray perpendicular to the limb axis being radiographed.

> **TECHNICIAN NOTES** *ALWAYS* keep the three principles of radiation safety in mind—time, distance, and shielding—when imaging large animals. Also remember to collimate, collimate, collimate.

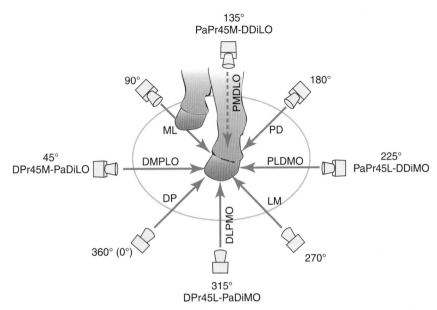

FIG. 24.5 Terminology of the Equine Proximal Limb Views. *Inner circle:* Common terminology and angles. *Outer circle:* Proper directional terms for the oblique views taken at the level of the metacarpus. *P* and *Pa,* Palmar; *D,* dorsal; *Pr,* proximal; *Di,* distal; *M,* medial; *L,* lateral; *O,* oblique.

Equipment

- Of the types of x-ray machines available—portable, mobile, and ceiling mounted—the portable unit is the most practical for those in ambulatory practices. Portable units are small and can be set up wherever there is a power supply. If there is not an adequate power supply, line voltage may vary, causing inconsistency in the exposures. These units are generally adequate for radiography of the equine distal limbs, skull, and cranial cervical vertebrae.
- Keep cords well away from feet to prevent tangling or damage from being stepped on. Position the horse so the cords can reach both the left and right sides. Although the portable equipment is built to withstand a certain amount of rough handling, transportation and frequent movement of radiographic equipment increase the opportunity for damage to x-ray equipment. Units should never be left in the vehicle overnight during below-freezing temperatures unless a sufficient warm-up time is taken into consideration before the first exposure.
- Depending on the type of unit, the kilovoltage (kV) and milliampere (mA) are generally preset, giving power anywhere from 40 to 120 kV and 15 to 100 mA. Time is usually the variable control, providing values of 0.3 to generally 50 milliampere-seconds (mAs). Newer units have variable kV and mAs. The digital displays allow adjustments of 1- to 5-kV increments. Because of the relatively low mA capacity, movement is a concern. Mobile units can be wheeled from room to room in the same premises, but are generally too cumbersome to be easily moved and transported. The kV and mA capacity is higher, allowing for shorter exposure times and less chance of motion artifacts than with the portable units.
- Veterinary specialty referral practices commonly use large units permanently mounted on a set of ceiling rails to allow horizontal and vertical movement. These high-capacity

units have the greatest output range (between 800 and 1000 mA), capable of obtaining high-quality radiographs of regions such as the thorax, pelvis, and thoracolumbar vertebrae. It may be difficult to obtain parallel views of the feet because the unit may not reach the ground close enough to prevent obliquity. A supplementary portable unit is often used in these situations. Exposure factors vary for each machine, so contact the generator manufacturer for a technique chart that can be used as a starting point. See Chapters 5 and 8 for suggested equine charts.
- Regular maintenance and calibration of all x-ray units are essential to the consistent production of quality radiographs and maintenance of a safe working environment. Inspections should be implemented as per local regulations. See Chapter 8 for further information on digital equipment.

> ✎ **TECHNICIAN NOTES** Electrical power may vary in different barn settings. Power may not be consistent (brownouts) to produce quality radiographs. Have suitable and safety-approved extension cord(s) for exterior use as part of your equipment list. Proper-length cords are best—the shorter the better—but make sure that cords used in digital radiography can reach both sides of the horse.

Equine Radiography

Radiographic Interpretation and Diagnosis

- You should have an understanding of the normal equine anatomy. Use a systematic approach, making sure to view the whole image. Review the radiography checklist found in Chapter 15.

- The purpose of most radiographs taken in equine practice is to evaluate the bones of the skeleton; thus, any response of the bone to insult or disease is relevant. Any changes such as sclerosis (causing more of a radiopaque image) or demineralization (radiolucent appearance) may not be visible on the radiograph, as a change of at least 30% in the bone mineral matrix is required before radiographic changes are evident.[1]

- Common indications for imaging the equine foot include localized lameness by clinical examination (pain on pressure from hoof testers, increased digital pulses, etc.) or by diagnostic analgesia (nerve block), laminitis, penetrating wounds, or as required for a prepurchase examination.[1]

- The main indications for radiography of the middle and proximal phalanx and proximal interphalangeal joint (pastern) are lameness localized with clinical examination or diagnostic analgesia and penetrating wounds. Specific views of this area are best obtained with the horse bearing weight squarely on all four limbs. The distal phalanx and the navicular bone comprise the digit or foot.

- The carpus consists of three principal joints with articulation between adjacent bones in each row of carpal bones. This causes overlying images, which may confuse interpretation. Consequently, it is recommended to obtain a minimum of five standard views.[2]

- Additional imaging may be required for accurate diagnosis and prognosis. This would include ultrasonography as well as cross-sectional imaging modalities such as computerized tomography (CT), magnetic resonance imaging (MRI), scintigraphy, and further diagnostic testing. CT and MRI show the most detail in all structures, indicating actual soft tissue and cartilage within the foot. Modalities such as nuclear scintigraphy and thermography show problem areas to the bone and soft tissue, such as ligaments, tendons, and articular cartilage that are poorly imaged on radiographs (see Fig. 24.57).

> **✎ TECHNICIAN NOTES**   A human middle finger is equivalent to the front foot of the horse, whereas the hind foot is a human's middle toe (Fig. 24.6). Imagine standing on your middle toes all day. It is no wonder the foot is the most frequently imaged for equine lameness issues. See Table 24.1 for comparative terminology of the human and equine limbs.

Prepurchase Examinations

- Equine clients often request a prepurchase examination of a horse before buying a competitive or breeding prospect. This examination is done to reduce the buyer's risk and assess the current health and athletic soundness of the horse. The examination is not a guarantee of the

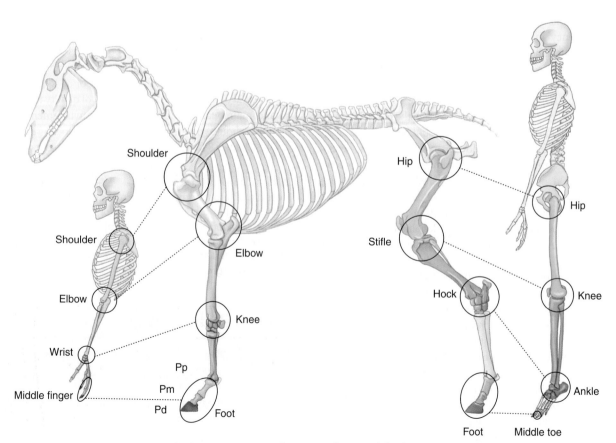

FIG. 24.6 Comparison of Human and Equine Skeletal Structures.

TABLE 24.1	Comparative Terminology of the Human and Equine Limbs		
ANATOMICAL TERM	**FURTHER TERM/ABBREVIATION**	**COMMON LAY TERM**	**HUMAN EQUIVALENT**
Distal phalanx (Pd)	Third phalanx (P3)	Coffin or pedal bone	Distal phalanx (fingertip)
Distal interphalangeal joint		Coffin joint	Distal interphalangeal joint
Distal sesamoid		Navicular bone	
Middle phalanx (Pm)	Second phalanx (P2)	Short pastern	Middle phalanx
Middle interphalangeal joint		Pastern joint	Middle interphalangeal joint
Proximal phalanx (Pp)	First phalanx (P1)	Long pastern	Proximal phalanx
Proximal sesamoid bones		Fetlock	
Metacarpal interphalangeal joint		Fetlock joint	Metacarpal interphalangeal joint—knuckle
Metacarpus/metatarsus	Third metacarpal/metatarsal bone (M3)	Cannon bone	Metacarpus /Metatarsus
	Second metacarpal bone/ metatarsal bone (M2)	Short splint bone	
	Fourth metacarpal bone/ metatarsal bone (M4)	Long splint bone	
Carpometacarpal/ carpometatarsal joint		Knee joint/hock joint	Wrist joint/ankle joint
Carpus/tarsus		Knee/hock	Wrist/ankle
Brachioantebrachial/ femorotibial joints	Elbow/stifle	Elbow/stifle	Elbow/knee
Shoulder/pelvis		Shoulder/hip	Shoulder/pelvis

Data from Butler JA, Colles CM, Dyson SJ, et al. *Clinical Radiology of the Horse.* Osney Mead, Oxford: Blackwell Science Ltd; 1993; Morgan JP. *Techniques of Veterinary Radiography.* Ames, IA: Iowa State University Press; 1993; Thrall DE. *Textbook of Veterinary Diagnostic Radiology.* 7th ed. St. Louis: Elsevier; 2018; Weaver M, Barakzai S. *Handbook of Equine Radiography.* London: Saunders; 2010.

health or soundness of the horse, but an interpretation of the ability of the horse to meet the intended purpose of the procurer. Depending on the level of expected performance or value of the purchase, this examination may include extensive radiographs.

- It is critical for all parties to identify any potential conflict of interest that may exist. The veterinarian requested to perform such an examination must clearly identify his or her relationship with, or prior knowledge of, the horse to be purchased and its owners or trainers. It is recommended to have a legal agreement prepared and signed that clearly identifies any relationship or knowledge to protect the interest of the performing veterinarian.

> ✎ **TECHNICIAN NOTES** Unless otherwise indicated, when the limb is described in this chapter, the forelimb terminology is used, but it is understood that the same principles apply to the hindlimb.

Labeling and Terminology

- For proper diagnosis and legal requirements, correct labeling is mandatory. As with radiography of small animals, permanent identification of the patient and owner (or purchaser for a prepurchase examination) is required. Identify both the specific limb (including front or hind) and the actual position, especially distal to the carpus/tarsus.

- As in small-animal radiography, the proximal end of the extremity is at the top of the viewer for DP/PD/CrCd/CdCr views. In lateral or oblique radiographs, the proximal end points up, with the cranial or dorsal aspect of the limb to your left.

- Conventionally, limb markers should be placed dorsally or laterally. Place directional markers (right/left, front/rear) on the lateral aspect of the limb for DP(CrCd) and oblique views and at the dorsal/cranial aspect for lateromedial views. Use Velcro tabs or duct tape to affix to plate. If there is a swelling on the limb, a marker such as a BB pellet taped on the skin might be useful.

- If using a digital plate, take images in the order of DP, DLPMO, DMPLO, and LM to move the markers only once. Alternatively, start with the LM and then proceed to DP and obliques.

- Because equine skeletal structures are large and complex, multiple views are required. In small animals, generally two views perpendicular to each other are taken. Horses generally require a minimum of four views for most positions, and six in some instances.

- Refer to Chapter 15 for a review of some of the basic terminology.

> ✎ **TECHNICIAN NOTES** Be consistent when viewing a series of radiographs from the same patient so that the images are oriented in the same direction.

✎ **TECHNICIAN NOTES**   Here is a short review of the terms you should be familiar with, especially in reference to large animals (see Fig. 24.1):

1. Dorsal, palmar and plantar, cranial, and caudal: Remember these terms take precedence when combined with other terms.
2. Describe radiographic projections from the point of entrance of the beam to the point of beam exit.
3. Technically, a lateromedial limb view should be termed *medial* if applying the rules, but the view is commonly referred to as *lateral*.
4. Proximal to the tarsus and carpus terminology is cranial (the part of the body facing the head) or caudal (the part of the body facing the tail).
5. Distal to and including the carpus and tarsus: The terms are *dorsal* (the part of the body facing the head) and *palmar* (front limb facing the tail) or *plantar* (hindlimb facing the tail).
6. Oblique: Not parallel to one of the two major directional axes (Fig. 24.5).
7. Tangential or skyline: Refers to the central ray entering and exiting the same side of the limb so that the bone is in profile.
8. In those views requiring a combination of directional terms: A hyphen should be inserted to separate the point of entry and point of exit. Example: palmaroproximal–palmarodistal (PaPr–PaDi).

Equine Radiographic Positioning

Table 24.2 lists the views that are used in equine limb examination.

✎ **TECHNICIAN NOTES**   Keep the principles of good radiographic imaging in mind every time. The body part should be close to and parallel to the image receptor, and the central ray is perpendicular to both. Think radiation safety for each exposure.

✎ **TECHNICIAN NOTES**   Minimizing obliquity is a concern for the lateral view, so it is important to make sure that the floor is level and the central ray lined up so that the bulbs of the heel are superimposed.

✎ **TECHNICIAN NOTES**   A common cause of nondiagnostic radiographs of the foot is lack of preparation. Artifacts need to be eliminated—remove the shoe; remove dirt, debris, and excess horny tissue; and pack the sulcus (Play-Doh, methylcellulose, or softened soap) to eliminate air artifacts.

TABLE 24.2	Views of the Equine Limb Examination	
STRUCTURES EVALUATED/ COMMENTS	**VIEWS/COMMENTS***	**COMMON TERMINOLOGY**
P3	Lateromedial (LM) with foot on block (ancillary).	Lateral (L)
	Dorsal 65-degree proximal–palmarodistal oblique (D65Pr–PaDiO); beam angled to ground, high coronary or upright pedal routes.	Dorsopalmar (DP)
	Dorsoproximal–palmarodistal (DPr–PaDi) with horizontal beam	
	Oblique views, especially if a P3 fracture is suspected:	
	1. Dorsal 65-degree proximal, 45-degree lateral–palmarodistomedial oblique (D65Pr–45L–PaDiMO)	(1) DLPMO
	2. Dorsal 65-degree proximal, 45-degree medial–palmarodistolateral oblique (D65Pr–45M-PaDiLO)	(2) DMPLO
Distal interphalangeal joint	Dorsal 65-degree proximal–palmarodistal oblique (D65Pr–PaDiO) high coronary route with beam angled to ground	Dorsopalmar (DP)
	Lateromedial (LM) with foot on block to include solar margin of P3 and soft tissues of sole on the radiograph	Lateral (L)
Ancillary views	Oblique views:	
	1. Dorsal 65-degree proximal, 45-degree lateral–palmarodistomedial oblique (D65Pr–45L–PaDiMO)	(1) DLPMO
	2. Dorsal 65-degree proximal, 45-degree medial–palmarodistolateral oblique (D65Pr–45M-PaDiLO)	(2) DMPLO

TABLE 24.2	Views of the Equine Limb Examination—cont'd	
STRUCTURES EVALUATED/ COMMENTS	**VIEWS/COMMENTS***	**COMMON TERMINOLOGY**
Navicular	Lateromedial (LM)	Lateral (L)
	Dorsoproximal–palmarodistal oblique (DPr–PaDiO):	Dorsopalmar (DP)
	1. High coronary stand-on route: 45 degrees: projects proximal border and extremities (D45Pr–PaDiO) 65 degrees: projects both borders and extremities (D65Pr–PaDiO)	
	OR	
	2. Upright pedal route (on a block): D90Pr–PaDiO Projects proximal border and extremities D80Pr–PaDiO: Projects both borders and extremities	Dorsopalmar (DP)
	OR	
	3. Dorsoproximal-palmarodistal (DPr–PaDi) with horizontal beam (True DP)	
	Palmaroproximal–palmarodistal oblique view (PaPr–PaDiO):	Flexor or skyline
	D65Pr45L–PaDiMO	DLPMO
	D65Pr45M–PaDiLO	DMPLO
Pastern P1, proximal interphalangeal joint, P2	Lateromedial (LM)	Lateral (L)
	Dorsoproximal–palmarodistal oblique (D30-45Pr–PaDiO)	Dorsopalmar (DP)
	Dorsal 35-degree proximal, 35-degree lateral–palmarodistomedial oblique (D35Pr-35L–PaDiMO)	DLPMO
	Dorsal 35-degree proximal, 35-degree medial–palmarodistolateral oblique (D35Pr-35M–PaDiLO)	DMPLO
Metacarpophalangeal/ metatarsophalangeal joint/proximal sesamoid bones (fetlock)	Dorsal 10-degree proximal–palmarodistal oblique (D10Pr–PaDiO)	Dorsopalmar (DP)
	Lateromedial (LM) extended	Lateral (L)
	Lateromedial (LM) flexed	Flexed lateral (L)
	Dorsoproximal 45-degree lateral–palmarodistomedial oblique (DPr45L–PaDiMO)	DLPMO
	Dorsoproximal 45-degree medial–palmarodistolateral oblique (DPr45M–PaDiLO)	DMPLO
Ancillary views	Palmaroproximal–palmarodistal oblique view (PaPr–PaDiO)	Flexor/skyline/caudal tangential
	Dorsoproximal–dorsodistal oblique (DPr–DDiO)	Extensor surface/skyline
Metacarpal/metatarsal cannon bone (M3)	Dorsoproximal–palmarodistal (DPr–PaDi)	Dorsopalmar (DP)
	Lateromedial (LM)	Lateral (L)
Lateral splint bone (M4)	Dorsoproximal 45-degree lateral–palmarodistomedial oblique (DPr45L–PaDiMO)	DLPMO
Medial splint bone (M2)	Dorsoproximal 45-degree medial–palmarodistolateral oblique (DPr45M–PaDiLO)	DMPLO
Carpus	Dorsoproximal–palmarodistal (DPr–PaDi)	Dorsopalmar (DP)
	Lateromedial extended (LM)	Lateral (L)
	Lateromedial flexed (LM)	Flexed lateral (L)
	Dorsoproximal 45-degree lateral–palmarodistomedial oblique (DPr45L–PaDiMO)	DLPMO
	Dorsoproximal 45-degree medial–palmarodistolateral oblique (DPr45M–PaDiLO)	DMPLO
Ancillary views	Dorsoproximal–dorsodistal oblique flexed (DPr–DDiO)	Skyline

Continued

TABLE 24.2	Views of the Equine Limb Examination—cont'd	
STRUCTURES EVALUATED/ COMMENTS	**VIEWS/COMMENTS***	**COMMON TERMINOLOGY**
Tarsus	Dorsoproximal–plantarodistal (DPr–PlDi)	Dorsoplantar (DP)
	Lateromedial (LM) extended	Lateral (L)
	Lateromedial flexed (LM)	Flexed lateral (L)
	Dorsoproximal 45-degree lateral–plantarodistomedial oblique (DPr45L–PlDiMO)	DLPMO
	Dorsoproximal 45-degree medial–plantarodistolateral oblique (DPr45M–PlDiLO)	DMPLO
Tuber calcaneus	Flexed plantaroproximal–plantarodistal (PlPr–PlDi)	Skyline
Radius	Cranioproximal–caudodistal (CrPr–CdDi)	Craniocaudal (CrCd)
	Lateromedial (LM)	Lateral (L)
Ancillary views	Caudoproximal–craniodistal (CdPr–CrDi)	Caudocranial (CdCr)
	Cranioproximolateral–caudodistomedial oblique (CrPrL–CdDiMO)	CrLCdMO
	Cranioproximomedial–caudodistolateral oblique (CrPrM-CdDiLO)	CrMCdLO
Elbow joint	Cranioproximal–caudodistal (CrPr–CdDi)—standing	Craniocaudal (CrCd)
	Mediolateral standing (ML)	Lateral (L)
Ancillary views	Cranioproximal–craniodistal oblique (CrPr–CrDiO) of olecranon	Skyline or flexor
	Lateromedial (LM)	Lateral (L)
	Mediolateral through the thoracic cavity	Mediolateral (ML)
	Cranioproximal–caudodistal (CrPr–CdDi)—recumbent	Craniocaudal (CrCd)
	Mediolateral (recumbent) (ML)	Lateral (L)
	Craniomedial-caudolateral oblique	CrMCdLO
Shoulder	Mediolateral (ML)	Lateral (L)
Ancillary views	Cranioproximal 45-degree medial–caudodistolateral oblique (CrPr45M–CaDiLO)	CrMCdLO
	Cranioproximal 45-degree lateral–caudodistomedial oblique (CrPr45L–CaDiMO)	CrLCdMO
Stifle	Lateromedial (LM)	Lateral (L)
	Caudoproximal–craniodistal (CdPr–CrDi)	Caudocranial (CdCr)
Lateral trochlear ridge and medial femoral condyle (stifle)	Caudoproximal 60-degree lateral–craniodistomedial oblique (Cd60L–CrMO)	CdLCrMO
Ancillary stifle	Cranioproximal–caudodistal (CrPr–CdDi)	Craniocaudal (CrCd)
	Cranioproximal–craniodistal oblique (CrPr–CrDiO)	Skyline patella
	Lateromedial flexed (LM)	Flexed lateral (L)

*Palmar is used in this chart and chapter with the understanding that plantar can be substituted when referring to the hindlimb.
Data from Weaver M, Barakzai S. Handbook of Equine Radiography. London: Saunders Elsevier; 2010; Butler JA, Colles CM, Dyson SJ, et al. Clinical Radiology of the Horse. Osney Mead, Oxford: Wiley-Blackwell; 2008; Thrall DE. Textbook of Veterinary Diagnostic Radiology. 7th ed. St. Louis: Elsevier; 2018.

Routine Lateromedial Views of the Limb (Table 24. 3)

The lateromedial view is routine and relatively consistent for most areas. What changes is the actual placement of the beam, the borders, and purpose. All these views also apply to the hindlimb, with the term *plantar* being substituted for palmar (Figs. 24.7–24.19).

Patient: Is weight bearing in a natural position. Make sure the hair coat is clean.

For the lower digit, it is especially essential to aim for a square stance on a level surface, unless the horse is painful or almost non–weight bearing, in which case the affected foot can be pulled forward.

Place the Foot/Limb: On a block (lower limb) or the ground.

Image Receptor: Vertically placed on the medial side of the area of interest either in the positional slot of a block (Fig. 24.7A) for the lower limb or supported with the cassette holder for the remainder views (Fig. 24.9A).

Beam: Always parallel to the ground. Aim 90 degrees to the midsagittal plane on the area of interest and keep the beam perpendicular to the vertically placed image receptor.

Label: Dorsal/Cranial aspect of limb.

> ✎ **TECHNICIAN NOTES** The technique is similar for imaging all lateral views of the lower limbs. What differs is the centering and what is included.

TABLE 24.3	Routine Lateromedial Views of the Various Parts of the Limb			
BODY AREA	**CENTRAL RAY**	**INCLUDE**	**COMMENTS**	
Digit and Navicular (Distal Sesamoid) (Fig. 24.7)	Below the coronary band so the bulbs of the heel are visually superimposed and in a straight line with the central ray. Wings of the coffin bone and distal sesamoids should be superimposed when viewing the radiograph.	The entire foot—whole foot wall, distal phalanx (P3), middle phalanx (P2), distal portion of P1, navicular bone, and distal interphalangeal and proximal interphalangeal joints	Digit: • Best to position affected limb on a block. To make it easier to visualize if there has been any rotation or sinking of the P3 in laminitis, consider taping radiodense wire or a line of barium paste placed on the dorsal wall of the hoof, beginning at the coronet band and working down. If using barium, always complete the other views before the barium is applied. • Care must be taken when assessing the foot pastern axis, which may be altered if the horse is not fully weight bearing on a level surface. • The purpose is to see the relationship between the dorsal foot wall and the dorsal border of the distal phalanx. The palmar processes may appear to be irregular, with separate bony fragments. They are normally separated from the distal phalanx cartilages by a prominent parietal *sulcus*.[2]	
(Fig. 24.7)			Navicular (Distal Sesamoid): • Evaluates the changes in the shape of the bone that are often associated with chronic degenerative changes of navicular disease.[1,2] • If only a lateral view is required, the shoe does not have to be removed; only cleaning and brushing of the wall are required. • There will be a foreshortened projection along the axis of the bone. Both borders and both surfaces will be projected in profile.	
Pastern (Fig. 24.8)	On proximal pastern joint (interphalangeal joint) or the joint of interest.	P2, the proximal interphalangeal joint, P1, and the interphalangeal-metacarpal joint.	• The lateromedial view of the pastern provides information on the integrity of the foot axis and the bones and joints in the digit. • Look at the foot from the front to see whether there is angulation of the digit. • If there is a conformation problem, the angle of the beam may need to be adjusted.	

Continued

Routine Lateromedial Views of the Limb (Table 24. 3)—cont'd

TABLE 24.3	Routine Lateromedial Views of the Various Parts of the Limb—cont'd		
BODY AREA	**CENTRAL RAY**	**INCLUDE**	**COMMENTS**
Fetlock Extended (Fig. 24.9)	Medial aspect of the proximal sesamoid bones	P1, the fetlock, and a third of the cannon bone.	• Aligning the beam parallel to a line tangential to the bulbs of the heel, results in a true lateromedial view. Palpation of the medial and lateral epicondyles of the third metacarpal bone may be helpful.[4] • If there is not a clear image of the joint space, the horse may need to be repositioned. • This view contains the fetlock joint and a portion of the bones proximal and distal. A true lateromedial view displays the metacarpal condyles and superimposed sesamoids, with a visible joint space.[3]
Fetlock - Flexed (Fig. 24.10)	Metacarpal interphalangeal joint	P1, the fetlock, and the proximal cannon bone.	• Affected limb is supported off the ground. Completely flex the fetlock, avoiding any obliquity by pointing the midsagittal ridge at the ground. Do not abduct the foot laterally. • The flexed lateromedial view allows for greater visualization of the spatial area of the metacarpophalangeal joint. The distal articular surface of metacarpal/tarsal bone is shown.
Metacarpus (Mc)/ Metatarsus (Mt) (Fig. 24.11)	On the midshaft of the cannon bone (MIII)	From the carpus/tarsus to the fetlock.	• The image receptor must be large enough to include at least one joint to provide orientation.
Carpus Extended (Fig. 24.12)	On the carpus	Entire carpus.	• A true LM view displays all carpal bones superimposed over one another, allowing for a clear view of the dorsal surfaces. A small portion of the distal and proximal bones, along with a full view of the carpus, should be visible. The carpus is a very complex joint. Multiple views may be required. • Consideration must be given to mature versus immature development.
Carpus Flexed (Fig. 24.13)	Center over the carpus.	Entire carpus.	• Important to keep the limb of interest elevated and the carpus flexed to approximately three-quarters of full flexion. Support the foot at the level of the carpus of the opposite limb so the carpus is slightly dorsal to the limb. Keep the carpus under the body, and prevent abduction. • The flexed lateromedial view displaces the patella distally to better visualize the proximal femoral trochlear ridges, medial femoral condyle proximal tibia, and apex of the patella.
Tarsus Extended (Fig. 24.14)	Middle of the tarsal joint.	Entire tarsal joint and calcaneus.	• Keep the tarsus under the body and prevent abduction.

Routine Lateromedial Views of the Limb (Table 24. 3)—cont'd

TABLE 24.3	Routine Lateromedial Views of the Various Parts of the Limb—cont'd		
BODY AREA	**CENTRAL RAY**	**INCLUDE**	**COMMENTS**
Tarsus Flexed (Fig. 24.15)	Lateral aspect of the limb at the talus.	Point of the hock, distal tibia, and proximal metatarsal bones.	• Limb of interest is elevated, and the tarsus is as flexed as the horse will allow. Support the foot at the level of the tarsus of the opposite limb with the affected tarsus slightly dorsal to the limb. Keep the tarsus under the body and prevent abduction. • Care must be taken when flexing the tarsus to monitor the comfort level of the patient. • It may be beneficial to have a different person flexing the tarsus than supporting the receptor plate. All must wear PPE.
Radius/Ulna (Fig. 24.16A) or Tibia/Fibula (Fig. 24.16B,C)	On the radius/ulna or tibia/fibula at the point of injury or pain.	At least one joint to provide orientation.	• If the affected limb can be pulled forward to position the plate laterally, the beam can be directed in a medial-to-lateral direction, though this is more difficult and not common. • A cassette holder should be utilized to decrease both physical and radiation danger.
Elbow (Brachioantebrachial Joint) ML (Mediolateral) (Fig. 24.17)	On the elbow joint, parallel to the ground, toward the medial side of the elbow joint just cranial to the opposite forelimb.	Entire joint.	With the patient standing, the mediolateral view is the easiest positioning for the elbow and is often suitable for a portable x-ray unit. • Affected limb is elevated and pulled cranially as far as possible so the radius is parallel to the ground. • Forward extension is required for an adequate projection. • It may be beneficial to have a different person flexing the carpus than supporting the receptor plate, but ensure all wear PPE. • If the limb cannot be extended, the patient may need to be bearing weight on the limb and a lateromedial view obtained with the image receptor positioned against the medial aspect (see Fig. 24.37C). The distal humerus or olecranon is not as well visualized in this position.
Stifle Extended Lateral (Fig. 24.18)	5 to 7 cm (2 inches) proximal to the tibial plateau between cranial and middle third of the stifle region.[4]	The entire patellae and proximal tibia.	• Image receptor is angled so it is aligned with the tibia and cautiously placed against the medial side of the stifle joint. • Sedation is highly recommended, especially if kicking seems likely. • Gently touching the medial stifle region and the flank, push the flat edge of the image receptor as far into the medial aspect of the stifle (flank) as possible. Patients may object to this image receptor placement. Gentle, calm movements are needed. All personnel involved must be prepared to respond to the patient at any moment. • If the limb being imaged is slightly caudal to the opposite limb, the space may open up on the medial side of the stifle for the receptor. • This view visualizes the articular surfaces of the femorotibial joints.

Continued

Routine Lateromedial Views of the Limb (Table 24. 3)—cont'd

TABLE 24.3	Routine Lateromedial Views of the Various Parts of the Limb—cont'd		
BODY AREA	**CENTRAL RAY**	**INCLUDE**	**COMMENTS**
Stifle Flexed	5 to 7 cm (2 inches) proximal to the tibial plateau between cranial and middle third of the stifle region.[4]	The entire patellae and proximal tibia.	• Position as for the extended lateral. In addition either lift the limb or rest the toe on the ground, creating a "dropped" stifle position. • The horse may prefer to rest the toe over a full weight-bearing position of the opposite limb. • It may be beneficial to have a different person flexing the tarsus than supporting the receptor plate, but ensure all wear PPE.
Shoulder Mediolateral (Fig. 24.19)	Beam: Parallel to the ground and perpendicular to the image receptor, centered on the joint.	The proximal humerus and distal spine of the scapula.	Aim the central ray on the scapulohumeral joint, palpate the distal aspect of the spine of the scapula of the opposite limb and aim cranial and proximal 10 cm (4 inches).[1] The image receptor is firmly placed against the lateral aspect of the shoulder joint of the neck. The affected limb is elevated forward and pulled cranially with the radius parallel to the ground. Superimpose the humeral head over the soft tissue The x-ray tube is on the opposite side of the patient. • If injury to the supraglenoid process is suspected, direct the central ray more dorsocaudally. • If there is injury to the tubercles, direct the central ray more ventrocaudally.[2] To obtain quality projections of the shoulder joint, the use of general anesthesia and placement of the patient in lateral recumbency are recommended. The standing position may be possible if the patient tolerates manipulation. The easiest and maybe only views of the shoulder that can be obtained are the mediolateral and an oblique view.

See patient and foot/limb position, image receptor, beam, and label as described above.
Use cassette holders or other positioning devices whenever possible.
In each case, the view also applies to the hindlimb, with the term plantar being substituted for palmar.

Routine Lateromedial Views of the Limb (Table 24. 3)—cont'd

FIG. 24.7 A, Positioning for the lateromedial view of the navicular bone standing on a block. **B,** Lateromedial radiograph of the navicular bone. (**B** courtesy Carolyn Bennett, Diagnostic Imaging, OVC, University of Guelph, ON.)

FIG. 24.8 A, Positioning for the lateromedial view of the middle and proximal phalanx and proximal interphalangeal joint (pastern). **B,** Radiographic anatomy of the middle and proximal phalanx and proximal interphalangeal joint (pastern). **C,** Radiograph of lateromedial middle and proximal phalanx and proximal interphalangeal joint (pastern). (**A** courtesy Shannon Brownrigg; **C** courtesy Carolyn Bennett, Diagnostic Imaging, OVC, University of Guelph, ON.)

FIG. 24.9 A, Positioning for the lateromedial view of the metacarpophalangeal/metatarsophalangeal joint/proximal sesamoid bones (fetlock). B, Radiograph of the lateromedial view of the metacarpophalangeal proximal sesamoid bones (fetlock). (A courtesy Shannon Brownrigg; B courtesy Carolyn Bennett, Diagnostic Imaging, OVC, University of Guelph, ON.)

FIG. 24.10 A, Positioning for the lateromedial flexed view of the metacarpophalangeal joint/proximal sesamoid bones or fetlock. B, Radiograph of the lateral flexed view of the fetlock. (A courtesy Shannon Brownrigg; B courtesy Carolyn Bennett, Diagnostic Imaging, OVC, University of Guelph, ON.)

Routine Lateromedial Views of the Limb (Table 24. 3)—cont'd

FIG. 24.11 A, Positioning for the lateral extended (lateromedial) view of the third metacarpus (cannon bone), M2, and M4 (splint bones). **B,** Anatomy of the lateral extended (lateromedial) view of the third metacarpus (cannon bone), M2, and M4 (splint bones). **C,** Radiograph of the lateral extended (lateromedial) of the third metacarpus (cannon bone), M2, and M4 (splint bones). **(A** courtesy Shannon Brownrigg; **B** courtesy Carolyn Bennett, Diagnostic Imaging, OVC, University of Guelph, ON.)

FIG. 24.12 A, Positioning for the lateromedial view of the carpus. **B,** Anatomy of the lateromedial view of the carpus. **C,** Radiograph of the lateromedial view of the carpus. **(A** courtesy Shannon Brownrigg; **C** courtesy Carolyn Bennett, Diagnostic Imaging, OVC, University of Guelph, ON.)

Routine Lateromedial Views of the Limb (Table 24. 3)—cont'd

FIG. 24.13 **A,** Positioning for lateromedial flexed view of the carpus. **B,** Radiograph of the lateromedial flexed view of the carpus. (**A** courtesy Shannon Brownrigg; **B** courtesy Carolyn Bennett, Diagnostic Imaging, OVC, University of Guelph, ON.)

FIG. 24.14 **A,** Positioning for the lateromedial (LM) view of the tarsus. **B,** Radiograph of lateromedial (LM) view of the tarsus. (**A** courtesy Shannon Brownrigg; **B** courtesy Carolyn Bennett, Diagnostic Imaging, OVC, University of Guelph, ON.)

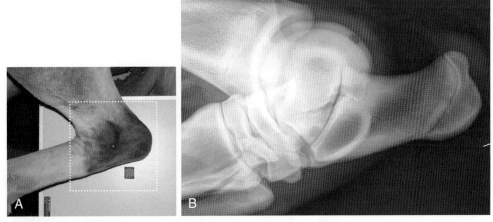

FIG. 24.15 A, Positioning for the lateromedial flexed view of the tarsus. **B,** Radiograph of the lateromedial flexed view of the tarsus. (**A** courtesy Shannon Brownrigg; **B** courtesy Carolyn Bennett, Diagnostic Imaging, OVC, University of Guelph, ON.)

FIG. 24.16 A, Positioning for the lateral view of the radius and ulna. **B,** Positioning for the lateromedial view of the tibia/fibula. **C,** Radiograph of the lateromedial view of the tibia/fibula. (Courtesy Stacey Thompson, BSc, RVT, McKee-Pownall Equine Services.)

Routine Lateromedial Views of the Limb (Table 24. 3)—cont'd

FIG. 24.17 A, Positioning for the mediolateral view of the elbow. **B,** Radiograph of the mediolateral view of the elbow. **C,** Lateromedial view of the elbow. (**A** courtesy Dr. Usha Knabe, Knabe Equine Veterinary Services, Orangeville, ON; **B** courtesy Carolyn Bennett, Diagnostic Imaging, OVC, University of Guelph, ON; **C** courtesy Shannon Brownrigg.)

FIG. 24.18 A, Positioning for the lateromedial view of the stifle. Centering of the stifle is assisted if a piece of tape is placed at the proximal end of the tibia *(arrow)*. **B,** Radiograph of the lateromedial view of the stifle. (**B** courtesy Carolyn Bennett, Diagnostic Imaging, OVC, University of Guelph, ON.)

Routine Lateromedial Views of the Limb (Table 24. 3)—cont'd

FIG. 24.19 A, Positioning for the mediolateral view of the shoulder joint. **B,** Radiograph of the mediolateral view of the equine shoulder joint (courtesy Shannon Brownrigg).

Routine Dorsoproximal–Palmarodistal View

Dorsopalmar (DP): Dorsoproximal–Palmarodistal View of the Digit and Navicular

The three following views can be taken for the dorsoproximal–palmarodistal (DPr–PaDi) views of the foot. The terminology changes slightly depending on the actual positioning. Because the beam is perpendicular to the foot, which is at an angle to the ground for the lower digit, the high coronary and upright pedal routes are technically termed *DPr–PaDiO views*. Note that there is no lateral or medial distinction. Proper full preparation of the sole is essential. These views also apply to the hindlimb, with the term *plantar* being substituted for *palmar*.

1. High Coronary Stand-On Routes

1. Proper angulation of the central ray is important for the high coronary views.
2. The high coronary view requires less restraint but involves more geometric distortion because the beam is not perpendicular to the image receptor.
3. The foot needs to be properly trimmed and the sole cleaned for the DP views.
4. The frog should be packed to eliminate air artifact. This view tends to be most common

   Patient: Is weight bearing. Proper full preparation of the sole, including trimming and cleaning, is essential.

Foot: Placed on the cassette tunnel, which is flat on the ground. Position the foot near the center and the toe close to the front edge of the tunnel so the full foot shadow will be on the image. Wings of the coffin bone and distal sesamoids should be equidistant.

Central Ray: On the midsagittal plane just distal to the coronary band centered between the bulbs of the heel, which are level.

Collimate to include: All of P3, the navicular, and P2.

Label: Lateral aspect of limb.

The beam is directed either 65 degrees or 45 degrees to the ground:

Dorsal 65-Degree Proximal–Palmarodistal Oblique (D65Pr–PaDiO) (Fig. 24.20)

The D65Pr–PaDiO view projects both borders and extremities of the navicular, and the distal border can be seen through the distal and palmar (plantar) portions of the middle phalanx.

Beam: 65 degrees to the ground and at 110 degrees with the hoof wall.

D65Pr-PaDiO

FIG. 24.20 A, Positioning for the dorsoproximal (DP) view of the digit using a tunnel cassette for the high coronary stand-on view angled 65 degrees to the ground. The foot is best placed closer to the front of the cassette so that the foot shadow and thus relevant structures are included. **B,** Dorsoproximal–palmarodistal oblique (D65Pr–PaDiO) or DP high coronary view of the equine distal phalanx and distal sesamoid bone (navicular) made at 65 degrees proximal to the supporting surface. **C,** Radiograph of the dorsoproximal distal phalanx using the high coronary view route.

Dorsopalmar (DP): Dorsoproximal–Palmarodistal View of the Digit and Navicular—cont'd

FIG. 24.20, cont'd D, Radiograph of the DP (D60-65Pr–PaDiO)-high coronary navicular position. Note the air artifact along the clefts of the frog due to improper packing of the sole. (C courtesy Carolyn Bennett, Diagnostic Imaging, OVC, University of Guelph, ON.)

Dorsal 45-Degree Proximal–Palmarodistal Oblique (D45Pr–PaDiO)

The D45Pr–PaDiO view projects the proximal border and extremities.

Beam: 45 degrees to the ground and at 90 degrees with the foot wall.

Comments Regarding the Digit

The purpose of the high coronary study is to note the number, size, and character of the vascular channels. The *crena*, which is the large notch in the solar border; the palmar processes, or wings formed by the solar border; and the *ungular or collateral cartilages* are all noted.[2] This is the preferred view for the interphalangeal joint.

TECHNICIAN NOTES The high coronary stand-on route literally means stand on the cassette tunnel. The beam is at an angle to the ground.

In the upright pedal route, the pedal bone (digit) is pointing downward on the block and the sole is flat on the cassette so that both are perpendicular to the ground. The area of interest is at an angle to the ground, whereas the beam is parallel to the ground.

TECHNICIAN NOTES Because of the foot conformation, the central ray is angled to the ground but always perpendicular to the hoof wall. Thus, the DP views of the foot taken with an angled beam to the ground are correctly referred to as *dorsoproximal–palmarodistal oblique views* (e.g., D30-45Pr–PaDiO means that the beam is angled 30 to 45 degrees to the ground). Note the angle designation is between the dorsal (D) and proximal (Pr) designations, indicating beam direction from the front of the limb. There is no lateral or medial designation showing an angle away from the midline.

TECHNICIAN NOTES The 45-degree high coronary stand-on and the 90-degree upright pedal routes show the undistorted proximal navicular border.

The 65-degree high coronary stand-on and the 80-degree upright pedal routes show both the distal and proximal borders.

Dorsopalmar (DP): Dorsoproximal–Palmarodistal View of the Digit and Navicular—cont'd

2. Upright Pedal Route of the Digit and Navicular Bone Dorsoproximal–Palmarodistal Oblique (DPr–PaDiO)

1. Proper full preparation of the sole is essential, including hoof trimming and cleaning. The frog should be packed to eliminate air artifact.
2. The upright pedal route designates the extensor process, conformation, quality of hoof care, and relationship of foot to the surface. It is preferred for the bones.[1,2]

   Foot: Point the toe of the foot downward so it is resting on a block, or use a navicular block.

   The sole is perpendicular to the ground, and the dorsal hoof wall is 65 degrees to the horizontal for the coffin bone.

   A positioning block with a slot (see Fig. 24.4A) or the Redden navicular block (Fig. 24.4B) can be used to change the hoof angle.

   Beam: Horizontal and parallel to the ground (Fig. 24.21).

Central Ray: Midsagittal plane just distal to the coronary band, centered between the bulbs of the heel.

Collimate and include: All of P3, navicular, and P2.

Label: Lateral aspect of limb (Fig. 24.9).

The dorsal foot wall will either be 90 or 80 degrees with the ground:

Dorsal 90-Degree Proximal–Palmarodistal Oblique (D90Pr–PaDiO)

The D90Pr–PaDiO view projects the proximal border and extremities (equivalent to 45-degree high coronary view).

Foot: Placed on a block with the toe pointing downward, the sole perpendicular to the ground, and the dorsal foot wall 90 degrees to the horizontal.

Use of Special Navicular Block: Place the foot in the slot closest to the front of the block or the 45-degree slot.

FIG. 24.21 **A,** Upright pedal positioning for the dorsoproximal (DP) dorsal 65-degree proximal–palmarodistal oblique (D65Pr–PaDiO) of the digit and the navicular bone. The beam is horizontal and parallel to the ground. **B,** An alternate upright pedal route for navicular positioning where the hoof is placed in one of two slots that change the angle at which the central ray strikes the navicular. **C,** Diagram for the upright pedal route of the navicular with the foot tipped so that the dorsal wall is positioned 90 degrees from the horizontal to show the proximal border and extremities of the distal sesamoid. The arrow indicates the horizontally directed central ray. **D,** Radiograph of the DP equine upright pedal route for the navicular with the dorsal wall positioned 80 degrees. (**A** courtesy Shannon Brownrigg; **D** courtesy Vetel Diagnostics, San Luis Obispo, CA, and Seth Wallach, DVM, DACVR, AAVR, director and CEO of Veterinary Imaging Center of San Diego.)

Dorsopalmar (DP): Dorsoproximal–Palmarodistal View of the Digit and Navicular—cont'd

Dorsal 80-Degree Proximal–Palmarodistal (D80Pr–PaDiO) of the Navicular Bone

The D80Pr–PaDiO view projects both the proximal and distal borders and the extremities (equivalent to 65-degree high coronary view).

Foot: Placed on a block with the toe pointing downward, the sole perpendicular to the ground, and the dorsal foot wall 80 degrees with the ground.

Use of a Special Navicular Block: Place the toe in the position closest to the image receptor or the 65-degree slot (Fig. 24.16).

> **TECHNICIAN NOTES** If a radiodense wire is taped or barium paste is applied on the midsagittal plane of the dorsal hoof wall, it is easier to see the hoof wall axis on an image of the phalanx.

Comments

1. A Redden navicular x-ray block (Fig. 24.4B) can also be used, which utilizes a 65-degree DP. The central ray is directed horizontally.
2. Collimate the beam for better image quality to decrease scatter radiation.
3. A lead shield (navicular mask) can be cut so that only the area of interest is exposed. This shield, along with placement of a lead sheet under the cassette tunnel for the high coronary stand-on route or behind the image receptor for the upright pedal route, minimizes scatter radiation and fogging from reaching the image.
4. Wings of the coffin bone and distal sesamoids should be equidistant.

5. These views also apply to the hindlimb, with the term *plantar* being substituted for *palmar*.

> **TECHNICIAN NOTES** When using the cassette tunnel, keep in mind how the "shadow" or image will project onto the receptor. Proper placement on the image receptor is especially important for the oblique or DP views to prevent projection beyond the detector.

3. True Dorsopalmar View for the Digit

(Dorsoproximal-palmarodistal (DPr-PaDi) with horizontal beam) (Fig. 24.22)

1. The true DP has the foot weight bearing on a block to raise it to the level of the x-ray tube with the beam horizontal and parallel to the ground.
2. This view is slightly more limited than the high coronary view, but does assess lateromedial foot imbalance, some distal phalanx fractures, and ossification of the collateral cartilages of P3.[1,2]
   i. The image receptor is positioned vertically for the true DP and directly caudal to the foot on the ground or in the cassette holder groove. Wings of the coffin bone and distal sesamoids should be equidistant.

Central Ray: On the *midsagittal plane* (MSP) of the pedal bone (dorsal foot wall) 2 cm above the dorsal coronary band.

Collimate: The full digit—foot wall, pedal bone, superimposed navicular bone, middle phalanx (P2), and the distal part of the proximal phalanx (P1).

Label: Lateral aspect of limb.

FIG. 24.22 A, Diagram for positioning of the foot on a foot block to obtain a weight bearing true DP view of the digit. B, Radiograph of the true dorsopalmar view with the foot on a block. (Courtesy Stacey Thompson, BSc, RVT, McKee-Pownall Equine Services.)

Routine DP Views Distal to the Digit (Figs. 24.23–24.29)

Patient: Is weight bearing. Clean the hair coat.

Image Receptor: Placed vertically, caudal to the limb (palmar or plantar), keeping it parallel to the area of interest.

Beam: On the midsagittal plane perpendicular to the foot axis or MSP.

Central Ray: Varying angle to the ground but **always** perpendicular to the foot axis or MSP.

Collimate to include: The area of interest and either the accompanying joints (if a bone) or 1/3 of the bone proximal and distal to the joint.

Label: Lateral aspect of limb.

See Table 24.4.

> ✐ **TECHNICIAN NOTES** The lateromedial and dorsopalmar (plantar) views evaluate only 50% of the limb. Further views are required for proper diagnosis. These routine views are known as *oblique views* and are obtained with the radiographic beam at an angle to the midsagittal plane of the limb (between dorsal and lateral/medial).

TABLE 24.4	Routine DP/CrCd Views of Proximal Phalanges and Limb		
AREA	**VIEW**	**BEAM**	**COMMENTS**
Pastern (Fig. 24.23)	Dorsopalmar (DP): *Dorsoproximal–Palmarodistal Oblique (D30-45Pr–PaDiO) View*	About a 30-degree to 45-degree angle with the ground but always perpendicular to the foot axis aimed at middle interphalangeal joint.	• The dorsopalmar (D30-45Pr–PaDiO) view of the pastern is a standard view to evaluate the causes of forelimb and hindlimb lameness. Additional views of the opposite limb are indicated in patients less than 9 months of age. Comparison studies permit evaluation of physeal closure.[2] • Collimate to include: P2, the proximal interphalangeal joint, P1, and the interphalangeal-metacarpal joint. • The joint space appears narrowed on one side if the horse is not standing straight. Make sure the horse is standing squarely or elevate the opposite forefoot for full weight bearing.
Fetlock -Metacarpophalangeal/ Metatarsophalangeal Joint/ Proximal Sesamoid Bones (Fig. 24.24)	Dorsopalmar (DP): *Dorsal 10-Degree Proximal–Palmarodistal Oblique (D10Pr–PaDiO) View*	On the midsagittal plane of the fetlock joint parallel to the pastern. Perpendicular to the foot axis and approximately 10- to 20-degree angle with the ground.	Collimate to include: P1, the fetlock, and one-third of the cannon bone. Superimposition of the proximal sesamoid bones over the joint space can be avoided by angling the image receptor and central ray with the ground proximodistally 10 degrees for the dorsopalmar view and 15 degrees for the dorsoplantar view.[4] This view provides visibility of the fetlock joint and the proximal sesamoid bones. Additional views of the opposite limb are indicated in patients less than 12 months of age.[2]
Metacarpus/Metatarsus (Cannon Bone, MII, and MIV) (Fig. 24.25)	Dorsopalmar (DP): *Dorsoproximal–Palmarodistal (DPr–PaDi) View of the Metacarpus (Mc)/Metatarsus (Mt)*	On the midsagittal plane of the third metacarpus/third metatarsus (cannon bone). Beam: Is parallel to the ground and perpendicular to the limb and image receptor.	Collimate to include: Fetlock, cannon bone and carpal/tarsal joints. • Larger image receptors are recommended for this area. • This view may include both joints (distal and proximal to metacarpus). If the image receptor is not large enough, include one joint to provide orientation. Distortion is possible because of the length of the area.

Routine DP Views Distal to the Digit (Figs. 24.23–24.29)—cont'd

TABLE 24.4	Routine DP/CrCd Views of Proximal Phalanges and Limb—cont'd		
AREA	**VIEW**	**BEAM**	**COMMENTS**
Carpus (Fig. 24.26)	Dorsopalmar (DP): *Dorsoproximal– Palmarodistal (DPr–PaDi)* View of the Carpus	Central Ray: Middle of carpus at a true DP plane, centering on an imaginary line from the middle of the foot wall to the radius. Beam: Parallel to the ground and perpendicular to the carpus and image receptor.	Opposite Limb may have to be elevated. Collimate to include the entire carpus and a portion of each of the metacarpal bones and radius/ulna. • To see whether there is closure of the distal radial physis in young horses, the other limb may be required for comparison. • The orientation of the central ray is perpendicular to the limb in question, not to the body of the horse. • On the radiograph, the intercarpal space between the radial and intermediate carpal bones should be visible with no superimposition.
Tarsus (Fig. 24.27)	Dorsoplantar (DP): *Dorsoproximal– Plantarodistal (DPr–PlDi)* View of the Tarsus	Central Ray: Centered mid-joint on the midsagittal plane at a true DP plane, centering on an imaginary line from the middle of the foot wall to the radius or tibia/ fibula.	Collimate to include the entire tarsus, a portion of each of the metatarsal bones, and the medial and lateral malleoli of the tibia. The beam is parallel to the ground and perpendicular to the tarsus and image receptor. • This view demonstrates the tarsal joint and a portion of the bones proximal and distal to it. • The primary beam is usually directed horizontally, but in some horses, it is best to direct the beam 5 to 10 degrees proximodistally to visualize the joint more clearly.
Radius/Ulna (Fig. 24.28A)	Craniocaudal (CrCd): *Cranioproximal– Caudodistal (CrPr– CdDi)* View of the Radius/Ulna	Central Ray: Cranio- proximally on the midsagittal plane of the radius/ulna at the point of injury or the location of pain or swelling. Beam: Directed slightly downward so it is perpendicu- lar to the limb and image receptor.	Collimate to include at least one joint for orientation. • Studies made of the area generally require a long image receptor. It is difficult to include the entire bone on a single radiograph. • A cassette holder should be utilized to decrease radiation exposure to personnel. • If the affected limb is uppermost in a re- cumbent patient, either a craniocaudal or caudocranial view is possible.
Tibia/Fibula (Fig. 24.28B)	Caudocranial (CdCr): *Caudioproximal– Cranioodistal (CdPr–CrDi)* View	Central Ray: On the midsagittal plane of the tibia/fibula at the point of injury or the location of pain or swelling. Beam: Slightly directed downward so it is perpendicu- lar to the limb and image receptor.	Collimate to include at least one joint for orientation. • Studies made of the area generally require a long image receptor. It is difficult to include the entire bone on a single radiograph. • A cassette holder should be utilized to de- crease both physical and radiation danger. • The study can be made as the cranio- caudal view, with the image receptor against the caudal aspect of the limb and the x-ray tube positioned cranially. However, there is increased OFD and concern with positioning safety.

Continued

Routine DP Views Distal to the Digit (Figs. 24.23–24.29)—cont'd

TABLE 24.4	Routine DP/CrCd Views of Proximal Phalanges and Limb—cont'd		
AREA	**VIEW**	**BEAM**	**COMMENTS**
Elbow (Brachioantebrachial Joint) (Fig. 24.29)	Craniocaudal (CrCd): *Cranioproximal–Caudodistal (CrPr–CdDi)* View	Central Ray: In a cranioproximal–caudodistal direction through the cranial aspect of the joint. Beam: Perpendicular to the image receptor and the limb	Patient is in standing position; extend the limb as far cranial as possible and elevate foot off the ground. Collimate to include the olecranon and a portion of the radius and ulna. • If positioned correctly, this is not a difficult view in spite of proximity to the ventral body wall. It may be beneficial to have a different person flexing the tarsus than supporting the receptor plate, but ensure all wear PPE. • This view shows the humeroradial joint space and medial and lateral aspects of the humerus and radius. • Lifting the foot off the ground partially separates the elbow from the chest wall. • If the patient is weight bearing, the central ray will be more horizontal to the ground. Place the image receptor with the long edge pressed firmly against the ventrolateral thorax at the caudal aspect of the elbow. Extend the lower inner corner ventral to the thorax to include the distal humerus.

See patient and limb position, image receptor, beam, borders and label as described above.
Use cassette holders or positioning devices whenever possible.
In each case, the view also applies to the hindlimb, with the term plantar being substituted for palmar.

Routine DP Views Distal to the Digit (Figs. 24.23–24.29)—cont'd

Proximal phalanx
Pastern joint
Middle phalanx

FIG. 24.23 A, Positioning for the dorsopalmar/dorsoplantar view of the middle and proximal phalanx, and proximal interphalangeal joint (pastern). **B,** Radiographic anatomy of the dorsal aspect of the middle and proximal phalanx and proximal interphalangeal joint (pastern). **C,** Radiograph of the dorsopalmar/dorsoplantar view of the middle and proximal phalanx and proximal interphalangeal joint (pastern). (**A** courtesy Shannon Brownrigg; **C** courtesy Carolyn Bennett, Diagnostic Imaging, OVC, University of Guelph, ON.)

FIG. 24.24 A, Positioning for the dorsopalmar view of the metacarpophalangeal/metatarsophalangeal joint/proximal sesamoid bones (fetlock). **B,** Radiograph of dorsopalmar view of the metacarpophalangeal joint/proximal sesamoid bones (fetlock). (**A** courtesy Shannon Brownrigg; **B** courtesy Carolyn Bennett, Diagnostic Imaging, OVC, University of Guelph, ON.)

Routine DP Views Distal to the Digit (Figs. 24.23–24.29)—cont'd

FIG. 24.25 **A**, Positioning of the DP—dorsoproximal–palmarodistal (DPr–PDi)—of the third metacarpals (cannon bone), M2, and M4 (splint bones). **B**, Anatomy of the third metacarpus (cannon bone), M2, and M4 (splint bones). **C**, Radiograph of the dorsopalmar view of the third metacarpus (cannon bone), M2, and M4 (splint bones). (**C** courtesy Carolyn Bennett, Diagnostic Imaging, OVC, University of Guelph, ON.)

FIG. 24.26 **A**, Positioning for the DP (dorsoproximal–palmarodistal) (DPr–PaDi) view of the carpus. **B**, Radiograph of the DP (dorsoproximal–palmarodistal) (DPr–PaDi) view of the carpus. **C**, Schematic diagrams of the bones of the carpal skeleton in carnivore *(Car)*, horse *(Eq)*, cattle *(Bo)*, and pig *(Su)*. (**A** courtesy Shannon Brownrigg; **B** courtesy Carolyn Bennett, Diagnostic Imaging, OVC, University of Guelph, ON.)

Routine DP Views Distal to the Digit (Figs. 24.23–24.29)—cont'd

FIG. 24.27 A, Positioning for the DP (dorsoproximal–plantarodistal) (DPr–PlDi) view of the tarsus. **B,** Radiograph of the DP view of the tarsus. **C,** Schematic diagrams of the bones of the tarsal skeleton in carnivore (*Car*), horse (*Eq*), cattle (*Bo*), and pig (*Su*). (**A** courtesy Shannon Brownrigg; **B** courtesy Carolyn Bennett, Diagnostic Imaging, OVC, University of Guelph, ON.)

Routine DP Views Distal to the Digit (Figs. 24.23–24.29)—cont'd

FIG. 24.28 A, Positioning for the craniocaudal (CrCd) (cranioproximal–caudodistal) view of the radius and ulna. **B,** Positioning for the CdCr view of the tibia/fibula. **C,** Radiograph of the CdCr view of the tibia/fibula. (**A** and **B** Courtesy Dr. Usha Knabe, Knabe Equine Veterinary Services, Orangeville, ON; **C,** Courtesy Stacey Thompson, BSc, RVT, McKee-Pownall Equine Services.)

Routine DP Views Distal to the Digit (Figs. 24.23–24.29)—cont'd

FIG. 24.29 A, Positioning for the craniocaudal view of the elbow (brachioantebrachial joint). B, Diagram of craniocaudal view of the elbow. C, Radiograph of the craniocaudal view of the elbow. (C courtesy Carolyn Bennett, Diagnostic Imaging, OVC, University of Guelph, ON.)

Oblique Views of the Equine

Overview

Oblique views are considered routine for most limb areas. The x-ray tube head is aimed perpendicular to the area of interest away from the MSP either toward the lateral or medial side. The view is correctly described first from where the beam enters on the limb and then where it exits.

Nomenclature

DLPMO- Dorsoproximal 45-Degree Lateral Palmarodistomedial Oblique [DPr45L-PaDiMO]

- Remember "point of entry to point of exit."
- The central ray enters the dorsal part of the limb proximally and is aimed 45 degrees laterally to the palmarodistomedial aspect of the limb and the image receptor. This angle is oblique to the MSP. The marker is placed along the lateral aspect of the image receptor.
- The simplified version of this is referred to as a dorsolateral–palmaromedial oblique (DLPMO) (Fig. 24.30B) or *medial* oblique (the medial aspect is against the film).
- The highlighted portion on this DLPMO projection (Fig. 24.30B) is the side that is not against the film—specifically the lateral sesamoid in Fig. 24.30B. Note that because this is taken at an oblique angle, the image of the medial proximal sesamoid is obstructed by the distal metacarpus (see Technician Notes). Thus, an oblique projection allows the portion of the bone farther from the film to be in profile.

- The radiograph is like a shadow: Because of beam direction, the body part on the film is superimposed in the oblique, and the opposite edges are highlighted.
- To help remember which views are highlighted in the oblique views, look at the abbreviation for the view and ignore the "O." Take the outer two letters and then the middle two letters. In the case of DLPMO, the outer two letters are (DM) and the middle two letters are (LP). So you are looking at the dorsomedial and lateropalmar surfaces of the bone (the red lines in Fig. 24.30B). Because of the angle of the beam, the lateral portion, not the medial aspect, is more in profile. The medial portion is hidden.
- Using point of entry to point of exit, the DLPMO is correctly termed a *medial oblique* because it is the medial aspect which is against the film. However, because the lateral portion of the bone is in profile in a DLPMO, practicing veterinarians may refer to the position as a *lateral oblique*, which is technically incorrect.

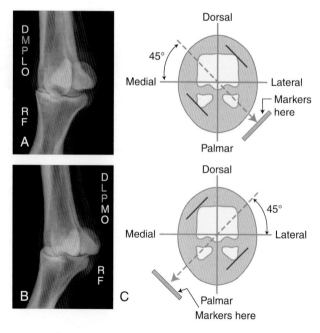

FIG. 24.30 **A,** DMPLO or dorsoproximal 45-degree medial–palmarodistolateral oblique (DPr45M–PaDiLO). Following the rule and taking the middle two and outer two letters, you are looking at the dorsolateral and palmaromedial surfaces of the limb/medial sesamoid. **B,** DLPMO or dorsoproximal 45-degree lateral–palmarodistomedial oblique (DPr45L–PaDiMO). Following the rule and taking the middle two and outer two letters, you are looking at the dorsomedial and palmarolateral surfaces of the limb/lateral sesamoid. **C,** Description of the terminology of the oblique views on a fetlock radiograph. The dotted lines are the direction of the beam and the red lines are the surfaces of the limbs being imaged. (**A** and **B** courtesy Carolyn Bennett, Diagnostic Imaging, OVC, University of Guelph, ON.)

Nomenclature

Dorsoproximal 45-Degree Medial–Palmarodistolateral Oblique (DPr45M–PaDiLO) DMPLO

- Point of entry to point of exit: The central ray proximally enters the dorsal part of the limb and is aimed 45 degrees medially from the midline to the palmarodistolateral aspect of the limb. The image receptor is on the palmarolateral aspect of the limb and is perpendicular to the beam. The marker is at the lateral aspect of the image receptor.
- The simplified version is dorsomedial–palmarolateral oblique (DMPLO) (Fig. 24.30A) or a lateral oblique because the beam travels from dorsomedial (point of entry) and exits at the palmarolateral portion, which is against the image receptor.
- Again, taking the two outer and two middle letters once the "O" is removed tells us that the dorsolateral and mediopalmar surfaces (*red lines* on Fig. 24.30A) will be highlighted. The medial proximal sesamoid is in profile. Because the medial portion of the bone is in profile in a DMPLO, practicing veterinarians may refer to the position as a *medial oblique*, but this is incorrect if proper terminology is used.

- In practice, you may hear common terms that are used in place of the correct anatomical terms (Table 24.1) or different modes of describing the beam. Anterior posterior (AP), a human term, is still sometimes used in practice; however, the correct nomenclature is *dorsopalmar* or *dorsoplantar* (DP). Common terms are listed here for the purpose of further understanding but are not necessarily the proper nomenclature.

> **✎ TECHNICIAN NOTES** To demonstrate that opposite projections are in profile, tape two different width objects, such as a pen and pencil, to an empty paper towel roll. Label four sides dorsal, palmar, lateral, and medial, and place a piece of paper behind your "limb." Using a flashlight or your fingers as the x-ray beam, take oblique views. Notice that the opposite protrusion away from the paper (receptor) is in profile—the pen or pencil closer to the paper (receptor) is superimposed by the paper towel roll, with the opposite object being highlighted.

Routine Oblique Views of the Limb (Figs. 24.31–24.37)

Patient: Is weight bearing.

Ensure that the foot and hair coat is cleaned, the sole picked.

Remove shoes for phalanx views.

Foot: Placed on cassette tunnel, block, or on the ground, depending on the body area and distance to the ground.

Image Receptor: Placed perpendicular to the ground, vertical to the area of interest against the lateral side of the limb for the DMPLO view and against the medial side for the DLPMO.

Central Ray: On the area of interest.

Beam: First, angle the beam perpendicular to the foot axis or MSP. (This may be at an angle to the ground depending on the confirmation of the site of interest.)

Secondly, rotate the tube head from the MSP the degrees listed:

- Example: D65Pr45L–PaDiMO: The tube head would be angled 65-degrees to the ground and then positioned 45-degrees on the lateral aspect of the limb.
- The image receptor is on the medial aspect of the limb, where the beam exits.

Borders: Include area of interest.

Bones: Include joints distal and proximal if possible

Joints: Include 1/3 bone distal and proximal

Label: Lateral aspect of limb.

See Table 24.5.

> **✎ TECHNICIAN NOTES** The same principles apply to both the front and hindlimb. Substitute the term *plantar* for *palmar* when referring to the hindlimb.

> **✎ TECHNICIAN NOTES** As with small-animal imaging, plan to minimize retakes. Your mental checklist includes but is not limited to the following: machine ready and settings correct, correct SID, PPE donned, use of a cassette holder or positioning device if possible, proper location of markers, patient properly prepared and restrained, correct body part and view, properly centered and borders included, with the central ray perpendicular to the body part and the image receptor.

Routine Oblique Views of the Limb (Figs. 24.31–24.37)—cont'd

TABLE 24.5	Routine Oblique Views of the Various Parts of the Limb		
AREA	OBLIQUE VIEW	BEAM	COMMENTS
Digit and Navicular See Fig. 24.31	DLPMO –Medial Oblique D65Pr45L–PaDiMO. *Dorsal 65-degree proximal, 45-degree lateral–palmarodistomedial oblique*	Angled 65 degrees on the dorsal surface downward on the DP line just below the coronary band and 45 degrees lateral to MSP just distal to the coronary band, half the distance between the dorsal wall and the heels.	• Ensure that the foot is clean, the sole packed, and shoes have been removed. • Foot is placed on the tunnel cassette with the foot off-center, slightly toward the side to be studied. The angle to be projected is closer to the edge of the image receptor. • Limb can be positioned as for a DP view, with the image receptor directly caudal to the limb if a cassette slot is used, but there will be distortion of the limb. • The medial oblique aspect of the limb is against the film. • The DLPMO view visualizes the lateral wing of the coffin bone, which appears larger due to increased OFD. Because there is no superimposition, the lateral wing of the coffin bone appears grayer.
See Fig. 24.32	DMPLO–Lateral Oblique D65Pr45M–PaDiLO *Dorsal 65-degree proximal, 45-degree medial–palmarodistolateral oblique*	Angled 65 degrees on the dorsal surface downward on the DP line just below the coronary band and 45 degrees medial to MSP.	• The oblique views help detect nondisplaced fractures in the quarters of the solar border and in the plantar or palmar processes of the distal phalanx. The oblique views do not superimpose the wings, so fractures are more easily diagnosed. • The DMPLO view visualizes the medial wing of the coffin bone, which appears larger due to increased OFD. Because there is no superimposition, the medial wing of the coffin bone appears grayer. • Keep the beam perpendicular to the foot axis.
Pastern (Fig. 24.33)	DLPMO–Medial Oblique D35Pr35L–PaDiMO; *Dorsal 35-degree proximal, 35-degree lateral–palmarodistomedial oblique*	35-degree angle with the ground, perpendicular to the foot axis and 35 degrees lateral to MSP.	• Limb for both pastern obliques can be positioned as for a DP view, with the image receptor directly caudal to the limb if a cassette slot is used, but there will be distortion of the limb. • These oblique views detect areas of new bone production located medially and laterally from the palmar/plantar and dorsal borders of the phalanges, as well as indicating new bone formation around the joints.[4]
	DMPLO–Lateral Oblique D35Pr35M–PaDiLO; *Dorsal 35-degree proximal, 35-degree medial–palmarodistolateral oblique*	35-degree angle with the ground, perpendicular to the foot axis and 35 degrees medial to MSP.	• Both oblique views detect areas of new bone production that are located medially and laterally from the palmar/plantar and dorsal borders of the phalanges, as well as indicating new bone formation around the joints.[4] • Chip fractures of the phalanges are best visualized on oblique views.[4]

Routine Oblique Views of the Limb (Figs. 24.31–24.37)—cont'd

TABLE 24.5	Routine Oblique Views of the Various Parts of the Limb—cont'd		
AREA	**OBLIQUE VIEW**	**BEAM**	**COMMENTS**
Fetlock (Fig. 24.34)	DLPMO–Medial Oblique *Dorsoproximal 30–45-degree lateral–palmarodistomedial oblique (DPr30-45L–PaDiMO)*	Angled 30 degrees to 45 degrees to ground, perpendicular to MSP in the lateral direction.	The DLPMO view is used to view the lateral sesamoid on the palmar/plantar aspect of the limb (see Fig. 24.5).
	DMPLO–Lateral Oblique *Dorsoproximal 45-degree medial–palmarodistolateral oblique (DPr45M–PaDiLO)*	Angled 30 degrees to 45 degrees to ground, perpendicular to MSP in the medial direction.	The DMPLO views the medial sesamoid on the palmar/plantar aspect of the limb (see Fig. 24.5). • The receptor should be angled slightly and the central ray is similarly tipped to elevate the sesamoids away from the joint space for better visualization.
Splint Bones To view M4 (Fig. 24.35B,C)	DLPMO–Medial Oblique *Dorsoproximal 45-degree lateral–palmarodistomedial oblique (DPr45L–PaDiMO)*	Is centered on the mid-shaft of the cannon bone parallel to the ground as follows: DLPMO view: Central ray: directed 35 degrees to 45 degrees laterally from the MSP.	The DLPMO view is used to provide an unobstructed view and evaluate the lateral splint bone (M4).
To view M2 (Fig. 24.35A,B,D)	DMPLO–Lateral Oblique *Dorsoproximal 45-degree medial–palmarodistolateral oblique DPr45M–PaDiLO*	Central ray: directed 35 degrees to 45 degrees medially from the MSP.	DMPLO view is taken to provide an unobstructed view and to evaluate the medial splint bone (M2).
Carpus	DLPMO–Medial Oblique *Dorsoproximal 45-degree lateral–palmarodistomedial oblique (DPr45L–PaDiMO)*	Parallel to the ground, perpendicular to the carpus and position the central ray laterally 45 degrees to 60 degrees from the dorsal midline (with the image receptor against the palmaromedial aspect).	Include the dome of the carpus.
(Fig. 24.36)	DMPLO–Lateral Oblique *Dorsoproximal 45–60 degree medial–palmarodistolateral oblique (DPr45-60M–PaDiLO)*	Position the central ray on middle of carpus medially 45 degrees to 60 degrees from the dorsal midline (with the image receptor against the palmarolateral aspect).	Include the dome of the carpus.
Tarsus (Fig. 24.37).	DLPMO–Medial Oblique *Dorsoproximal 45-degree lateral–plantarodistomedial oblique (DPr45L–PlDiMO)*	Position the central ray laterally 45 degrees to 60 degrees from the dorsal midline (with the image receptor against the plantaromedial aspect).	• The actual position of the central ray in relation to the dorsal midline may vary depending on the conformation. • There will be greater magnification with the DLPMO view due to increased OFD, which is caused by the angulation of the distal tibia.

Continued

Routine Oblique Views of the Limb (Figs. 24.31–24.37)—cont'd

TABLE 24.5	Routine Oblique Views of the Various Parts of the Limb—cont'd		
AREA	OBLIQUE VIEW	BEAM	COMMENTS
(Fig. 24.35C)	DMPLO–Lateral Oblique *Dorsoproximal 45-degree medial–plantarodistolateral oblique (DPr45M–PlDiLO)*	Position the central ray medially 45 degrees to 60 degrees from the dorsal midline (with the image receptor against the plantarolateral aspect).	• The actual position of the central ray in relation to the dorsal midline may vary depending on the conformation.
Shoulder (Fig. 24.37D)	CrMCdLO[1]: *Cranio-proximal 45-degree medial–caudodistolateral oblique (CrPr45M–CaDiLO)*	Beam: Parallel to the ground directed cranio-medial to caudolateral aimed at the shoulder joint.	• Patient is standing with the affected limb in a normal position, slightly cranial to the opposite limb. An assistant should pull the distal aspect of the affected limb cranially as far as possible. • Image receptor is placed cranial and lateral to the affected shoulder joint against the pectoral muscle mass. • Collimate to include the proximal humerus and distal spine of the scapula. • Because the central ray hits the image receptor at an angle, there is distortion of the underlying bones. • It is difficult to adequately evaluate the shoulder joint space with this view. • These views are used to evaluate an area of suspected injury at the point of the shoulder, such as tubercles.

Use cassette holders or positioning devices whenever possible.
In each case, the view also applies to the hindlimb, with the term plantar being substituted for palmar.

Routine Oblique Views of the Limb (Figs. 24.31–24.37)—cont'd

FIG. 24.31 A, A D65Pr45L–PaDiMO (DLPMO) view of the left equine distal phalanx made at 65 degrees proximal to the supporting surface and 45 degrees lateral to the dorsopalmar line or the midsagittal plane. The blue arrow indicates the side the beam is directed from. **B,** Positioning for the D65Pr45L–PaDiMO radiograph of the left front distal phalanx to view the lateral wing of the coffin bone. **C,** Radiograph of the DLPMO position of the digit as described in **A** and **B**. (**A** and **B** courtesy Dr. Usha Knabe, Knabe Equine Veterinary Services, Orangeville, ON; **C** courtesy Carolyn Bennett, Diagnostic Imaging, OVC, University of Guelph, ON.)

FIG. 24.32 A, Positioning for the DMPLO (D65Pr45M–PaDiLO) view of the left front distal phalanx with the beam 65 degrees to the ground and 45 degrees medial to the MSP. Note placement of foot to ensure the full image will be shown. **B,** DMPLO radiograph of the distal phalanx to view the medial wing of the coffin bone. (**A** courtesy Dr. Usha Knabe, Knabe Equine Veterinary Services, Orangeville, ON; **B** courtesy Carolyn Bennett, Diagnostic Imaging, OVC, University of Guelph, ON.)

Routine Oblique Views of the Limb (Figs. 24.31–24.37)—cont'd

FIG. 24.33 A, Positioning for the DLPMO view of the right front pastern. **B,** Radiograph of the DLPMO view of the pastern. **C,** Positioning of the DMPLO view of the right front pastern. **D,** Radiograph of the DMPLO view of the pastern. (**A** and **C** courtesy Stacey Thompson, BSc, RVT, McKee-Pownall Equine Services; **B** and **D** courtesy Carolyn Bennett, Diagnostic Imaging, OVC, University of Guelph, ON.)

Routine Oblique Views of the Limb (Figs. 24.31–24.37)—cont'd

FIG. 24.34 A, Positioning for the DLPMO (dorsoproximal 45-degree lateral–palmarodistomedial oblique [DPr45L-PaDiMO]) view of the left fetlock. **B,** DLPMO view of the proximal sesamoids or fetlock joint. **C,** Positioning for the DMPLO view of the left front proximal sesamoids or fetlock joint. **D,** Radiograph of the DMPLO (DPr45M–PaDiLO) view of the proximal sesamoids or fetlock joint. (**A** courtesy Dr. Usha Knabe, Knabe Equine Veterinary Services, Orangeville, ON; **B** and **D** courtesy Carolyn Bennett, Diagnostic Imaging, OVC, University of Guelph, ON.)

Routine Oblique Views of the Limb (Figs. 24.31–24.37)—cont'd

FIG. 24.35 A, Positioning for the DMPLO (dorsoproximal 45-degree medial–palmarodistolateral oblique [DPr45M-PaDiLO]) view of the third metacarpus (cannon bone), M2, and M4 (splint bones). B, Diagram of the DLPMO (a) and DMPLO (b) radiographic views of the third metacarpus (cannon bone), M2, and M4 (splint bones). C, Radiograph of the DLPMO view of the third metacarpus (cannon bone), M2, and M4 (splint bones), to show the lateral splint bone or M4. D, DMPLO radiograph to show the medial splint bone or M2. (A courtesy Dr. Usha Knabe, Knabe Equine Veterinary Services, Orangeville, ON; C and D courtesy Carolyn Bennett, Diagnostic Imaging, OVC, University of Guelph, ON.)

Routine Oblique Views of the Limb (Figs. 24.31–24.37)—cont'd

FIG. 24.36 **A,** Positioning for the DMPLO (dorsoproximal 45-degee medial–palmarodistolateral oblique [DPr45M-PaDiLO]) view of the carpus. Place the limb as close as possible to the image receptor. **B,** Radiograph of the DMPLO view of the carpus. **C,** Radiograph of the DLPMO view of the carpus. (**A** courtesy Dr. Usha Knabe, Knabe Equine Veterinary Services, Orangeville, ON; **B** and **C** courtesy Carolyn Bennett, Diagnostic Imaging, OVC, University of Guelph, ON.)

Routine Oblique Views of the Limb (Figs. 24.31–24.37)—cont'd

FIG 24.37 A, The DLPMO (dorsoproximal 45-degree lateral–plantarodistomedial oblique [DPr45L–PlDiMO]) of the tarsus **B,** Radiograph of the DLPMO view of the tarsus. **C,** Radiograph of the DMPLO view of the tarsus. **D,** Radiograph of the CrPr45M–CaDiLO of the shoulder joint. (**A** courtesy Shannon Brownrigg; **B** and **D** courtesy Carolyn Bennett, Diagnostic Imaging, OVC, University of Guelph, ON.)

Ancillary and Further Views

Navicular Bone

In addition to the 4 routine views dorsopalmar lateromedial, or DLPMO and DMPLO, the following flexor view is also taken to show the flexor surface, palmar cortex, and medulla of the navicular bones.[2]

Flexor/Caudal Tangential/Skyline (Palmaroproximal–Palmarodistal Oblique) View of the Navicular Bone

Image Receptor: Is placed directly under the foot slightly toward the back of the tunnel to project the image slightly forward.

Position: The affected navicular bone more caudally than the contralateral foot.

Extend: The fetlock, causing the middle phalanx to be vertical and isolating the navicular bone (Fig. 24.38).

Central Ray: On the midpoint between the bulbs of the heel at the distal–palmar (or distal–plantar) fetlock. The central ray must be angled tangentially in the same plane as the flexor cortex.

Beam: Along the palmar or plantar surface on the midsagittal plane at about 65 degrees with the ground.

Collimate: To include area of interest.

Label: Lateral aspect of limb.

Comments

1. Decrease the SID to 20 inches and adjust the exposure factors accordingly.
2. Full patient preparation is required.
3. Take advantage of any nerve blocks and perform the study before the anesthetic wears off, if possible.
4. Keep a small field of exposure to minimize scatter radiation.
5. Extending the affected hoof caudally while leaning the limb and fetlock slightly forward keeps the fetlock out of the field of view.

6. This view also applies to the hindlimb. For radiographing the rear feet, it is physically safer for the machine and restrainer if the hindlimbs are kept in a normal position.

> **TECHNICIAN NOTES** Common problems for imaging the skyline of the navicular bone of the forelimb include not extending the foot far enough backward, improper foot preparation (cleaning and packing), and not angling the central ray proximally enough.

> **TECHNICIAN NOTES** The restrainer should never be within the beam direction and always wear proper PPE.
> Always collimate.

> **TECHNICIAN NOTES** The precise position of the central ray may vary depending on the patient conformation. It is important to be perpendicular to the area of interest and the image receptor.

Flexor/Caudal Tangential/Skyline (Palmaroproximal–Palmarodistal Oblique) View of the Navicular Bone—cont'd

FIG. 24.38 **A,** Positioning for the palmaroproximal–palmarodistal oblique (flexor/caudal tangential/skyline) view of the navicular bone. **B,** Diagram of the skyline view of the navicular bone. This view highlights the flexor surface of the navicular bone and allows the distinction between the cortex and medulla to be visualized. **C,** Radiograph of the palmaroproximal skyline of the navicular bone. (**A** courtesy Stacey Thompson, BSc, RVT, McKee-Pownall Equine Services; **C** courtesy Carolyn Bennett, Diagnostic Imaging, OVC, University of Guelph, ON.)

Metacarpophalangeal/Metatarsophalangeal Joint/Proximal Sesamoid (Fetlock) Bones

In addition to the 4 required views—dorsopalmar, lateromedial, DLPMO and DMPLO:

Flexor/Skyline/Caudal Tangential (Palmaroproximal–Palmarodistal Oblique [PaPr–PaDiO]) View of the Fetlock

Patient: Is weight bearing (Fig. 24.39).

Foot: Placed as far back under (or behind for the hind foot) the horse as possible.

Image Receptor: Positioned in the tunnel with the foot centered on the tunnel.

Central Ray: In between the proximal sesamoid bones.[1]

Beam: Should be perpendicular to the ground caudal to the front limb.

Collimate: To include the area of interest.

Label: Lateral aspect of limb.

Comments

- This view allows visualization of the axial surface and abaxial recess of the proximal sesamoid bone.[1,2]
- SID is decreased because there is minimal space caudal to the front limb when the x-ray tube is placed under the horse.
- This study can also be made using an oblique view with the tube shifted either medially or laterally.
- This view also applies to the hindlimb, with the term *plantar* being substituted for *palmar*.

Extensor Surface/Skyline (Dorsoproximal–Dorsodistal [DPr–DDi]) View of the Fetlock

Fetlock Joint: Fully flexed and leg is positioned forward.

Image Receptor: Positioned against the dorsal surface of the proximal phalanx and parallel to the ground.

Central Ray: On the dorsodistal end of the third metacarpal (tarsal) bone.

Beam: Positioned directly above the distal end of the third metacarpal (tarsal) bone almost perpendicular to the ground.

Collimate: To include the area of interest.

Label: Lateral aspect of limb.

Comments

- The extensor surface/skyline study evaluates lesions dorsal to the distal end of the third metacarpal bone, as well as soft tissue mineralization. It also detects the character of intraarticular fracture lines of the distal metacarpal bone.[1,2]

- The SID is decreased to 50 cm (20 inches).
- This study can be performed on the hindlimb, but positioning is more difficult.

> ✎ **TECHNICIAN NOTES** When taking radiographs, mark the center of the area to be examined with a radiolucent indicator such as tape. This maneuver may minimize repeat radiographs due to inaccurate centering and also gives a reference point if the position is to be repeated.

FIG. 24.39 Flexor (Skyline/Caudal Tangential) Diagram of the Fetlock. The proper term is palmaroproximal–palmarodistal oblique (PaPr–PaDiO).

Carpus Ancillary Views

In addition to the five standard views which includes both extended and flexed laterals:

Skyline: Flexed Dorsoproximal–Dorsodistal Oblique (DPr–DDiO) Views of the Distal Radius, Proximal Row of Carpal Bone, and the Distal Carpal Row[1,3]

Limb: Elevated with carpus flexed so the metacarpals are horizontal and parallel to the ground for all the views.

Image Receptor: Placed firmly against the dorsal surface of the proximal metacarpus, parallel to the ground (Fig. 24.40).

Central Ray: Aimed toward the midsagittal plane of the dorsal surface of the carpus.

Location and angle of the beam to the image receptor depend on the row of carpal bones being imaged:

1. **Flexed D65Pr–DDi-skyline view of the dorsodistal radius:**
   - The radius is vertical to the ground at the level of the opposite carpus.
   - The central ray is angled 65 degrees to the image receptor.
2. **Flexed D45Pr–DDi-skyline view of the dorsal aspect of the proximal row of the carpal bones:**
   - The radius is angled at 45 degrees with the ground and slightly cranially so the flexed carpus is slightly in front of the opposite carpus.
   - The central ray is angled to 45 degrees to the cassette.

3. **Flexed D30Pr–DDi-skyline view of the dorsal aspect of the distal carpal row:**
   - The carpus is maximally flexed so that the radius is angled 60 degrees to the ground and positioned cranial and proximal the opposite carpus.
   - The central ray is angled 30 degrees with the image receptor.

   Collimate: To include carpus.

   Label: Lateral aspect of limb.

Comments

- Keep the image receptor perpendicular to the carpal bones to avoid distortion.
- Avoid abducting the flexed carpus.

FIG. 24.40 A, Beam angles for the skyline views of the carpus (dorsoproximal–dorsodistal oblique flexed views [DPr–DDiO]). **B,** Radiograph of a 60-degree, dorsoproximal–dorsodistal oblique flexed (skyline) view (D60Pr–DDiO) of the distal row of carpal bones. **C,** Radiograph of the distal row of carpal bones with a 30-degree angle. (**A** courtesy Dr. Usha Knabe, Knabe Equine Veterinary Services, Orangeville, ON; **B** and **C** courtesy Carolyn Bennett, Diagnostic Imaging, OVC, University of Guelph, ON.)

Pelvic Limb Ancillary Views

> **TECHNICIAN NOTES** If joint space is not properly visible on the radiograph, try repositioning the horse. Minor adjustments to stance can greatly affect the ability to properly image joint spaces.

Tarsus Ancillary Views

In addition to the required five views (extended and flexed laterals, DPr–PlDi, DLPMO, and DMPLO), the skyline or flexed view may be required. The skyline flexed view provides evaluation of the calcaneus and the sustentaculum tali from a proximal-to-distal direction without overlying bony shadows.[1,2]

Skyline: Flexed Plantaroproximal–Plantarodistal (PlPr–PlDi) View of the Tuber Calcaneus and Sustentaculum Tali

Limb: Elevated with tarsus flexed so that the metatarsal bones are parallel and horizontal with the ground for all views.

Image Receptor: Placed horizontally and firmly against the plantar surface of the calcaneus, parallel to the ground (Fig. 24.41).

Central Ray: On the tuber calcaneus.

Beam: Directly above the tarsus, perpendicular to the ground, and aimed straight down, being as perpendicular to the image receptor as possible.

A slight cranial angulation may be required to avoid the thigh musculature.

Include: Only the calcaneus and sustentaculum tali.

Collimate: To include the area of interest.

Label: Lateral aspect of limb.

Comments

- Two people may be required, with one person flexing the tarsus and the other supporting the receptor plate. All must wear PPE.
- The use of a ceiling-mounted x-ray unit is preferred because of the height of the positioning of the tube head required, though most clinics use a hand-held portable unit.

FIG. 24.41 A, Positioning of the tuber calcaneus for the skyline flexed or plantaroproximal–plantarodistal (PlPr–PlDi) view. B, Radiograph of the tuber calcaneus for the skyline flexed or plantaroproximal–plantarodistal (PlPr–PlDi) view. (A courtesy Shannon Brownrigg; B courtesy Carolyn Bennett, Diagnostic Imaging, OVC, University of Guelph, ON.)

Stifle (Femorotibial Joint) Ancillary Views

Safety is paramount in radiography of the hind region of the horse. Radiographs of this region should be attempted only if the patient is sedated and cooperative. Sedation and/or a twitch should be used.

Radiography of the femorotibial joint (stifle) is difficult because of the thickness of the surrounding tissue and the sensitive nature of this region. The caudocranial projection demonstrates little above the joint space due to muscle depth. The extended or flexed lateromedials are generally completed first (see Table 24.3).

Caudocranial (CdCr): Caudoproximal–Craniodistal (CdPr–CrDi) View of the Stifle

Patient: In natural weight-bearing position.

Image Receptor: Placed cranially to the stifle and tilted so that the long edge is snug against the body wall (Fig. 24.42). Extend the hindlimb caudally and angle the central ray 10 to 20 degrees proximodistally[1,2] (downward) to increase the ease of image receptor placement (Fig. 24.42).

X-ray Tube: Positioned caudally to the stifle joint.

Beam: Almost perpendicular to the image receptor.

Central Ray: Over the stifle joint approximately 10 cm (4 inches) distal to the patella angled 10 to 15 degrees proximodistally so the ray exits at the proximal cranial tibia level.[1]

Collimate to include: The entire patella and proximal tibia.

Label: Cranial aspect of limb.

Comments

- This view helps detect changes indicative of secondary joint disease and evaluates the joint width. The distal femoral growth center closes at 20 to 30 months of age.

The apophyseal center of the tibial tuberosity joins the proximal tibial growth center at 9 to 12 months, and the combined growth centers join the tibial shaft at 20 to 30 months.[1,4]

- Personal preference may require the image receptor to be tipped to the angle of the tibia or directly perpendicular to the ground, provided the central ray is perpendicular to the receptor.
- Human safety is a major issue. Have the receptor in position before moving in with the x-ray tube.

> ✎ **TECHNICIAN NOTES**   A firm touch is less irritating than a light touch for the patient. Introduce a gloved hand before introducing the image receptor. Try not to come in contact with the sheath of a male horse (sometimes this is unavoidable). Keep alert to any signs of agitation displayed by the patient.

FIG. 24.42 A, Positioning for caudocranial (caudoproximal–craniodistal) view of the stifle. **B,** Radiograph of the caudocranial view of the stifle.

CdLCrMO: Caudoproximal 60-Degree Lateral–Craniodistomedial Oblique (CdPr60L–CrDiMO) View of the Stifle

Patient: In natural weight bearing position (Fig. 24.43).

Image Receptor: Pushed as far into the flank as possible, resting it against the medial ridge of the trochlea.[1,4]

Central Ray: Approximately 10 cm (4 inches) on the caudal aspect of the limb at the level of the femorotibial joint[2] at a downward angle of 10 degrees.[1]

Beam: Directed horizontally, positioned caudally and laterally 60 degrees.[1,3]

Collimate to include: The entire patella and proximal tibia.

Label: Cranial aspect of limb.

FIG. 24.43 **A,** Positioning of the caudolateral–craniomedial oblique view of the stifle. **B,** Radiograph of the caudolateral–craniomedial oblique view of the stifle. (**A** courtesy Shannon Brownrigg; **B** courtesy Carolyn Bennett, Diagnostic Imaging, OVC, University of Guelph, ON.)

Skyline: Cranioproximal–Craniodistal Oblique (CrPr–CrDiO) View of the Stifle

Patient: In natural weight-bearing position. Lift the distal hindlimb, flex, and retract it caudally to place the tibia horizontally.

Image Receptor: Positioned horizontal to the ground facing the stifle—the caudal part of the plate touches the tibial crest.

Beam: Positioned dorsally and angled down to the stifle (Fig. 24.44).

Central Ray: Downward distally and 10 degrees lateral to medial.

Collimate to include: Cranial patella.

Label: Lateral aspect of limb.

Comments

- Two people may be required, with one person flexing the tarsus and the other supporting the receptor plate. All must wear PPE.
- This view is used to access fractures of the patella. The medial and lateral trochlear ridges, as well as the intertrochlear groove of the femur, are visualized.[1]

FIG. 24.44 **A,** Diagrammatic positioning for the skyline view of the stifle joint. **B,** Skyline radiographic view of the patella. (**B** courtesy Carolyn Bennett, Diagnostic Imaging, OVC, University of Guelph, ON.)

Pelvis and Hip Joints

General anesthesia is required for the pelvic radiographic study of a large animal patient. Young foals (or calves) can be successfully radiographed in the field, whereas larger patients (horses or cows) must be radiographed in the hospital setting because of the specific high-powered radiographic equipment required, such as a mobile or ceiling-mounted unit, to provide proper output (high kV exposure). Views may be segmented to obtain a complete pelvic view (multiple images used for a single view). If using film, the use of a table with an embedded cassette tunnel is preferred to increase ease of positioning and cassette exchange. Due to the thickness of this region, the use of a grid is suggested.

Special consideration must be given to the anesthesia recovery process for patients with pelvic fractures or luxation. As a result, a pelvic radiographic study may be contraindicated.

Ventrodorsal (VD) View of the Pelvis

Patient: In dorsal recumbency with the hindlimbs flexed in a "frog-leg" position (Fig. 24.45). Evacuation of the rectum may be required to minimize artifacts for pelvic symphysis evaluation.

Image Receptor: Under the pelvis.

Limbs: Positioned about 20 to 30 degrees above the surface, not touching the ground or table.

Beam: Directly vertical to the pelvis with the beam centered over the image receptor. Multiple views may be required, depending on the size of the patient.

Central Ray: Over specific areas of interest and perpendicular to the image receptor to minimize distortion.

Collimate to include: Entire pelvis if possible.

Label: Affected side.

Comments

- To maintain symmetry of the pelvic joints, it is important that both legs are positioned at the same angle and flexion.
- If more than one projection is necessary, each centering point should be marked with a marker or tape. Marking the centering points allow adjustments to be made from the previously exposed site.
- For a thorough assessment, five to seven overlapping radiographs may be required.

FIG. 24.45 **A,** Positioning for the VD view of the pelvis and coxofemoral joint. The arrow is the direction of the central ray. **B,** Radiograph of the acetabulum of an anesthetized patient in a ventrodorsal view. (**B** courtesy Carolyn Bennett, Diagnostic Imaging, OVC, University of Guelph, ON.)

Ventrodorsal Oblique View of the Pelvis (for Each Hip)

Patient: Placed in a ventrodorsal position, with the hindlimbs flexed (frog-leg) and pelvis then shifted 10 degrees to 20 degrees to elevate the unaffected side away from the tabletop. Rectal evacuation is not required for this position.

Image Receptor: Positioned under the patient.

Beam: Angled perpendicular to the image receptor.

Central Ray: Directly vertical to the hip joint and laterally from the midline over the hip joint of interest.[1,2]

Include: The entire pelvis if possible.

Label: Affected side.

Comments

- The oblique views isolate and evaluate individual hip joints. Comparative radiographs are recommended.

- A specific angle is not critical, provided it is possible to repeat the same angle on the opposite side.
- X-ray positioning devices may be helpful to maintain and repeat the angle of the pelvis. Ensure that both the hind and front ends of the horse are rotated.
- Secure the patient to prevent injury and unexpected movement. The use of ropes is critical to secure the patient on the tabletop.
- Protective padding is recommended with the use of ropes to prevent tendon and ligament injuries.
- The use of a cassette tunnel is preferred for ease of changing image receptors.
- The proximal femur can also be radiographed if the beam is centered more laterally.

Head, Neck, Thorax, and Abdomen

Note that for all positions:

Image Receptor: Is placed against the side of the skull (see Fig. 24.46) closest to the area of interest (i.e., lesion).

X-ray Tube: Is positioned on the opposite lateral side.

Position: The patient is in a natural standing posture.

Central Ray: On the area of interest and perpendicular to the image receptor.

Collimate: Tightly to include the area of interest, ensuring that labels are included and borders are visible.
See Table 24.6 for further specifics.

FIG. 24.46 **A,** Positioning for the lateral view of the skull. **B,** Diagram of the view of the lateral skull. Radiographs of the lateral skull, cranial aspect (C) and caudal aspect (D). (**A** courtesy Shannon Brownrigg; **C** and **D** courtesy Carolyn Bennett, Diagnostic Imaging, OVC, University of Guelph, ON.)

Head, Neck, Thorax, and Abdomen—cont'd

TABLE 24.6	Imaging of the Equine Head, Neck, Thorax, and Abdomen				
BODY PART	**PROJECTION**	**IMAGE RECEPTOR PLACEMENT**	**X-RAY TUBE**	**CENTRAL RAY**	**FURTHER COMMENTS**
Skull	Lateral (Fig. 24.46)	Against the affected side.	Opposite lateral side.	From the opposite side on area of interest.	
Skull	Dorsoventral (DV) (Fig. 24.47)	Horizontal ramus against the ventral aspect of the mandible.	At the dorsal aspect.	Along the midline of dorsal skull on area of interest, perpendicular to the horizontal ramus of mandible.	Easier to note asymmetry. Will need increased exposure.
Maxillary sinuses, nasal passage	Oblique views: Dorso 45-degree lateral–ventrolateral oblique (D45L–VLO) (Fig. 24.48)	Ventral, against affected side. Plate is angled 45 degrees.	Dorsolateral above the head on the opposite unaffected side.	On third and fourth cheek teeth and 45 degrees from parallel plane directed downward.	Avoids superimposition of cheek teeth. Best views for maxillary sinuses, frontal sinuses, and both dental arcades. Bilateral recommended.
Incisor	D45L–VLO	Below affected jaw and laterally.	Above affected jaw and opposite lateral.	45-degree angle directed downward on area of interest.	
Upper dental arcade	D45L–VLO	Against affected side laterally.	Position laterally against unaffected side on the dorsal head.	Downward 45 degrees from horizontal on area of interest.	Can reverse so image receptor is against unaffected side and beam is aimed upward 45 degrees (V45L-DLO).
Lower dental arcade	D45L–VLO	Unaffected side ventrally.	Laterally to affected side of head dorsally.	Downward 45 degrees from horizontal on area of interest.	
Frontal region	D30L–VLO	Affected side slightly ventrally.	Opposite unaffected side, slightly above head.	30 degrees centered on midline behind eye on the affected side.	Avoid inadvertent rostrocaudal angulation. Will need less exposure than if imaging teeth.
Teeth	V45L–DLO (Fig. 24.49)	Above affected jaw (dorsally) and laterally.	Below affected jaw (ventrally) and from opposite lateral.	45-degree angle directed upward.	Alternative view for oblique teeth. For upper dental arcade, the image receptor is placed against the unaffected side.
Teeth	Occlusal (Fig. 24.50)	In the mouth as far caudal as the patient will allow.	Maxillary: dorsal to head. Mandibular: ventral to head.	Maxillary: direct beam downward. Mandibular: direct beam upward at 60–80 degrees from vertical, depending on the conformation of incisors.	Difficult as patient not likely to cooperate without chemical restraint. Need lower exposure than for cheek teeth.

Continued

Head, Neck, Thorax, and Abdomen—cont'd

TABLE 24.6	Imaging of the Equine Head, Neck, Thorax, and Abdomen—cont'd				
BODY PART	**PROJECTION**	**IMAGE RECEPTOR PLACEMENT**	**X-RAY TUBE**	**CENTRAL RAY**	**FURTHER COMMENTS**
Guttural pouch/ larynx/ pharynx/ hyoid bones	Lateral (Fig. 24.51)	Lateral side of the caudal skull.	Horizontal beam opposite lateral side of the skull.	Caudal to vertical ramus of mandible (over guttural pouch region). At caudoventral angle of the mandible for the nasopharynx, larynx, and proximal trachea.	Portable unit may be used due to soft tissue density. Position as for routine skull views. Oblique views can be taken with 10- to 20-degree caudorostral angle.[1] Endoscopy is preferred for nasopharynx, larynx, and proximal trachea.
	Dorsoventral (DV)	Ventral: under the mandible.	Dorsal to the head.	Midline of the skull over the area of interest.	Sedation is highly recommended.
Cervical spine	Lateral (Fig. 24.52)	Side of the cervical region.	Opposite side of neck.	Centered on region of choice: C2 C4 C6	Because of the size of the patient, the cervical spine must be exposed in three views. The patient can be standing or recumbent.
Thoracic spine	Lateral	Side of the patient on area of interest.	Opposite side.	Area of interest is perpendicular to the image receptor.	Often completed for the dorsal spinous processes (withers).
Thorax	Lateral (Fig. 24.53)	Affected side	Horizontal beam on opposite side.	See comments later for specifics: 1. Midcraniodorsal 2. Midcaudodorsal 3. Midcranioventral 4. Midcaudoventral	Patient standing. Portable unit not powerful enough.
Abdomen	Lateral (Fig. 24.54)	On side (most lesions on midline).	Opposite side.	Last rib for small horses: 1. Midcranioventral 2. Midabdominal 3. Midcaudodorsal	Multiple laterals required for larger patients.

FIG. 24.47 A, Positioning for the dorsoventral view of the skull. **B,** Radiograph of the dorsoventral view of the skull. (**A** courtesy Shannon Brownrigg; **B** courtesy Carolyn Bennett, Diagnostic Imaging, OVC, University of Guelph, ON.)

FIG. 24.49 A, Positioning for the oblique view of the teeth. Also referred to as a lateral 30-degree dorsal–lateroventral oblique. **B,** Radiograph of the oblique projection of the skull. (**A** courtesy Shannon Brownrigg; **B** courtesy Carolyn Bennett, Diagnostic Imaging, OVC, University of Guelph, ON.)

FIG. 24.48 Positioning for the Oblique View of the Skull. (Courtesy Shannon Brownrigg.)

Head, Neck, Thorax, and Abdomen—cont'd

FIG. 24.50 **A,** Diagrammatic positioning for an intraoral rostrocaudal oblique radiograph to evaluate the rostral aspect of the incisive bone and the incisors. The downward arrow is the direction of the central ray for radiography of the maxilla, and the upward arrow indicates the direction of the central ray for the mandibular structures. **B,** Radiograph of the intraoral rostrocaudal mandibular incisors. Note the fractured incisor.

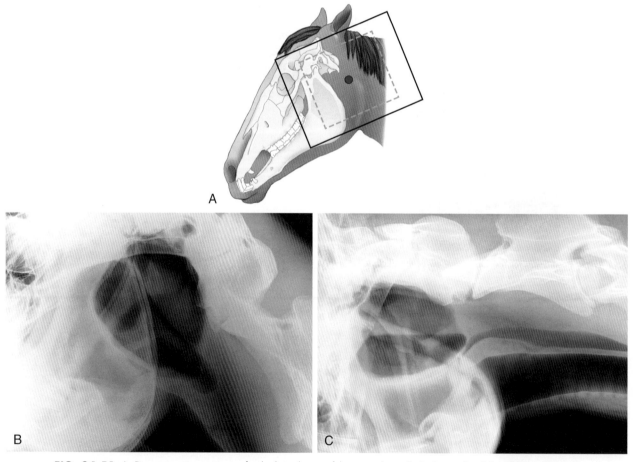

FIG. 24.51 **A,** Diagrammatic positioning for the lateral view of the guttural pouch. Radiographs of the **(B)** lateral guttural pouch; **(C)** larynx/pharynx. (B and C courtesy Carolyn Bennett, Diagnostic Imaging, OVC, University of Guelph, ON.)

Head, Neck, Thorax, and Abdomen—cont'd

FIG. 24.52 **A,** Positioning of the cervical vertebrae. Note the three areas of centering, C2, C4, and C6. Radiographs of the lateral cervical spine series: **B,** C1 and C2; **C,** C3 and C4; **D,** C4 and C5; **E,** C6 and C7. (**A** courtesy Dr. Usha Knabe, Knabe Equine Veterinary Services, Orangeville, ON; **B–E** courtesy Carolyn Bennett, Diagnostic Imaging, OVC, University of Guelph, ON.)

Head, Neck, Thorax, and Abdomen—cont'd

FIG. 24.53 A, Thorax areas of centering for the four main views. Lateral radiographs of the cranioventral thorax **(B)** craniodorsal thorax **(C)** caudoventral thorax

Head, Neck, Thorax, and Abdomen—cont'd

D   E   R

L

FIG. 24.53, cont'd (D) and caudodorsal thorax (E). (B–E courtesy Carolyn Bennett, Diagnostic Imaging, OVC, University of Guelph, ON.)

FIG 24.54 Radiographic Quadrants of the Equine Abdomen.

Head, Neck, Thorax, and Abdomen—cont'd

Skull Comments

- Isolate the area of interest due to skull density and multiple areas of interest. For best results, multiple views are recommended, including oblique views. Keep the plate closest to the area of interest.
- It is difficult to minimize movement of the skull. Sedation is crucial for most horses to obtain high-quality radiographs with minimal retakes.
- Removal of the nylon halter is required to avoid artifacts. A commercial or homemade rope halter should be used. Inspect the rope for small metal clips, which are often present in manufactured rope products.
- The head is held without rotation. A lead rope placed under the chin and pulled upward may help stabilize the head. **Resting the chin on a tall stool or upside-down trash can provides better stability and less movement.** Placing a cover over the patient's eyes may be helpful. Maintaining constant contact will keep the horse at ease and prevent reaction to changes in positioning.
- Lowering the level of the head by extension or mild pressure allows for easier positioning of the unit and the image receptor.
- The weight of the x-ray unit may make it difficult and awkward to hold the unit motionless at the level of the skull. The use of a stand or ceiling-mounted unit is suggested.
- Flush the oral cavity to remove any foodstuffs to prevent artifacts.
- If the patient is sedated, an oral gag may be used to improve the isolation of the selected arcade for oblique views. An incisor block can be used for oblique views.
- Barium or malleable metal may be used to mark draining facial tracts.

> ✎ **TECHNICIAN NOTES** The dental formula (see Chapter 22 for further explanation) of the horse is:
> - Deciduous: 2(di3/3, dc 0/0, dp 3/3) = 24
> - Permanent: 2(I3/3, *C1/1, *P3-4/3, M3/3) = 36 to 42

*Mares often do not have canine teeth; the first premolars, called *wolf teeth*, may not be present in either gender.

Cervical Spine Comments

- Remember that the cervical spine is located in the ventral portion of the neck. If the patient is in lateral recumbency, positioning devices are required to position the spine parallel to the table.
- An increase in exposure factors is needed. Flexed lateral, ventrodorsal, and oblique views are optional. Collimate to the bones (Fig. 24.52).
- Consider placing radiopaque markers dorsal to the vertebrae for identification and repeat radiographs.

Thoracic Spine Comments

- A lower-powered unit can be used to visualize the dorsal spinous processes (withers) of the thoracic spine. Mobile equipment may be used with smaller patients (i.e., foals). For the ventral portion of the thoracic vertebrae, a high-powered x-ray apparatus and a grid are needed.
- Patient positioning is similar to that for radiographs of the thorax, except that the central ray is over the thoracic spine.

Thorax Comments

- High kVp with a grid is used and the SID is usually increased to 200 cm (80 inches). The caudodorsal region could be imaged with low-output equipment, short SID, and fast intensifying screens.
- Radiographs are generally taken at full inspiration.
- In a natural standing position, the elbows of a horse are superimposed over the cranial region of the thorax. Extend the forelimbs to prevent superimposition.
- Center for the following regions in an average-size horse. Use a large image receptor and collimate to within the margins[1] (Fig. 24.53):
  - Craniodorsal: 10 to 15 cm (4 to 6 inches) ventral to the most caudal point of the scapula.
  - Caudodorsal: 20 cm (8 inches) caudal to and 15 cm (6 inches) ventral to the most caudal part of the scapula.
  - Cranioventral: 15 cm (6 inches) caudal to the shoulder joint.
  - Caudoventral: 20 cm (8 inches) ventral to and 10 cm (4 inches) caudal to most caudal point of the scapula.

Abdomen Comments (Fig. 24.54)

- Equipment and preparation are as for the thorax, with high-powered equipment being needed to penetrate the thick tissue.
- The abdomen of the horse can be radiographed in standing or recumbent position.
- Diagnostic ultrasound is generally used in lieu of abdominal radiographs.

Other Large-Animal Radiography

Bovine

Even if they are frequently handled, bovine patients have little to no experience of manipulation of their lower extremities, which poses a challenge to perform these radiographs. Maintaining image receptor placement close to the limb without proper restraint devices is almost impossible in most conditions. It is because of these challenges, as well as economic concerns, that radiographs are generally completed only in high-quality or high-producing livestock.

The use of stocks, ropes, and pulley, or ideally, a tilt table, will aid in the production of quality radiographs of cattle. The use of stocks provides reduced mobility of the patient; however, they do not limit the mobility of the limbs. Securing the affected limb or, if weight bearing, rigging an alternate limb through ropes, may be required. The use of a tilt table enables the limbs to be secured in a motionless fashion and increases positioning options because the patient can be lifted and tilted off the ground. The lifting of the alternate limb may increase the safety of maneuvering around distal extremities. Sedation or rapid general anesthesia may be used with the bovine patient. The combined use of restraint devices and sedation can significantly increase the safety of personnel, equipment, and the patient for bovine radiographs. Care must be taken to consider the stage of gestation, if applicable, and the potential for recovery trauma.

Equipment requirements and positioning techniques for bovine radiography are the same as those for equine radiography. Handling restrictions may hinder the options and available positions. Pelvis, skull, spine, thorax, and abdomen radiographs are completed much like those in horses following the procedures for centering, inclusion and collimation. In the case of a small calf, radiographs may be performed in the clinic with use of positioning and techniques similar to those used for a large dog. A mobile x-ray machine can be used to take thoracic or abdominal radiographs in a small calf.

See Table 24.7 for the common views of the skeleton and keep these principles in mind:

Center: On the area of interest (Fig. 24.55).
Include: Distal joint: Up to one-third of the bones proximal and distal.
Bone: Include the joints proximal and distal.
Collimate: Tightly to include the area of interest, ensuring that labels are included and borders are visible.

TABLE 24.7   Suggested Views for the Bovine Limb Examination

STRUCTURES	COMMON NAME	SPECIFIC TERMINOLOGY*	POSITION†	CENTRAL RAY IS POSITIONED
Digit/foot: P-III (distal phalanx, coffin bone) P-II (middle phalanx) P-I (proximal phalanx-pastern) Proximal interphalangeal joint (pastern joint) joint	DP (Standard) (Fig. 24.55)	Dorsal 45-degree proximal–palmarodistal (D45Pr–PaDi)	Foot slightly forward on image receptor.	Perpendicular to foot axis at MSP (midsagittal plane) at area of interest with beam angled ~45 degrees to ground
	Lateral (Standard) (Fig. 24.55C)	Lateromedial	On a block to elevate limb for P-III; resting on ground for other views.	90 degrees lateral to MSP, parallel to ground on area of interest: coronary band for PIII
	Lateral-interdigit (Ancillary)	Lateromedial (mediolateral) with interdigital film	Receptor between digits. Easiest with patient in lateral recumbency but can be completed standing with foot raised.	90 degrees laterally from MSP to radiograph the lateral claw. 90 degrees medially from MSP medially to radiograph the medial claw.
	DLPMO (Ancillary) (Fig. 24.55D)	Dorsoproximal 45-degree lateral–palmarodistomedial oblique (DPr45L–PaDiMO)/(DPr45M–PDiLO)	As for the lateral view for P-III.	45 degrees to ground on the area of interest
	DMPLO (Ancillary)	Dorsoproximal 45-degree medial–palmarodistolateral oblique (DPr45M–PaDiLO) (DMPLO)	As for the DP view for P-II and P-I	45 degrees lateral to MSP directed either laterally (DLPMO) or medially (DMPLO)
Fetlock joint and proximal sesamoid bones	Dorsopalmar: DP (Standard)	Dorsoproximal–palmarodistal (DPr–PaDi)	Foot on ground, full weight bearing and cassette against palmar aspect.	On MSP parallel to the ground, centered at the fetlock

Continued

TABLE 24.7	Suggested Views for the Bovine Limb Examination—Cont'd			
STRUCTURES	**COMMON NAME**	**SPECIFIC TERMINOLOGY***	**POSITION†**	**CENTRAL RAY IS POSITIONED**
Metacarpophalan-geal/metatarsophalan-geal articulation	Lateral (Standard)	Lateromedial extended (LM).	Foot on ground, full bearing and cassette against medial aspect.	90 degrees laterally from MSP parallel to the ground directed toward the fetlock joint.
	DLPMO (Ancillary)	Dorsoproximal 30-degree lateral–palmarodistomedial oblique (DPr30L–PaDiMO) (DLPMO).	Foot on ground, full weight bearing and cassette against medial aspect of palmar surface	45 degrees lateral to MSP directed either laterally (DLPMO).
	DMPLO (Ancillary)	Dorsoproximal 30-degree medial–palmarodistolateral oblique (DPr30M–PaDiLO) (DMPLO)	Foot on ground, full weight bearing and cassette against lateral aspect of palmar surface	Or medially (DMPLO) and parallel to ground on the fetlock joint or the proximal sesamoid bones.
Carpus‡	DP (Standard)	Dorsoproximal–palmarodistal (DPr–PaDi)	Weight bearing with limbs evenly on ground and cassette on palmar aspect of limb.	Parallel to the ground, centered on palpable intercarpal joint space; slightly lateral to MSP as legs are slightly rotated externally when standing.
	Lateral (Standard)	Lateromedial extended (LM)	Weight bearing with limbs evenly on ground and cassette against medial aspect of limb.	90 degrees lateral to MSP; parallel to ground just distal and dorsal to prominence of accessory carpal bone.
Elbow joint	CdCr (Standard)	Caudoproximal–cranio-distal–standing (CdPr–CrDi)	Weight bearing with limbs evenly on ground and cassette against cranial aspect of joint at angle to the x-ray beam.	Caudal to joint; parallel to ground so beam perpendicular to radius.
	Lateral (Standard)	Lateromedial standing (LM)	Weight bearing with limbs evenly on ground; cassette against medial aspect of joint at angle to the x-ray beam.	90 degrees lateral to MSP, parallel to ground on either the elbow joint or olecranon if required.
	CrCd (Ancillary)	Cranioproximal–caudodistal standing (CrPr–CdDi)	Weight bearing with limbs evenly on ground and cassette parallel against caudal aspect of olecranon and per-pendicular to the lateral chest wall.	Directed upward at 20–30 degrees craniodistal to caudoproximal.
Shoulder	Tangential oblique (Standard)	Caudomedial–Craniolateral oblique**	Weight bearing with limb in normal position and image receptor placed vertically cra-nial to shoulder and pushed medially to en-sure that the lateral tu-berosity of the humerus will be imaged.	Caudally and is lateral and slightly dorsal to middle of thorax, angled downward, centered at the craniolateral aspect of the proximal humerus.

TABLE 24.7	Suggested Views for the Bovine Limb Examination—Cont'd			
STRUCTURES	**COMMON NAME**	**SPECIFIC TERMINOLOGY***	**POSITION†**	**CENTRAL RAY IS POSITIONED**
	Lateral (Ancillary since lateral recumbency required).	Mediolateral recumbent (ML).	In lateral recumbency with affected limb down and pulled cranially. with the humeral head superimposed over the soft tissue of the neck.	Above the patient with the beam perpendicular to the ground and centered on the shoulder joint or area of interest.
Tarsus	DP (two views) (Standard).	Horizontal dorsoplantar (1) 10 degrees dorsoproximal–plantarodistal (2).	For both views: full weight bearing with digit pointing slightly outward so beam is not under the patient. Image receptor against plantar aspect of tarsus parallel with calcaneus.	Dorsally and slightly laterally on MSP centered on palpable trochlea. For view 1: beam is parallel to ground (shows tarsometatarsal joint space). For view 2: angle 10 degrees downward in dorsoproximal to plantarodistal angle (for intertarsal joint space).
	Lateral (Standard).	Lateromedial.	Weight bearing with limbs evenly on ground and cassette against medial aspect of limb.	10 cm (4 inches) distal to point of hock.
Stifle	Caudocranial CdCr (Standard).	Caudoproximal–craniodistal standing (CdPr–CrDi).	Weight bearing with limbs evenly on ground and vertical cassette against cranial aspect of patella at right angle to body wall, placed as far proximal and pushed as far medially as abdomen permits.	Caudal to the joint and directed downward to obtain a "tunnel" view of the distal femur.
	Lateral (Standard).	Lateromedial.	Weight bearing with limbs evenly on ground and cassette against medial aspect of joint.	Laterally, parallel to the ground and centered distal and caudal to the patella.
	Lateral patella (Ancillary).	Lateromedial (LM) patella.	Weight bearing with limbs evenly on ground and cassette against medial aspect of patella further proximally and cranially than for regular LM view.	Parallel to the ground and centered on the patella.

**Palmar(o)* is used with the understanding that *plantar(o)* can be substituted when referring to the hindlimb.

†Further specifications with preparation and positioning for the digit: Before a digit radiograph is taken in the bovine patient, the interdigital space and both claws should be cleansed thoroughly and lightly trimmed. If this step is not taken, false images or shadows may mask abnormalities present in the claws. The digits can be viewed radiographically using four angles or projections.[4]

‡Ancillary views for the carpus include the lateromedial flexed, dorsolateral–palmaromedial oblique (DLPMO), and dorsomedial–palmarolateral oblique (DMPLO). The oblique views are also possible for the elbow joint.

**Usually only the area of the acromion process of the scapula and lateral tubercles of the humerus are visualized on the oblique views and not the character of the shoulder joint. There is extensive scatter radiation due to increased soft tissue. The oblique view is best combined with the lateral view in a recumbent patient.

Further studies of the bovine include pelvis (dorsal recumbency only with hindlimbs extended laterally as much as possible); the head (please see the equine for similar positioning); and the spine, thorax, and abdomen (also see as per the equine patient).

FIG. 24.55 A, Positioning for the dorsopalmar (plantar) (dorsoproximal–palmarodistal oblique [DPr–PaDiO]) view of the distal phalanx (PIII). Positioning is similar to that used in equine limb studies. The accurate description is D45Pr–PaDiO because the beam is 45 degrees to the ground. B, Radiograph of cattle DP view of the foot. C, Radiograph of cattle lateral view of phalanx. As per the equine limb, the beam is parallel to the ground and 90 degrees to the MSP (midsagittal plane). D, Oblique view of a cattle foot. (B–E courtesy Carolyn Bennett, Diagnostic Imaging, OVC, University of Guelph, ON.)

Ovine/Caprine/Porcine

Small ruminant patients (sheep/goats) and swine can be radiographed much like small animals following the same principles of positioning, centering, inclusion, and collimation (Fig. 24.56). Small ruminant patients are often radiographed within a clinic setting because they can be easily transported. Care must be taken to prevent injury due to patient response to fear (i.e., thrashing of limbs), as they have minimal handling experience. If the patient is horned, special precautions to prevent injury to staff must be taken. Sedation is recommended to produce quality radiographs in an efficient manner.

The fleece of the ovine patient is dense and may contain dirt and debris (i.e., twigs, clumps of mud/stones). Before imaging, carefully inspect and remove debris that may produce artifacts within the image.

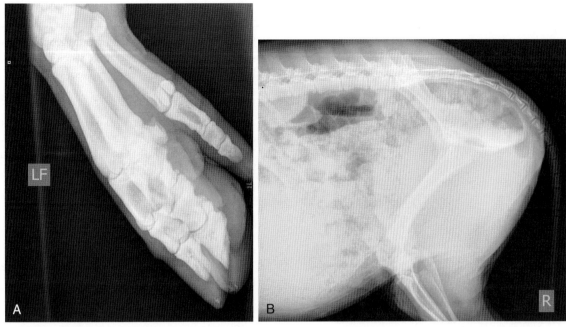

FIG. 24.56 A, Radiograph of lateral view of digits/metacarpus of a swine. **B,** Radiograph of caprine abdomen. (Courtesy Carolyn Bennett, Diagnostic Imaging, OVC, University of Guelph, ON.)

> ✏ **TECHNICIAN NOTES** Think of positioning cattle for x-rays as being similar to horses with exceptions due to limb angles or anatomy; positioning of sheep and swine is similar to the dog. Restraint is different for all species.

Alternate Modality Images

It is beyond the scope of this section to discuss alternate modalities (Fig. 24.57). Please see Part A, Chapters 10–14 for alternate imaging such as ultrasonography, nuclear scintigraphy, infrared thermal imaging, and MRI. These modes are more diagnostic but are considerably more expensive than radiography.

Fig. 24.58 is a mystery radiograph. Review it and answer the question presented with it.

FIG. 24.57 A, Nuclear scintigraphy of the front limbs indicating dark areas known as "hot spots" or inflammation on the carpus. **B,** Infrared thermal image of another horse. The red areas indicate "hot spots" or inflammation. (**A** courtesy Jill McFadden Surette, Toronto Equine Hospital, Mississauga, ON; **B** courtesy Vetel Diagnostics San Luis Obispos, CA; and Seth Wallack, DVM, DACVR, AAVR, director and CEO.)

FIG. 24.58 Mystery Radiograph. What body part and position is this? Where is the image receptor placed?

⁕ KEY POINTS

1. Patience, planning, proper preparation, and knowledge of anatomy and directional terms are all required for diagnostic large-animal radiographs.
2. Large animals are generally weight bearing when imaging, which necessitates the use of a horizontal beam.
3. Radiation, patient, and human safety need to be kept in mind at all times.
4. A minimum of four views is required because of the unique anatomy of the equine limb. These views are dorsopalmar/dorsoplantar, lateromedial, and two oblique views (one on either side of the midsagittal plane [MSP] taken between the DP and lateromedial positions).
5. If joints are to be examined, further positions may include a flexed lateral, skyline, or flexor view.
6. The same principles of radiography apply to all species, including the angle of the beam always being perpendicular to the area of interest. In the equine patient, the angle of the beam to the ground for dorsopalmar/dorsoplantar and oblique radiographs may vary according to the foot trimming and anatomy. For lateromedial views, the beam is always parallel to the ground.
7. Standard radiographs for cloven-footed large animals are generally the dorsopalmar/dorsoplantar and lateromedial views with occasional oblique projections for joints.

REVIEW QUESTIONS

1. Safety is a priority when taking radiographs. To keep personnel away from the central ray when the metacarpus of large animals is being radiographed, you should:
   a. Use a cassette tunnel
   b. Use a foot block with a cassette slot
   c. Use a cassette holder with a clamp and long handle
   d. Hold the cassette
2. When viewing a DMPLO radiograph of the equine fetlock, you should place the image on the viewer so that the proximal cannon bone is positioned:
   a. Down with the dorsal aspect to your left
   b. Up with the dorsal aspect to your left
   c. Up with the dorsal aspect to your right
   d. Down with the dorsal aspect to your right
3. To prevent air artifacts when radiographing the equine foot, it is best to use:
   a. Play-Doh
   b. Sand
   c. Styrofoam
   d. Plaster
4. The dorsal 65-degree proximal–palmarodistal oblique (D65Pr–PaDiO) view of the distal phalanx means that the beam is angled:
   a. To the ground, 65 degrees palmaroproximal
   b. 65 degrees from the MSP and to the ground
   c. 65 degrees to the limb, dorsoproximal
   d. To the ground, 65 degrees dorsoproximal
5. The dorsal 65-degree proximal–palmarodistal oblique (D65Pr–PaDiO) view of the digit is also known as a:
   a. True DP view
   b. Lateral oblique view
   c. High coronary view
   d. Upright pedal view
6. A human wrist is equivalent to the equine:
   a. Proximal phalanx
   b. Metacarpal interphalangeal joint
   c. Carpus
   d. Fetlock joint
7. For the upright pedal route of the navicular bone, the foot will be:
   a. Pointed on a block with the beam parallel to the ground
   b. Placed flat on the tunnel cassette with the beam angled
   c. Placed flat on a block with the beam angled to the ground
   d. Placed flat on the tunnel cassette with the beam parallel to the ground

8. For a true DP view of the navicular bone, you need to include:
   a. Navicular only
   b. P3, navicular, and P2
   c. P1, navicular, and P2
   d. Coffin bone, navicular, and long pastern

9. The descriptive terminology for a DLPMO is:
   a. Dorsal 45-degree proximal lateral–palmarodistomedial oblique
   b. Dorsoproximal 45-degree lateral–palmarodistomedial oblique
   c. Dorsoproximal 45-degree medial–palmarodistolateral oblique
   d. Dorso 45-degree proximal medial–palmarodistolateral oblique

10. You are preparing to image the DMPLO of the digit of a Thoroughbred. The image receptor should be placed at the _____ oblique aspect of the limb and the beam directed dorsal 65 degrees proximal and _____
    a. lateral; 45 degrees at the lateral
    b. lateral; 45 degrees at the medial
    c. medial; 45 degrees at the medial
    d. medial; 45 degrees at the lateral

11. The veterinarian will request that you complete the DMPLO view of the digit to visualize the _____ wing of the coffin bone, which will appear _____ on the image.
    a. lateral; smaller and denser
    b. lateral; larger and less dense
    c. medial; smaller and denser
    d. medial; larger and less dense

12. To image the fetlock, the image receptor should be placed against the:
    a. Medial aspect of the limb, perpendicular to the ground for a flexed lateral view
    b. Medial aspect of the limb, perpendicular to the ground for a DP view
    c. Medial aspect of the limb, parallel with the ground for a flexed lateral view
    d. Lateral side of the limb, perpendicular to the ground for a lateromedial view

13. The splint bones are the:
    a. First and fifth metacarpus/metatarsus
    b. Second and fourth metacarpus/metatarsus
    c. Second and third metacarpus/metatarsus
    d. Third and fourth metacarpus/metatarsus

14. You are required to complete a lateromedial view of the metacarpals of an Arabian. The central ray is:
    a. On the medial aspect and angled 90 degrees from the MSP
    b. Angled to the ground and 90 degrees from the MSP
    c. Parallel to the ground and angled 90 degrees from the MSP
    d. Parallel to the ground and angled 45 degrees from the MSP

15. To position for the craniocaudal view of the elbow, place the image receptor on the:
    a. Palmar aspect of the joint
    b. Plantar aspect of the joint
    c. Cranial aspect of the joint
    d. Caudal aspect of the joint

16. Oblique views are necessary for an equine dental survey to avoid:
    a. Increased amount of soft tissue on the head
    b. Superimposition of the guttural pouch
    c. Superimposition of the frontal sinuses
    d. Superimposition of the opposite arcade

17. Pelvic radiographs may be contraindicated in equine patients with a pelvic injury because:
    a. Anesthesia poses a risk to the equine patient
    b. Patient recovery may cause additional injury
    c. Pelvic radiographs are often unsuccessful
    d. Pelvic radiographs are never contraindicated

18. The SID for large animals is generally:
    a. The same as for small animals
    b. Not of concern
    c. Shorter than for small animals
    d. Longer than for small animals

19. You are required to complete a carpus DP view for a Holstein cow (dairy). You should position the central ray:
    a. Parallel to the ground and slightly lateral to the MSP
    b. Parallel to the ground on the MSP
    c. Parallel to the ground slightly medial to the MSP
    d. At a slight angle to the ground on the MSP

20. The view that is completed for cattle but not performed on an equine P3 is the:
    a. Lateromedial view
    b. Dorsal 45-degree proximal–palmarodistal view
    c. Lateromedial (mediolateral) view with interdigital image receptor
    d. Dorsal 45-degree lateral–palmaromedial oblique

Chapter Review Question answers are located in the Instructor Resources on Evolve and can be provided to students at the discretion of the instructor.

References

1. Weaver M, Barakzai S. *Handbook of Equine Radiography.* London: Saunders Elsevier; 2010.
2. Butler JA, Colles CM, Dyson SJ, et al. *Clinical Radiology of the Horse.* Osney Mead, Oxford: Wiley-Blackwell; 2008.
3. Aiello, S.E, Moses,M. *The Merck Veterinary Manual,* 11 ed. Kenilworth, NJ: Wiley; 2016.
4. Thrall DE. *Textbook of Veterinary Diagnostic Radiology.* 7th ed. St. Louis: Elsevier; 2018.

Bibliography

American College of Veterinary Radiology (ACVR). *Radiology 2—Equine*. ACVR; 2009.

Aspinall V, Cappello M. *Introduction to Veterinary Anatomy*. London: Butterman-Heineman; 2009.

Colville T, Bassert J. *Clinical Anatomy and Physiology for Veterinary Technicians*. 3rd ed. St. Louis: Mosby; 2016.

Crawford SJ. *Equine Radiography: Positioning Techniques and Tips for Acquiring Good Images*. August 2012. Available at: http://www.slideshare.net/ShalynCrawfordGarman/equine-radiography-positioning-techniques-tips-for-acquiring-good-images.

Done SH, Goody PC, Evans S, Stickland NC. *Color Atlas of Veterinary Anatomy, the Dog and Cat*. London: Mosby; 2009.

Garrett KS, Berk JT. *How to Properly Position Thoroughbred Repository Radiographs*. December 6, 2006. Available at: https://www.ivis.org/library/aaep/aaep-annual-convention-san-antonio-2006/how-to-properly-position-thoroughbred-repository-radiographs

Radiology of the equine limbs. n.d. Available at: http://www.quia.com/files/quia/users/medicinehawk/2407-Vet/Radiology-2.pdf.

Redden RF. Radiographic imaging of the equine foot. *Vet Clin North Am Equine Pract*. 2003;19(2):379-392, vi. doi: 10.1016/

Romich J. *An Illustrated Guide to Veterinary Medical Terminology*. 4th ed. Stamford, CT: Cengage Learning; 2015.

Singh B. *Dyce, Sack and Wensing's Textbook of Veterinary Anatomy*. 5th ed. St. Louis: Elsevier; 2018.

Smallwood JE, Shively MJ, Rendano VT, et al. A standardized nomenclature for radiographic projections used in veterinary medicine. *Vet Radiol*. 1985;24:2-9.

CHAPTER 25

Avian and Exotic Radiography*

Marg Brown, RVT, BEd Ad Ed

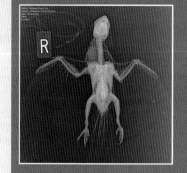

The bird dares to break the shell, then the shell breaks open and the bird can fly openly. This is the simplest principle of success. You dream, you dare, and you fly.
—Israelmore Ayivor (1989), Author

OUTLINE

LEARNING OBJECTIVES

When you have finished this chapter, you will be able to:

1. Produce diagnostic high-quality images of birds, exotic companion mammals, and reptiles with special emphasis on nonmanual restraint.
2. Position the body part parallel to the image receptor with the central ray perpendicular to both.
3. Focus on patient and machine preparation, centering and inclusion when positioning.
4. Describe reasons for imaging, normal views, and protocols for various species.
5. Identify normal avian and exotic species anatomy found on a radiograph.

*Special thanks to Lorelei D'Avolio, LVT, VTS (Exotics), CVPM, from The Center for Avian and Exotic Medicine, NYC for her meticulous editing and assistance of this chapter.

Key terms are defined in the Glossary on the Evolve website.

Amphibian	Coelom	Horizontal beam	Positional terminology
Cloacagram	Gavaging	Orthogonal	Testudine

TECHNICAL NOTE: To preserve space, the radiographic images presented in this chapter do not show collimation. For safety, always collimate so that the beam is limited to within the image receptor edges. In film radiography, there should be a clear border of collimation (frame) on every radiograph. In some jurisdictions, evidence of collimation is required by law. In digital imaging, the algorithm depends on proper collimation.

Introduction

- Medical imaging is an important diagnostic tool in avian and exotic veterinary medicine (Table 25.1) because anatomy of the respiratory tract limits auscultation, and palpation of the viscera is difficult.
- Radiographs are often required by the veterinarian for avian patients that show obscure clinical signs. Fortunately, the bird's system of air sacs provides enhanced contrast in areas that are not well visualized in mammals.
- Very small variations in x-ray output are more noticeable in the avian patient than in mammals because of their smaller size; thus an x-ray unit with uniform output is required. The machine should be capable of producing at least 300 milliamperes (mA) and have an exposure time of 1/120 seconds or shorter with a kilovolt (kV) range from a minimum of 40 kV that should be adjustable in 1-kV increments. Short exposure times are essential to minimize the motion artifacts associated with a rapid respiratory rate and muscle tremors that are common in birds as well as in some exotic companion mammals.
- Because of lower bone density than in reptiles or mammals, less exposure is needed for birds of the same thickness. Wing radiographs are often overpenetrated, making this area appear excessively dark with low contrast. Unlike with dogs and cats, most exposure charts for exotics are based on species and size and not on measurement.
- If there is not a specific avian or exotic small mammal chart, the cat abdomen chart for that thickness is useful, especially for the larger small exotics such as rabbits. Decrease the milliampere-seconds (mAs) by at least 50%. Alternatively, the feline extremity chart can be used by halving the exposure. If a measurement is required, do so at the thickest body part of the area to be examined.
- The general positioning principles of canine and feline radiography apply to avian and exotic companion mammal imaging—two orthogonal views should be taken. A shorter scale of contrast, associated with lower kV in the 40 to 60 kV range, is preferred.

TABLE 25.1	Recommended Views of Exotic Species for Complete Body Study	
SPECIES	**RECOMMENDED VIEW**	**OPTIONAL**
Avian	VD: coelom (whole body) Lateral: coelom (whole body) with wing superimposition	Modified lateral: whole body; wings not superimposed Wing: CdCr and mediolateral Lateral and VD Foot: lateral and CrCd Contrast study for GI tract Urography for urinary tract
Smaller exotic companion mammals	VD: whole body or site of interest Lateral: whole body or site of interest Skull: DV and lateral Extremities: lateral and ventral recumbency	Contrast study for GI Further skull views
Lizards	Whole body: DV with vertical beam Whole body: lateral with horizontal beam	Extremities: vertical beam Contrast study for GI
Chelonian	DV with vertical beam Lateral: horizontal (preferred). Craniocaudal: horizontal beam (preferred)	Contrast study for GI
Snakes	DV: whole body for GI, cranial 2/3 for respiratory Whole body for GI: lateral view, with horizontal beam	Contrast study for GI

Cd, Caudal; *Cr,* cranial; *DV,* dorsoventral; *GI,* gastrointestinal; *VD,* ventrodorsal.

- Nonscreen film (larger dental film, size 4) is useful, and high-detail film/screen systems produce images with good detail. If available, a mammography cassette with a single screen and with single emulsion film is especially diagnostic. As a guide, about four times the mAs will be required over a regular 400-speed system, 1/120 sec or shorter, with a kilovolt range from a minimum of 40 kV.
- Digital radiography systems often use higher kV techniques than the film/screen systems, possibly leading to lower contrast, but incremental changes of 1 kV will help with adjustments to achieve the proper contrast. However, a greater image contrast range, resulting in improved image quality, is more possible in digital radiography than with film imaging. Special algorithms for digital units are required. These are often provided by the manufacturers.[1]
- Further detail can also be achieved with smaller focal spots. Grids are not typically used because even for those patients over 10 cm, the air within the air sacs of birds, for example, does not generate noteworthy scatter radiation.
- The tube stand should have source-image distance (SID) adjustments that can compensate for changing the mAs to decrease the exposure time. The minimum SID used should be 76 cm (30 inches) unless a magnification study is required. Recall from Chapter 6 that mAs are inversely proportional to the square of the distance from the x-ray source (focal spot) and that as you decrease the distance from the source, you can also decrease the mAs. In addition, as SID decreases, magnification increases, also affecting penumbra.
- Dental units can be used, but due to lower mAs settings, respiratory movement will be more noticeable than regular units. It is best if the patient is anesthetized, small (typically less than 20 g for birds), and the area localized. Portable units used for large animals also typically do not produce sufficient mA values at the required short exposure times without drastically reducing the SID.

- Ultrasound, computerized tomography, and magnetic resonance imaging are more diagnostic modalities but are very expensive and not always readily available.

Avian Radiography

Patient Preparation

- A bird is best fasted so that the crop (for those species that possess one) feels empty on palpation. The time varies greatly with species and can range from 1 to multiple hours. The crop and proventriculus emptying times may be prolonged in dehydrated birds. Digestive tract contents may obscure the radiographic appearances of the internal organs, possibly leading to misdiagnosis.[1]
- Recall that in canine and feline patients, thorax radiographs should be taken at peak inspiration. In the avian patient, the effect of the respiratory cycle on the radiographic appearance is less noticeable, as the lungs are nonexpansile, and air is continuously moving into the pulmonary parenchyma and the air sac. Distention of the abdominal air sacs may enhance the contrast of the abdominal viscera, especially those with abundant coelomic fat.
- Respiratory movements should be minimized, if possible, by trying to coordinate the exposure time during a pause in the respiratory cycle. Positive-pressure ventilation can be applied to an intubated, anesthetized bird for air sac inflation, and radiographic exposure can then be timed accordingly to correspond with increased air in the sacs.
- Bird-positioning devices or restraint boards may simplify and reduce the time required for correct positioning (Fig. 25.1). Extensions such as intravenous (IV) tubing, Velcro, rope, or gauze can be used in lieu of tape to attach the limbs to the positioner or to the table. Alternatively, sandbags can be gently placed over the extensions.

A B

FIG. 25.1 Two Types of Avian Restrainers. **A,** VSP Avian Neck Restraint and VSP Avian Restraint Board (Veterinary Specialty Products, Shawnee, KS). Different-sized collars or suction cups are available. **B,** VSP Miami Vise Avian Restraint. Another type of positioner is the Auspex Avian Positioner (Jorgensen Laboratories, Inc., Loveland, CO; not shown).

FIG. 25.2 Three Types of Tape Used for Avian and Exotic Restraint. *Left,* Transparent medical tape is best, as it does not pull the feathers off birds. *Center,* Paper masking tape or autoclave tape also minimizes hair and feather loss. *Right,* Adhesive tape could pull off feathers and hair and is not suggested. Floral tape is also effective. (Courtesy Rick Axelson, Links Road Animal Clinic, North York, ON.)

- If using tape to secure extremities, ensure that the tape will not rip out feathers. Using masking tape or a floral Millipore tape causes less damage to the skin and feathers (Fig. 25.2) than porous medical tape. Always remove tape in the direction the feathers are pointed.

Sedation and Anesthesia

- Providing sedation and anesthesia while imaging will decrease the stress of obtaining radiographs. Sedation alone may be preferable to full anesthesia, especially in sick birds. Combining midazolam (1–2 mg/kg intranasal [IN] or intramuscular [IM]) and butorphanol (1–2 mg/kg IN or IM) is often enough to decrease stress and position birds properly. Sedatives will also decrease minimum alveolar concentration (MAC), which will decrease the amount of anesthetic gas required if needed.
- Anesthetizing a healthy bird with sedation and inhalation gas anesthesia is generally safe and will be less stressful for the patient than taking radiographs without chemical restraint. Radiographs are generally of higher quality, and fewer images need to be taken because there is less chance of motion artifacts when the patient is anesthetized. Positioning is easier and there is less potential for patient struggling and consequent iatrogenic fractures.
- If anesthetizing, have everything prepared ahead of time, working quickly and accurately to minimize the anesthetic time. It is recommended to preoxygenate birds with 100% oxygen for 3 to 5 minutes prior to exposing them to anesthetic gas. Intubation is ideal to both insufflate the air sacs for diagnostic purposes, as well as being able to address any apnea that may occur as a result of anesthesia.
- An anesthetized or chemically restrained bird should be monitored very closely for respiration, mentation/reflexes, and be kept warm. In longer radiographic procedures, use SpO2 to monitor heart rate and saturated oxygen will aid patient monitoring. Lingual probes attached to the talons/toes will provide fairly accurate readings and not interfere with images. Make sure that the images and the number of views are satisfactory before recovering the patient.
- In between imaging and during recovery, ensure that the avian patient is placed in a sternal position to aid breathing efforts. A towel "donut" (twisted towel to support the bird) can help reduce sternal pressure and make breathing easier. Do not place the bird on a perch until the patient is fully recovered. Because recovery can be rapid, keep hands on the patient to prevent a fall.
- Sedation and anesthesia may further compromise debilitated patients and there will be cases where birds will need to have radiographs obtained without chemical restraint. The following suggested precautions apply to pet and wild birds (and other exotic animals) that are fully conscious[2] for radiography:
  - Minimize manual restraint.
  - Have everything organized beforehand to minimize the time required for the procedure.
  - Wear protective clothing, gloves, and headgear as appropriate with the species. Wear protective eyewear and long protective gloves over the lower arms for raptor restraint. Never leave talons unrestrained. Once the feet have been radiographed, it is advisable to wrap the talons of raptors for added handler safety. A full-face shield is suggested for water birds with long beaks. Never leave dangerous beaks, such as those of herons, unrestrained.
  - Work in a dimly lit room and minimize unnecessary noise and movement.
  - Ensure that the area is contained, avoiding escape routes and areas for the patient to hide or injure itself. Have capture devices, such as nets, on hand in case of escape.
  - Cover the bird's head and torso with a towel.
- Another option for debilitated birds that will not tolerate anesthesia or restraint is to use a lateral horizontal beam. The bird can either perch or be placed in a small radiolucent box or plastic container to prevent excessive movement. Make sure the patient's breathing is not compromised in any container in which it is placed. These images are not ideal, but they may be diagnostic enough to indicate a problem. If horizontal beam is not available, radiolucent containers can be used to hold birds on the dorsoventral (DV) vertical line. This position is considered nondiagnostic except in instances where the practitioner is concerned about a shelled egg, evaluating bone density/pathology, or metal foreign body (see VD positioning).

Radiographic Views

Avian Coelom

Lateral View of the Avian Coelom

Positioning

Place the patient in right lateral recumbency. If using film, use a radiolucent or cardboard sheet on the image receptor to tape the patient and to facilitate moving the patient if another exposure is required (Fig. 25.3B). Gently extend the bird, and with precut strips of tape, carefully tape the patient on the radiolucent Plexiglas or cardboard sheet in the following order:

Head: Tape/Velcro is gently placed across the neck at the base of the skull with neck extended to reduce curvature of the neck.

Use fingers to position the trachea ventrally to avoid superimposition over the vertebral column.

Wings: Extend the wings dorsally in full extension; tape the dependent wing first, and then superimpose the upper wing.

Avoid excessive pressure to the upper wing to prevent rotation.

Pelvic Limbs: Extend and superimpose the pelvic limbs slightly caudally, secure the tape or gauze to the distal tarsometatarsal bones, and extend the limbs.

Tape the dependent limb first.

Tail: Taping of the tail is optional but should be close to the base. Include the correct positional marker and place it on the cranial aspect of the film.

- *If a bird positioner (commercial or homemade guillotine device) is being used:* Place the neck in the cervical restraint portion; then gently move the body caudally to reduce the curvature of the neck (Fig. 25.3A). Position the trachea and immobilize the rest of the body as needed to obtain positioning as described previously, using tape, gauze, Velcro, or tubing to secure the limbs to the cleats (Figs. 25.3 and 25.4).

Comments and Tips

1. Be gentle; luxation of the shoulder can result if the position is forced, especially in awake birds.
2. Superimposition of the extremities helps minimize rotation (Fig. 25.4). If pelvic limb or wing images are required, the limbs are not superimposed. Instead, they are positioned as described later for the modified whole-body/pectoral limb lateral view (Fig. 25.5).
3. The pelvic limbs need to be securely pulled and fastened to straighten the femur.
4. The sternum and vertebral column can be palpated and should be on the same plane.
5. The tail can be taped, and more tape/Velcro can be placed on either the humeral portions of the wings or on the body if needed.
6. Be careful to avoid pressure over the chest area when applying restraint.
7. If the lungs are to be examined, it may be beneficial to deliberately underexpose a lateral view. Make sure that the wings are drawn away from the torso.
8. A species and size exposure chart will likely be used; otherwise, measure at the thickest part of the chest (over the keel).

> ✎ **TECHNICIAN NOTES** When working with raptors, make sure to tape the talons or use vet wrap to keep them restrained once the feet have been imaged.

CENTRAL RAY: At the level of the xiphoid (caudal tip of keel), between the spine and keel.
BORDERS:
Small Birds: The whole body should be included.
Large and Medium Birds: Include the coelom, proximal extremities, and caudal cervical regions or the area of interest.
Multiple exposures are needed for larger birds, especially long-necked patients such as swans.

Lateral View of the Avian Coelom—cont'd

FIG. 25.3 A, Positioning technique for a right lateral radiograph of the avian coelom with the use of a positioning device.[5] B, Positioning for a lateral whole-body radiograph of a Caique with the use of tape. C, Image of the lateral view of an adult bird with the limbs superimposed. (A courtesy Deven Graves; B and C courtesy Lorelei D'Avolio, The Center for Avian and Exotic Medicine, NYC).

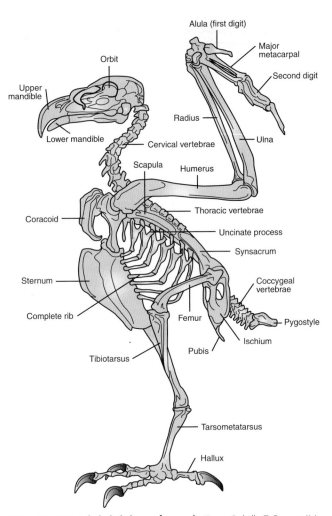

FIG. 25.3D Labeled Skeleton of a Hawk. (From Colville T, Bassert JM. *Clinical Anatomy and Physiology for Veterinary Technicians.* 3rd ed. St. Louis: Elsevier; 2016.)

Lateral View of the Avian Coelom—cont'd

FIG. 25.4 Radiographic Anatomy of the Lateral View of the Adult Lovebird. Projection: Laterolateral (right lateral recumbency). *1,* Trachea; *2,* crop; *3,* brachiocephalic artery and aorta; *4,* brachiocephalic artery; *5,* aorta; *6,* pulmonary artery; *7,* pulmonary vein; *8,* heart; *9,* left atrium; *10,* esophagus; *11,* liver; *12,* lung; *13,* syrinx; *14,* gonad; *15,* ovary; *16,* testes; *17,* proventriculus; *18,* ventriculus; *19,* intestines; *20,* cloaca; *21,* cervical air sac; *22,* clavicular air sac; *23,* thoracic air sac; *24,* abdominal air sac; *25,* apex of heart; *26,* interface between caudal thoracic and abdominal air sacs; *27,* kidneys; *28,* spleen.

FIG. 25.5 **A,** Modified positioning technique for a right lateral radiograph of the avian (Sun Conure) if separation of the extremities is required. **B,** Radiograph of the modified lateral view of an adult pigeon with the wings separated. (**A** courtesy Rick Axelson, Links Road Animal Clinic, North York, ON; **B** courtesy Sue Carstairs, Kawartha Turtle Trauma Centre, ON.)

Lateral View of the Avian Coelom—cont'd

Avian Coelom: Modified Whole-Body/Pectoral Limb Lateral View

Comments and Tips

1. If the pectoral or pelvic limbs of small birds need to be radiographed, the limbs and wings can be separated in the lateral view to minimize the number of images needed (see Fig. 25.5).
2. Position in lateral recumbency as described previously, with the following exceptions:
   a. Do not superimpose the limbs; instead, separate both the wings and the legs.
   b. The extremities on the dependent side should be pulled and taped cranially, with padding placed between the perspective limbs to avoid rotation of the body.
   c. Secure the contralateral limbs caudally (leg) and dorsally (the wing) to minimize superimposition.

3. In this view, the contralateral wing is in a lateromedial view, and there will be increased object-film distance (OFD).
4. The patient is best placed in a VD position for true mediolateral pectoral limb.
5. The body is more rotated when the limbs are not superimposed.

> **TECHNICIAN NOTES**   To ensure that a lateral coelom or whole-body view is symmetrical:
> 1. The head is slightly extended.
> 2. The acetabula, ribs, coracoids, femoral heads, and kidneys are superimposed.
> 3. The sternum and vertebral column are on the same plane.

Ventrodorsal View of the Avian Coelom

Positioning

Place the patient in dorsal recumbency. Have precut paper tape ready.

If the positioning board is used, the Velcro or IV tubing found on the board can be attached to the cleats or suction cups in lieu of tape (Fig. 25.6).

Gently extend and carefully secure the patient in the order described below if the bird is not chemically restrained:

Head: If using a bird-positioning board, gently place the head in the cervical restrainer portion in a true rostrocaudal position.

   If not using a bird-positioning board, place tape at the mandibular articulation at the base of the skull.

Wings: Open the wings at a 90-degree angle to the body with two pieces of tape crossed at the carpal region of each wing.

   Never tape over the chest; because of the delicate air sacs, respiration could be affected.

Pelvic limbs: Apply tape or tubing separately around each tarsometatarsus and pull caudally and symmetrically.

Tail: Tape close to the base of the tail if needed.

Comments and Tips

1. Place an indicator marker on the appropriate side.
2. If the patient is anesthetized, the order of taping or positioning is not important.
3. To position the leg caudally without moving the bird's body:
   a. Gently place a finger at the tip of the sternum for release, making sure not to press dorsally on the sternum while doing so; otherwise, the bird could suffocate.
4. A species and size exposure chart will likely be used; otherwise, measure at the thickest part of the chest (over the keel).

CENTRAL RAY: Over the midline at the caudal tip of the sternum.

BORDERS:

Small Bird: Include the whole body.

Large or Medium-Sized Bird: Include the coelom, proximal extremities, and caudal cervical regions or the area of interest.

   Multiple exposures are needed for larger birds, especially long-necked patients such as swans.

> **TECHNICIAN NOTES**   To ensure that a VD coelom or whole-body view will appear symmetrical:
> 1. The keel (sternum) is directly over the spine.
> 2. The scapula, acetabula, and femurs are parallel, equidistant, and symmetrical.
> 3. The wings are open at 90 degrees to the body.

Ventrodorsal View of the Avian Coelom

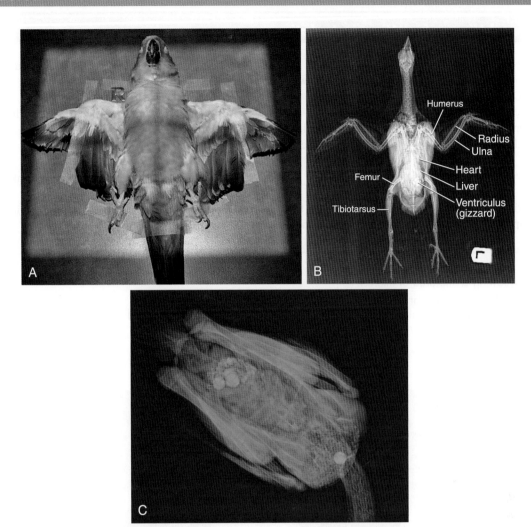

FIG. 25.6 A, Positioning for the ventrodorsal view of a Sun Conure with the use of tape. **B,** Radiographic anatomy of a ventrodorsal view of an adult pigeon. **C,** A vertical beam with the avian patient in DV position. This view is normally nondiagnostic but the veterinarian wished only to determine what might have caused an obstruction in the Mallard Duck—the patient had swallowed marbles. (**A** courtesy Rick Axelson, Links Road Animal Clinic, North York, ON; **B** courtesy Sue Carstairs, Kawartha Turtle Trauma Centre, ON; **C** courtesy L orelei D'Avolio, The Center for Avian and Exotic Medicine, NYC.)

Wing

Mediolateral View of a Wing in Isolation

Positioning

Dorsal recumbency: True mediolateral view of the wing with decreased OFD.

1. Position the body as in the VD view of the coelom.
2. Place the body to the side of the image receptor to allow the affected wing and area of interest to be centered (Fig. 25.7).
3. Tape at the mandibular articulation at the base of the skull.
4. Open the wings at a 90-degree angle to the body, with two pieces of tape crossed at the carpal region of each wing.
5. Separate and tape the pelvic limbs at the tarsometatarsal bones.
6. Tape the tail close to the base.
7. Additional tape can be applied to the proximal and distal portions of the affected wing if needed.

Comments and Tips

1. Positioning of affected wing is more crucial, but consider the patient's injuries.
2. Decrease 2 to 4 kV from the coelomic view to prevent overexposure.

CENTRAL RAY: Midwing or the area of interest.

BORDERS: Include the entire wing, including the scapulohumeral joint.

Large Birds: Position wings diagonally across the image receptor to maximize the x-ray field.

FIG. 25.7 Positioning for a Mediolateral View of Avian Wing in Isolation. (Courtesy Sue Carstairs, Kawartha Turtle Trauma Centre, ON.)

Caudocranial View of the Avian Wing

This view allows a true orthogonal view, as the lateral and VD coelom positions show the wings in a lateral projection. This caudocranial (CdCr) view is also referred to as a *"leading edge"* or *"hanging drop view"*[2] because the cranial edge of the wing is placed just above the image receptor. The patient should be sedated or anesthetized. Unfortunately, to obtain a true caudocranial view, the patient needs to be held (Fig. 25.8).

Positioning

1. Carefully position the patient upside down with the head directed to the floor.
2. Have the long axis of the body parallel to the vertically directed x-ray beam.
3. Extend the wing fully with its cranial edge in contact with the image receptor.

Comments and Tips

1. Keep the wing close and parallel to the image receptor to minimize OFD.
2. Distortion may occur toward the edges of the image of birds with large wings because of beam divergence.
3. Depending on the sensor size in direct digital units, the CdCr view may not be fully captured in large birds.

CENTRAL RAY: On the area of interest.

FIG. 25.8 A, Demonstrating placement of a patient in position for a caudocranial (CdCr) wing. **B,** The patient does need to be sedated and is held to ensure the proper orientation. **C,** Image of a CdCr (hanging view) wing. (**A** and **C** courtesy Lorelei D'Avolio, The Center for Avian and Exotic Medicine, NYC; **B,** Deven Graves.)

Avian Head—Ancillary

Lateral View of the Avian Head

Positioning

1. Place the patient in right lateral recumbency with the head either positioned through the cervical restrainer of the acrylic positioning board or taped to a sheet or image receptor (Fig. 25.9).
2. Collimate and keep the head on the plate, carefully supporting the rest of the body with a towel or other positioner, depending on patient size.
3. Secure the head by separately applying tape to the mandible and maxilla.

4. A species and size exposure chart will likely be used; otherwise, measure at the thickest part.
5. Depending on the patient size or the radiographic need, imaging of the head in addition to routine body views may not be required.

CENTRAL RAY: Ventral to the eye.
BORDERS: Include the entire head extending to the cervical region.

FIG. 25.9 Positioning for a Lateral View of the Avian Head. (Courtesy Deven Graves.)

Ventrodorsal View of the Avian Head

Positioning

1. Place the patient in dorsal recumbency as for the VD view of the coelom. Ensure the head is in a true rostro-caudal position.
2. Apply radiolucent tape to the ventral aspect of the rhinotheca to bring the maxilla closer to the image receptor (Fig. 25.10).

3. Depending on the patient size or the radiographic need, imaging of the head in addition to routine VD view may not be required.

CENTRAL RAY: Midline between the eyes.
BORDERS: Include the entire head.

FIG. 25.10 Ventrodorsal Positioning for a Radiograph of the Avian Head. (Courtesy Deven Graves.)

Avian Limb—Ancillary

Mediolateral View of the Avian Foot

1. Depending on the patient size or the radiographic need, imaging of the limb in addition to routine lateral views may not be required (Fig. 25.11A).

Positioning

1. Place the patient in lateral recumbency on an acrylic positioning board or tape to a sheet or image receptor directly with the affected limb down.
2. If the positioning board is utilized, use Velcro or tape, not the cleats, to secure the feet directly to the board.

3. Apply radiolucent tape to each toe to separate the digits of the affected limb to minimize superimposition. The tape allows for more precise positioning than gauze.
4. Tie and secure the unaffected limb caudally.
5. Extend the dependent limb cranially to prevent superimposition.

Comments and Tips

1. A decrease of 2 to 4 kV from the coelomic view prevents overexposure.

CENTRAL RAY: On the condyles of the tarsometatarsal bone.
BORDERS: Include all of the phalanges.

FIG. 25.11 A, Positioning for a lateral view of the pelvic limb and foot.

Craniocaudal View of the Avian Pelvic Limb

Positioning

1. Place the patient in dorsal recumbency.
2. Position as for the VD view of the coelom, securing the head and pectoral limbs.
3. Separate and use tape, gauze, or tubing at the tarsometatarsal bones of the pelvic limbs; caudally extend the pelvic limbs.
4. Separate the toes with tape or cotton to prevent superimposition, being careful of any injury (Fig. 25.11B).

Comments and Tips

1. Place the R or L marker on the appropriate limb.
2. Center accordingly.
3. If needed, tape the tail close to the base.
4. Additional tape can be applied to the proximal portions of the affected limb.

CENTRAL RAY: On the affected limb(s).

BORDERS: Include just beyond the affected area.

FIG. 25.11, cont'd B, Craniocaudal view of the pelvic limb of an Amazon Parrot. (A courtesy Deven Graves; B from Silverman A, Tell L. *Radiology of Birds: An Atlas of Normal Anatomy and Positioning.* St. Louis: Elsevier; 2010.)

Contrast Study of the Gastrointestinal Tract

Due to anatomy and variable rapid digestive tract transit time, a single protocol for a contrast study is limited. Oral contrast media highlights the digestive tract from the esophagus to the large intestine and occasionally the cloaca. For true cloacal studies, contrast medium should be retrogradely administered directly into the cloaca.

Preparation

- If the bird can tolerate fasting, the crop and the proventriculus should be empty. The fasting period depends on the size, metabolic requirements, and health of the bird. Food in the ingluvies (crop) decreases the volume of contrast media that can be safely administered. Food in the gastrointestinal (GI) tract prevents full contact of the contrast medium with the digestive tract mucosa and may delay passage of the contrast medium.
  - Birds weighing more than 300 g should not be fed pelleted foods within 4 hours of the contrast study. When food is mixed with the contrast medium, the patterns shown on images are unpredictable.

Anesthesia and Contrast Media

If the health of the bird permits, anesthesia is suggested. Tracheal intubation is ideal to prevent aspiration of possibly regurgitated contrast media.

- Watch for regurgitation. If this occurs, remove the medium immediately from the oropharynx with cotton-tipped applicators to prevent the contrast medium from passing through the choanal slit into the nasal cavity. Monitor the oral cavity carefully for any regurgitated contrast medium. In all situations, the cranial portion of the body should be raised.
- Barium sulfate 30% weight to volume (w/v) is recommended at a general calculation of 0.025 to 0.05 mL/g body weight, depending on the species and presence or absence of a crop. The lower dose range is used in larger birds. It is better to estimate the volume of food that can be safely administered via crop gavage and to give the contrast medium at only 50% to 75% of this amount.[1]
- Warm the medium to room temperature by immersing the syringe in warm water. Mix the warmed liquid well and test the temperature before administration to prevent crop burn, which can precipitate severe metabolic and fluid imbalances as well as decrease the mucosal detail.
- Slowly administer the contrast media via a rigid or soft gavage tube passed into the crop. Verify that the tube is correctly palpated and placed. Keeping a finger over the distal portion of the cervical esophagus may help prevent aspirating barium sulfate during administration. Do not place excessive pressure on the full crop, and slowly remove the tube.

- Increase 2 to 4 kV due to the greater opacity of the contrast medium.

Technique for Antegrade GI

- Produce survey ventrodorsal and right lateral radiographs just before the contrast study to indicate the current status of the digestive tract.
- If the esophagus, crop, and proventriculus are of interest, lateral and ventrodorsal radiographs should be taken immediately. There are significant species variations in transit time, so depending on the type of bird, further lateral and ventrodorsal radiographs can be taken at 15 minutes and 30 minutes. Further 30-minute radiographs can be taken as needed and if continued anesthesia allows.
  - The procedure is technically finished when the contrast medium has entered the colon. Digestive transit time is generally more rapid than in mammals.

Positioning

BORDERS: Include the caudal cervical area and the entire coelom.
POSITION: as for the lateral and ventrodorsal coelom.

- To prevent retrograde flow of contrast medium, either raise the cranial portion of the body with a translucent positioning device or apply a bandage to the cervical esophagus. A bandage can partially occlude the cervical esophagus to minimize retrograde flow of contrast medium. Ensure bandage material does not occlude the trachea.
- Diligently monitor the anesthesia level, hypothermia, and any regurgitation.

Double-Contrast Study

- A double-contrast study gives superior mucosal detail and generally a shorter transit time.
- Anesthesia is frequently required, as gas infused into the crop is immediately expelled in most awake birds.
- Less contrast medium is used than in positive-contrast studies, lessening the potential for aspiration into the respiratory tract. If air is regurgitated, further air can be administered to distend the crop.[1]

Cloacagram

Hollow organs are best viewed if properly distended; thus retrograde administration of barium into the vent is best implemented to fully visualize the cloaca (Fig. 25.12).

Procedure

- Before administering the barium, gently flush the cloaca with isotonic saline.
- Positive- and double-contrast cloacagrams can be performed. The common dosage of barium sulfate is 0.025 to 0.05 mL per gram body weight.

FIG. 25.12 Gastrointestinal Barium Study with Contrast Medium Administered About 3 Hours Previously. **A,** Right lateral. **B,** Ventrodorsal view. Barium is in the crop, proventriculus, ventriculus, intestines, and cloaca. (Courtesy Rick Axelson, Links Road Animal Clinic, North York, ON.)

- If a double-contrast study is to be completed, perform the positive-contrast study first and then remove all of the barium pooled in the cloaca before introducing the negative-contrast medium (room air or carbon dioxide). The cloacal mucosal surface is better visualized in this way.
- Research indicates that carbon dioxide creates less potential for intravascular air emboli to occur. Fecal matter can be refluxed into the ureters when retrograde vent procedures are performed.[1]

CENTRAL RAY: Cranial to the cloaca (vent).

BORDERS: Include the cranial third of the coelom.

Positioning

As described for VD and lateral views of the coelom.

Urography

- Urography can also be completed through the use of an intravenous contrast medium to evaluate the urinary tract.
- This may be warranted if the patient is polyuric/polydipsic, has increased blood uric acid levels, changes in the color and consistency of the urates in the droppings, or unilateral or bilateral lameness, especially if these symptoms are in conjunction with a coelomic mass of unknown origin.
- Because of the requirement of an indwelling IV catheter or injection, it is not recommended to perform this study if sedation or anesthesia cannot be used.

- Iohexol 3–5 mg/kg IV given slowly over 5 seconds is injected IV. VD and lateral radiographs are rapidly imaged at 10, 60, and 120 seconds after administration. Repeated radiographs can be taken at 5 to 7 minutes to show the contrast agent at the cloaca or rectum.

Radiographic Anatomy

Radiographic anatomy of the avian skeleton (see Fig. 25.3D) is very straightforward, but radiographic anatomy and interpretation of the internal structures is more complicated. The viscera are tightly packed together, soft tissue density is similar and there is a minimal amount of perivascular fat, making differentiation difficult.

There is no diaphragm and thus no true division of thoracic and abdominal structures. The advantage for birds and reptiles in not having a diaphragm is the ability to expand abdominal contents into the respiratory system without any major compromise.

Anatomically, the coelom is not divided in birds, but for discussion purposes, it is often separated into the thoracic and abdominal regions.

Please see Figs. 25.13 and 25.14 as well as Appendix D on the Evolve website for avian anatomy and further radiographic concerns.

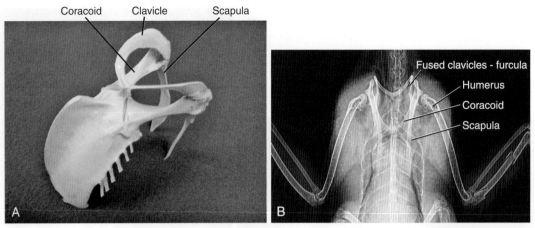

Coracoid   Clavicle   Scapula

Fused clavicles - furcula
Humerus
Coracoid
Scapula

FIG. 25.13 **A,** Anatomy of the pectoral girdle of a Rough-Legged Hawk. **B,** Radiograph showing the pectoral girdle of a Red-Tailed Hawk. (**B** courtesy Sue Carstairs, Kawartha Turtle Trauma Centre, ON.)

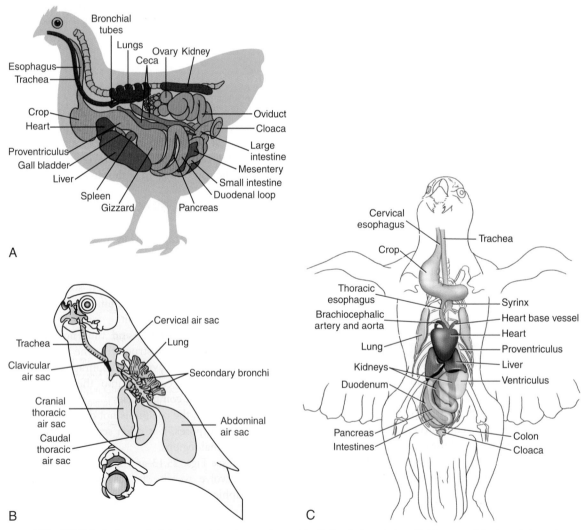

Bronchial tubes
Lungs
Ovary Kidney
Ceca
Esophagus
Trachea
Crop
Heart
Oviduct
Cloaca
Large intestine
Proventriculus
Gall bladder
Mesentery
Liver
Small intestine
Spleen
Duodenal loop
Gizzard
Pancreas

A

Cervical esophagus
Trachea
Crop
Thoracic esophagus
Syrinx
Brachiocephalic artery and aorta
Heart base vessel
Heart
Lung
Proventriculus
Kidneys
Liver
Duodenum
Ventriculus
Pancreas
Colon
Intestines
Cloaca

Cervical air sac
Lung
Trachea
Clavicular air sac
Secondary bronchi
Cranial thoracic air sac
Abdominal air sac
Caudal thoracic air sac

B   C

FIG. 25.14 **A,** Anatomical drawing of the viscera of an adult chicken in lateral view. **B,** Diagram of the lateral view of the avian respiratory system. **C,** Anatomical drawing (ventrodorsal view) of the viscera of an adult bird. (**B** from Colville T, Bassert JM. *Clinical Anatomy and Physiology for Veterinary Technicians.* 3rd ed. St. Louis: Elsevier; 2016; **C** from Silverman S. *Radiology of Birds: An Atlas of Normal Anatomy and Positioning.* Philadelphia: Saunders; 2010.)

Exotic Companion Mammals

The two orthogonal views used in exotic small mammal are the same as for other small mammal patients; the ventrodorsal (VD) and lateral.

In severely debilitated patients that cannot tolerate sedation, anesthesia, or positioning, information may be gathered with a lateral decubitus view (dorsoventral position with a horizontal beam) where the image receptor is placed vertically behind the patient and the beam directed perpendicular to both. These images will not yield traditionally diagnostic images due to overlaying of extremities and hunching of the body preventing the true symmetry required to properly evaluate visceral content. However, they may provide some basic information such as the presence of fetuses, foreign body, urinary calculi, or basic integrity of the lung fields.

Sedation, Anesthesia, and Positioning Concerns

- Due to the deleterious effects of stress on prey species, it is strongly recommended to use sedation in order to safely position small mammals for diagnostic imaging. Some healthy but nervous animals may only need some anxiolytics such as midazolam to decrease anxiety. If there is anticipated pain, partial or pure mu opioids such as buprenorphine, butorphanol, or hydromorphone may be warranted to both address the pain and provide added sedation. If deeper sedation is required, fast -acting drugs such as alfaxalone can be used in rabbits. Dexmedetomidine is also safe for healthy rabbits and may be desirable due to the benefits of having a reversal agent.[3]
- Following these sedatives with inhalant anesthesia such as isoflurane or sevoflurane induction can be achieved via a small face mask over the nose. Using an induction chamber or box is not recommended due to the stress of the patients when gassed in a box, and the risks to personnel of exposure. With proper sedatives, use of box induction should not be necessary.
- More jumpy, smaller mammals such as rats, mice, or hamsters may be best sedated first with anxiolytics, analgesics if needed, and then induced with a small isoflurane or sevoflurane mask. These patients can be taped to either the image receptor or a plastic positioner, radiographed, and then allowed to recover.
- It is important to keep these patients warm and monitor regularly because they can quickly become hypothermic due to their small size and rapid metabolism. Plastic containers, paper positioning tape, Velcro, foam props, gauze, and IV tubing are all simple positioning devices that are extremely useful for positioning of exotic companion mammals (Fig. 25.15). Masking tape or transparent medical tape is less likely to remove the animal's fur and is less likely to be radiodense at lower kV settings.

- As with the avian patient, it is important to be quick and efficient to minimize stress and anesthesia time.
- For most exotic small mammals, radiographs should encompass both the thoracic and the abdominal cavities on the same image. Because of their small size, the densities of these cavities are similar enough that the technique will not vary. It also saves time imaging two views of the entire body, as well as minimizing their stress and anesthesia length. Large rabbits and long-bodied ferrets, however, may require separate thoracic and abdominal VD and lateral views.
- Species variation can dictate different techniques when determining the best methods to restrain. For example, the dorsal half of a hedgehog's body is covered by a thick coat of long protective spines. When threatened, hedgehogs roll into a tight ball. If not anesthetized, radiography will not be a useful diagnostic tool. When anesthetized, the spines must be pulled away to allow the thoracic and abdominal cavity to be imaged without the overlay of the spines.
- Positioning for radiography is fairly consistent with other mammalian species. Depending on the site of interest, variations occur where the patient is measured, centered, and with the peripheral borders. Table 25.2 indicates the differences. See the particular views for how to position.

> ✎ **TECHNICIAN NOTES** It is important to keep these patients warm and monitored regularly, because they can quickly become hypothermic due to their small size.

Species Considerations

Small Rodent (Rat, Hamster, Mouse, Gerbil, Degu)

Small rodents have several common illnesses that may indicate the need for radiographic diagnostic imaging. Traumatic injuries can cause fractures of the extremities or spine, as well as crushing injuries causing damage to the diaphragm or viscera. Rats, mice, and hamsters frequently have tumors, malignant and benign, both soft tissue and related to internal organs. Respiratory disease is very common, often caused by mycoplasma, and can result in thoracic abscesses, pneumonia, and scarring of the lungs.

Rabbit

Common reasons for radiographing rabbits are fractures or dislocations of the extremities, pelvis, or spine. Dental disease is of concern, and radiographs are often required to evaluate coronal elongation as well as tooth root integrity. Though there are exceptions, most middle ear infections in rabbits appear radiographically normal. Rabbits suffer many gastrointestinal problems requiring imaging, such as ileus, dilation of the stomach and/or cecum, and liver lobe

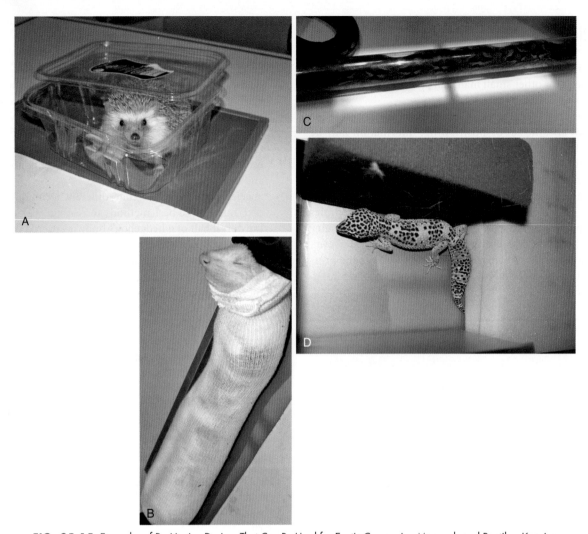

FIG. 25.15 Examples of Positioning Devices That Can Be Used for Exotic Companion Mammals and Reptiles, Keeping in Mind That True Symmetry May Not Be Achieved Depending on the Device Used. **A,** Hedgehog in a deli container for a dorsoventral (DV) or horizontal beam lateral. **B,** Utilizing a stockinet for a ventrodorsal (vd) view of an unanesthetized ferret. Sandbags can be placed at either end and the patient placed on a v-trough. **C,** A snake tube, which allows for proper symmetry. **D,** Positioning of a gecko, using foam devices to keep it in place. (C courtesy Ryan Cheeck, Veterinary Technology, Gwinnett Technical College, Lawrenceville, GA.)

TABLE 25.2	Where to Measure an Center, and What to Include When Radiographing Slightly Larger Exotic Companion Mammals			
SPECIES	**VIEW**	**WHERE TO MEASURE**	**WHERE TO CENTER**	**WHAT TO INCLUDE**
Guinea pig, chinchilla, and small rabbits	Ventrodorsal (VD) of full body	Last rib (thickest part of the body)	Thoracolumbar (TL) junction	Minimum of shoulder joint to caudal to ilium, including the limbs
	Lateral of full body	Last rib (thickest part of the body)	TL junction for a full-body view	Depends on size (similar to small cat)
Ferrets and larger rabbits	VD of abdomen	Last rib (thickest part of the body)	Caudal to last rib	Cranial from xiphoid process to caudal to pubis
	Lateral of abdomen	Last rib (thickest part of the body)	Caudal to last rib	Cranial from xiphoid process to caudal to pubis
	VD of thorax	Last rib (thickest part of the body)	At xiphoid of sternum	Shoulder joint to slightly caudal to last rib
	Lateral of thorax	Last rib (thickest part of the body)	Caudal sternum	Shoulder joint to slightly caudal to last rib

torsions. Cranial mediastinal masses such as thymoma are also common, as is primary heart and lung disease. Rabbits also commonly have urinary tract problems that cause calcium "sludge" in the bladder, often in conjunction with uroliths and/or renolithiasis. Intact female rabbits frequently suffer from reproductive tract cancers and hyperplasia.

To minimize radiation exposure for the radiographer and prevent stress to the rabbit, a healthy patient is best sedated as previously described. Rabbits are not fasted before sedation or anesthesia because they cannot regurgitate or vomit, and because fasting in the rabbit can contribute to ileus. Rabbits are generally docile and can be easily handled; however, many prey species are very nervous. A panicking, kicking rabbit can easily injure itself or a restrainer when afraid.

Ferret

Radiographic imaging will benefit ferrets in many ways. Ferrets are active, curious, playful animals and can get underfoot and experience limb fractures, or fall out of windows like cats. Especially when young, they tend to eat anything they find on the floor and frequently suffer from GI obstruction. Ferrets also present with various congenital and acquired heart diseases, with cardiomyopathy being the most common. The two most common diseases seen in older ferrets, adrenal disease and insulinoma, are best diagnosed with ultrasound.

Dental radiographs may be needed in ferrets. Occlusal dental film is preferred, but oblique extraoral projections can be made. Follow the same procedure as suggested for the dental radiography of cats (see Chapter 22). At least four views should be taken.

Ferrets are relatively easy to handle because they are friendly and inquisitive, but, as with rabbits, healthy ferrets are best sedated for positioning of radiographs or ultrasound. They can be extremely flexible and squirmy, and will not remain still for very long. If anesthetized, a ferret should be fasted for 3 to 4 hours before to prevent vomiting and aspiration. Check for hidden food in the cage of a ferret that is to be fasted.

Guinea Pig and Chinchilla

The most common reasons for diagnostic imaging of guinea pigs and chinchillas are for GI -related ileus and bloating of the stomach or cecum. Like rabbits, they also suffer commonly from urinary calculi and reproductive disease of intact females. Additionally, dental disease is frequently seen, requiring imaging of the tooth roots. Chinchillas, more than guinea pigs, suffer from tooth root elongation which causes severe pain and anorexia. Both species can also easily be dropped, stepped on, or fall off edges, causing traumatic injuries.

Guinea pigs and chinchillas are not aggressive but do become stressed easily. They will wiggle, nip, and try to escape when scared. They are best sedated or anesthetized as previously described for radiography. Like rabbits, they are not fasted prior to anesthesia.

Whole-Body View of Exotic Companion Mammals

Ventrodorsal View of Whole Body/Abdomen/Thorax of Exotic Companion Mammal

Positioning

- Place the patient in dorsal recumbency, preferably with the patient being chemically restrained.
- Gently extend the pectoral limbs cranially.
- Slightly rotate the pelvic limbs medially and caudally, keeping the limbs equidistant.
- Tape/Velcro the legs keeping them symmetrical.
- Alternatively, place gauze or tubing around the hocks and elbows, extending to either a cleat at each end of the table or a positioning device.
- A sandbag can be placed over the gauze, stretching the limbs, or on the hindlimbs for larger patients.
- Keep the head straight and secure with tape if needed.
- Collimation should include the entire thorax from the top of the manubrium to the base of the pelvis, including genitals of patients suspected of urinary tract disease (Figs. 25.16–25.19).

> ### ✎ TECHNICIAN NOTES
> To ensure that the ventrodorsal view is symmetrical on the image:
> - The sternebrae are over the vertebrae on the same vertical plane.
> - The spinous processes are aligned in the center of the vertebral bodies.
> - The acetabula are symmetrical and the femurs parallel, if possible.
> - The patient is as straight as possible from the head to its tail, avoiding any rotation.

Comments and Tips

- An acrylic or foam positioning device similar to that used for cats can also be utilized.
- The exposure factors may have to be increased by 2 to 4 kV if a positioning device is used.
- The extended VD can be painful if there is any injury. This pain can be slightly alleviated by not fully extending the legs and by placing the patient on a medium-density foam pad.
- If limb studies are required, slightly rotate the patient to the opposite side to minimize soft tissue superimposition. Extend the affected forelimb cranially and the hindlimb caudally and tape/Velcro separately.
- Keep the patient warm and monitor if anesthetized.

FIG. 25.16 A, Positioning for the ventrodorsal view of a rat. B, Ventrodorsal image of a rat. (Courtesy Lorelei D'Avolio, The Center for Avian and Exotic Medicine, NYC.)

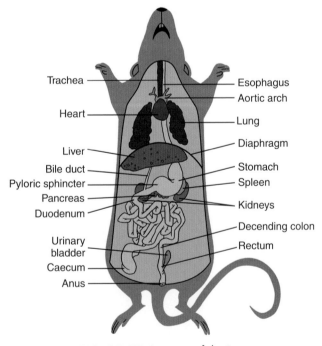

FIG. 25.17 Anatomy of the Rat.

Ventrodorsal View of Whole Body/Abdomen/Thorax of Exotic Companion Mammal—cont'd

Humerus
Clavicle
Scapula
Rib
Cecum
Transverse process of the lumbar vertebra
Sacrum
Acetabulum and femoral head
Ischium
Pubis

Lung
Heart
Lung
Liver
Stomach
Left kidney
Spinous process of the lumbar vertebra
Mammillary process of the lumbar vertebra
Iliac crest
Ilium
Greater trochanter of femur
Obturator foramen
Femur

A

R   L

B

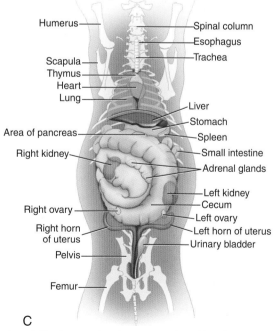

Humerus
Scapula
Thymus
Heart
Lung
Area of pancreas
Right kidney
Right ovary
Right horn of uterus
Pelvis
Femur

Spinal column
Esophagus
Trachea
Liver
Stomach
Spleen
Small intestine
Adrenal glands
Left kidney
Cecum
Left ovary
Left horn of uterus
Urinary bladder

C

FIG. 25.18 **A,** Positioning for a full-body ventrodorsal (VD) view of a rabbit. The same positioning applies for abdomen, thorax, VD skull, pelvis, and proximal limbs. **B,** Radiographic anatomy of the VD view of the rabbit. **C,** Anatomical drawing of the viscera of the thorax and abdomen of an adult female rabbit in VD view (**A** courtesy Rick Axelson, Links Road Animal Clinic, North York, ON.)

Ventrodorsal View of Whole Body/Abdomen/Thorax of Exotic Companion Mammal—cont'd

FIG. 25.19 **A,** Positioning for a full body ventrodorsal (VD) of a ferret. **B,** VD image of the ferret. **C,** Positioning for a VD view of a chinchilla. Place the central ray over the area of interest and collimate appropriately. (**A** and **B** courtesy Lorelei D'Avolio, The Center for Avian and Exotic Medicine, NYC; **C** courtesy Rick Axelson, Links Road Animal Clinic, North York, ON.)

Lateral View of the Whole Body/Abdomen/Thorax of Exotic Companion Mammal

Positioning

- Place the patient in lateral recumbency (Figs. 25.20–25.22).
- A right lateral view is often preferred but be consistent to minimize misdiagnosis.
- Position the head cranially and secure with tape/Velcro if needed.
- Place a small foam wedge under the sternum to keep the sternum and vertebrae on the same horizontal plane.
- Fully extend and tape the dependent limbs—the pelvic limbs caudally and pectoral limbs cranially.
- Superimpose the contralateral pelvic and pectoral limbs and tape separately.
- Use padding between the legs if needed.

Comments and Tips

- If limb radiographs are required and two extra views are not practical, separate the limbs when completing a whole-body view. The dependent limb will be pulled slightly cranial in each case.
- Applying and securing tape around the contralateral limb and rotating the body slightly minimizes superimposition.

- Though not ideal, a lateral decubitus (dorsoventral view with a horizontal beam) can be completed if necessary and if the machine permits (Fig. 25.23).

> **⌨ TECHNICIAN NOTES** To ensure that the lateral view appears symmetrical on the image:
> - Sternebrae and vertebrae are on the same plane.
> - The ribs are superimposed and straight.
> - Intervertebral foramina are the same size.
> - The acetabula are superimposed.
> - Ventral processes are superimposed.

> **⌨ TECHNICIAN NOTES** Be sure to fully extend the front limbs cranially on the lateral projection, especially for a rabbit, so that you have optimum radiographic detail of the cranial thorax. Hindlimbs not properly extended interfere with the caudal abdomen viscera.

FIG. 25.20 **A,** Positioning for the lateral view of the full body of a rat. **B,** Lateral image of a rat. (Courtesy Lorelei D'Avolio, The Center for Avian and Exotic Medicine, NYC.)

Lateral View of the Whole Body/Abdomen/Thorax of Exotic Companion Mammal—cont'd

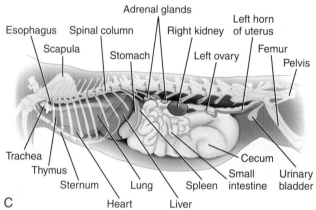

FIG. 25.21 **A,** Positioning for the lateral full-body view of the rabbit. The same positioning applies for abdomen, thorax, skull, pelvis, and limbs (if separated). **B,** Radiograph of the lateral abdomen of a rabbit. **C,** Anatomical drawing of the lateral view of the rabbit. (**A** courtesy Rick Axelson, Links Road Animal Clinic, North York, ON.)

Lateral View of the Whole Body/Abdomen/Thorax of Exotic Companion Mammal—cont'd

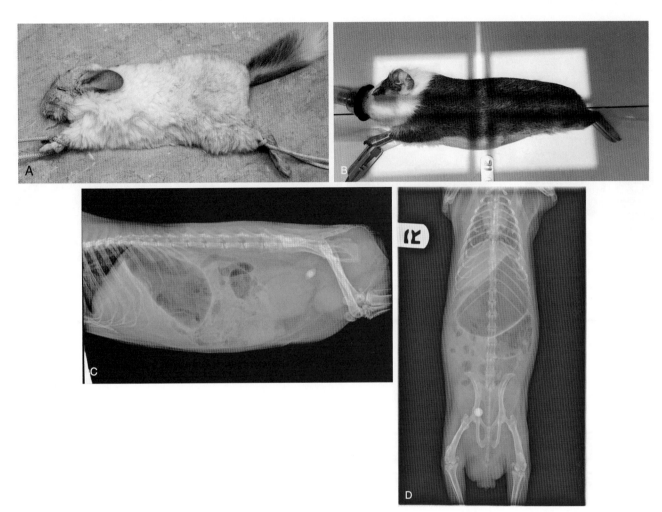

FIG. 25.22 A, Positioning for a lateral view of a chinchilla. Place the central ray over the area of interest and collimate appropriately. **B.** Positioning for the lateral view of a guinea pig. **C,** Image of the lateral view of a guinea pig showing urinary calculi (compare to Fig. 25.23B). **D,** The ventrodorsal of this guinea pig. (**A** courtesy Rick Axelson, Links Road Animal Clinic, North York, ON; **B–D** courtesy Lorelei D'Avolio, The Center for Avian and Exotic Medicine, NYC.)

Lateral View of the Whole Body/Abdomen/Thorax of Exotic Companion Mammal—cont'd

FIG. 25.23 A, Lateral decubitus (dorsoventral with horizontal beam) of a guinea pig. **B,** Image of a lateral guinea pig with the horizontal beam. The urinary calculi may be misdiagnosed with this view. Compare to Fig. 25.22C. (Courtesy Lorelei D'Avolio, The Center for Avian and Exotic Medicine, NYC.)

Skull of Exotic Companion Mammal

Lateral View of the Skull of Exotic Companion Mammal

Positioning

- Place the patient in lateral recumbency with affected side down (Figs. 25.24 and 25.25).
- Position the head so that the mandible is parallel to the long edge of the image receptor.
- Use a foam pad or cotton under the nose and neck to superimpose the rami and to prevent rotation of the skull. Tape in place to align the skull parallel to the table.
- Keep the ears dorsal and caudal so they are out of the field of view.
- Place the label dorsal to the nose.

Comments and Tips

- How to ensure a symmetrical image:
  - Draw an imaginary line between the medial canthi and make sure this line is perpendicular to the table.
  - The left and right halves of a normal skull should be superimposed.
- Malocclusion is common in rabbits. Dental abscesses and resultant osteomyelitis are also of concern.

MEASURE: The thickest part of the skull.
CENTRAL RAY: Midskull just rostral and ventral to the eye.
BORDERS: Include from the tip of the nose to C2 (the base of the skull).

Lateral View of the Skull of Exotic Companion Mammal—cont'd

FIG. 25.24 Comparisons of Skulls of Exotic Companion Mammals. Right lateral views of a rat **(A)**, hamster **(B)**, guinea pig **(C)**, ferret **(D)**, rabbit **(E)**, and chinchilla **(F)**. (A to D from Silverman S, Tell L. Radiology of Rodents, Rabbits and Ferrets: An Atlas of Normal Anatomy and Positioning. St. Louis: Saunders; 2005. E courtesy Lorelei D'Avolio, The Center for Avian and Exotic Medicine, NYC; F courtesy Rick Axelson, Links Road Animal Clinic, North York, ON.)

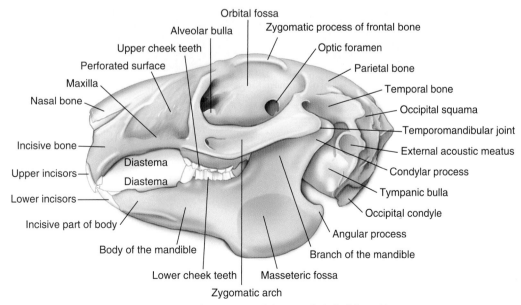

FIG. 25.25 The Anatomy of the Lateral Skull of the Rabbit.

Dorsoventral or Ventrodorsal View of the Skull of Exotic Companion Animals

Positioning

For the DV view (place in ventral recumbency directly on the table):

- Position the head flat on the image receptor.
- Place tape/Velcro across the nasal septum and the cranium to keep the sagittal plane of the head perpendicular to the image receptor.

For the VD view (place in dorsal recumbency directly on the table) (Fig. 25.26):

- Position a foam pad or cotton under the neck, keeping the hard palate parallel with the image receptor.
- Put tape/Velcro over the head caudal to the ears.
- Place tape across the mandible to keep the head aligned with the table.

Comments and Tips

- Sandbags or foam pads can be placed on either side to prevent rotation.
- Keep radiopaque devices out of the field of view. Place the label lateral to the nose.
- Make sure the ears are positioned laterally, equidistant from the head.
- To ensure that the image will be symmetrical:
  - An imaginary line drawn between the medial canthi must be parallel to the table.
  - The left and right halves of a normal skull should be a mirror image of each other when looking at the image.

MEASURE: The thickest part of the skull.

CENTRAL RAY: Midline between the eyes.

BORDERS: Include the tip of the nose to C2 (base of the skull).

FIG. 25.26 Ventrodorsal View of the Skull of a Chinchilla. (Courtesy Rick Axelson, Links Road Animal Clinic, North York, ON.)

Lateral Oblique (Oblique Dorsoventral) Views of the Skull for Tympanic Bullae, Dental Arcade, and Temporomandibular Joint of a Larger Exotic Companion Mammal

Positioning

- Place the patient in left or right lateral recumbency and place a label dorsal to the nose.
- Place sponges under the skull, creating a 30-degree angle[4] to the table or receptor, with the nose pointing down and touching the surface.
- Keep the ears out of the field of view.
- With the patient lying on its right side, the position is technically termed the *LeD30-RtVO* or *right oblique DV view.* (Fig. 25.27; see Chapter 21 for a review of oblique terminology.)
- This position also produces a radiograph of the lower dental arcade.

Comments and Tips

- If the upper dental arcade is of interest, place foam pads under the nose, creating a 30- to 45-degree angle to the table, with the back of the skull touching the image receptor and the nose pointing upwards. Secure with tape if needed.
- If the patient is lying on its right side, the position is technically named the *LeV30-RtDO* or *right oblique VD view.*
- A complete radiographic study of the skull should include extraoral lateral, oblique, dorsoventral (or ventrodorsal), and rostrocaudal head views as well as intraoral views (Table 25.3).[5]
- See Chapters 21 and 22 for further information on radiographing the canine or feline skull and teeth, which can also be applied to smaller mammals.
- Magnification of rodent and rabbit skulls may be required. This can be obtained by using a small focal spot and increased OID/decreased SID. The patient can be positioned on a radiolucent foam sponge on top of the image receptor. If the OFD is 12 inches and the SID is 20 inches, the magnification is about 2.0.[4]

MEASURE: The thickest part of the skull.
CENTRAL RAY: Midskull, just rostral and ventral to the eye.
BORDERS: Include the tip of the nose to C2 (the base of the skull).

TABLE 25.3	Dentition of Some Common Rodents and the Rabbit*				
	PERMANENT	PERMANENT INCISORS	PERMANENT CANINES	PERMANENT PREMOLARS	PERMANENT MOLARS
Hamsters, gerbils, rodents	16	2/2	0/0	0/0	6/6
Guinea pigs	20	2/2	0/0	2/2	6/6
Rabbits	28	4/2	0/0	6/4	6/6

*Number before slash indicates maxillary teeth; number after indicates mandibular teeth.

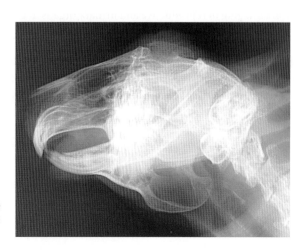

FIG. 25.27 Oblique (30-degree) Ventrodorsal View of the Skull of an Adult Rabbit. (From Silverman S, Tell L. *Radiology of Rodents, Rabbits and Ferrets: An Atlas of Normal Anatomy and Positioning.* St. Louis: Saunders; 2005.)

Normal Guinea Pig, Chinchilla, Rabbit, and Ferret Anatomy

See Appendix D on the Evolve website and Figs. 25.18, 25.19, 25.21, and 25.25 for some common radiographic anatomy of these species.

Ultrasonography Restraint

- Ultrasonography is a useful diagnostic tool for exotic companion mammals. Guinea pigs, rabbits, and small rodents are difficult to examine with ultrasound because of their small size and reluctance to keep still.
- They are often best restrained in an upright position in the lap of, or against the body of, a restraining assistant. The restrainer will support the upper limbs and head with one hand and the rear limbs with the other.
- If further support for a larger patient is needed for ultrasonography, the lower limbs can be grasped by another person. If patients are showing stress during this restraint, sedation should be used as described previously.

Reptiles

Radiographic imaging is frequently required in pursuing reptile diagnostics. Knowledge of reptiles' unique anatomical characteristics is essential for providing a technically proficient image. Traumatic injuries, gravidity evaluation, impactions, lung evaluation for pneumonia, and urinary calculi are common reasons that a radiograph may need to be acquired in a reptile.

The fused ribs and sternum form the carapace and plastron in chelonians (tortoises and turtles), making coelomic detail difficult to view. Some lizard species have particularly dense scales that are radioopaque, making visualization of the organs challenging. A symmetrical lateral view in snakes may be difficult to obtain because of constant movement.

Ultrasound and endoscopy are other imaging tools commonly used in reptilian medicine. Because of shells and scales, there are also significant limitations with ultrasound. Placing the probe at the prefemoral fossa in chelonians can yield imaging of reproductive and urinary organs. If chelonians are large enough, imaging of the liver and heart is possible. Use of water and copious ultrasound gel can make visualization past scales possible.

Endoscopy is particularly useful. Coelioscopy, or internal examination of the coelomic cavity, provides a direct view of the liver, lungs, kidneys, heart, spleen, bladder, GI tract, pancreas, and gonads, although it requires anesthesia and an incision. In lizards, the incision for coelioscopy is generally made in the lateral body wall just caudal to the last rib. In chelonians, the incision is at the center of the prefemoral fossa, and in snakes, at the junction of the ventral and lateral scales at the expected site of interest. Endoscopy can also be used in reptiles to visualize the trachea and bronchi for evaluation of respiratory disease, to retrieve foreign bodies from the GI tract, and to obtain tissue specimens of diseased organs.

Chelonians/Testudines: Turtle, Tortoise, and Terrapin

Positioning Concerns of Chelonians (Testudines)

- The terms *chelonian* and *testudine* are generally interchangeable and refer to shelled reptiles. Although most chelonians will readily sit still long enough to expose a radiograph, keeping the limbs in extension can be a challenge. Consider using a round device under the plastron so the limbs are out of the shell and not touching the plate (see Fig. 25.28B). Alternatively, tape/Velcro over the shell caudally to keep the patient from wandering and to encourage chelonians to pull against the force of the tape to extend their limbs (see Fig. 25.28A). The chelonian can be turned on its back and then flipped upright just before taking the image. This may disorient the patient so as to cause momentary extension of the appendages and head. A short-acting anesthetic agent such as alfaxalone can also facilitate proper positioning.
- With turtles, it is important to obtain a craniocaudal (rostrocaudal) view in addition to dorsoventral and lateral views. The craniocaudal view enables unobstructed vision of both lungs. The horizontal beam should be considered for the craniocaudal as well as lateral views if the machine and plate positioning allow. A grid is not likely needed except for the larger species over 10 cm.
- Nonscreen dental film or a digital dental unit can be used for smaller patients, and a high-detail system should be used for the larger patients. A positive-contrast study can be completed if the GI tract is of concern. If GI contrast studies are completed, the time scale for passage of the medium is significantly longer than in mammals, lasting several days in some species. See Fig. 12.13 for a CT scan of a chelonian.

Radiographic Views

Dorsoventral View of Chelonians/Testudines

Positioning

- Position the patient on its plastron and use tape at the caudal aspect if required, or place on a round object (Fig. 25.28).

Comments and Tips

- As long as the central ray is in the center of the shell, most chelonian images show symmetry.

MEASURE: The thickest part of the body.
CENTRAL RAY: The center of the shell.
BORDERS: Include the whole body.

FIG. 25.28 A, Strategic use of tape keeps this turtle in position and may encourage it to extract its limbs as it tries to walk away. B, The use of a round positioning device under this Indian Star Tortoise (*Geochelone elegans*) is ideal.

Dorsoventral View of Chelonians/Testudines—cont'd

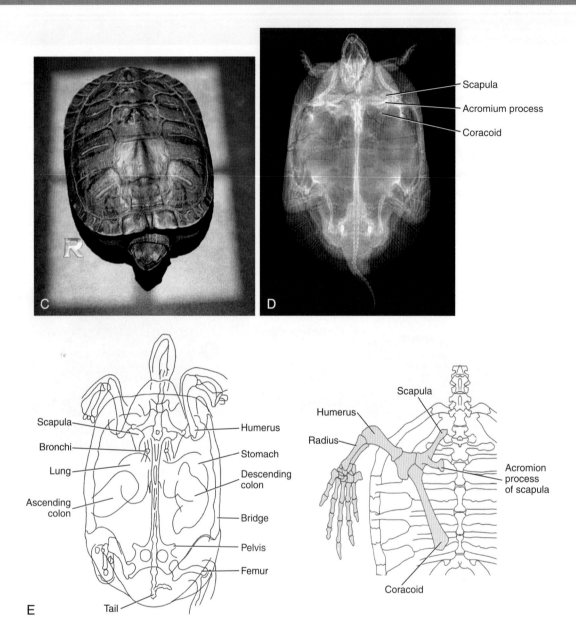

Scapula

Acromium process

Coracoid

Scapula
Bronchi
Lung
Ascending
colon

Humerus
Stomach
Descending
colon
Bridge
Pelvis
Femur
Tail

Scapula
Humerus
Radius
Acromion
process
of scapula
Coracoid

E

FIG. 25.28, cont'd C, Dorsoventral view of a Painted Turtle. **D**, Dorsoventral radiograph of a Painted Turtle. **E**, Radiographic anatomy of the Snapping Turtle. (**A** and **D** courtesy Sue Carstairs, Kawartha Turtle Trauma Centre, ON; **B** courtesy Ryan Cheeck, Veterinary Technology, Gwinnett Technical College, Lawrenceville, GA; **C** courtesy Rick Axelson, Links Road Animal Clinic, North York, ON.)

Lateral View of Chelonians/Testudines

Positioning for a Lateral View with a Horizontal Beam of Chelonians/Testudines

- Use of the lateral decubitus view (dorsoventral position with a horizontal beam) is preferred for the lateral view of a chelonian.
- Place the chelonian in ventral recumbency on top of a foam pad or acrylic positioning device or on a small radiolucent object so the legs are exposed (Fig. 25.29).
- Tape/Velcro over the shell caudally or place over round foam to prevent the patient from wandering.
- Place the image receptor perpendicular to the table directly behind the turtle's lateral side opposite to the beam.
- Position the beam parallel to the table so that the central ray is midway between the plastron and carapace, in full view of the image receptor.
- The beam should bisect the plastron and carapace for the image to be symmetrical.

> **✎ TECHNICIAN NOTES** As with other positions, the lateral decubitus view is labeled according to the side against the image receptor. In a right lateral, the right side is against the plate. Technically this is called a *left to right lateral decubitus view* (dorsoventral position with a horizontal beam).

Positioning for a Lateral View with a Vertical Beam of Chelonians/Testudines

- Place the chelonian in ventral recumbency on its plastron, and securely tape the patient to a foam pad or acrylic positioning device, or secure between two devices (Fig. 25.29).
- Turn the pad so that the lateral side of the chelonian is positioned on the image receptor.
  - The chelonian is lying laterally on its "side."
  - The beam passes vertically between the carapace and plastron.
  - The beam should bisect the plastron and carapace for the image to be symmetrical.

MEASURE: The thickest part of the shell.

CENTRAL RAY: The center of the body between the carapace and plastron.

BORDERS: Include the whole body.

FIG. 25.29 A, Positioning for a lateral view of an Indian Star Tortoise with the use of a horizontal beam.

Lateral View of Chelonians/Testudines—cont'd

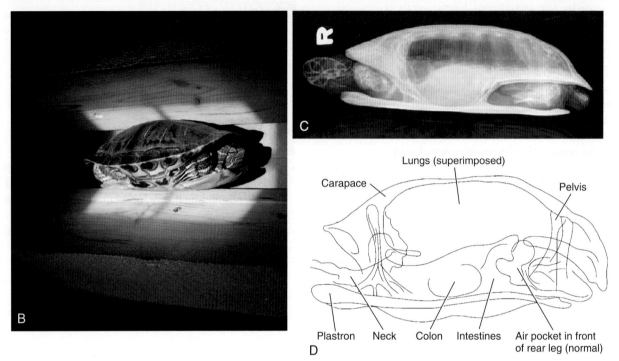

FIG. 25.29, cont'd B, Positioning for a lateral view of a Painted Turtle with the use of a vertical beam. C, Radiograph of a lateral view with the use of the horizontal beam of a Painted Turtle. D, Lateral radiographic anatomy of a Painted Turtle. (A courtesy Ryan Cheeck, Veterinary Technology, Gwinnett Technical College, Lawrenceville, GA; B and C courtesy Sue Carstairs, Kawartha Turtle Trauma Centre, ON.)

Craniocaudal View of Chelonians/Testudines

Positioning for a Craniocaudal View with a Horizontal Beam

- Place the chelonian in ventral recumbency on a circular foam block.
- Have the image receptor caudal to and as close to the patient as possible.
- Direct the beam horizontally from a cranial direction through to the tail (Fig. 25.30A).

Positioning for Craniocaudal View with a Vertical Beam of Chelonians/Testudines

- Place the chelonian in ventral recumbency and tape the patient to a foam pad or block.
- Place and position the chelonian and block so that the caudal portion of the body is resting on the cassette and table and the head is pointing up to the beam (Fig. 25.30B).

- Direct the beam vertically from the head through the tail.

See Appendix D on the Evolve website and Figs. 25.28–25.31 for normal anatomy and radiographic concerns of chelonians.

> **TECHNICIAN NOTES** In female turtles, the caudal vertebrae are short and decrease in size distally, whereas in males, the lateral and dorsal processes are stout. As a general rule, the vent of a female is found at or within the carapace perimeter. The male generally has a long tail, and the vent (cloacal opening) is generally more caudal (nearer the tip of the tail) than in the female. In some tortoises, males have a curved plastron to facilitate mating. Some male aquatic turtles have very long front toenails.

MEASURE: The thickest area of the body.
CENTRAL RAY: Through the middle of the head.
BORDERS: Include the whole body.

FIG. 25.30 A, Craniocaudal view of an Indian Star Tortoise with the use of a horizontal beam.

Craniocaudal View of Chelonians/Testudines—cont'd

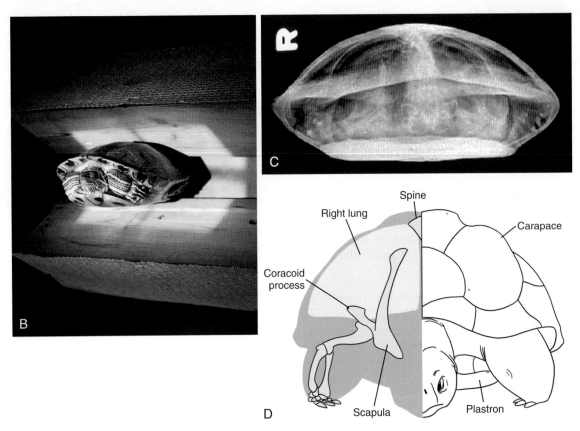

FIG. 25.30, cont'd **B**, Craniocaudal view of a Painted Turtle using a vertical beam. The patient is positioned between two blocks. **C**, Craniocaudal radiograph of a Painted Turtle. **D**, Radiographic anatomy and overlay of the craniocaudal view of a Painted Turtle. (**A** courtesy Ryan Cheeck, Veterinary Technology, Gwinnett Technical College, Lawrenceville, GA; **B** and **C** courtesy Sue Carstairs, Kawartha Turtle Trauma Centre, ON.)

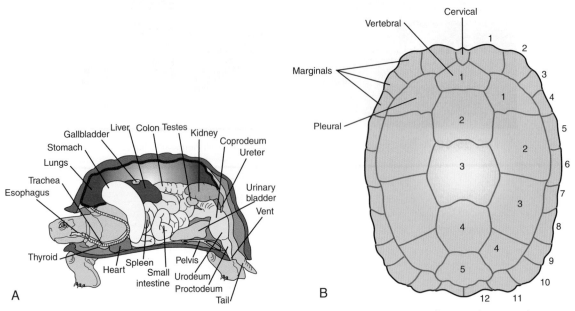

FIG. 25.31 **A**, Cross-section of the internal anatomy of a chelonian. **B**, Chelonian carapace illustrating the nomenclature of scutes. (**A** from Colville T, Bassert JM. *Clinical Anatomy and Physiology for Veterinary Technicians.* 3rd ed. St. Louis: Elsevier; 2016.)

Lizards—Radiography Concerns

- Positioning of lizards (order *Squamata*) for radiography employs the conventional DV and lateral views. They are the most straightforward of the reptiles to image, and many of the concepts employed for small mammal radiography can be utilized. Many species can be radiographed awake, although anesthesia aids in obtaining diagnostic radiographs. Strategically placed tape can be employed to stabilize the patient on the image receptor.
- Placing a blindfold of some sort over the eyes of the lizard may minimize movement. This can be achieved by placing eye lubricant in the eyes and wrapping the head with vet wrap. Applying pressure over both eye orbits through closed lids can also be effective. The response to this pressure is the vasovagal reflex, which can induce a drop in heart rate and blood pressure and induce a catatonic state.
- Be careful not to pull the patient by the tail, as tail autonomy can occur in some species. Take appropriate precautions with venomous lizards.

Dorsoventral View of the Lizard

Positioning

- Place the lizard in sternal recumbency with limbs lateral to the body (Fig. 25.32).
- Put masking tape/Velcro over the neck, caudal to the pectoral limbs and over the pelvis, if needed. Use a vertical beam.

Comments and Tips

- The limbs are naturally positioned lateral to the body, so superimposition with viscera does not usually occur.
- Be aware of the level of stress of the patient.
- If only the extremities are of interest, tape as described and extend the limb of interest with masking tape, gauze, or Velcro.

MEASURE: The thickest point of the body.

CENTRAL RAY: Over the midline of the body about the level of the TL junction, unless the tail is of interest.

BORDERS: Include the whole body.

> **TECHNICIAN NOTES** How to tell whether the image will appear symmetrical in a DV:
> - The spine is superimposed over the sternum.
> - The patient is straight from head to tail.

FIG. 25.32 A, Simplified internal anatomy of a lizard. **B,** Dorsoventral positioning for a bearded dragon prior to imaging. To minimize skull magnification, use tape or Velcro to keep the head and neck more parallel to the cassette. **C,** Dorsoventral radiograph of the bearded dragon. (**A** from Colville T, Bassert JM. *Clinical Anatomy and Physiology for Veterinary Technicians.* 3rd ed. St. Louis: Elsevier; 2016.)

Lateral View of the Lizard

The lateral decubitus (dorsoventral position with horizontal beam) is less stressful for the patient and may yield more anatomically accurate radiographs (Fig. 25.33).

Positioning with the Use of a Horizontal Beam

- Place the patient in ventral recumbency on a raised sponge block or plastic sheet.
- Tape/Velcro the neck, shoulders, and pelvis if needed.
- Position the beam so it is horizontal with the table and perpendicular to the image receptor, which is placed as close as possible to the side of the lizard that is being radiographed
- Mark the side placed against the image receptor.

Comments and Tips

- Keep the body of the patient close to the cassette and the spine straight and parallel to minimize OFD and distortion.
- The tails of larger lizards can be taped.
- To ensure that the image will be symmetrical:
  - The patient should have equal weight on its feet, with the spine parallel to the receptor.
  - The central ray is perpendicular to both.

MEASURE: The thickest part of the body if not using a species chart.
CENTRAL RAY: Over the midline of the body.
BORDERS: Include the whole body.

FIG. 25.33 A, Horizontal beam for the right lateral view of a gecko. **B,** Lateral view of a Bearded Dragon on positioning devices with use of a horizontal beam and the patient in ventral recumbency. **C,** Radiograph of a lizard in regular lateral position with the use of a vertical beam.

Lateral View of the Lizard—cont'd

Normal Anatomy of the Lizard

See Fig. 25.32A and Appendix D on the Evolve website for normal anatomy and radiographic concerns of the lizard.

Ultrasound Concerns of the Lizard

- Ultrasound can be used to evaluate various systems, such as the reproductive, as well as the heart and other viscera. The heart, as in most reptiles, is three-chambered. In most lizards, it is situated in the pectoral girdle. Place the transducer in the axillary region and rotate it to evaluate all three chambers.

- The viscera in the caudal coelom can be examined, and ultrasound can be used to help collect fine-needle biopsy specimens or aspirates. Ovulation can be determined by placing the transducer over the ovary on the lateral body wall just caudal to the last rib and noting the follicle measurement. Both ovaries should be examined. Depending on the species, this comparison may help determine when the male and female should be placed together for breeding.

Snakes[2,6,7]—Radiography Concerns

- Snake species (order *Squamata*) are extremely variable in size, and thus various sized restraint devices are required. The snake is best placed in a tube (Fig. 25.34A) or stretched and taped to a long plastic sheet or supported in a tubed stockinet. If the stockinet or a tube is used, the position will be fairly well maintained, provided that the patient is not able to rotate its head inside the tube. Keeping the body elongated and not coiled is especially important for the lateral view. It is important to have the body in a straight line, and thus multiple exposures may be required to allow the entire body to be imaged.

- Small snakes can be coiled on the image receptor or in a radiolucent container. However, true symmetry will not be obtained with the oblique view.

- Placing metallic pellets laterally may assist with "dividing" the body for easier identification.

- Manual restraint may be needed for some of the larger species in order to position the body correctly. Consider the use of the bird positioner, especially if the snake is venomous or aggressive.

- Knowledge of organ location is essential for proper positioning. The dorsoventral view is more useful for imaging the spine and ribs, and lateral recumbency is more useful for proper visualization of the organs. Reptiles do not tolerate being placed in lateral position, so if this view is required, a horizontal beam for the lateral radiograph with the patient in a tube is recommended.

Dorsoventral View of the Snake

Positioning

- Keep the patient in true sternal recumbency, ideally in a plastic tube. Use a vertical beam.
- For true symmetry, there should be no overlapping of the vertebrae, and the ribs should appear equidistant on each side of the vertebrae (Figs. 25.34 and 25.35).

- Multiple handlers may be required for safe radiography of a large snake.
  Center over the area of interest.
  Include the area of interest (cranial, middle, caudal).

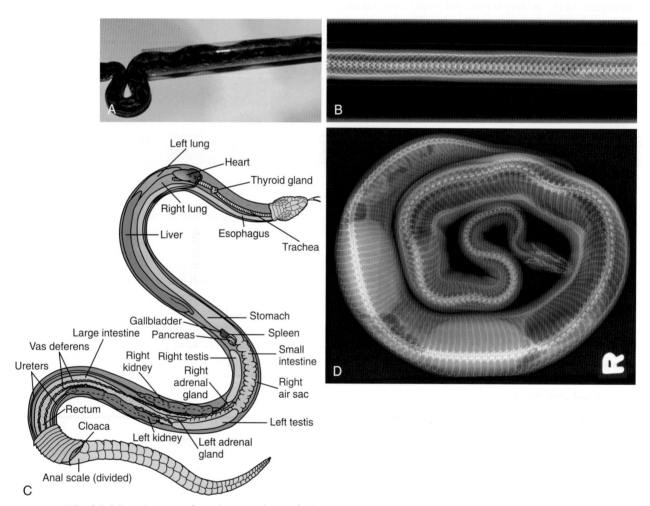

FIG. 25.34 A, Positioning for a dorsoventral view of a boa constrictor. The same positioning can be used for the lateral with the use of a horizontal beam. **B,** Radiograph of a dorsoventral view of a boa constrictor. **C,** Ventral view of a male snake showing internal anatomy. **D,** When the patient is allowed to coil naturally, an oblique view, rather than a true DV will be obtained, as in this image. (**A** and **B** courtesy Ryan Cheeck, Veterinary Technology, Gwinnett Technical College, Lawrenceville, GA; **C** from Colville T, Bassert JM. *Clinical Anatomy and Physiology for Veterinary Technicians.* 3rd ed. St. Louis: Elsevier; 2016.)

Lateral View of the Snake

Lateral decubitus (dorsoventral view with horizontal beam) (preferred)

- Place the patient in a DV position as described earlier. Use a horizontal beam, placing the image receptor vertically on the side of interest.

Lateral view with a vertical beam

- If the horizontal beam is not available, the snake will need to be placed in lateral position with the aid of a tube or multiple handlers, depending on the snake size. A vertical beam is used.

For the lateral views: Center over the area of interest. **Include** the area of interest (cranial, middle, caudal)

How to tell whether the body is symmetrical:

- The snake is stretched out, with no coiling of the body.
- The vertebrae appear on the dorsal aspect.

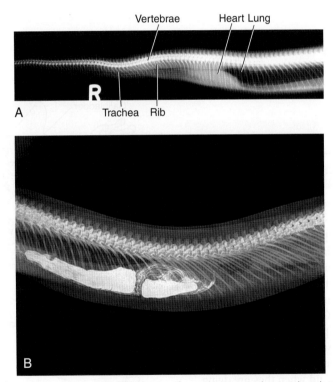

FIG. 25.35 A, Radiographic anatomy of the lateral view of a snake. **B,** Lateral view taken during a contrast study of a snake. (**A** courtesy Sue Carstairs, Kawartha Turtle Trauma Centre, ON; **B** courtesy Rick Axelson, Links Road Animal Clinic, North York, ON.)

FIG. 25.36 **A,** Dorsoventral views of South American Tree Frogs in Petri dishes. **B,** Dorsoventral view of a Red-Spotted Newt (*Caudata* species of amphibian).

Normal Snake Anatomy

See Appendix D on the Evolve website and Fig. 25.34C for normal anatomy and radiographic concerns of the snake.

Amphibians

Radiography Comments and Tips

- Amphibians such as toads and frogs (order *Anura*), salamanders, and newts (order *Caudata*) can be imaged much like other species. Depending on the size of the species, Petri dishes or containers can be used.
- When handling amphibians, make sure to use wet, powder-free gloves. Gloves protect the wet mucosal surface on the skin of aquatic amphibians, which is quite sensitive to the chemicals on hands. Gloves also prevent allergic reactions for humans and protects the handler from transmission of bacterial diseases. Anurans are able to prolapse the stomach after eating undesirable food, after some methods of anesthesia, and when they are dying.
- The most commonly used view is the DV (Fig. 25.37). If required and if available, lateral views are completed with the patient in a DV position with the use of a horizontal beam if available. See Fig. 25.37 for Anura anatomy.

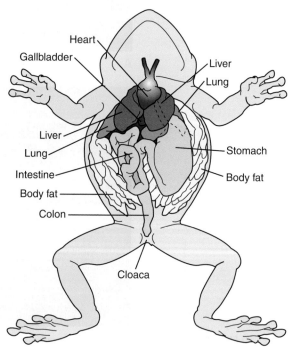

FIG. 25.37 Ventral View of the Frog Showing Internal Anatomy. (From Colville T, Bassert JM. *Clinical Anatomy and Physiology for Veterinary Technicians.* 3rd ed. St. Louis: Elsevier; 2016.)

Fish

Radiography and Positioning Concerns

- Fish medicine is a fast-growing area in veterinary medicine, with ever-increasing knowledge in the area of diagnostics. As such, radiography is more commonly performed. Common reasons for radiography include trauma, swim bladder issues, and neoplasia.

- When handling fish, keep in mind that the skin and scales provide a protective barrier and are quite sensitive to handling. Scales grow continuously throughout the life of the fish and are not regenerated if lost. They must continuously be kept moist using water from its aquarium and not exposed to air for more than a few seconds. If a temporary aquarium or bucket with some of the aquarium water is used, it will be difficult to keep the fish stationary and there will likely be movement artifacts. As with amphibians, make sure to use powder-free gloves.

- Generally, fish require anesthesia with an agent such as tricaine methanesulfonate (MS-222) with appropriate buffering in the water to enable proper positioning. Using a moist plastic bag with the MS-222 for the procedure will keep the patient comfortable and minimize movement. It is vital that the patient be handled as minimally as possible and returned to its environment as quickly as possible.

Dorsoventral and Lateral Views of Fish

- Place the fish in a bag with water from its aquarium (Fig. 25.38A).
- Complete the procedure quickly. For both views, use a vertical beam.
- The lateral view is more practical, but if the DV is required, support the bag so the fish is upright.
- Center over the middle of the body and include the whole body.

Normal Radiographic Anatomy of Amphibians and Fish[3,7]

See Appendix D on the Evolve website and Figs. 25.38 and 25.39 for normal anatomy and radiographic concerns of the amphibian and fish.

Fig. 25.39 is a mystery radiograph. Review it and answer the question presented with it.

FIG. 25.39 Mystery Radiograph. What view is this for this Red-Footed tortoise? Explain the internal contents and their likely cause. (Courtesy Lorelei D'Avolio, The Center for Avian and Exotic Medicine, NYC.)

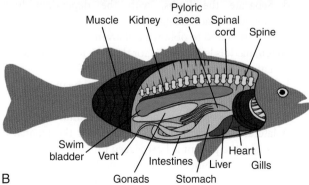

Pyloric
caeca
Muscle Kidney   Spinal
                      cord   Spine

Swim
bladder Vent   Heart
         Intestines   Liver   Gills
    Gonads   Stomach
B

FIG. 25.38 A, Lateral view of a fish radiographed in a bag of water. B, Anatomy of the lateral view of a fish. (B from Colville T, Bassert JM. *Clinical Anatomy and Physiology for Veterinary Technicians.* 3rd ed. St. Louis: Elsevier; 2016.)

Image Gallery

eFigs. 25.1 to 25.16 are additional images to supplement avian and exotic radiographic positioning.

✳ KEY POINTS

1. Generally, avian radiography requires chemical restraint for diagnostic results. Fasting time before anesthesia is variable and species specific.
2. Ensure handler safety when radiographing patients by always restraining their particular weapons, which vary by species.
3. For proper diagnosis, the positions must be exactly perpendicular, especially with the avian ventrodorsal view, to avoid misinterpretation of the radiograph.
4. Exotic companion mammals also generally require chemical restraint for adequate radiographs, but they are not usually fasted before sedation or anesthesia.
5. Dental concerns are extremely common in rodents and rabbits, so excellent skull radiographs are essential.
6. Good coelomic detail is difficult to visualize during radiography of chelonians. A craniocaudal view is essential to obtain an unobstructed view of the lungs.
7. Lateral radiographs of snakes are necessary to adequately visualize internal structures. Consider use of a horizontal beam if available.
8. Almost any species can be radiographed if the behavior and important radiographic principles are kept in mind.

REVIEW QUESTIONS

1. You are required to obtain an image of a budgerigar. 2.5 mAs is best obtained with:
   a. 300 mA and 1/120 of a second
   b. 200 mA and 1/80 s
   c. 100 mA and 1/40 s
   d. Whatever you can set on your machine

2. A budgerigar is being positioned for a VD whole-body view. To ensure there will be symmetry on the image, the:
   a. Acetabula, ribs, coracoids, and kidneys are superimposed
   b. Keel is directly over the spine, and the scapulae, acetabula, and femurs are parallel
   c. Sternum and vertebral column are on the same plane
   d. Patient is in true ventral recumbency

3. You should center for this VD whole-body view of the budgerigar:
   a. Over the midline at the caudal tip of the sternum
   b. Slightly to the left side of the keel
   c. Slightly to the right side of the keel
   d. Over the midline at the cranial part of the sternum

4. An ill cockatoo needs to be gavaged and radiographed. You should obtain a radiograph for this patient:
   a. After the gavaging
   b. Before the gavaging
   c. At any time, as gavaging is not an issue
   d. While gavaging

5. For the VD survey of the cockatoo coelom, you should take the image:
   a. At maximum inspiration
   b. At maximum expiration
   c. Whenever there is movement to assist in showing contrast
   d. At any point, as distension of the abdominal air sacs may enhance abdominal viscera

6. A full contrast study is required for the cockatoo patient noted earlier. The images will likely be taken:
   a. Immediately, 15 minutes, 30 minutes, and then half-hourly as needed
   b. Immediately and then half-hourly as needed
   c. Immediately and then hourly as needed
   d. At 15 minutes and then every 15 minutes as needed

7. A Blue Heron suspected of lead poisoning is to be imaged. When restraining this species, it is particularly important to:
   a. Tape the talons
   b. Wear a full-face shield
   c. Keep the room bright
   d. Measure at the thickest part

8. The minimum source-image distance (SID) that should be used when radiographing birds is:
   a. 30 inches
   b. 40 inches
   c. 50 inches
   d. 60 inches

9. To obtain a mediolateral view of the right wing of a swan, the patient should be positioned in:
   a. Dorsal recumbency
   b. Ventral recumbency
   c. Right lateral recumbency
   d. Left lateral recumbency

10. The dorsoventral as opposed to the ventrodorsal position is best utilized for:
    a. All exotic companion mammals and reptiles
    b. Reptiles
    c. Small animals such as dogs and cats
    d. Larger exotic companion mammals such as rabbits and ferrets

11. You are looking at the orthogonal image of the rat and know that the image is symmetrical because the:
    a. Acetabula are square and the femurs are bent 90 degrees
    b. Vertebrae and sternebrae are on the same horizontal plane
    c. Spinous processes are to the left of the vertebral bodies
    d. Sternebrae are superimposed over the vertebrae on the same vertical plane

12. A lateral view is needed of a male ferret abdomen. You should center:
    a. Cranial to the xiphoid
    b. Cranial to the pubis
    c. Caudal to the last rib
    d. At the TL junction

13. For this lateral view of the male ferret abdomen, you should include cranial from the:
    a. Shoulder joint and slightly caudal to the last rib
    b. Shoulder joint and caudal to the pubis
    c. Xiphoid process and caudal to the last rib
    d. Xiphoid process and caudal to the pubis

14. When positioning the limbs for this lateral abdomen of the ferret, it is best to:
    a. Superimpose the limbs and pull toward the center as much as possible
    b. Superimpose the limbs, pulling the pectoral limbs cranially and the pelvic limbs caudally
    c. Separate the limbs, with the dependent limb positioned more caudally
    d. Separate the limbs, with the dependent limb positioned more cranially

15. You are required to obtain a dorsoventral (DV) view for an iguana. It is less stressful for the patient to position in:
    a. Lateral recumbency and use a vertical beam
    b. Lateral position and use a horizontal beam
    c. Ventral recumbency and use a vertical beam
    d. Ventral recumbency and use a horizontal beam

16. A lateral radiograph is also required for the iguana. If available, the patient is best placed in:
    a. Lateral recumbency and use a vertical beam
    b. Lateral recumbency and use a horizontal beam
    c. Ventral recumbency and use a vertical beam
    d. Ventral recumbency and use a horizontal beam

17. The view that best illustrates both lung fields when radiographing chelonians is the:
    a. Craniocaudal
    b. Dorsoventral
    c. Lateral
    d. Ventrodorsal

18. The veterinarian wants you to obtain a craniocaudal radiograph of a turtle, but the machine does not allow a horizontal view. After taping the turtle in ventral recumbency to a foam pad or block, you should position both so that the:
    a. Caudal portion is pointing to the beam
    b. Head is pointing to the beam
    c. Lateral surface is pointing to the beam
    d. Beam is horizontal from a cranial direction to the tail.

19. A lateral view is required of a ball python. If available, it is best to:
    a. Use a bird positioner to place it in lateral position and use a vertical beam
    b. Place it in lateral position in a tube and use a vertical beam
    c. Place it in a tube and use a horizontal beam
    d. Allow it to coil in a natural position and use a horizontal beam

20. Fish are best radiographed in position by:
    a. Being taped to a plastic sheet
    b. Placement in a container with tap water
    c. Placement in a moistened small bag
    d. Placement in a small dry container

Chapter Review Question answers are located in the Instructor Resources on Evolve and can be provided to students at the discretion of the instructor.

References

1. Silverman A, Tell, L. *Radiology of Birds, an Atlas of Normal Anatomy and Positioning.* St. Louis: Elsevier; 2010.
2. Farrow C. *Diagnostic Imaging*: Birds, *Exotic Pets and Wildlife.* St. Louis: Elsevier; 2009.
3. Mayer J. Clinical anatomy and physiology of fish. CVC in Kansas City proceedings. Aug 1, 2012.
4. Silverman S, Tell L. *Radiology of Rodents, Rabbits and Ferrets: An Atlas of Normal Anatomy and Positioning.* St. Louis: Saunders; 2005.
5. Gracis MD. Clinical technique: normal dental radiography of rabbits, guinea pigs, and chinchillas. *J Exotic Pet Med.* 2008; 17:78-86.
6. Mitchell MA, Tully TN. *Manual of Exotic Pet Practice.* St. Louis: Saunders; 2009.
7. Colville T, Bassert J. *Clinical Anatomy and Physiology for Veterinary Technicians.* 3rd ed. St. Louis: Elsevier; 2016. http://veterinarycalendar.dvm360.com/avhc/Veterinary1Exotics/.

Bibliography

Aspinall V, Cappello M. *Introduction to Veterinary Anatomy.* London: Butterworth Heinemann; 2009.
Avian respiration. n.d. Retrieved March 2020. Available at: http://people.eku.edu/ritchisong/birdrespiration.html.
Ballard B, Cheek R. *Exotic Animal Medicine for the Veterinary Technician.* Ames, IA: John Wiley and Sons; 2017.
Dyce KM, Sack WO, Wensing CJG. *Textbook of Veterinary Anatomy.* 5th ed. St. Louis: Saunders; 2018.
Hernandez-Divers S. Snake radiology: the essentials. In: *NAVC Conference: Small Animal and Exotics.* Orlando, FL: North American Veterinary Conference; 2008:1772-1774.
Mitchell M. Diagnostic imaging of lizards. In: *NAVC Conference: Small Animal and Exotics.* Orlando, FL: North American Veterinary Conference; 2007:1590-1591.
Quesenberry K, Mans C, Orcutt C, Carpenter J. *Ferrets, Rabbits and Rodents.* 4th ed. Philadelphia: Saunders; 2020.
Tighe M, Brown M. *Mosby's Comprehensive Review for Veterinary Technicians.* 5th ed. St. Louis: Mosby; 2019.

15% Rule States that changing the kilovoltage peak by 15% has the same effect on image receptor exposure as doubling or halving the mAs (within the 60–90 kV range).

A

Abduction The movement of the limb away from the midline.

Absorbed Dose The transfer of radiation energy into matter (e.g., tissue).

Acoustic Impedance The effect of interference with the passage of sound waves, such as those generated by ultrasound equipment, by objects in the path of the sound waves.

Activator Something that activates a catalyst.

Active Layer The radiation/light sensitive layer of the film.

Actual Focal Spot Size The size of the area on the anode target that is exposed to electrons from the tube current. Actual focal spot size depends on the size of the filament producing the electron stream.

Added Filtration The filtration that is added to the port of the x-ray tube.

Air Gap Technique Based on the simple concept that much of the scatter will miss the image receptor if there is an increased distance between the patient and the image receptor (increased OID).

Air Kerma The amount of energy deposited in a unit mass of air.

ALARA (Principle) As Low As Reasonably Achievable.

Algorithm A process or set of rules used in calculations or problem-solving operations.

Alternating Current An electric current that reverses its polarity many times a second.

Ambient Lighting The level of light in the room when viewing images.

Ammonium Thiosulfate An inorganic compound used in photographic fixer. It is a rapid fixer.

Amperage The strength of an electric current, measured in amperes.

Amphibian A cold-blooded vertebrate class that comprises frogs, toads, newts, and salamanders, distinguished by having an aquatic gill-breathing larval stage, generally followed by a terrestrial lung-breathing adult stage.

Analog A substance, tissue, or organ that is similar in appearance or function to another but differing in origin or development.

Angiocardiography Radiography of the heart and great vessels after the introduction of an opaque contrast medium into a blood vessel or a cardiac chamber (from Greek *angeion* [vessel] + *kardia* [heart] *graphein* [to record]).

Angiography Radiographic examination of the vascular system after the intravenous injection of positive-contrast medium.

Annihilation The breaking apart of a positron and electron when they collide. The collision produces two gamma ray photons which depart 180 degrees away from each other.

Anode A positively charged electrode within the x-ray tube. Composed of molybdenum, copper, tungsten and graphite. It consists of a target and, in rotating anode tubes, a stator and rotor.

Anode Heel Effect The x-ray beam has greater intensity (number of x-rays) on the cathode side of the tube, with the intensity diminishing toward the anode side. The heel effect occurs because of the angle of the target.

Antegrade Radiographic examination of a body part in which positive-contrast medium is injected vascularly (from Latin *ante* [before] and *gradi* [to go]).

Antifroth A chemical that is added to a liquid to reduce or hinder formation of foam or froth.

Antisludge A chemical composition used to minimize or prevent the formation of sludge. A term used in automatic film processing.

Aperture Diaphragm A flat piece of lead (diaphragm) containing a hole (aperture) for beam restriction.

Apical Towards the apex or tip of the root of a tooth.

Arch Crescent arrangements of teeth on the mandible and on the maxilla that together constitute the dentition.

Archive A collection of historical documents or records, i.e., transfer of data to a less frequently used storage medium.

Arthrography Radiographic examination of the articular cartilage, joint space, and joint capsule after the sterile injection of contrast medium.

Articular Margin The area where the joint attaches (from Latin *articulus* [small connecting part]).

Artifact Accidental or unintentional image on a radiographic image.

Atalectasis The collapse of alveolar tissue affecting part or all of one lung. It can occur in the dependent lung during lateral recumbency in awake patients (from Greek *atel* [incomplete] + *ectasis* [extension]).

Atom The smallest division of an element that exhibits all the properties and characteristics of the element.

Atomic Theory The concept that all matter is composed of submicroscopic atoms that are in turn composed of protons, electrons, and neutrons.

Attenuation Reduction in the radiation intensity that results from absorption and scattering.

Attenuation Profile A calculation used to approximate the absorption of radiation by denser tissues such as bone. This is used in PET imaging to create actual images.

Automatic Brightness Control (ABC) A function of the fluoroscopic unit that maintains the overall appearance of the fluoroscopic image (contrast and density) by automatically adjusting the kilovoltage peak (kVp) or milliamperage (mA) or both.

Automatic Collimator/Positive Beam-Limiting Device Automatically limits the size and shape of the primary beam to the size and shape of the image receptor.

Automatic Exposure Control (AEC) A system used to consistently control the amount of radiation reaching the image receptor by terminating the length of exposure.

Automatic Film Processor A device that encompasses chemical tanks, a roller transport system, and a dryer system for the processing of radiographic film.

Automatic Rescaling Occurs during histogram analysis and is employed to maintain consistent image brightness despite overexposure or underexposure of the digital image receptor.

Average Gradient The slope of the straight-line region of a film's sensitometric curve.

Axial Rotation Rotation of an object around its own axis; improper positioning causing false narrowing on the image.

B

Backup Time The maximum length of time for which the x-ray exposure continues when using an AEC system.

Barium Sulfate Positive-contrast medium that is often used as a suspension in a radiographic contrast study to evaluate the gastrointestinal tract.

Base Plus Fog (B + F) The lowest amount of density on the radiographic film due to the tint added to its base and any slight amount of fog added during processing.

Beam-Restricting Device Changes the shape and size of the primary beam, located just below the x-ray tube housing.

Beam Restriction/Collimation Interchangeably used terms that refer to a decrease in the size of the projected radiation field.

BIPS Inert, low-density, radiopaque, barium-impregnated polyethylene spheres designed for evaluation of gastric dysmotility and intestinal transit time in dogs and cats.

Bisecting Angle A method used in dental radiography to image teeth that do not allow placement of the receptor directly behind the tooth. The central ray is perpendicular to the bisecting angle, which is formed by the intersection of the plane of the film and the long axis of the tooth.

Bit 0 or 1 that refers to the computer's basic unit of information.

Bit Depth Number of bits.

Blur Unsharpness resulting from patient motion.

B-mode or 2D Mode or Brightness Mode It is a two-dimensional ultrasound image display composed of bright dots representing the ultrasound echoes. The brightness of each dot is determined by the amplitude of the returned echo signal.

Brachycephalic Dogs with short and wide heads such as bulldogs (from Greek *brachy* [short] + *cephal* [head]).

Bremsstrahlung Radiation Occurs during the production of x-rays when a projectile electron completely avoids the orbital electrons of the tungsten atom and travels very close to its nucleus. The very strong electrostatic force of the nucleus causes the electron to suddenly "slow down." As the electron loses energy, it suddenly changes its direction and the energy loss then reappears as an x-ray photon.

Brightness The amount of luminance (light emission) of a display monitor.

Brightness Gain The product of both flux gain and minification gain, which results in a brighter image on the output phosphor.

Buccal The portion of the tooth or root that is closest to the cheek (from Latin *bucca* [cheek]).

Bucky It is more accurately called the Potter-Bucky diaphragm and is located directly below the radiographic tabletop. The grid is positioned just above the tray that contains the image receptor. It is normally replaced by a grid tray or receptor tray in veterinary medicine because the release of the spring holding the grid makes a loud noise which startles the patient.

Byte A collection of 8 bits.

C

Cachexia A complex syndrome state associated with an underlying illness causing ongoing muscle loss in which there is loss of weight, muscle atrophy, fatigue, weakness, and significant loss of appetite (from Greek *kakos* [bad] and *hexis* [condition]).

Calcium tungstate Occurs in nature as scheelite and is among the most important luminophores, i.e., when exposed to x-rays it appears blue. It is chiefly used in radiographic screens and in digital imaging.

Caliper A device that measures part thickness.

Camera Tube A device used to convert the light emitted from the output phosphor to an electrical signal sent to the television monitor.

Canthi (s. canthus, palpebral commissure) The outer corner of the eye where the upper and lower eyelids meet (from Greek *cantos* [corner of the eye]).

Carnassial Tooth The fourth upper premolars of dogs used for breaking up and crushing hard food.

Cassette A container for both intensifying screen and film.

Cathartic A purgative; an agent for purging the bowels, especially a laxative (from Greek *kathairein* and Latin XXX [to purge]).

Cathode A negatively charged electrode within the x-ray tube. It is comprised of a filament and a focusing cup.

Caudal (Cd) The parts of the body positioned toward the tail from any given point. Caudal also refers to the parts of the limb above (proximal to) the carpal and tarsal joints that face toward the tail (from Latin *cauda* [tail]).

Caudocranial (CdCr) The x-ray beam passes from the caudal surface to the cranial surface of a structure. Technically used for radiographing extremities that are proximal to the carpus or tarsus.

Caudoproximal–Craniodistal (CdPr–CrDi) The central ray is directed slightly downward perpendicular to the midsagittal plane from the back of the limb to the front of the limb. This is in reference to anatomy proximal to and including the carpus and tarsus.

Cavitation The formation of bubbles in a liquid.

Celiography Evaluation of the abdominal cavity generally used to determine the integrity of the diaphragm.

Cementoenamel Junction (CEJ) The area where the enamel, which is the outer covering of the crown, and the cementum, which is the outer covering of the root, meet.

Central Ray The portion of an x-ray beam that is directed towards the center of the film or the object being radiographed.

Chairside Radiography Manual processing of dental film images in small jars with sealed lids in the regular darkroom that allows the operator to process the films in close proximity to where they are being exposed. The chairside darkroom has a red translucent cover and light-tight arm holes.

Characteristic Radiation or Interactions Produced when a projectile electron interacts with an electron from the inner (K) shell of the tungsten atom. When the K-shell electron is ejected from its orbit, an outer shell electron drops into the open position and thereby creates an energy difference. The energy difference is emitted as an x-ray photon.

Charge Coupled Device (CCD) Detectors used in direct digital radiography that record flashes of light produced by the exit x-rays interacting with a screen that scintillates.

Chondrodystrophic Refers to breeds such as Dachshund, Bulldog, Corgi, Pug, French Bulldog, etc. with abnormal cartilage formation.

Cine Loop A period of images stored digitally as a sequence of individual frames.

Circuit A course or pathway through which an electric current passes.

Circuit Breaker An automatic safety device for stopping the flow of current in an electrical circuit.

Cloacogram Study of the cloaca, best accomplished with contrast media injected retrograde.

Cloud Storage A model of computer data storage in which digital data is stored remotely in logical pools. The physical storage spans multiple servers and the physical environment is typically owned and managed by a hosting company.

Coelom The body cavity in metazoans (all animals other than protozoans and sponges), located between the intestinal canal and the body wall.

Coherent Scattering An interaction that occurs with low-energy x-rays, typically below the diagnostic range. The incoming photon interacts with the atom, causing it to become excited. The x-ray does not lose energy but changes direction.

Coincidence A remarkable concurrence of events or circumstances without apparent causal connection. In imaging, two images may superimpose or relate to one another concurrently. They are said to be in coincidence.

Collimator A device for limiting particles of radiation to a particular path, used to restrict the beam of radiation to a specific area.

Collimator Indicator The notation table on the front/side of the collimator that indicates the various cassette sizes and positions at which the leaves should be set to open or close to the correct size at a selected distance.

Collimator Shutters/Leaves Two sets of adjustable lead shutters located 3–7 in (4–18 cm) below the tube that consist of longitudinal and lateral leaves or blades, each with its own control; this makes the collimator adjustable in terms of its ability to produce projected fields of varying sizes.

Color Flow Doppler A method for noninvasively imaging blood flow through the heart by displaying flow data on the two-dimensional echocardiographic image.

Commissure The corner of the mouth where the upper lip meets the labium lower lip.

Comparative Anatomy Concept stating that different parts of the same size can be radiographed using the same exposure factors, provided the minimum kVp value needed to penetrate the part is used in each case.

Compensating Filter Special filters added to the primary beam to alter its intensity. These types of filters are used to image anatomic areas that are nonuniform in makeup and assist in producing more consistent exposure to the image receptor.

Compton Effect The loss of energy of the incoming photon when it ejects an outer-shell electron from the atom. The remaining lower-energy x-ray photon changes direction and may leave the anatomic part.

Compton Electron/Secondary Electron The ejected electron resulting from the Compton effect interaction.

Computerized Tomography Creation of a cross-sectional tomographic section of the body with a rotating fan beam, a detector array, and computer reconstruction.

Concave In reference to the surface curving inward inside the dental film packet. Used to assist in determining correct identification of the tooth.

Cone An aperture diaphragm that has an extended flange attached to it. The flange can vary in length and is shaped as a cone. The flange can also be made to telescope, increasing its total length.

Coned-Down View Narrowing in on a particular area of the body part with the x-ray beam.

Congruency Agreement, harmony, compatibility. If two bones are congruent, it means there is no difference from one to the other.

Continuous Fluoroscopy The x-ray exposure continues without interruption while the exposure pedal is activated.

Continuous Wave Doppler Ultrasound that uses spectral Doppler in a constant series of echoes both originating and being received by the same transducer.

Contralateral Pertaining to the opposite side (from Latin *contra* [against]).

Contrast Degree of difference between the light and dark areas of a radiograph.

Contrast Medium A substance that can be radiolucent or radiopaque and is administered to increase the radiographic contrast within an organ or system.

Contrast Resolution The ability of the image receptor to distinguish between objects having similar subject contrast.

Contrast to Noise Ratio A method of describing the contrast resolution with the amount of noise apparent in a digital image.

Convergent Line If points were connected along the length of the grid, they would form an imaginary line.

Convergent Point If imaginary lines were drawn from each of the lead lines in a linear focused grid, these lines would meet to form an imaginary point.

Conversion Efficiency Rate at which x-ray energy is transformed into light in an intensifying screen.

Conversion Factor An expression of the luminance at the output phosphor divided by the input exposure rate; its unit of measurement is candela per square meter per milliroentgen per second.

Convex Having an outline or surface curved like the exterior of a circle or sphere in reference to the dot on dental film.

Coronal Towards the crown of the tooth.

Coxofemoral Joint Another word for the hip joint in which the head of the femur fits into the acetabulum.

Cranial (Cr) The parts of the neck, trunk, and tail positioned toward the head from any given point. In limbs, cranial refers to the parts above (proximal to) the carpal and tarsal joints that face toward the head (from Latin *cranio* [head]).

Craniocaudal (CrCd) Passing of the x-ray beam from the cranial surface to the caudal surface of a structure. Technically, the craniocaudal projection is used for radiographing extremities that are proximal to the carpus or tarsus.

Cranioproximal–Caudodistal (CrPr-CdDi) The central ray is directed slightly downward, perpendicular to the midsagittal plane from the front of the limb to the back of the limb. This is in reference to anatomy proximal to and including the carpus and tarsus.

Crena The large notch in the solar border of the equine sole.

Crossed/Cross-hatched Grid A grid containing lead lines that are perpendicular to one another. Crossed grids remove more scattered photons than linear grids because they contain more lead strips, oriented in two directions.

Crossover Effect Light that has been produced by an intensifying screen that exposes one emulsion and then "crosses over" the base layer of the film to expose the other emulsion.

Crossover Rollers An assembly that moves the film from one tank to another and into the dryer assembly during automatic processing.

CT Number Value related to the attenuation characteristics of the tissue in the voxel.

Current A flow of electrons along a conductor in a closed circuit.

Cusp Raised points *or* projections on the crowns of the teeth in animals.

Cyclotron A type of particle accelerator that is used to produce nuclides used in nuclear medicine and PET scans.

Cylinder An aperture diaphragm that has an extended flange attached to it. The flange can vary in length and is shaped as a cylinder.

Cystography Radiographic contrast studies evaluating the urinary bladder (from Greek *cyst/o* [urinary bladder]).

D

Darkroom Integrity The ability of the darkroom to maintain a fog or light-free environment by light tight seals around processors, doors, pass boxes, ceiling tiles, or cracked safe lights.

Decubitus The act of lying down or the position assumed. Lateral decubitus is lying on the side, and dorsal decubitus is lying on the back.

Degenerative Joint Disease A type of arthritis caused by inflammation, breakdown, and eventual loss of the cartilage of the joints. Also known as osteoarthritis.

Densitometer A device used to numerically determine the amount of blackness on the radiograph.

Density The degree to which a substance is dense; mass per unit volume. Usually in reference to the level of darkness on a radiograph which can be measured with a densitometer. The darkest portion of a radiograph contains the most silver atoms and is the blackest area.

Dependent The side that the patient is lying on (from French *dépendre* [to hang down]).

Depth Control The setting on an ultrasound unit that controls the level of tissue imaged by the signals from the transducer.

Detector The portion of a radiation measuring device that transmits the amount of radiation to the unit which will display the levels in roentgens, milliroentgens, or sieverts.

Detective Quantum Efficiency (DQE) A measure of the efficiency of the image receptor in digital imaging converting the x-ray exposure it receives to a quality radiographic image.

Developer Agents that reduce the silver halide to metallic silver during film processing. The common chemicals are hydroquinone and phenidone.

Diaphragmatic Crura Tendinous structures that extend caudally from the diaphragm to attach to the vertebral column (singular: crus; from the Latin for leg).

Diffusion The process by which the x-ray film is developed, fixed, and washed. The chemicals are diluted in water and saturate the emulsion of the film.

Digital Imaging A method of imaging whereby the remnant radiation is converted into electrical signals which are then converted into an image within a computer.

Digital Imaging and Communications in Medicine (DICOM) An international communication language through which healthcare institutions are able to review images and data, no matter how the images were acquired. At this point, all images, both veterinary and medical, are converted to DICOM images

Dimer A compound formed by the union of two radicals or two molecules of a simpler compound.

Direct Current An electric current flowing in one direction only.

Direct Radiation Radiation traveling in a straight line from source to receptor. Typically, this is the central ray.

Distal (Di) The area farthest from the midline or the beginning of a structure (from Latin *dist/o* [distant]).

Distance The length of the space between two points.

Distolateral Oblique A projection used in dental radiography where the tube head is directed from the distal to mesial aspect, approximately 30 degrees from the initial position, demonstrating the SLOB rule.

Distortion Radiographic misrepresentation of either the size or shape of the anatomic part.

Distraction Index A measurement of hip joint laxity.

Diverge X-rays travel in straight lines and a beam of x-rays separates away from its source. This means that the most accurate image will be represented closest to the midline (from Latin *dis* [in two ways] + *vergere* [to turn or incline]).

D_{max} The point on the sensitometric curve demonstrating the maximum density achieved on the radiograph.

D_{min} The point on the sensitometric curve that shows the minimum optical density of the image.

DNA Molecule A molecule that carries the genetic instructions used in the growth, development, functioning, and reproduction of all known living organisms and many viruses.

Dolichocephalic Dogs that have long, narrow heads and tapered muzzles, such as Collies (from Greek *dolich/o* [long] + *cephal* [head]).

Dorsal (D) Toward the back; thus, dorsal describes the upper aspect of the head, neck, trunk, and tail. In limbs, dorsal refers to those areas of the legs distally from the carpus and tarsus joints that face cranially or towards the head (from Latin *dors/o* [back]).

Dorsal Plane Divides the body into back and ventral (belly parts).

Dorsolateral–Palmaromedial Oblique (DLPMO) The beam enters the cranial or front of the front limb at an angle lateral to the midline and exits on the caudal or back of the limb at an angle medial to the midline.

Dorsolateral–Ventrolateral Oblique (DLVLO) Projection usually referring to the teeth and skull where the central ray is directed in an angle downward on the area of interest laterally.

Dorsomedial–Palmarolateral Oblique (DMPLO) The beam enters the cranial or front of the front limb at an angle medial to the midline and exits the caudal or back of the limb at an angle lateral to the midline.

Dorsopalmar (DPa) Radiographs that are taken distal to and including the carpus of the front limb. The central ray passes from the cranially facing surface to the caudal or hind surface of the forelimb.

Dorsoplantar (DPl) Radiographs that are taken distal to and including the tarsus of the hindlimb. The central ray passes from the front surface of the hindlimb to the back or plantar surface.

Dorsoproximal–Dorsodistal Oblique (Dpr–DDiO) The central ray enters and exits in a slightly downward perpendicular direction, toward the midsagittal plane of the front of the limb. Usually in reference to the carpus.

Dorsoproximal–Palmarodistal (DPr–PaDi) The central ray enters perpendicular to the front of the front limb and exits at the back of the front limb.

Dose Creep A term used in digital radiography to describe incremental increases in exposure in an attempt to reduce the amount of "noise" affecting the image quality. This will increase patient dose.

Dosimeter A device that is used to measure x-ray exposure.

Double Contrast A radiographic contrast technique that uses a combination of positive- and negative-contrast media to better evaluate organs.

Dynamic Motion studies such as flexion and extension of the cervical and lumbosacral vertebrae (from Greek *dynamis* [power, might, strength]).

Dynamic Range Refers to the range of exposure intensities an image receptor can accurately detect.

Dyschezia Difficult or painful defecation (from Greek *dys* [bad or difficult] + *chezein* [stool]).

E

Echo Time (in ultrasound) A measure of time from the emission of sound from the transducer until the echo is received back to the transducer.

Effective Focal Spot Size Focal spot as measured directly beneath the anode target of the x-ray tube.

Electricity A form of energy resulting from the existence of charged particles either statically as a buildup of a charge or dynamically as a current.

Electrolysis Chemical decomposition produced by passing an electric current through a conducting liquid.

Electromagnetic Radiation Radiation that has both electrical and magnetic properties. All radiations that are electromagnetic make up the electromagnetic spectrum.

Electromagnetic Spectrum A method of ordering the intensities of all radiations.

Electronic Masking Also known as shuttering. A postprocessing function in digital imaging that removes portions of the digital image. Mainly used to eliminate areas of nonexposure, which contribute to high-contrast glare.

Electrostatic Focusing Lenses Focuses and accelerates the electrons through the image intensifier towards the anode.

Elements The simplest substances that cannot be broken down using chemical reactions. They are primary constituents of matter.

Elongation Distortion of the image due to lack of parallelism. The image appears longer than the true size. In dental imaging, the beam is aimed too directly at the long axis of the tooth instead of the bisecting angle.

Emulsion The radiation and light sensitive layers of film and intensifying screens spread evenly across a polyester or Mylar base.

Enamel Bulge A circumferential widening at the base of every crown of the tooth.

Energy The quantitative property that must be transferred to an object in order to perform work.

Esophagography Examination of the esophageal function and morphology following the administration of contrast medium.

Excretory Urography Radiographic examination of the kidneys and ureters following an injection of an intravenous positive-contrast medium. Originally referred to as intravenous urogram (IVU) or intravenous pyelogram (IVP).

Exit Radiation The attenuated x-ray beam that leaves the patient. Also called remnant radiation. It is composed of both transmitted and scattered radiation.

Expiration Date The last day a product is safe to use or consume according to its manufacturer.

Exposure Indicator The numeric value that is displayed on the processed image to indicate the level of x-ray exposure received on the digital receptor.

Exposure Intensity The amount and energy of the x-rays reaching an area of the image receptor.

Exposure Latitude The range of exposures along the straight-line portion of the sensitometric curve.

Exposure Switch The switch that allows the current to flow to the x-ray tube. A remote-control device that permits current to flow through the circuit.

Exposure Technique Charts Preestablished guidelines used by the radiographer to select standardized exposure factors for each type of radiographic image.

Exposure Time The length of the time that the x-ray tube produces x-rays.

Extension Arm The portion extending from the dental x-ray generator that moves 180 degrees.

Extraoral Outside the mouth (from Latin *extra* [outside]).

Extrapolated Mathematically estimated; the mathematical process used to create technique charts.

F

Facial The surface of a tooth that faces the buccal or labial mucosa of the vestibule of the mouth.

Feed Tray In a film processor, a flat metal surface with an edge on either side that permits the film to enter the processor easily and align correctly.

Field of View (FOV) The area of the detector that will result in an anatomical image when the exposure is made.

FIFO (First In First Out) The product storage system whereby the inventory that arrives first will be the first to be put into service.

Filament A coiled tungsten wire within the x-ray tube that is the source of electrons during x-ray production.

Fill Factor The percentage of the x-rays reaching the sensitive area of the detector element (DEL).

Filling Defect Anything that occupies space within the lumen of an organ, thus preventing normal filling from occurring, such as a blood clot.

Film Base A transparent substrate which acts as a support medium for the photosensitive emulsion that coats it.

Film/Screen Contact The amount of direct contact between the film and intensifying screens within a cassette.

Filtration A process that is used to separate solids from liquids or gases using a medium that allows fluid but not the solid to pass through.

Fistulography A positive or negative radiographic contrast study generally used in equine radiography to determine the depth and origin of a fistulous tract (abnormal tube-like passage within body tissue).

Fixer The second step in film processing that clears the undeveloped silver halide from the film base and hardens the emulsion. It is highly acidic, with a pH of 4–4.5.

Fixing Agent In processing chemistry, the main agent of the fixer is sodium thiosulphate.

Flat Panel Detectors (FPD) Solid-state imaging receptors using a large-area active matrix array of electronic components ranging in sizes from 35 × 43 cm to 43 × 43 cm.

Flexed To bend or put in a state of flexion.

Flexed Lateral A lateral radiograph with the joint bent rather than straight.

Flexor View Imaging the flexor or palmar/dorsal portion of the bone such as the knee or navicular. Also referred to as skyline or caudal tangential.

Fludeoxyglucose The radioactive positron particle used in PET imaging. Otherwise called "FDG." The isotope gathers in sites of increased or decreased metabolic activity.

Fluoroscopy Real-time imaging of internal structures using a continuous beam of x-rays.

Focal Distance The distance from the focal spot to the detector.

Focal Length The most effective grids are constructed of material that is angled specifically to absorb scattered radiation from the divergent x-ray beam. The various angulations are specific to the range of distances that the grid is positioned from the focal spot.

Focal Range The recommended range of distances that can be used with a focused grid of a specific focal length.

Focusing Cup Installed around the cathode within the x-ray tube. It is open at one side to allow electrons to flow freely from the cathode to the anode. It is made of nickel and absorbs electrons that are not aimed directly at the anode.

Focal Radiograph Separation of tissues to better enhance imaging.

Focal Spot The area of the anode that is most efficient when bombarded by electrons during x-ray production.

Focal Spot Bloom An increase in the effective size of the focal spot when the anode is overused due to the focal spot heating the area immediately adjacent. The larger-sized focal spot will contribute to unsharpness of the image.

Fog Increased density on the radiographic image caused by extraneous heat, light, or chemical fumes. The contrast of the image is reduced as the fog eliminates the minimum density (D_{min}) of the image.

Foreshortening Refers to images that appear on the image to be shorter than the true objects. In dental imaging, the beam is aimed too directly at the imaging receptor rather than the bisecting angle.

Frenulum A fold of skin beneath the tongue, or between the lip and the gum, that secures or restricts the motion.

Frequency The number of waves passing a given point per given unit of time. Values are measured in Hertz.

Frog-Leg VD A radiographic position of the hips in which the patient is in dorsal recumbency and the hindlimbs are in a relatively natural flexed position.

Functional Study Contrast radiographic studies that evaluate the activity, purpose, or reason; relating to the way something works or operates (from Latin *funct/o* [to perform]).

Furcation The areas where teeth with multiple roots separate. Bone loss that is specific to the branching of a tooth's roots is known as a *furcation defect*.

G

Gain Control A closed-loop feedback regulating circuit, the purpose of which is to provide controlled signal amplitude at its output, despite variation of the amplitude in the input signal.

Gantry The frame housing the x-ray tube, collimators, and detectors in a computed tomography (CT) machine with a large opening in the center. The patient table is supported by the gantry. The table moves forward into the gantry as the CT examination progresses.

Gastrography Radiographic examination of the size, shape, position, and morphology of the stomach following administration of contrast media.

Gavaging Force feeding or irrigation into the stomach via a tube. In birds, the tube is passed into the crop.

Generator In radiography, an x-ray generator is a device that energizes the electrical circuit that produces x-rays based upon the technical factors chosen by the operator. It is also a device that converts mechanical energy into electrical energy.

Gonadal Shields Lead shields that protect the gonadal area of the patient from radiation during radiographic procedures.

Gradient Point The slope along any portion of the sensitometric curve.

Granuloma A tumor composed of granulation tissue produced in response to chronic infection, inflammation, a foreign body, or unknown causes (from Latin *granulum* [granular] + *oma* [lump, tumor, or mass]).

Gray Scale The number of different shades of gray that can be stored and displayed by a computer monitor. In film radiography, it is the number of shades of gray that are displayed on the film image.

Grid A device that has very thin lead strips with radiolucent interspaces. It is located between the tabletop and the image receptor and is used to absorb scatter radiation.

Grid Cutoff A decrease in the number of photons reaching the receptor because of misalignment of the grid. A decrease in the number of photons reaching the receptor due to an overincrease or decrease of the focal length of the x-ray tube.

Grid Deterioration Older grids will deteriorate over time as the interspace material dissolves. An irregular pattern of the deterioration will overlay the anatomical image.

Grid Lines A linear pattern on the image of the lines of the grid. The grid lines are usually parallel to the length of the table.

Grid Ratio The ratio of the height of the lead strips to the distance between them. Typical grid ratios are 8:1 and 10:1.

Grid Tray The tray that holds the cassette beneath the grid and the table top for film radiography. The tray that is positioned under the table top in which the digital plate is positioned in direct digital radiography.

Ground A protective measure to neutralize an electrical charge by connecting the electrical device to the earth via a conductor.

Guide Shoes A part of the crossover roller assembly that transports the film between the developer, fixer, and wash tank in an automatic processor. Guide shoes are now small indentations in the crossover assembly that steer the film as it travels through the processor.

H

Halation When the image is produced by light in a film screen system, the light may be reflected back from the film base. The light forms a diffuse halo appearance on the image. This effect is resolved by adding an antihalation layer to the film base.

Half-Life The time required for a quantity to reduce to half of its normal value. The term is commonly used in nuclear physics to describe how quickly unstable atoms undergo decay.

Half-Value Layer The amount of filtration required to reduce the intensity of the x-ray beam to half its original value. Usually expressed in mm of aluminum. It is the best method for determining the quality of the x-ray beam.

Hardener A chemical that is added to the fixer to adhere the emulsion to the base following fixation.

Heat Bloom Another term for focal spot bloom that occurs if the anode of the x-ray tube becomes over heated.

Heat Dissipation Process of becoming cooler; a temperature reduction.

Heat Unit The amount of heat produced from any given exposure. Heat unit charts are supplied with every x-ray tube so that excessive heat units can be prevented.

Heel Effect Due to the geometry of the angled anode target, the radiation intensity is greater on the cathode side because the radiation of the anode side is "cut off" and reabsorbed into the material of the anode. The anode angle is typically 11–15 degrees.

Hemithorax One side of the chest; the cavity lateral to the mediastinum.

Hertz The SI unit of frequency equal to one cycle per second. A measurement of electromagnetic waves

Heterogeneous Beam The x-ray beam contains various wave lengths.

High Contrast An image with few densities but great differences in density between them.

High Coronary View Refers to imaging of the digit where the beam is angled to the ground in a dorsoproximal direction with the foot standing on the image receptor. Also referred to as a stand-on route.

High Frequency The range of electromagnetic waves between 3 and 30 Mhz.

Hilar Region The hilum of the lung found on the medial aspect of each lung, and the only site of entrance or exit of structures associated with the lungs.

Hip Dysplasia An abnormal formation of the hip socket that, in its more severe form, can eventually cause crippling lameness and painful arthritis of the joints. It is a genetic (polygenic) trait that is affected by environmental factors and is particularly common in larger dog breeds.

Histogram An approximate representation of the distribution of numerical or categorical data. In digital radiography, it is used to approximate the ideal representation of each anatomical image.

Histogram Analysis Graphic display of individual pixel values. An analysis of the various densities demonstrated on individual examples of anatomical images. For example, the thorax is represented by high-contrast images. Abdominal images have many low contrast densities.

Horizontal Beam The x-ray tube is repositioned at 90 degrees from the normal vertical projection. The x-ray beam now travels parallel to the tabletop. It is commonly used to display fluid levels in upright patients.

Hounsfield Unit A quantitative scale for describing radiodensity particularly in CT examinations. It is also known as the CT number.

Hydroquinone A reducing agent found in the film developer chemistry that produces the black (higher) densities.

Hyperextension Extension of a joint beyond its normal range of motion.

Hyperflexion Flexion of a joint beyond its normal range of motion.

I

Iatrogenesis Inadvertent and preventable induction of disease or complications caused by medical treatment by medical treatment, such as an infection or a complication (from Greek *iatro* [healer, medicine] + *genic* [producing]).

ICRP (International Commission on Radiological Protection) An international committee that oversees all types of radiation, mainly referred to by countries that do not have their own commission. Most commissions use the ICRP guidelines when developing their own rules and regulations.

Illuminator Light box for viewing radiographs.

Illuminator Mask The device to close off some areas of the illuminator for viewing. Usually a blackened x-ray film with a window cut out.

Image Data The digital array of CT numbers, based on the image matrix that results from raw data being reconstructed.

Image Intensifier An electronic device that receives the image forming the x-ray beam and converts it into a visible light image of high intensity.

Imaging Plate (IP) The flexible plate inside the computed radiography cassette that receives the remnant radiation and converts it by means of a photostimulable phosphor into an image that can be read by a laser.

Imaging Receptor (IR) The device that transforms the remnant radiation from the patient to a visible image, e.g., x-ray film, PSP, digital plate.

Incident Radiation The radiation produced at the x-ray tube after it has reached the patient.

Incisal The biting edge of the canines and incisors furthest from the apex of the root.

Inert A chemical deficient in active properties; chemically inactive.

Inherent Filtration The filtration built into the structure of the x-ray tube such as the glass envelope, the collimation mirror.

Input Phosphor Converts incoming radiation into visible light energy.

Intensification Factor A formula that represents the degree to which exposure factors are reduced when intensifying screens are used.

Intensifying Screens Phosphors are coated onto a flexible medium and installed in x-ray cassettes. The phosphors convert x-ray energy into light, which then exposes the radiographic film.

International Commission on Radiological Protection (ICRP) A commission that oversees radiation protection for those countries that do not have their own commissions. All countries base their policies on the ICRP rulings.

Intervertebral Foramen An opening between two spinal vertebrae through which nerves and blood vessels pass. Every pair of cervical, thoracic, and lumbar vertebrae have intervertebral foramen (singular) The plural is foramina (from Latin *forare* [to bore a hole]).

Intraoral Inside the mouth (from Latin *intra* [inside]).

Inverse Square Law The relationship between the intensity of the x-ray beam and its source. The intensity of the x-ray beam is inversely proportional to the square of the distance from the source.

Ionic Iodine Iodinated contrast media whose molecules dissociate into anions and cations, causing changes in osmolality.

Ionization A property of x-rays that has the ability to remove electrons from their rings about the nucleus.

Ipsilateral Belonging to or occurring on the same side of the body (from Latin *ipse* [self])

K

Kilovoltage (kV) The potential difference applied to the x-ray tube that determines the speed at which the electrons in the tube current move.

Kyphosis The curvature of the thoracic vertebrae. Dogs and cats have a natural kyphosis in the mid to caudal thoracic vertebrae (from Greek *kyphos* [bent]).

L

Labial The surface of the teeth facing the lips in reference to the canines and incisor (from Latin *labium* [lip]).

Lamina Dura The wall of the alveolar socket that surrounds the tooth, appearing as a dense white line adjacent to the periodontal ligament space on dental images.

Latent Image The invisible image that exists on the exposed film before it has been chemically processed. Also, the image that exists on the PSP before it is read.

Latent Image Centers Several sensitivity specks with many silver ions attached to them.

Latent Image Formation The Gurney-Mott theory, used to explain what happens to the silver halide crystals when exposed to x-rays and light.

Lateral (L) The side that the patient is lying when in recumbency is designated as that lateral, e.g., a "left lateral" limb means that the patient is lying on its left side. Also refers to limbs in which lateral is the outer portion of the limb (from Latin *later/o* [side]).

Lateral Oblique When referring to the head, the patient is lying in lateral recumbency with the nose either raised or lowered from a true lateral position.

Lateromedial (LaM) Projection in which the x-ray beam enters a limb through the lateral side and exits on the medial side, usually in reference to equine radiography but are referred to as lateral.

Laxity Slackness or displacement in the motion of a joint; a lack of tautness, firmness, or rigidity.

Legg-Calve-Perthes (LCP) Disease This is believed to be an inherited disorder of hip joint conformation occurring in dogs, most often seen in the miniature and toy breeds between the ages of 4 months to a year.

Light Spectrum The portion of the electromagnetic spectrum that is visible to the human eye.

Linear Energy Transfer (LET) A term used in dosimetry. It describes how much energy an ionizing particle transfers to the material transversed per unit distance.

Linear Grid Contains lead lines that are oriented in one direction only.

Line Focus Principle Describes the relationship between the actual and effective focal spots in the x-ray tube. By angling the face of the anode, the actual focal spot can remain relatively large, whereas the effective focal spot is reduced in size.

Line Pairs/Inch The number of bars and interspaces of equal width per inch.

Line Pairs/Millimeter The number of bars and interspaces of equal width per millimeter.

Line Voltage Compensator A device that monitors electric power for medical devices such as x-ray equipment and adjusts for incoming line voltage fluctuations.

Lingual The surface of the mandibular teeth directed toward the tongue (from Latin *lingua* [tongue]).

Log Book A record book (may be digital) in which all cases are entered along with the technical factors used to produce the image.

Long Scale/Low Contrast A radiograph with a large number of densities with small differences between the densities; many shades of gray between black and white.

Lookup Tables (LUP) Provides a method of altering the digital image to change the display of the digital image, e.g., increase contrast; decrease brightness.

Lower Gastrointestinal (LGI) Study Radiographic examination of the rectum, colon, and cecum following the administration of contrast medium, often given as a barium enema.

Luminescence The emission of light from the screen when stimulated by radiation.

M

Magnet An object having polarity and capable of attracting iron.

Magnetic Field The sphere of influence of a magnet.

Magnification An increase in the image size of the object compared with its true or actual size. Also known as size distortion.

Magnification Factor (MF) Indicates how much size distortion or magnification is shown on a radiograph or display image. Formula: MF = SID / SOD.

Malocclusion Imperfect positioning of the teeth when the jaws are closed.

Main Drive In this context, it is twofold: a) it can refer to the drive motor on an automatic processor; or b) it can also refer to one of the drives on a computer central processing unit (CPU).

Manifest Image The visible image on film after processing.

mAs Milliampere seconds—the time of the exposure. The "A" is capitalized.

Matrix A digital image is displayed as a combination of rows and columns (array) of small square "picture elements" or pixels.

Matter Any substance that has mass and takes up space by having volume.

Maximum Contrast The greatest difference in optical densities.

Measurement The size, length, or amount of something as determined by measuring.

Medial (M) The direction toward the animal's midline. In reference to limbs, it is the inside of the limb (from Latin *medi/o* [middle]).

Mediastinum Divides the thorax into right and left sides and is formed by the parietal pleura of the right and left hemithoraces. It contains important structures including the trachea, esophagus, heart, aorta and its major branches, thoracic duct, lymph nodes, and nerves.

Mediolateral The beam enters from the medial side and exits the lateral side. Technically, in small animal limbs, this should be called a mediolateral, though lateral is the common term.

Meiosis Process of germ cell division that reduces the chromosomes in each daughter cell to half the number of chromosomes in the parent cell.

Mental Foramina Openings located on the ventral surface of the mandible that transmit the terminal branches of nerves. They appear as lucent defects in imaging.

Mesaticephalic Describes the majority of dogs with medium or average head shape (from Greek *mesi* [middle]" + *cephal* [head]). Sometimes also referred to as mesocephalic.

Mesial The surface that is closest to the midline of the face and considered to be in between the surface of the tooth next to it.

Mesiobuccal The angle formed by the junction of the mesial and buccal surfaces of a tooth.

Mesiolateral Oblique In dental radiography, the tube head is directed from mesial to distal approximately 30 degrees from the initial position, demonstrating the SLOB rule.

Mesiolingual The angle formed by the mesial and lingual surfaces of a tooth.

Microconvex Refers to the shape of the footprint of the transducer used in ultrasound; in this case, the transducer has a reduced "footprint" size.

Midsagittal Plane A vertical plane through the midline of the body; divides the body into right and left halves. Also called the median plane (from Latin *sagitta* [arrow]).

Milliamperage The x-ray tube current during an exposure.

Milliampere (mA) The unit used to measure tube current. 1/1000 of an ampere.

Milliampere Seconds (mAs) Product of exposure time (s) and x-ray tube current (mA).

Millicuries .001 of a curie. A curie is a unit of radioactivity, named after Marie Curie.

Mitosis Process of somatic cell division wherein a parent cell divides to form two daughter cells identical to the parent cell.

Modulation Transfer Function (MTF) A measure of the imaging systems ability to display contrast of anatomic objects varying in size.

Moire Effect An artifact that can occur when a stationary grid is used during computed radiography if the grid frequency is similar to the scanning frequency.

M-mode Motion modulation in diagnostic ultrasound.

Monomer A molecule that forms the basic unit for polymers. Iodinated monomers can be ionic or nonionic.

Morphological Studies Contrast studies looking at the form and structure, including size and shape (from Greek *morpho* [shape or form]).

Motion Blurring of the image that results from movement within the imaging components; may be the patient, the receptor, or the tube stand.

Must/Should Within the Radiation Emitting Devices Act: Must is a legal requirement; should denotes a suggestion to be put into a protocol.

Myelography Radiographic examination of the subarachnoid space surrounding the spinal cord following the administration of contrast medium (from Greek *myel/o* [spinal cord or bone marrow, white substance]).

N

National Council on Radiation Protection and Measurements (NCRP) This is the council responsible for producing the federal radiation legislation guidelines in the USA

Negative-Contrast Agents Gases that are more radiolucent to x-rays than soft tissues and will thus appear black on a radiograph. Air, carbon dioxide, and nitrous oxide are such agents.

Nephrogram A phase of an excretory urogram characterized by the diffuse opacification of the functional renal parenchyma which show the vascular supply and kidney perfusion. It is immediately noted in a normal contrast study of the kidneys (from Greek *nephr/o* [kidney]).

Nonionic Iodine Iodinated contrast media whose molecules remain whole in solution so as not to cause changes in osmolality.

Nonradiation Worker A worker within the practice who does not work with radiation.

Nonstochastic Effects Biologic effects of ionizing radiation that are delivered in measurable units; demonstrate the existence of a threshold.

Nuclear Energy Energy contained within the nucleus of an atom.

Nuclear Scintigraphy A diagnostic method that uses very small tracer amounts of radioactive molecules to diagnose diseases involving bone, vessels, and soft tissue.

O

Object Receptor Distance The distance from the body part being imaged to the image receptor. Also referred to as Object Image Distance (OID).

Object to Image Distance (OID) Object to receptor distance. Initially referred to as object film distance (OFD).

Oblique (O) Positioning in which the primary beam enters the body at an angle other than 90 degrees to the anatomical area of interest. It is used primarily in dental and large-patient limb radiographs (from Latin *obliquus* [slanting, sidelong, indirect]).

Occlusal Relating or involved in the occlusion of teeth. Denoting the surface of a tooth that comes into contact with a tooth on the opposite jaw. The image receptor is placed inside the mouth.

Occlusion The contact of the teeth when the mandible and maxillae are closed.

Occult Hidden (from Latin *celare* [to hide]).

Odor Masks Substances added to processing chemicals to eliminate the natural odor of the developer and fixer.

OFA Orthopedic Foundation of Animals Organization that maintains genetic databases to promote the health and welfare of companion animals through a reduction in the incidence of genetic disease.

Off-Focus Radiation X-rays produced at the anode but not at the focal spot.

Opaque/Radiopaque Clear images on the receptor where areas of the anatomy are not penetrable by the radiation used to create the image. Radiopaque is a term usually in connection with contrast media or positioning devices not penetrated by the x-rays.

Optical Density A numeric calculation that is read by a densitometer. It compares the intensity of light transmitted through an area on the film to the intensity of light originally striking the film with zero density.

Optimal kV The kV value that is high enough to ensure penetration of the anatomy but not too high to diminish radiographic contrast.

Optimized Image Occurs when all the factors align to create the perfect image.

Organogenesis Production and development of the organs of a plant or animal.

Orthogonal Pertaining to or involving right angles or perpendiculars (from Greek *ortho* [straight] + *gonia* [angle]).

Osmolality The concentration of an osmotic solution, usually in terms of osmoles. The osmolality of blood or the osmotic pressure of blood is usually expressed in terms of osmoles. This measures the amount of solute concentration per unit of total volume of a particular solution (from the Greek *ōsmos* [impulsion or pushing]).

Osteoblastic Activity The body's activity of building new bone.

Osteochondritis Dissecans (OCD) Inflammation of the bone and cartilage whereby a variable amount of bone and its adjacent cartilage loses its blood supply, resulting in the splitting of a piece of articular cartilage into the joint space. Most common in the humeral head and distal condyles of the femur in large, fast-growing breeds of dogs.

Output Phosphor Light-emitting material in the image intensifier that converts accelerated electrons into visible light.

P

Palatal Surface The surface of the maxillary teeth directed towards the palate.

Palmar (Pa) The caudal surface of the forelimb from the carpal joint distally (from Latin *palmar* [hollow of hand]).

Palmarodorsal (PaD) Describes radiographs that are taken distal to the carpus of the front limb. The x-ray beam passes from the palmar (towards the tail) surface of the forelimb to the dorsal (toward the head) surface.

Palmaroproximal–Palmarodistal Oblique (PaPr–PaDi O) The beam enters and exits from the back of the front limb at an oblique angle pointing downwards as in imaging the navicular. Also known as a flexor or skyline view.

Parallel Technique Direction of x-ray beam perpendicular to the image when the dental receptor is placed directly behind and parallel to the tooth.

Parasympatholytic Agents Drugs that reduce the activity of the parasympathetic nervous system, sometimes referred to as anti-cholinergics.

Parenchyma The essential parts of the organ that are concerned with its function.

Particles A minute portion of matter distinct from x-rays alpha particles; electrons, neutrons, protons.

Patient Dose The unit of radiation dose or effective dose measured in millisieverts.

PennHIP A multifaceted radiographic screening method for hip evaluation. The technique assesses the quality of the canine hip and quantitatively measures canine hip joint laxity.

Periapical Of, relating to, occurring in, affecting, or being the tissues surrounding the apex of the root of a tooth.

Phased Array An electronically scanned array which creates a beam of radio waves which can be electronically directed to point in different directions without moving the antenna.

Phenidone Secondary constituent in the chemical composition of developing agents used in manual processing of x-ray film.

Photocathode Converts the visible light in the image intensifier into electrons.

Photodiode Solid-state device that converts light into an electrical current.

Photoelectrical Effect Complete absorption of the incoming x-ray photon occurs when it has enough energy to remove (eject) an inner shell electron. The ionized atom has a vacancy or electron hole in its inner ring, and an electron from an outer shell drops into place to fill the vacancy.

Photoelectron The ejected electron resulting from ionization during the photelectric effect.

Photoemission Electron emission after light stimulation.

Photomultiplier Tube An electronic device that converts visible light energy into an electrical signal.

Photon Electromagnetic radiation that has neither mass nor electric charge but interacts with matter as though it is a particle; x-rays and gamma rays.

Photostimulable Luminescence The release of energy from trapped electrons by a laser during the scanning of a photostimulable phosphor plate.

Photostimulable Phosphor (PSP) A plate made of several layers that stores x-ray energy as a latent image for cassette-based digital systems. Used in computerized radiography.

Picture Archival and Communications System (PACS) A medical imaging technology which provides economical storage and convenient access to images from multiple modalities. A method of archiving images either remotely or locally into a file system that can be read universally.

Pitch Identifies the relationship between slice thickness and the distance the table travels every time the tube rotates in spiral computed tomography.

Pixel The smallest component of the matrix—a picture element.

Pixel Density The number of pixels per unit area.

Pixel Pitch The pixel spacing, or distance measured from the center of a pixel to the center of an adjacent pixel.

Plantar (Pl) The caudal surface of the hindlimb from the tarsal joint distally (from Latin *plantar* [sole of the foot]).

Plantarodorsal (PlD) Radiographs that are taken distal to and including the tarsus of the hindlimb. The x-ray beam passes from the plantar (towards the tail) surface of the hindlimb to the dorsal (toward the head) surface.

Plantaroproximal–Plantarodistal (PlPr–PlDi) The central ray is directed straight down at the back of the hindlimb.

Pneumocystogram Radiographic examination of the urinary bladder following the administration of a radiolucent or negative-contrast medium (from Greek *pneum/o* [air]).

Pneumoperitoneography The radiographic examination of the peritoneal cavity following the administration of negative-contrast medium or gas (from Greek *pneum/o* [air]).

Position Indicating Device The lead-lined cone or cylinder that directs the x-ray beam during a dental radiographic exposure to guide the direction of the x-ray beam.

Positional Terminology Common position descriptions include lateral, medial, distal, proximal, caudal, cranial, caudocranial, craniocaudal, dorsal, ventral, dorsoventral, ventrodorsal, palmar, dorsopalmar, palmarodorsal, plantar, plantarodorsal, dorsoplantar, oblique. See Chapter 15 for definitions.

Positioning The study of radiographic positions that best demonstrate the designated anatomy.

Positive-Contrast Agents Substances that contain elements of high atomic number that are more radiopaque to x-rays than they are to tissue or bone so they appear white on a radiograph.

Positron Emission Tomography (PET) An imaging technique that uses radioactive substances to observe metabolic processes in the body. It is usually paired with a nuclear medicine camera or a magnetic resonance imaging unit. The images are registered together so that the final image shows form and function.

Positron A radioactive particle, the antimatter of an electron.

Potential Difference The difference of electrical potential between two points.

Power The product of Volts times Time. It is expressed in Watts and describes the function of a generator. Current $\times$ Volts = Watts ($I \times V = W$).

Preservative In reference to processing solutions, a chemical additive that maintains the chemical balance of the developer and fixer.

Presets The factory settings of the digital imaging plate in order to produce an image. In some cases, they can be reset at the time of installation.

Primary Beam The x-ray beam upon exiting the collimator and reaching the patient. Often associated with the central ray.

Processing Chemical treatment of the emulsion of a radiographic film to change a latent image to a visible image.

Proximal (Pr) Nearer to the middle or the point of origin of a structure (from Latin *proxim/o* [next]).

Pulsed Doppler Employs elements of the transducer that sends as well as receives signals in ultrasonography.

Pulsed Radiation Exposure An imaging technique turns the radiation on and off during fluoroscopy in order to reduce the dose to the patient.

Pulses (Timer) The timer limits the length of the exposure time in x-rays. In a 60-cycle unit, there will be 60 positive and 60 negative pulses. When the unit is rectified, there will be 120 bursts of radiation.

Pyelogram A phase of an excretory urogram showing the opacification of the renal collection system (the renal pelvis, pelvic recesses, and ureters).

Q

Quadrant Any lines that divide the anatomy into four sections. In dental radiography, formed in the mouth by the midline which passes between the central incisors in the maxillary and mandibular arches. The four quadrants are upper right, upper left, lower left, and lower right.

Quality The standard of something as measured against other things of a similar kind. The degree of excellence.

Quality Assurance All planned and systematic actions necessary to provide adequate confidence that a facility, system, or administrative component will perform safely and satisfactorily in service to a patient. It includes scheduling, preparation, and promptness in examination or treatment, reporting of results, and quality control.

Quality Control All actions necessary to control and verify the performance of equipment; part of quality assurance.

Quantity A certain amount or number defined by the object(s) counted.

R

RAD (Radiation Absorbed Dose) A unit of absorbed dose of any type of radiation defined as 1 rad = 0.01 Gray = 0.01 J/kg. This can refer to the human body or silicon chip.

Radiation Dosimeter Device that measures radiation dose in sieverts. This is a shielded meter that reads X and gamma radiation.

Radiation Emitting Devices Act An act by the government of Canada that regulates all radiation emitting devices. Also referred to as Safety Code SC20A.

Radiation Worker Someone who works with radiation in all forms.

Radicular Groove Longitudinal grooves present on some teeth that correspond with alveolar ridges in the alveoli, providing extra retentive surfaces and preventing rotation.

Radioactive Decay Naturally occurring process whereby an unstable atomic nucleus relieves its instability through the emission of one or more energetic particles.

Radioactive Disintegration Process by which the nucleus spontaneously emits particles and energy and transforms itself into another atom to reach stability.

Radioactivity Unstable atoms spontaneously emitting particles and energy from the nucleus in an effort to attain stability.

Radiofrequency Any of the electromagnetic wave frequencies that lie in the range extending from 3 kHz to 300 GHz.

Radiographic Contrast The degree of difference or ratio between adjacent densities on an x-ray film.

Radiography Imaging modality that uses x-ray film or digital detector and an x-ray tube to provide fixed images (from Greek *graphy* [to write]).

Radiology The study of radiographic images of any and all imaging disciplines (from Latin *ology* [knowledge of]).

Radioisotopes Radioactive atoms that have the same number of protons. They are changed into a different atomic species by disintegration of the nucleus accompanied by the emission of ionizing radiation.

Radiolucent Invisible to x-rays. A radiolucent surface will not absorb radiation. Air, carbon dioxide, and nitrous oxide may be used as negative contrast in radiographic studies as they will appear black on an image (from Latin *radiare* [to emit rays] + *lucere* [to shine]).

Radionuclide An atom that has excess nuclear energy, making it unstable. Radionuclides are mainly used in nuclear medicine studies.

Radiopaque A positive-contrast agent of high atomic number which contains elements that will absorb more x-rays than tissue or bone. Any element that absorbs radiation and therefore does not allow it to pass through anatomy during radiographic examination, so they appear white or clear on a radiograph (from Latin *radiare* [to emit rays] + *opacus* [to obscure]).

Rare Earth Elements Chemical compounds that are relatively difficult to extract from the earth and range in atomic number from 57 to 71 on the periodic table of elements. They are used in intensifying screens in radiography.

Raw Data Data that has been accepted from a source and that has not been processed for use.

Recirculation System A system within the automatic processor designed to stabilize temperature, pH of the chemicals, dilution of the chemicals, and filter the solutions. Each separate tank contains one pump.

Rectifier Electronic device that converts alternating current, which periodically reverses, to direct current, which flows in only one direction. These are positioned in the x-ray circuit so that the current flows in one way through the x-ray tube.

Recumbent Lying down or reclining. Most radiographs of the dog and cat are made in this position. In small animals, it is the assumed position unless otherwise noted (from Latin *recumbere* re-[back] + *cumbere* [to lie down]).

RED Act This legislation outlines the legal requirements concerning the radiation produced during diagnostic imaging. Also known as Safety Code 20A.

Reducing Agents Developing agents that reduce silver halide into metallic silver and add electrons to the exposed silver halide during film processing.

Reflux A backward flow of the contents (from Latin *re* [back, again] + *fluxus* [a flowing]).

Relative Speed Results of comparing the film screen systems on the basis of the amount of light produced for a given exposure.

REM (Radiation Equivalent Man/Matter) A unit measuring the biologic effect of x, alpha, beta, and gamma radiation on humans and animals.

Remnant Radiation The attenuated x-ray beam leaves the patient and is composed of both transmitted and scattered radiation. Also known as exit radiation.

Repetition Time The time it takes to repeat a function.

Replenishment Replacement of fresh developer and fresh fixer after the loss of chemicals during either manual or automatic film processing.

Reproducibility The ability to produce again—in radiography, it refers to the product of mitosis and meiosis as well as the repeatability of the output of the x-ray generator.

Resistance That property of an element in a circuit that resists or impedes the flow of electricity.

Resolution The ability of the imaging system to distinguish between two adjacent structures and can be expressed in the unit of line pairs per millimeter.

Resonance An echo or other sound produced by percussion.

Restrainer A chemical added to the processing solution that stops the unexposed crystals from developing or to prevent fog.

Restrainers slow the development of exposed crystals to a certain extent to slow down the overall processing speed.

Retrograde Infusion of either a positive- or negative-contrast agent that is in reverse order of how the discharge normally flows; going backwards (from Latin *retr/o* [behind or backwards] + *gradi* [to go]).

Roentgen A measure of the ionization produced in air by x-rays or gamma radiation. 1 Roentgen = 1 RAD = 1 REM in comparative doses.

ROI (Region of Interest) Specifically, the area on the patient's body that is of interest in the diagnosis of the patient's disease.

Rollers Principal film transport system in an automatic film processor.

Rostral (R) Parts of the head positioned toward the nares from any given point on the head (from Latin *rostrum* [beak]).

Rostrocaudal In reference to skull radiography where the central ray enters at the nose and exits at the back of the head. The patient is in dorsal recumbency.

Rostrodorsal–Caudoventral Oblique A rostrocaudal position in which the central ray enters the body from the top of the head and exits at the back and bottom of the head in an oblique angle. The nose is pointing caudally.

Rostroventral–Caudodorsal Oblique A rostrocaudal position in which the central ray enters the body from the nose ventrally and exits in a caudal direction obliquely toward the patient's back.

Rotating Anode A method of dissipating heat in general purpose x-ray tubes which must be capable of producing high intensity x-ray beams in a short time.

Rotor Causes the target to rotate rapidly during x-ray production.

S

Safe Light Incandescent lamp with a colored filter that provides sufficient illumination in the darkroom while ensuring that the film is not fogged during handling.

Sagittal Plane The plane that divides the body into equal right and left parts (from Latin *sagitta* [arrow]).

Sampling Frequency The frequency with which the analog signal is reproduced in its discrete digitized form.

Sampling Pitch The distance between sampling points.

Scale of Contrast The range of densities visible in a film image.

Scattered Radiation Upon integration with atoms of tissue, incoming photons that are not absorbed lose energy during interactions, change direction, and are scattered within the anatomic part. They may have enough energy to leave the patient's anatomy and affect the image receptor, where they can also be called secondary radiation.

Scintigraphy The mapping of radioactive particles using a scintillating camera attached to a computer. Mainly used in nuclear medicine.

Scintillator A phosphor material that converts exit radiation into visible light. Used in nuclear medicine.

Scissor Arm The portion at the end of the extension arm of a dental x-ray unit to assist in positioning.

Screen Characteristics The physical characteristics of modern radiographic screen-film systems.

Screen Film Film sensitive to light, in this case that emitted by the intensifying screens.

Screen Speed Refers to the speed with which the intensifying screen emits light during a radiographic procedure. The speed refers to the reaction time of the screen. Rare earth screens are the most commonly used phosphors today.

Secondary Radiation The ejected electron resulting from the Compton interaction. Also known as the Compton electron. Scattered reaction produced within the subject being radiographed.

Sector Probe A probe that generates a sector or pie-shaped image in ultrasound.

Sensitometer A electronic device designed to produce consistent stepped wedge densities. It is used in conjunction with an x-ray film and is processed in an automatic processor. It is meant to be used every operational day in order to assess processing activity.

Sensitometric Curve A graph of stepped wedge optical densities that visually represent the relationship between the intensity of radiation exposure (x-axis) and the resultant optical densities (y-axis).

Sensitometry The study of the relationship between the intensity of radiation exposure to a film and the amount of blackness produced by processing in chemistry (density).

Shape Distortion Images of objects that appear differently on the image than they are actually shaped. They may be longer, shorter, or visually distorted.

Shielding A material, such as concrete or lead, which absorbs radiation or prevents the transmission of radiation. Radiation protection may be in the form of a leaded apron, lead in the walls of the x-ray room, and/or a leaded screen. One factor in the safety triumvirate of time, distance, shielding.

Short-Scale Contrast A film radiograph with few densities but great differences between them is said to have high contrast. There are few steps between black and white.

Shoulder Region A point on the sensitometric curve where an increase in exposure no longer has an effect on the density of the film.

Signal Intensity The relative brilliance of a radiographic image on the monitor.

Signal to Noise Ratio (SNR) A method of describing the strength of the radiation exposure compared with the amount of noise apparent in a digital image.

Silver Halide A component of the film emulsion that will be affected by radiation exposure and film processing, eventually becoming metallic silver and forming the image on film.

Silver Recovery The removal of metallic silver from the fixer solution.

Size Distortion/Magnification An increase or decrease in the image size of the object on film as opposed to the actual size of the object.

SLOB Rule In reference to imaging teeth in dental radiography. The acronym means "same lingual opposite buccal."

Slope Steepness of the sensitometric curve indicated by the ratio of the change in *y* (optical density) for a unit change in *x* (log relative exposure).

Source to Image Receptor Distance (SID) The distance between the x-ray tube and the detector, either film or digital plate. Also referred to as source-image distance (SID).

Source to Object Distance (SOD) The distance from the x-ray source to the object being radiographed.

Skyline Tangential radiographic view of any structure; taken to provide more information than the standard projections. Refers to the central ray entering and exiting the same side of the limb so the bone is in profile.

Soft Copy Viewing Assessing the image on a viewing monitor as opposed to hard copy viewing from a film.

Solvent A liquid into which various solids and powders can be dissolved; the most common solvent is water.

Space Charge Effect The phenomenon of the space charge restricting the number of electrons boiled off the filament due to electrostatic repulsion.

Spatial Frequency Variation in anatomic details imaged as black to white brightness levels that can be defined by the unit of line pairs per millimeter (lp/mm).

Spatial Resolution Refers to the smallest detail that can be detected in an image. The term is typically used in digital imaging.

Specific Absorption A measure of the rate at which energy is absorbed by the body when exposed to radio frequency, electromagnetic, or ultrasound energy.

Spectral Emission The color of light produced by a particular intensifying screen.

Spectral Matching Correctly matching the color sensitivity of the film to the color emission of the intensifying screen.

Spectral Sensitivity The color of light to which the film is particularly sensitive.

Speed A film's sensitivity to radiation exposure.

Spinous process A bony dorsal projection on the vertebrae that projects backwards in animals. The spinous process protrudes where the laminae of the vertebral arches join and provide the point of attachment for muscles and ligaments of the spine.

Stance Phase The patient is lying in dorsal recumbency with its hindlimbs in a neutral or standing orientation as if it were weight bearing.

Standby Control An electric circuit that shuts off power to an electric motor when the unit is not in use.

Stationary Anode A fixed (nonrotating) anode in the x-ray tube.

Stator An electric motor that turns the rotating anode at a very high speed during x-ray production.

Stepped Wedged Densities A radiograph of uniform densities resembling a stepped wedge.

Stir Rods Stainless steel poles used to stir chemicals in a darkroom.

Stochastic Effects Probability or frequency of the biologic response to radiation as a function of radiation dose delivered intermittently over a period of time; there is no dose threshold.

Storage Phosphor Screen Screens that capture the latent image produced by ionizing radiation.

Stress Radiographs Involves application of traction, rotation, or a wedge to the joint and is useful for sprains to show subluxation, evaluation of ligamentous tears, joint stability, or fracture unions that might not be demonstrated on standard radiographic views.

Subject Contrast A result of the absorption characteristics of the anatomic tissue radiographed and the quality of the x-ray beam.

Subluxation A partial dislocation of the joint.

Sulcus On the foot of a horse, the central groove of the frog that extends up between the bulbs (plural, sulci) (from Latin/Greek *furrow*).

Supercoat A durable protective layer on film that is intended to prevent damage to the sensitive emulsion layer underneath it.

Survey In reference to radiographs in which an initial inspection or examination is conducted to determine if further diagnostic tools are needed before treatment can be initiated.

T

Tabletop The top of the radiographic table or bed.

Tangential Diverging from a previous course or line. Most commonly referred as "at an angle from the vertical or the perpendicular as commonly used."

Target In radiography, the target is the anode. When the exposure switch is closed, the electrons boiled off the cathode are magnetically drawn to the target anode, which abruptly decelerates the electrons and thereby allows the production of x-rays.

Technique Chart A radiographic exposure chart that identifies reliable exposure factors (mA, kV, and exposure time) for a known tissue thickness.

Tenesmus Generally referred to as painful or ineffective defecation but can also refer to painful, ineffective urination (from Greek *teinesmos* [to stretch]).

Testudine Formerly referred to as Chelonian. A reptile order that includes turtles, tortoise, and terrapins. Testudines/Chelonii lack teeth and usually have a special bony or cartilaginous shell developed from the ribs.

Thermal Energy Energy of molecular motion; heat; infrared radiation.

Thermionic Emission The process of heat supplied to the cathode resulting in electrons energized off the cathode filament.

Thermoluminescent Dosimeters A type of radiation dosimeter that measures ionizing radiation exposure by measuring the intensity of visible light emitted from a crystal in the detector when the crystal is heated.

Thermostat A device that senses the temperature of a system and controls the unit so that temperature can be maintained at a desired set point.

Thin Film Transistor Components layered onto a glass substrate that include the readout, charge collector, and light-sensitive elements.

Timer A device for counting time intervals, usually in seconds.

Tissue Density Matter per unit volume or the compactness of the anatomic particles comprising the anatomic part.

Tissue Fluence The density of tissue that is to be radiated.

Toe Region The area of lowest density on a sensitometric curve.

Total Filtration The sum of the x-ray tubes and added inherent filtration.

Transducer A device that converts energy from one form to another.

Transformer A device used to increase or decrease voltage (or current) through electromagnetic induction.

Transmission The incoming x-ray photon passes through the anatomic part without any interaction with the atomic structures.

Transverse Plane The plane that divides the body into cranial and caudal parts. This is also called the horizontal plane or cross-sectional plane and can describe a perpendicular cross section to the long axis of the limb (from Latin *transversus*, "turned or directed across").

Transverse Process Small bony projections off the lateral sides of each vertebrae that function as the site of attachment for muscles and ligaments of the spine, as well as the point of articulation of the ribs (in the thoracic spine).

Triiodinated Compounds A common component of iodinated positive-contrast media that contains three atoms of iodine per molecule.

U

Umbra/Penumbra The fully shaded inner region of a shadow cast by an opaque object is called the umbra and the region of diffuse shadow is called the penumbra.

Ungual Cartilage The medial and lateral cartilages of the distal phalanx that extend from the palmar processes of the bone to the coronary region of the hoof (from Latin *unguis* [nail]).

Unsharpness Loss of spatial resolution in a radiographic image.

Upper Gastrointestinal (UGI) Study Radiography of the stomach and small intestines following ingestion of contrast medium, usually barium sulfate.

Upright Pedal Route In reference to the digit with a horizontal beam parallel to the ground and the toe pointing down.

Urethrography Radiography of the urethra following administration of a contrast agent.

V

Vaginocystourethrography Radiographic examination of the vagina, bladder, and urethra following retrograde administration of a radiopaque medium.

Values of Interest (VOI) Determines the range of the histogram data set included in the displayed digital image.

Ventral (V) Lower or toward the lower aspect of the body (from Latin *venter* [belly, stomach]).

Ventrodorsal Extended Leg View A routine radiographic view of the pelvis in which the patient is in dorsal recumbency and the hindlimbs are equally extended.

Ventrolateral–Dorsolateral Oblique Refers to imaging of the skull where the central ray is directed upward from the opposite lateral side to the affected area.

Vertebral Body The thick oval segment of bone forming the front of the vertebra as distinct from the arches. The cavity of the vertebral body consists of cancellous bone tissue and is encircled by a protective layer of compact bone.

Vertebral Formula The formula indicates the number of each vertebra in each segment of the spinal column for each species.

Viscosity Refers to the resistance of fluid to flow, which influences the injectability or delivery of the contrast agent. It is commonly perceived as thickness, or resistance to pouring.

Voltage An electromotive force or potential difference expressed in volts.

Voltage Ripple The amount of voltage consistency in the voltage waveform during x-ray production as read by a voltmeter.

W

Wash Stage Stage of film processing during which the fixer is removed from the film.

Watt A measure of current. One ampere of current that flows through an electric potential of one volt. 1 Amp × 1 Volt = 1 Watt.

Waveform Graphic representation of a wave. Used mainly in the measurement of electricity and how it is applied to the voltage and current of the x-ray tube.

Wavelength The distance between two successive crests or troughs. Wavelength is represented by the Greek letter lambda and values are given in units called angstroms. X-rays used in radiography range in wavelength from about 0.1 to 1.0 angstrom.

Weight Bearing The limbs are firmly on the ground with the weight of the body supported only by the limbs without accessories such as splints, etc.

Window Level Location of the midpoint (center) of the number scale at which the levels of grays are assigned. It regulates the optical density of the image displayed on the monitor and identifies the type of tissue to be imaged. Window level controls the brightness of the image.

Window Width Specific number of gray scale levels assigned to an image. It determines the gray scale rendition of the imaged tissue. The higher the number of gray levels on the image, the lower the contrast. Window width controls the image contrast.

X

Xiphoid The pointed process of the cartilage, supported by the core of bone and connected with the posterior end of the body of the sternum.

X-Ray Penetrating ionizing electromagnetic radiation that has a wavelength much shorter than that of visible light.

X-Ray Emission Spectrum The range and intensity of emitted x-rays.

X-Ray Quality Penetrability of the x-ray beam.

X-Ray Quantity Output intensity of the x-ray imaging system. Measured in roentgens.

X-Ray Tube Rating Charts Supplied with each x-ray tube, graphically outlining the maximum allowable use of the x-ray tube before it overheats.

X-Ray Tube The device where the electrical energy is converted into x-radiation and heat.

Y

Y-Axis The vertical portion of a graph.

Z

Zonography Thick-slice tomography with a tomographic angle of less than 10 degrees.

Index